CASARETT AND DOULL'S

ESSENTIALS
OF TOXICOLOGY

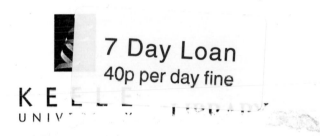

CASARETT AND DOULL'S

ESSENTIALS OF TOXICOLOGY

EDITORS

Curtis D. Klaassen, Ph.D.

Professor of Pharmacology and Toxicology
Department of Pharmacology, Toxicology, and Therapeutics
University of Kansas Medical Center
Kansas City, Kansas

and

John B. Watkins III, Ph.D.

Professor of Pharmacology and Toxicology
Medical Sciences Program
Indiana University School of Medicine
Bloomington, Indiana

McGraw-Hill
Medical Publishing Division

New York / Chicago / San Francisco / Lisbon / London / Madrid
Mexico City / Milan / New Delhi / San Juan / Seoul / Singapore
Sydney / Toronto

Casarett and Doull's Essentials of Toxicology

67890 DOC DOC 0987

ISBN 0-07-138914-8

This book was set in Times Roman by The GTS Companies/York, PA Campus.
The editors were Andrea Seils, Kathleen McCullough, and Lester A. Sheinis.
The production supervisor was Richard C. Ruzycka.
The text designer was Marsha Cohen/Parallelogram.
The cover designer was Janice Bielawa.
The indexer was Alexandra Nickerson.
RR Donnelley was printer and binder.

This book is printed on acid-free paper.

Library of Congress Cataloging-in-Publication Data is on file for this title at the Library of Congress.

CONTENTS

UNIT 4

TARGET ORGAN TOXICITY / 161

UNIT 5

TOXIC AGENTS / 331

UNIT 6

ENVIRONMENTAL TOXICOLOGY / 405

UNIT 7

APPLICATIONS OF TOXICOLOGY / 429

CONTRIBUTORS

DANIEL ACOSTA, JR., PH.D.
Dean and Professor
College of Pharmacy
University of Cincinnati
Cincinnati, Ohio
CHAPTER 18

TODD A. ANDERSON, PH.D.
Assistant Section Leader
The Institute of Environmental and Human Health (TIEHH)
Associate Professor, Department of Environmental Toxicology
Texas Tech
Lubbock, Texas
CHAPTER 29

DOUGLAS C. ANTHONY, M.D., PH.D.
Associate Professor of Pathology
Harvard Medical School
Department of Pathology
Children's Hospital
Boston, Massachusetts
CHAPTER 16

ROBERT J. BAKER, PH.D.
Adjunct Professor
The Institute of Environmental and Human Health (TIEHH)
Horn Professor
Department of Biological Sciences
Texas Tech University
Lubbock, Texas
CHAPTER 29

CATHERINE M. BENS, M.S.
Senior Research Associate
The Institute of Environmental and Human Health (TIEHH)
Texas Tech
Lubbock, Texas
CHAPTER 29

JOHN C. BLOOM, V.M.D., PH.D.
Director, Diagnostic and Experimental Medicine
Eli Lilly and Company
Indianapolis, Indiana
CHAPTER 11

WILLIAM K. BOYES, PH.D.
Neurophysiological Toxicology Branch
Neurotoxicology Division
National Health and Environmental Effects Research Laboratory
U.S. Environmental Protection Agency
Research Triangle Park, North Carolina
CHAPTER 17

JOHN T. BRANDT, M.D.
Senior Clinical Research Pathologist
Eli Lilly and Company
Indianapolis, Indiana
CHAPTER 11

JAMES V. BRUCKNER, PH.D.
Professor of Pharmacology and Toxicology
College of Pharmacy
University of Georgia
Athens, Georgia
CHAPTER 24

GEORGE A. BURDOCK, PH.D., D.A.B.T.
Burdock and Associates, Inc.
Vero Beach, Florida
CHAPTER 30

LEIGH ANN BURNS-NAAS, PH.D.
Senior Toxicology Specialist
Health, Environmental, and Regulatory Affairs
Dow Corning Corporation
Midland, Michigan
CHAPTER 12

LOUIS R. CANTILENA, JR., M.D., PH.D.
Associate Professor of Medicine and Pharmacology
Director, Division of Clinical Pharmacology and Medical
    Toxicology
Uniformed Services University of the Health Sciences
Bethesda, Maryland
CHAPTER 32

CHARLES C. CAPEN, D.V.M., PH.D.
Professor and Chairperson
Department of Veterinary Biosciences
Ohio State University
Columbus, Ohio
CHAPTER 21

JAMES A. CARR, PH.D.
Adjunct Associate Professor
The Institute of Environmental and Human Health (TIEHH)
Associate Professor, Department of Biological Sciences
Texas Tech University
Lubbock, Texas
CHAPTER 29

ENRIQUE CHACON, PH.D.
Vice President of Business Development
Cedra Corporation
Austin, Texas
CHAPTER 18

LOUIS A. CHIODO, PH.D.
Assistant Director
The Institute of Environmental and Human Health (TIEHH)
Professor of Pharmacology
Texas Tech University Health Sciences Center
Lubbock, Texas
CHAPTER 29

THOMAS W. CLARKSON, PH.D.
J. Lowell Orbison Distinguished Alumni Professor
Department of Environmental Medicine
University of Rochester School of Medicine
Rochester, New York
CHAPTER 23

GEORGE P. COBB III, PH.D.
Division Leader
The Institute of Environmental and Human Health (TIEHH)
Associate Professor
Department of Environmental Toxicology
Texas Tech
Lubbock, Texas
CHAPTER 29

DAVID E. COHEN, M.D., M.P.H.
Director of Occupational
  and Environmental Dermatology
Assistant Professor of Dermatology
New York University School of Medicine
New York, New York
CHAPTER 19

DANIEL L. COSTA, SC.D.
Chief, Pulmonary Toxicology Branch
Experimental Toxicology Division
National Health and Environment Effects
  Research Laboratory
U.S. Environmental Protection Agency
Research Triangle Park, North Carolina
CHAPTER 28

RICHARD L. DICKERSON, PH.D.
Research Scientist
The Institute of Environmental and Human Health (TIEHH)
Associate Professor
Department of Environmental Toxicology
Texas Tech
Lubbock, Texas
CHAPTER 29

KENNETH R. DIXON, PH.D.
Section Leader
The Institute of Environmental and Human Health (TIEHH)
Professor
Department of Environmental Toxicology
Texas Tech
Lubbock, Texas
CHAPTER 29

YVONNE P. DRAGAN, PH.D.
Assistant Professor
Ohio State University
James Cancer Hospital and Solove Research Institute
  and the Environmental Molecular Science Institute
Columbus, Ohio
CHAPTER 8

DAVID L. EATON, PH.D.
Professor and Associate Dean for Research
School of Public Health and Community Medicine
Department of Environmental Health
University of Washington
Seattle, Washington
CHAPTER 2

DONALD J. ECOBICHON, M.D.
Professor
Department of Pharmacology and Toxicology
Queen's University
Kingston, Canada
CHAPTER 22

ELAINE M. FAUSTMAN, PH.D.
Professor
School of Public Health and Community Medicine
Department of Environmental Health
University of Washington
Seattle, Washington
CHAPTER 4

W. GARY FLAMM, PH.D., F.A.C.T., F.A.T.S.
Flamm Associates
Vero Beach, Florida
CHAPTER 30

DONALD A. FOX, PH.D.
Professor
College of Optometry
Department of Biochemical and Biophysical Sciences, and
Department of Pharmacology and Pharmaceutical Sciences,
  University of Houston
Houston, Texas
CHAPTER 17

LYNN T. FRAME, PH.D.
Senior Research Associate
The Institute of Environmental and Human Health (TIEHH)
Texas Tech
Lubbock, Texas
CHAPTER 29

MICHAEL A. GALLO, PH.D.
UMDNJ-Robert Wood Johnson Medical School
Piscataway, New Jersey
CHAPTER 1

ROBERT A. GOYER, M.D.
Professor Emeritus
University of Western Ontario
London, Ontario, Canada
CHAPTER 23

DOYLE G. GRAHAM, M.D., PH.D.
Professor and Chair of Pathology
Department of Pathology
Vanderbilt University Medical Center
Nashville, Tennessee
CHAPTER 16

ZOLTÁN GREGUS, M.D., PH.D., D.SC.
Professor
Department of Pharmacology and Pharmacotherapy
University of Pécs Medical School
Pécs, Hungary
CHAPTER 3

NAOMI H. HARLEY, PH.D.
Research Professor
New York University School of Medicine
Department of Environmental Medicine
New York, New York
CHAPTER 25

GEORGE R. HOFFMANN, B.A., M.S., PH.D.
Anthony and Renee Marlon Professor
Department of Biology
Holy Cross College
Worcester, Massachusetts
CHAPTER 9

MICHAEL J. HOOPER, PH.D.
Research Scientist
The Institute of Environmental and Human Health (TIEHH)
Associate Professor
Department of Environmental Toxicology
Texas Tech
Lubbock, Texas
CHAPTER 29

ROBERT J. KAVLOCK, PH.D.
Director, Reproductive Toxicology Division
National Health and Environmental Effects
    Research Laboratory
United States Environmental Protection Agency
Research Triangle Park, North Carolina
CHAPTER 10

RONALD J. KENDALL, PH.D.
Director
The Institute of Environmental and Human Health (TIEHH)
Professor and Chair
Department of Environmental Toxicology
Texas Tech
Lubbock, Texas
CHAPTER 29

CURTIS D. KLAASSEN, PH.D.
Professor of Pharmacology and Toxicology
Department of Pharmacology, Toxicology,
    and Therapeutics
University of Kansas Medical Center
Kansas City, Kansas
CHAPTERS 2, 3, 5

FRANK N. KOTSONIS, PH.D., D.A.B.T.
Corporate Vice President, Monsanto Company
Worldwide Regulatory Affairs
Skokie, Illinois
CHAPTER 30

JEROLD A. LAST, PH.D.
Professor
Pulmonary/Critical Care Medicine
School of Medicine
University of California, Davis
Davis, California
CHAPTER 15

CLYDE F. MARTIN, PH.D.
Special Assistant
The Institute of Environmental and Human Health (TIEHH)
Horn Professor
Department of Mathematics and Statistics
Texas Tech University
Lubbock, Texas
CHAPTER 29

SCOTT T. MCMURRY, PH.D.
Section Leader
The Institute of Environmental and Human Health (TIEHH)
Assistant Professor
Department of Environmental Toxicology
Texas Tech
Lubbock, Texas
CHAPTER 29

B. JEAN MEADE, D.V.M., PH.D.
Toxicologist
National Institute of Occupational Safety and Health
Morgantown, West Virginia
CHAPTER 12

MICHELE A. MEDINSKY, PH.D., D.A.B.T.
Toxicology Consultant
Durham, North Carolina
CHAPTER 7

RUSSELL B. MELCHERT, PH.D.
Assistant Professor
Department of Pharmaceutical Sciences
College of Pharmacy
University of Arkansas for Medical Sciences
Little Rock, Arkansas
CHAPTER 18

RICHARD A. MERRILL, L.L.B., M.A.
Professor of Law
University of Virginia
Charlottesville, Virginia
CHAPTER 34

THOMAS J. MONTINE, M.D., PH.D.
Associate Professor of Pathology and Pharmacology
Margaret and George Thorne Professorship
    in Pathology
Department of Pathology
Vanderbilt University Medical Center
Nashville, Tennessee
CHAPTER 16

ALBERT E. MUNSON, PH.D.
Director Health Effects Laboratory Division
National Institute of Occupational Safety and Health
Morgantown, West Virginia
CHAPTER 12

STATA NORTON, PH.D.
Emeritus Professor of Pharmacology and Toxicology
Department of Pharmacology, Toxicology,
  and Therapeutics
University of Kansas Medical Center
Kansas City, Kansas
CHAPTER 27

GILBERT S. OMENN, PH.D., M.D.
Executive Vice President for Medical Affairs
Professor of Internal Medicine, Human Genetics
  and Public Health
University of Michigan
Ann Arbor, Michigan
CHAPTER 4

ANDREW PARKINSON, PH.D.
CEO
XENOTECH
Kansas City, Kansas
CHAPTER 6

REYNALDO PATINO, PH.D.
Section Leader
The Institute of Environmental and Human Health (TIEHH)
Associate Professor
Department of Biological Sciences
Texas Tech University
Assistant Unit Leader
Texas Cooperative Fish and Wildlife Research Unit
United States Geological Survey
Lubbock, Texas
CHAPTER 29

HENRY C. PITOT III, M.D., PH.D.
Professor Emeritus
University of Wisconsin
McArdle Laboratory for Cancer Research
  and the Center for Environmental Toxicology
Madison, Wisconsin
CHAPTER 8

ALPHONSE POKLIS, PH.D.
Professor
Department of Pathology
Medical College of Virginia Campus
Virginia Commonwealth University
Richmond, Virginia
CHAPTER 31

R. JULIAN PRESTON, B.A., M.A., PH.D.
Director
Environmental Carcinogenesis Division
U.S. Environmental Protection Agency
Research Triangle Park, North Carolina
CHAPTER 9

KENNETH S. RAMOS, PH.D.
Professor
Department of Physiology and Pharmacology
College of Veterinary Medicine
Texas A&M University
College Station, Texas
CHAPTER 18

ROBERT H. RICE, PH.D.
Professor
University of California/Davis
Department of Environmental Toxicology
Davis, California
CHAPTER 19

JOHN M. ROGERS, PH.D.
Chief
Developmental Biology Branch
Reproductive Toxicology Division
National Health and Environmental Effects
  Research Laboratory
United States Environmental Protection Agency
Research Triangle Park, North Carolina
CHAPTER 10

KARL K. ROZMAN, PH.D.
Professor of Pharmacology and Toxicology
Department of Pharmacology and Toxicology
University of Kansas Medical Center
Kansas City, Kansas
CHAPTER 5

FINDLAY E. RUSSELL, M.D., PH.D.
Department of Pharmacology and Toxicology
College of Pharmacy
University of Arizona
Tucson, Arizona
Department of Neurology
University of Southern California
Los Angeles, California
Department of Neurological Sciences
Loma Linda University
Loma Linda, California
CHAPTER 26

RICK G. SCHNELLMANN, PH.D.
Professor and Chair
Pharmaceutical Sciences
Department of Pharmaceutical Sciences
Medical University of South Carolina
Charleston, South Carolina
CHAPTER 14

ERNEST E. SMITH, PH.D.
Research Scientist
The Institute of Environmental and Human Health (TIEHH)
Assistant Professor
Department of Environmental Toxicology
Texas Tech
Lubbock, Texas
CHAPTER 29

CHRISTOPHER W. THEODORAKIS, PH.D.
Assistant Section Leader
The Institute of Environmental and Human Health (TIEHH)
Assistant Professor
Department of Environmental Toxicology
Texas Tech
Lubbock, Texas
CHAPTER 29

JOHN A. THOMAS, PH.D.
Professor Emeritus
University of Texas Health Science Center—San Antonio
Department of Pharmacology
San Antonio, Texas
CHAPTER 20

MICHAEL J. THOMAS, M.D., PH.D.
Assistant Professor
University of North Carolina School of Medicine
Division of Endocrinology
Chapel Hill, North Carolina
CHAPTER 20

PETER S. THORNE, PH.D.
Professor of Toxicology
Professor of Environmental Engineering (secondary)
University of Iowa College of Public Health
Department of Occupational and Environmental Health
Iowa City, Iowa
CHAPTER 33

MARY TREINEN-MOSLEN, PH.D.
William C. Levin Professor of Environmental Toxicology
Toxicology Program
University of Texas Medical Branch
Galveston, Texas
CHAPTER 13

JOHN L. VALENTINE, PH.D.
Research Pharmacokineticist
Research Triangle Institute
Research Triangle Park, North Carolina
CHAPTER 7

WILLIAM M. VALENTINE, D.V.M., PH.D.
Associate Professor of Pathology
Department of Pathology
Vanderbilt University Medical Center
Nashville, Tennessee
CHAPTER 16

D. ALAN WARREN, M.P.H., PH.D.
Toxicologist
Terra, Inc.
Tallahassee, Florida
CHAPTER 24

HANSPETER R. WITSCHI, M.D.
Professor of Toxicology
Institute of Toxicology and Environmental Health
   and Department of Molecular Biosciences
School of Veterinary Medicine
University of California
Davis, California
CHAPTER 15

PREFACE

Essentials of Toxicology is a distillation of the major principles and concepts of toxicology that were described in detail in the sixth edition of *Casarett and Doull's Toxicology: The Basic Science of Poisons*. We are grateful to our colleagues who contributed to the sixth edition of *Casarett and Doull's Toxicology: The Basic Science of Poisons*; their contributions to the parent text served as the foundation of the chapters in *Essentials of Toxicology*.

Essentials of Toxicology was prepared to concisely present the broad science of toxicology to students in undergraduate and graduate courses in toxicology. Important basic concepts from anatomy, physiology, and biochemistry have been included to facilitate the understanding of the principles and mechanisms of toxicant action on specific organ systems. In addition, it is hoped that the book will be useful to students from other disciplines who want to have a strong foundation in toxicologic concepts and principles.

The book is organized into seven units: 1. General Principles of Toxicology; 2. Disposition of Toxicants; 3. Nonorgan-Directed Toxicity; 4. Target Organ Toxicity; 5. Toxic Agents; 6. Environmental Toxicology; and 7. Applications of Toxicology. A summary of important points is included at the beginning of each chapter, and a set of review questions is provided at the end of the book. We invite our readers to send us their suggestions of ways to improve this textbook.

We would like to acknowledge all individuals who were involved in this project. We particularly give a heartfelt and sincere thanks to our families for their love, patience, and support, which has sustained us making the completion of this book possible. We especially appreciate Abbie Berryman, who provided invaluable assistance on this project. The capable advice, guidance, and assistance of the McGraw-Hill staff, especially Andrea Seils, Kathleen McCullough, and Lester Sheinis, is gratefully acknowledged. Finally, we thank our students for their enthusiasm for learning and what they have taught us during their time with us.

CASARETT AND DOULL'S

ESSENTIALS
OF TOXICOLOGY

UNIT 1

GENERAL PRINCIPLES OF TOXICOLOGY

CHAPTER 1

HISTORY AND SCOPE
OF TOXICOLOGY

Michael A. Gallo

HISTORY OF TOXICOLOGY

  Antiquity
  Middle Ages
  Age of Enlightenment

MODERN TOXICOLOGY

AFTER WORLD WAR II

KEY POINTS

* Toxicology is the study of the adverse effects of xenobiotics on living systems.
* Toxicology assimilates knowledge and techniques from biochemistry, biology, chemistry, genetics, mathematics, medicine, pharmacology, physiology, and physics.
* Toxicology applies safety evaluation and risk assessment to the discipline.

HISTORY OF TOXICOLOGY

Modern toxicology extends beyond the study of the adverse effects of exogenous agents by assimilating knowledge and techniques from many branches of biochemistry, biology, chemistry, genetics, mathematics, medicine, pharmacology, physiology, and physics and applies safety evaluation and risk assessment to the discipline. In all branches of toxicology, scientists explore the mechanisms by which chemicals produce adverse effects in biological systems.

Antiquity

Knowledge of animal venoms and plant extracts for hunting, warfare, and assassination almost certainly predated recorded history. One of the oldest known writings, the Ebers papyrus (circa 1500 B.C.), contains information pertaining to many recognized poisons, including hemlock, aconite, opium, and metals such as lead, copper, and antimony. The Book of Job (circa 1400 B.C.) speaks of poison arrows (Job 6:4), and Hippocrates (circa 400 B.C.) added a number of poisons and clinical toxicology principles pertaining to bioavailability in therapy and

overdosage. Theophrastus (370–286 B.C.), a student of Aristotle, included numerous references to poisonous plants in *De Historia Plantarum*. Dioscorides, a Greek physician in the court of the Roman emperor Nero, made the first attempt at classifying poisons into plant, animal, and mineral poisons.

A legend tells of the Roman king Mithridates VI of Pontus, who was so fearful of poisons that he regularly ingested a mixture of 36 ingredients to protect himself against assassination. On the occasion of his imminent capture by enemies, his attempts to kill himself with poison failed because of his successful antidote concoction, and he was forced to use a sword held by a servant. Sulla issued the *Lex Cornelia* (circa 82 B.C.), which appears to be the first law against poisoning, and it later became a regulatory statute directed at careless dispensers of drugs.

Middle Ages

Come bitter pilot, now at once run on
The dashing rocks thy seasick weary bark!
Here's to my love! O true apothecary!
Thy drugs are quick. Thus with a kiss I die.
    Romeo and Juliet, act 5, scene 3

The writings of Maimonides (Moses ben Maimon, A.D. 1135–1204) included a treatise on the treatment of poisonings from insects, snakes, and mad dogs (*Poisons and Their Antidotes,* 1198). Maimonides described the subject of bioavailability, noting that milk, butter, and cream could delay intestinal absorption. In the early Renaissance, under the guise of delivering food to the sick and the poor, Catherine de Medici tested toxic concoctions, carefully noting the rapidity of the toxic response (onset of action), the effectiveness of the compound (potency), the degree of response of different parts of the body (specificity, site of action), and the complaints of the victim (clinical signs and symptoms).

Age of Enlightenment

All substances are poisons; there is none which is not a poison.
The right dose differentiates a poison from a remedy.

Paracelsus

Philippus Aureolus Theophrastus Bombastus von Hohenheim-Paracelsus (1493–1541) was pivotal, standing between the philosophy and magic of classical antiquity and the philosophy and science willed to us by figures of the seventeenth and eighteenth centuries. Paracelsus, a physician-alchemist, formulated many revolutionary views that remain integral to the structure of toxicology, pharmacology, and therapeutics today. He focused on the primary toxic agent as a chemical entity and held that (1) experimentation is essential in the examination of responses to chemicals, (2) one should make a distinction between the therapeutic and toxic properties of chemicals, (3) these properties are sometimes but not always indistinguishable except by dose, and (4) one can ascertain a degree of specificity of chemicals and their therapeutic or toxic effects. These principles led Paracelsus to articulate the dose–response relationship as a bulwark of toxicology.

Although Ellenbog (circa 1480) warned of the toxicity of mercury and lead from goldsmithing and Agricola published a short treatise on mining diseases in 1556, the major work on the subject, *On the Miners' Sickness and Other Diseases of Miners* (1567), was published by Paracelsus. That treatise addressed the etiology of miners' disease, along with treatment and prevention strategies. Occupational toxicology was advanced by the work of Bernardino Ramazzini when he published in 1700 the *Discourse on the Diseases of Workers,* which discussed occupations ranging from miners to midwives and including printers, weavers, and potters. Percival Pott's (1775) recognition of the role of soot in scrotal cancer among chimney sweeps was the first report of polyaromatic hydrocarbon carcinogenicity. Those findings led to improved medical practices, particularly in prevention.

Experimental toxicology accompanied the growth of organic chemistry and developed rapidly during the nineteenth century. Magendie (1783–1855), Orfila (1787–1853), and Bernard (1813–1878) carried out seminal research in experimental toxicology and laid the groundwork for pharmacology, experimental therapeutics, and occupational toxicology.

Orfila, a Spanish physician in the French court, used autopsy material and chemical analysis systematically to provide legal proof of poisoning. His introduction of this detailed type of analysis survives as the underpinning of forensic toxicology. In 1815, Orfila published a major work devoted expressly to the toxicity of natural agents. Magendie, a physician and experimental physiologist, studied the mechanisms of action of emetine and strychnine. His research determined the absorption and distribution of those compounds in the body. One of Magendie's more famous students, Claude Bernard, contributed the classic treatise *An Introduction to the Study of Experimental Medicine.*

The German scientists Oswald Schmiedeberg (1838–1921) and Louis Lewin (1850–1929) made many contributions to the science of toxicology. Schmeideberg trained approximately 120 students who later populated the most important laboratories of pharmacology and toxicology throughout the world. Lewin published much of the early work on the toxicity of narcotics, methanol, glycerol, acrolein, and chloroform.

MODERN TOXICOLOGY

Toxicology evolved rapidly during the twentieth century. Toxicology calls on almost all the basic sciences to test its hypotheses. This fact, coupled with the health and occupational regulations that have driven toxicology research since 1900, has made the discipline exceptional in the history of science.

Modern toxicology has drawn strength and diversity from its proclivity for borrowing. With the advent of anesthetics and disinfectants in the late 1850s, toxicology as it is currently understood began. The prevalent use of "patent" medicines led to several incidents of poisonings from those medicaments; that, coupled with the response to Upton Sinclair's exposé of the meat-packing industry in *The Jungle,* culminated in the passage of the Wiley Bill in 1906, the first of many U.S. pure food and drug laws.

During the 1890s and early 1900s, the discovery of radioactivity and the vitamins, or "vital amines," led to the use of the first large-scale bioassays (multiple animal studies) to determine whether those "new" chemicals were beneficial or harmful to laboratory animals.

One of the first journals expressly dedicated to experimental toxicology, *Archiv für Toxikologie,* began publication in Europe in 1930. In the same year, the National Institutes of Health (NIH) was established in the United States. As a response to the tragic consequences of acute kidney failure after the taking of sufanilamide in glycol solutions, the Copeland bill was passed into law in 1938. This was the second major bill involving the formation of the U.S. Food and Drug Administration (FDA). The first major U.S. pesticide act was signed into law in 1947. The significance of the initial Federal Insecticide, Fungicide, and Rodenticide Act was that for the first time in U.S. history, a substance that was neither a drug nor a food had to be shown to be safe and efficacious.

AFTER WORLD WAR II

You too can be a toxicologist in two easy lessons, each of ten years.

Arnold Lehman (circa 1955)

The mid-1950s witnessed the strengthening of the FDA's commitment to toxicology. The U.S. Congress passed and the President of the United States signed the additives amendments to the Food, Drug, and Cosmetic Act. The Delaney clause (1958) of these amendments stated broadly that any chemical found to be carcinogenic in laboratory animals or humans could not be added to the food supply. Delaney became a battle cry for many groups and resulted in the inclusion at a new level of biostatisticians and mathematical modelers in the field of toxicology. Shortly after the Delaney clause, the first American journal dedicated to toxicology, *Toxicology and Applied Pharmacology,* was launched. The founding of the Society of Toxicology followed shortly afterward.

The 1960s started with the tragic thalidomide incident, in which several thousand children were born with serious birth defects, and the publication of Rachel Carson's *Silent Spring* (1962). Attempts to understand the effects of chemicals on the embryo and fetus and on the environment as a whole gained momentum. New legislation was passed, and new journals were founded. Cellular and molecular toxicology developed as a subdiscipline, and risk assessment became a major product of toxicological investigations.

Currently, many dozens of professional, governmental, and other scientific organizations with thousands of members and over 120 journals are dedicated to toxicology and related disciplines. In addition, the International Congress of Toxicology, which is made up of toxicology societies from Europe, South America, Asia, Africa, and Australia, brings together the broadest representation of toxicologists.

Toxicology has an interesting and varied history. Perhaps as a science that has grown and prospered by borrowing from many disciplines, it has suffered from the absence of a single goal, but its diversity has allowed the interspersion of ideas and concepts from higher education, industry, and government. This has resulted in an exciting, innovative, and diversified field that is serving science and the community at large. Few disciplines can point to both basic sciences and direct applications at the same time. Toxicology—the study of the adverse effects of xenobiotics—may be unique in this regard.

BIBLIOGRAPHY

Bryan CP: *The Papyrus Ebers.* London: Geoffrey Bales, 1930.

Carson R: *Silent Spring.* Boston: Houghton Mifflin, 1962.

Gunther RT: *The Greek Herbal of Dioscorides.* New York: Oxford University Press, 1934.

Guthrie DA: *A History of Medicine.* Philadelphia: Lippincott, 1946.

Hays HW: *Society of Toxicology History, 1961–1986.* Washington, DC: Society of Toxicology, 1986.

Munter S (ed): *Treatise on Poisons and Their Antidotes.* Vol. II of *the Medical Writings of Moses Maimonides.* Philadelphia: Lippincott, 1966.

Pagel W: *Paracelsus: An Introduction to Philosophical Medicine in the Era of the Renaissance.* New York: Karger, 1958.

Thompson CJS: *Poisons and Poisoners: With Historical Accounts of Some Famous Mysteries in Ancient and Modern Times.* London: Shaylor, 1931.

PRINCIPLES OF TOXICOLOGY

David L. Eaton and Curtis D. Klaassen

KEY POINTS

- A *poison* is any agent capable of producing a deleterious response in a biological system.
- A *mechanistic toxicologist* identifies the cellular, biochemical, and molecular mechanisms by which chemicals exert toxic effects on living organisms.
- *Toxicogenomics* allows mechanistic toxicologists to identify and protect genetically susceptible individuals from harmful environmental exposures and to customize drug therapies on the basis of their individual genetic makeup.
- A *descriptive toxicologist* is concerned directly with toxicity testing, which provides information for safety evaluation and regulatory requirements.
- A *regulatory toxicologist* both determines from available data whether a chemical poses a sufficiently low risk to be marketed for a stated purpose and establishes standards for the amounts of chemicals permitted in ambient air, industrial atmospheres, and drinking water.
- *Selective toxicity* means that a chemical produces injury to one kind of living matter without harming another form of life even though the two forms may exist in intimate contact.
- The individual or "graded" dose–response relationship describes the response of an *individual* organism to varying doses of a chemical.
- A quantal dose–response relationship characterizes the distribution of responses to different doses in a *population* of individual organisms.
- Hormesis, a "U-shaped" dose–response curve, results with some xenobiotics that impart beneficial or stimulatory effects at low doses but have adverse effects at higher doses.
- Descriptive animal toxicity testing assumes that the effects produced by a compound in laboratory animals, when properly qualified, are applicable to humans and that exposure of experimental animals to toxic agents in high doses is a necessary and valid method of discovering possible hazards in humans.

INTRODUCTION TO TOXICOLOGY

Toxicology is the study of the adverse effects of chemicals on living organisms. A *toxicologist* is trained to examine the nature of those effects (including their cellular, biochemical, and molecular mechanisms of action) and assess the probability of their occurrence.

Different Areas of Toxicology

A *mechanistic toxicologist* identifies the cellular, biochemical, and molecular mechanisms by which chemi-

cals exert toxic effects on living organisms (see Chap. 3 for a detailed discussion of mechanisms of toxicity). Mechanistic data may be useful in the design and production of safer chemicals and in rational therapy for chemical poisoning and treatment of disease. *Toxicogenomics* allows mechanistic toxicologists to identify and protect genetically susceptible individuals from harmful environmental exposures and to customize drug therapies on the basis of their individual genetic makeup.

A *descriptive toxicologist* is concerned directly with toxicity testing, which provides information for safety evaluation and regulatory requirements. Toxicity tests (described later in this chapter) in experimental animals are designed to yield information that can be used to evaluate the risks posed to humans and the environment by exposure to specific chemicals.

A *regulatory toxicologist* has the responsibility for deciding, on the basis of data provided by descriptive and mechanistic toxicologists, whether a drug or another chemical poses a sufficiently low risk to be marketed for a stated purpose. Regulatory toxicologists also are involved in the establishment of standards for the amounts of chemicals permitted in ambient air, industrial atmospheres, and drinking water (see Chap. 4).

Forensic toxicology is a hybrid of analytic chemistry and fundamental toxicologic principles that focuses primarily on the medicolegal aspects of the harmful effects of chemicals on humans and animals (see Chap. 31).

Clinical toxicology is concerned with diseases caused by or uniquely associated with toxic substances (see Chap. 32).

Environmental toxicology focuses on the impacts of chemical pollutants in the environment on biological organisms, specifically studying the impacts of chemicals on nonhuman organisms such as fish, birds, and terrestrial animals. *Ecotoxicology,* a specialized area within environmental toxicology, focuses specifically on the impacts of toxic substances on population dynamics in an ecosystem (see Chap. 29).

Developmental toxicology is the study of adverse effects on the developing organism that occur any time during the life span of an organism that may result from exposure to chemical or physical agents before conception (either parent), during prenatal development, or postnatally until the time of puberty. *Teratology* is the study of defects induced during development between conception and birth (see Chap. 10).

Reproductive toxicology is the study of the occurrence of adverse effects on the male or female reproductive system that may result from exposure to chemical or physical agents (see Chap. 20).

Spectrum of Toxic Dose

A *poison* can be defined as any agent capable of producing a deleterious response in a biological system. Virtually every known chemical has the potential to produce injury or death if it is present in a sufficient amount. Table 2-1 shows the dosages of chemicals needed to produce death in 50 percent of treated animals (LD_{50}). It should be noted that measures of acute lethality such as LD_{50} may not reflect accurately the full spectrum of toxicity, or hazard, associated with exposure to a chemical. For example, some chemicals with low acute toxicity

Table 2-1
Approximate Acute LD_{50}s of Some Representative Chemical Agents

AGENT	LD_{50}, mg/kg*
Ethyl alcohol	10,000
Sodium chloride	4,000
Ferrous sulfate	1,500
Morphine sulfate	900
Phenobarbital sodium	150
Picrotoxin	5
Strychnine sulfate	2
Nicotine	1
d-Tubocurarine	0.5
Hemicholinium-3	0.2
Tetrodotoxin	0.10
Dioxin (TCDD)	0.001
Botulinum toxin	0.00001

*LD_{50} is the dosage (mg/kg body weight) causing death in 50 percent of exposed animals.

may have carcinogenic or teratogenic effects at doses that produce no evidence of acute toxicity.

CLASSIFICATION OF TOXIC AGENTS

Toxic agents are classified in accordance with the interests and needs of the classifier. Toxic agents may be discussed in terms of their target organs, use, source, and effects. The term *toxin* generally refers to toxic substances that are produced by biological systems such as plants, animals, fungi, and bacteria. The term *toxicant* is used in speaking of toxic substances that are produced by or are by-products of anthropogenic (human) activities. Toxic agents also may be classified in terms of their physical state, chemical stability or reactivity, general chemical structure, or poisoning potential.

CHARACTERISTICS OF EXPOSURE

Toxic effects in a biological system are not produced by a chemical agent unless that agent or its metabolic breakdown (biotransformation) products reach appropriate sites in the body at a concentration and for a length of time sufficient to produce a toxic manifestation. Whether a toxic response occurs is dependent on the chemical and physical properties of the agent, the exposure situation, how the agent is metabolized by the system, and the overall susceptibility of the biological system or subject.

Route and Site of Exposure

The major routes (pathways) by which toxic agents gain access to the body are the gastrointestinal tract (ingestion), lungs (inhalation), skin (topical, percutaneous, or dermal), and other parenteral (other than intestinal canal) routes. Toxic agents generally produce the greatest effect and the most rapid response when they are introduced directly into the bloodstream (the intravenous route). An approximate descending order of effectiveness for the other routes would be inhalation, intraperitoneal, subcutaneous, intramuscular, intradermal, oral, and dermal. The "vehicle" (the material in which the chemical is dissolved) and other formulation factors can alter absorption markedly. In addition, the route of administration can influence the toxicity of agents.

Duration and Frequency of Exposure

Toxicologists usually divide the exposure of experimental animals to chemicals into four categories: acute, subacute, subchronic, and chronic. *Acute* exposure is defined as exposure to a chemical for less than 24 h. Although acute exposure usually refers to a single administration, repeated exposures may be given within a 24-h period for some slightly toxic or practically nontoxic chemicals. Acute exposure by inhalation refers to continuous exposure for less than 24 h, most frequently for 4 h. Repeated exposure is divided into three categories: subacute, subchronic, and chronic. *Subacute exposure* refers to repeated exposure to a chemical for 1 month or less, *subchronic* for 1 to 3 months, and *chronic* for more than 3 months.

In human exposure situations, the frequency and duration of exposure usually are not defined as clearly as they are in controlled animal studies, but many of the same terms are used to describe general exposure situations. Thus, workplace or environmental exposures may be described as *acute* (resulting from a single incident or episode), *subchronic* (occurring repeatedly over several weeks or months), or *chronic* (occurring repeatedly for many months or years).

For many agents, the toxic effects that follow a single exposure are quite different from those produced by repeated exposure. Acute exposure to agents that are absorbed rapidly is likely to produce immediate toxic effects but also can produce delayed toxicity that may or may not be similar to the toxic effects of chronic exposure. Conversely, chronic exposure to a toxic agent may produce some immediate (acute) effects after each administration in addition to the long-term, low-level, or chronic effects of the toxic substance. The other time-related factor that is important in the temporal characterization of repeated exposures is the frequency of exposure. The relationship between elimination rate and frequency of exposure is shown in Fig. 2-1. A chemical that produces severe effects with a single dose may have no effect if the same total dose is given at several different times. For the chemical depicted by line B in Fig. 2-1, in which the half-life for elimination (the time necessary for 50 percent of the chemical to be removed from the bloodstream) is approximately equal to the dosing frequency, a theoretical toxic concentration of 2 U is not reached until the fourth dose, whereas that concentration is reached with only two doses for chemical A, which has an elimination rate that is much slower than the dosing interval (time between repeated doses). Conversely, for chemical C, for which the elimination rate is much shorter than the dosing interval, a toxic concentration at the site of the toxic effect will never be reached regardless of how many doses are administered. Of course, it is possible that residual cell or tissue damage occurs with each dose even though the chemical is not accumulating. The important consideration, then, is whether the interval between doses is sufficient to allow for complete repair of tissue damage. Chronic toxic effects may occur, therefore, if the chemical accumulates in the biological system (the rate of absorption exceeds the rate of biotransformation and/or excretion), if it produces irreversible toxic effects, or if there is insufficient time for the system to recover from the toxic damage within the exposure frequency interval. For additional discussion of these relationships, consult Chaps. 5 and 7.

SPECTRUM OF UNDESIRED EFFECTS

The spectrum of undesired effects of chemicals is broad. In therapeutics, for example, each drug produces a number of effects, but usually only one effect is associated with the primary objective of the therapy; all the other effects are referred to as *undesirable effects* or *side effects*. However, some of these side effects may be desired for another therapeutic indication. Some side effects of drugs are always deleterious to the well-being of humans. They are referred to as the *adverse, deleterious,* or *toxic* effects of a drug.

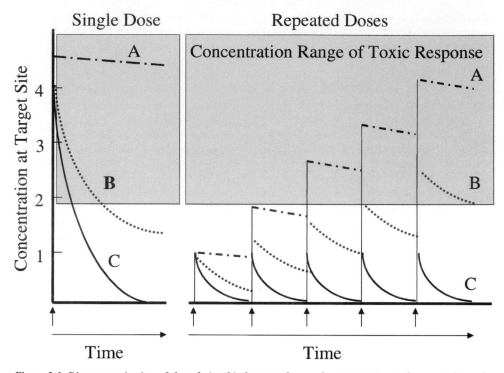

Figure 2-1. Diagrammatic view of the relationship between dose and concentration at the target site under different conditions of dose frequency and elimination rate.   Line A. A chemical with very slow elimination (e.g., half-life of 1 year). *Line B.* A chemical with a rate of elimination equal to frequency of dosing (e.g., 1 day). *Line C.* Rate of elimination faster than the dosing frequency (e.g., 5 h). The blue-shaded area is representative of the concentration of chemical at the target site necessary to elicit a toxic response.

Allergic Reactions

Chemical allergy is an immunologically mediated adverse reaction to a chemical resulting from previous sensitization to that chemical or to a structurally similar one. The terms *hypersensitivity, allergic reaction,* and *sensitization reaction* are used to describe this situation (see Chap. 12). Once sensitization has occurred, allergic reactions may result from exposure to relatively very low doses of chemicals; therefore, population-based dose–response curves for allergic reactions seldom have been obtained. However, for a given allergic individual, allergic reactions are dose-related. Sensitization reactions are sometimes very severe and may be fatal.

Most chemicals and their metabolic products are not sufficiently large to be recognized by the immune system as foreign substances and thus must first combine with an endogenous protein to form an antigen (or immunogen). This type of molecule is called a *hapten.* The hapten-protein complex (antigen) is then capable of elic-

iting the formation of antibodies. Subsequent exposure to the chemical results in an antigen–antibody interaction, which provokes typical manifestations of allergy that range in severity from minor skin disturbance to fatal anaphylactic shock.

Idiosyncratic Reactions

Chemical idiosyncrasy refers to genetically determined abnormal reactivity to a chemical. The response observed is usually qualitatively similar to that observed in all individuals but may take the form of extreme sensitivity to low doses or extreme insensitivity to high doses of the chemical.

Immediate versus Delayed Toxicity

Immediate toxic effects occur or develop rapidly after a single administration of a substance, whereas delayed toxic effects occur after the lapse of some period of time.

Carcinogenic effects of chemicals usually have long latency periods, often 20 to 30 years after the initial exposure, before tumors are observed in humans.

Reversible versus Irreversible Toxic Effects

Some toxic effects of chemicals are reversible, and others are irreversible. If a chemical produces pathological injury to a tissue, the ability of that tissue to regenerate largely determines whether the effect is reversible or irreversible. For liver, with its high regeneration ability, most injuries are reversible, whereas injury to the central nervous system (CNS) is largely irreversible because the differentiated cells in the CNS cannot be replaced. Carcinogenic and teratogenic effects of chemicals, once they occur, usually are considered irreversible toxic effects.

Local versus Systemic Toxicity

Another distinction between types of effects is made on the basis of the general site of action. Local effects occur at the site of first contact between the biological system and the toxicant. In contrast, systemic effects require absorption and distribution of a toxicant from its entry point to a distant site at which deleterious effects are produced. Most substances except highly reactive materials produce systemic effects. For some materials, both effects can be demonstrated.

Most chemicals that produce systemic toxicity usually elicit their major toxicity in only one or two organs, which are referred to as the *target organs* of toxicity of a particular chemical. The target organ of toxicity is often not the site of the highest concentration of the chemical.

Target organs, in order of frequency of involvement in systemic toxicity, are the CNS; the circulatory system; the blood and hematopoietic system; visceral organs such as the liver, kidney, and lung; and the skin. Muscle and bone are seldom target tissues for systemic effects.

INTERACTION OF CHEMICALS

Because of the large number of different chemicals an individual may come in contact with at any given time (workplace, medications, diet, hobbies, etc.), it is necessary to consider how different chemicals may interact with each other. Interactions can occur through various mechanisms, such as alterations in absorption, protein binding, and the biotransformation and excretion of one or both of the interacting toxicants. In addition to these modes of interaction, the response of the organism to combinations of toxicants may be increased or decreased because of toxicologic responses at the site of action.

An *additive* effect occurs when the combined effect of two chemicals is equal to the sum of the effects of each agent given alone (example: 2 + 3 = 5). The effect most commonly observed when two chemicals are given together is an additive effect. A *synergistic* effect occurs when the combined effects of two chemicals are much greater than the sum of the effects of each agent given alone (example: 2 + 2 = 20). For example, both carbon tetrachloride and ethanol are hepatotoxic compounds, but together they produce much more liver injury than the mathematical sum of their individual effects on liver at a given dose would suggest. *Potentiation* occurs when one substance does not have a toxic effect on a certain organ or system but when added to another chemical makes that chemical much more toxic (example: 0 + 2 = 10). Isopropanol, for example, is not hepatotoxic, but when it is administered in addition to carbon tetrachloride, the hepatotoxicity of carbon tetrachloride is much greater than is the case when it is given alone. *Antagonism* occurs when two chemicals administered together interfere with each other's actions or one interferes with the action of the other (example: 4 + 6 = 8; 4 + (−4) = 0; 4 + 0 = 1). There are four major types of antagonism: functional, chemical, dispositional, and receptor. *Functional antagonism* occurs when two chemicals counterbalance each other by producing opposite effects on the same physiologic function. For example, the marked fall in blood pressure during severe barbiturate intoxication can be antagonized effectively by the intravenous administration of a vasopressor agent such as norepinephrine or metaraminol. *Chemical antagonism* or *inactivation* is simply a chemical reaction between two compounds that produces a less toxic product. For example, chelators of metal ions decrease metal toxicity and antitoxins antagonize the action of various animal toxins. *Dispositional antagonism* occurs when the absorption, biotransformation, distribution, or excretion of a chemical is altered so that the concentration and/or duration of the chemical at the target organ are diminished. Thus, the prevention of absorption of a toxicant by ipecac or charcoal, increased activity of metabolizing enzymes with enzyme inducers, and the increased excretion of a chemical caused by the administration of a diuretic are examples of dispositional antagonism. *Receptor antagonism* occurs when two chemicals that bind to the same receptor produce less of an effect when given together than the addition of their separate effects (example: 4 +

6 = 8) or when one chemical antagonizes the effect of the second chemical (example: 0 + 4 = 1). Receptor antagonists often are termed *blockers*.

TOLERANCE

Tolerance is a state of decreased responsiveness to a toxic effect of a chemical resulting from prior exposure to that chemical or to a structurally related chemical. Two major mechanisms are responsible for tolerance: One is due to a decreased amount of toxicant reaching the site where the toxic effect is produced (*dispositional tolerance*), and the other is due to reduced responsiveness of a tissue to the chemical.

DOSE RESPONSE

The characteristics of exposure and the spectrum of effects come together in a correlative relationship customarily referred to as the *dose–response relationship*. Whatever response is selected for measurement, the relationship between the degree of response of the biological system and the amount of toxicant administered assumes a form that occurs so consistently that it is considered the most fundamental and pervasive concept in toxicology.

From a practical perspective, there are two types of dose–response relationships: (1) the individual dose–response relationship, which describes the response of an *individual* organism to varying doses of a chemical, often referred to as a "graded" response because the measured effect is continuous over a range of doses, and (2) a quantal dose–response relationship, which characterizes the distribution of responses to different doses in a *population* of individual organisms.

Individual, or Graded, Dose–Response Relationships

Individual dose–response relationships are characterized by a dose-related increase in the severity of the response. For example, Fig. 2-2 shows the dose–response relationship between different dietary doses of the organophosphate insecticide chlorpyrifos and the extent of inhibition of two different enzymes in the brain: acetylcholinesterase and carboxylesterase. In the brain, the degree of inhibition of both enzymes is clearly dose-related and spans a wide range, although the amount of inhibition per unit dose is different for the two enzymes. From the shapes of these two dose–response curves it is evident that in the brain, cholinesterase is more easily inhibited than carboxylesterase is. The toxicologic response that results is related directly to the degree of cholinesterase

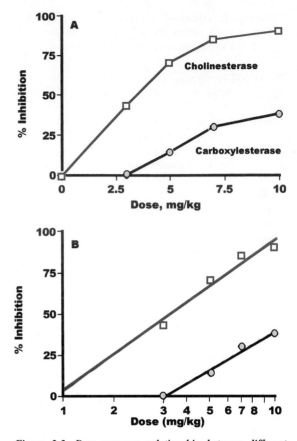

Figure 2-2. Dose–response relationship between different doses of the organophosphate insecticide chlorpyrifos and esterase enzyme inhibition in the brain. Open squares and blue lines represent acetylcholinesterase activity and closed circles represent carboxylesterase activity in the brains of pregnant female Long-Evans rats given five daily doses of chlorpyrifos. *A.* Dose–response curve plotted on an arithmetic scale. *B.* Same data plotted on a semilog scale. (Data derived from Lassiter et al: Gestational exposure to chlorpyrifos: Dose response profiles for cholinesterase and carboxylesterase activity. *Toxicol Sci* 52:92–100, 1999, with permission.)

enzyme inhibition in the brain. It should be noted that most toxic substances have multiple sites or mechanisms of toxicity, each with its own "dose–response" relationship and subsequent adverse effect.

Quantal Dose–Response Relationships

In contrast to the "graded" or continuous-scale dose–response relationship that occurs in individuals, the dose–response relationships in a *population* are by definition quantal—or "all or none"—in nature; that is, at any given dose, an individual in the population is classified as either a "responder" or a "nonresponder." Although these distinctions between "quantal population" and "graded individual" dose–response relationships are useful, the two types of responses are conceptually identical. The ordinate in both cases is simply labeled *the response,* which may be the degree of response in an individual or system or the fraction of a population responding, and the abscissa is the range in administered doses.

The LD$_{50}$ is the statistically derived single dose of a substance that can be expected to cause death in 50 percent of the animals tested. The top panel of Fig. 2-3 shows that quantal dose responses such as lethality exhibit a normal or gaussian distribution. The frequency histogram in this panel also shows the relationship between dose and effect. The bars represent the percentages of animals that died at each dose minus the percentages that died at the immediately lower dose. One can see clearly that only a few animals responded to the lowest dose and the highest dose. Larger numbers of animals responded to doses intermediate between those two extremes, and the maximum frequency of response occurred in the middle portion of the dose range. Thus, we have a bell-shaped curve known as a *normal frequency distribution.* The reason for this normal distribution is that there are differences in susceptibility to chemicals among individuals. Animals responding at the left end of the curve are referred to as *hypersusceptible,* and those at the right end of the curve are called *resistant.* If the numbers of individuals responding at each consecutive dose are added together, a cumulative, quantal dose–response relationship is obtained. When a sufficently large number of doses is used with a large number of animals per dose, a sigmoid dose–response curve is observed, as depicted in the middle panel of Fig. 2-3. With the lowest dose (6 mg/kg), 1 percent of the animals die. A normally distributed sigmoid curve such as this one approaches a response of 0 percent as the dose is decreased and approaches 100 percent as the dose is increased, but—theoretically—it never passes through 0 and 100 percent. However, the minimally effective dose of any chemical that evokes a stated all-or-none response is called the *threshold dose* even though it cannot be determined experimentally.

The sigmoid curve has a relatively linear portion between 16 percent and 84 percent. These values represent the limits of 1 standard deviation (SD) of the mean (and the median) in a population with truly normal or gauss-

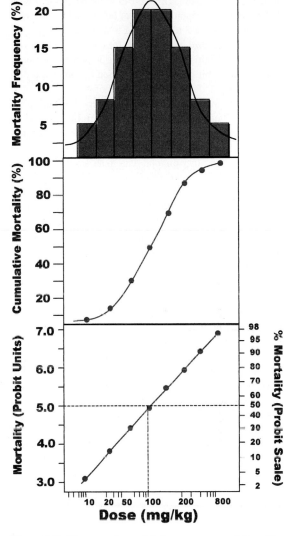

Figure 2-3. Diagram of quantal dose–response relationship. The abscissa is a log dosage of the chemical. In the top panel the ordinate is mortality frequency, in the middle panel the ordinate is percent mortality, and in the bottom panel the mortality is given in probit units (see text).

ian distribution. In a normally distributed population, the mean ± 1 SD represents 68.3 percent of the population, the mean ± 2 SD represents 95.5 percent of the population, and the mean ± 3 SD equals 99.7 percent of the population. Since quantal dose–response phenomena usually are normally distributed, one can convert the percent response to units of deviation from the mean or normal equivalent deviations (NEDs). Thus, the NED for a

50 percent response is 0; an NED of +1 is equated with an 84.1 percent response. Units of NED can be converted by the addition of 5 to the value to avoid negative numbers and called *probit units* (from the contraction of *probability unit*). In this transformation, a 50 percent response becomes a probit of 5, a +1 deviation becomes a probit of 6, and a −1 deviation is a probit of 4.

The data in the top two panels of Fig. 2-3 are replotted in the bottom panel with the mortality plotted in probit units to form a straight line. In essence, what is accomplished in a probit transformation is an adjustment of mortality or other quantal data to an assumed normal population distribution, resulting in a straight line. The LD_{50} is obtained by drawing a horizontal line from the probit unit 5, which is the 50 percent mortality point, to the dose–effect line. At the point of intersection, a vertical line is drawn, and this line intersects the abscissa at the LD_{50} point. In addition to the LD_{50}, the slope of the dose–response curve can be obtained. Figure 2-4 shows the dose–response curves for the mortality of two compounds. Compound A exhibits a "flat" dose–response curve, indicating that a large change in dosage is required before a significant change in response will be observed. However, compound B exhibits a "steep" dose–response curve in which a relatively small change in dosage will cause a large change in response. The LD_{50} for both compounds is the same (8 mg/kg); however, the slopes of the dose–response curves are quite different. At one-half of the LD_{50} of the compounds (4 mg/kg), less than 1 percent of the animals exposed to compound B would die but 20 percent of the animals given compound A would die.

One might view dosage on the basis of body weight as being less appropriate than other bases, such as surface area, which is approximately proportional to (body

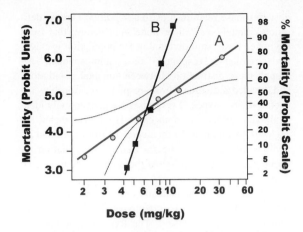

Figure 2-4. Comparison of dose–response relationships for two different chemicals, plotted on a log dose-probit scale. Note that the slope of the dose–response relationship is steeper for chemical *B* than for chemical *A*. Dotted lines represent the confidence limits for chemical *A*.

weight)$^{2/3}$. In Table 2-2, selected values are given to compare the differences in dosage by the two alternatives. Given a dose of 100 mg/kg, it can be seen that the dose (milligrams per animal), of course, is proportional to the dose administered by body weight. Surface area is not proportional to weight: Whereas the weight of a human is 3500 times greater than that of a mouse, the surface area of humans is only about 390 times greater than that of mice. The same dose given to humans and mice on a weight basis (mg/kg) would be approximately 10 times greater in humans than in mice if that dosage were expressed per surface area (mg/cm^2).

Table 2-2
Comparison of Dosage by Weight and Surface Area

	BODY WEIGHT g	DOSAGE mg/kg	DOSE mg/animal	SURFACE AREA cm^2	DOSAGE mg/cm^2
Mouse	20	100	2	46	0.043
Rat	200	100	20	325	0.061
Guinea pig	400	100	40	565	0.071
Rabbit	500	100	150	1,270	0.118
Cat	2,000	100	200	1,380	0.145
Monkey	4,000	100	400	2,980	0.134
Dog	12,000	100	1,200	5,770	0.207
Human	70,000	100	7,000	18,000	0.388

Shape of the Dose–Response Curve

Essential Nutrients The shape of the dose–response relationship has many important implications in toxicity assessment. For example, for substances that are required for normal physiologic function and survival (e.g., vitamins and essential trace elements such as chromium, cobalt, and selenium), the shape of the "graded" dose–response relationship in an individual over the entire dose range is actually U-shaped (Fig. 2-5). That is, at very low doses (or deficiency), there is a high level of adverse effect, which decreases with an increasing dose. As the dose is increased to a point where the deficiency no longer exists, no adverse response is detected and the organism is in a state of homeostasis. However, as the dose is increased to abnormally high levels, an adverse response (usually qualitatively different from that observed at deficient doses) appears and increases in magnitude with increasing doses.

Hormesis Some nonnutritional toxic substances also may impart beneficial or stimulatory effects at low doses, but at higher doses they produce adverse effects. This concept of "hormesis" also may result in a U-shaped dose–response curve. For example, chronic alcohol consumption is well recognized to increase the risk of esophageal cancer, liver cancer, and cirrhosis of the liver at relatively high doses, and this response is dose-related (curve A in Fig. 2-6). However, there is substantial clinical and epidemiologic evidence that low to moderate consumption of alcohol reduces the incidence of coronary heart disease and stroke (curve B in Fig. 2-6). Thus, when all responses are plotted on the ordinate, a U-shaped dose–response curve is obtained (curve C in Fig. 2-6).

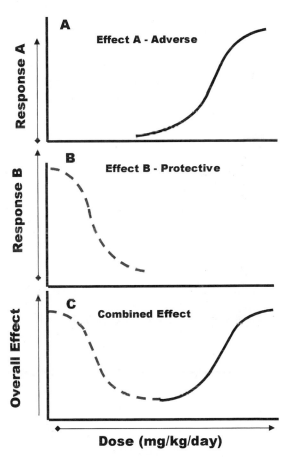

Figure 2-6. Hypothetical dose–response relationship depicting characteristics of hormesis. Hormetic effects of a substance are hypothesized to occur when relatively low doses result in the stimulation of a beneficial or protective response (*B*), such as the induction of enzymatic pathways that protect against oxidative stress. Although low doses provide a potential beneficial effect, a threshold is exceeded as the dose increases and the net effects will be detrimental (*A*), resulting in a typical dose-related increase in toxicity. The complete dose–response curve (*C*) is conceptually similar to the individual dose–response relationship for essential nutrients shown in Fig. 2-5.

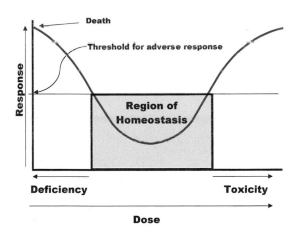

Figure 2-5. Individual dose–response relationship for an essential substance such as a vitamin or trace element. It generally is recognized that for most types of toxic responses, a threshold exists such that at doses below the threshold, no toxicity is evident. For essential substances, doses below the minimum daily requirement, as well as those above the threshold for safety, may be associated with toxic effects. The blue-shaded region represents the "region of homeostasis"—the dose range that results in neither deficiency nor toxicity.

Another important aspect of the dose–response relationship at low doses is the concept of the threshold: a dose below which the probability of an individual responding is zero. For the individual dose–response relationship, thresholds for most toxic effects certainly exist, although interindividual variability in response and qualitative changes in response pattern with dose make it difficult to establish a true "no effects" threshold for any chemical.

In evaluating the shape of the dose–response relationship in populations, it is realistic to consider inflections in the shape of the dose–response curve rather than absolute thresholds. That is, the slope of the dose–response relationship at high doses may be substantially different from the slope at low doses, usually because of dispositional differences in the chemical. Saturation of biotransformation pathways, protein-binding sites or receptors, and depletion of intracellular cofactors are some reasons why sharp inflections in the dose–response relationship may occur.

Assumptions in Deriving the Dose–Response Relationship

A number of assumptions must be considered before dose–response relationships can be used appropriately. The first is that the response is due to the chemical administered, a cause-and-effect relationship.

A second assumption is that the magnitude of the response is in fact related to the dose. This assumes that there is a molecular target site (or sites) with which the chemical interacts to initiate the response, which is related to the concentration of the agent at the target site, which in turn is related to the dose administered.

The third assumption is that there exists both a quantifiable method of measuring and a precise means of expressing the toxicity. A given chemical may have a family of dose–response relationships, one for each toxic endpoint. For example, a chemical that produces cancer through genotoxic effects, liver damage through inhibition of a specific enzyme, and CNS effects through a different mechanism may have three distinct dose–response relationships, one for each endpoint.

With a new substance, the customary starting point in toxicologic evaluation utilizes lethality as an index. Lethality provides an unequivocal measure of comparison among many substances whose mechanisms and sites of action may be markedly different. From these studies, clues to the direction of further studies come about in two important ways. The first is a detailed observation

of the intact animal while it is alive. The second is histologic examination of major tissues and organs for abnormalities after death. From these observations, one usually can obtain more specific information about the events leading to the lethal effect and the target organs involved and often a suggestion about the possible mechanism of toxicity.

Evaluating the Dose–Response Relationship

Comparison of Dose Responses   Figure 2-7 illustrates a hypothetical quantal dose–response curve for a desirable effect of a chemical effective dose (ED) such as anesthesia, a toxic dose (TD) effect such as liver injury, and the lethal dose (LD). Even though the curves for the effective dose and the lethal dose are nearly parallel, the mechanism by which the drug works is not necessarily that by which the lethal effects are caused. The same admonition applies to any pair of parallel "effect" curves or any other pair of toxicity or lethality curves.

Therapeutic Index   The hypothetical curves in Fig. 2-7 illustrate two other interrelated points: the importance of the selection of the toxic criterion and the interpretation of comparative effect. The *therapeutic index* (TI) is defined as the ratio of the dose required to produce a toxic effect and the dose needed to elicit the desired therapeutic response. Similarly, an index of comparative toxicity is

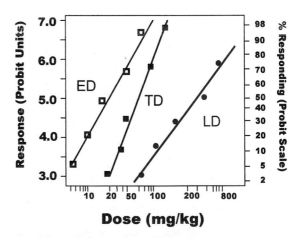

Figure 2-7. Comparison of effective dose (ED), toxic dose (TD), and lethal dose (LD).   The plot is of log dosage versus percentage of population responding in probit units.

obtained from the ratio of doses of two different materials to produce an identical response or the ratio of doses of the same material necessary to yield different toxic effects.

The most commonly used index of effect, whether beneficial or toxic, is the median dose, that is, the dose required to result in a response in 50 percent of a population (or to produce 50 percent of a maximal response). The therapeutic index of a drug is an approximate statement about the relative safety of a drug expressed as the ratio of the lethal or toxic dose to the therapeutic dose:

$$TI = LD_{50}/ED_{50}$$

From Fig. 2-7, one can approximate a therapeutic index by using these median doses. The larger the ratio, the greater the relative safety. The ED_{50} is approximately 20, and the LD_{50} is about 200; thus, the therapeutic index is 10, a number indicative of a relatively safe drug. However, median doses indicate nothing about the slopes of the dose–response curves for therapeutic and toxic effects.

Margins of Safety and Exposure   One way to overcome this deficiency is to use the ED_{99} for the desired effect and the LD_1 for the undesired effect. These parameters are used to calculate the margin of safety:

$$\text{Margin of safety} = LD_1/ED_{99}$$

For nondrug chemicals, the term *margin of safety* is an indicator of the magnitude of the difference between an estimated "exposed dose" to a human population and the NOAEL (no observable adverse effect level) determined in experimental animals.

Potency versus Efficacy   To compare the toxic effects of two or more chemicals, the dose response to the toxic effects of each chemical must be established. The potency and maximal efficacy of the two chemicals to produce a toxic effect can be explained by reference to Fig. 2-8. Chemical A is said to be more potent than chemical B, and C is more potent than D, because of their relative positions along the dosage axis. Potency thus refers to the range of doses over which a chemical produces increasing responses. Maximal efficacy reflects the limit of the dose–response relationship on the response axis to a certain chemical. Chemicals A and B have equal maximal efficacy, whereas the maximal efficacy of C is less than that of D.

VARIATION IN TOXIC RESPONSES

Selective Toxicity

Selective toxicity means that a chemical produces injury to one kind of living matter without harming another form of life even though the two may exist in intimate

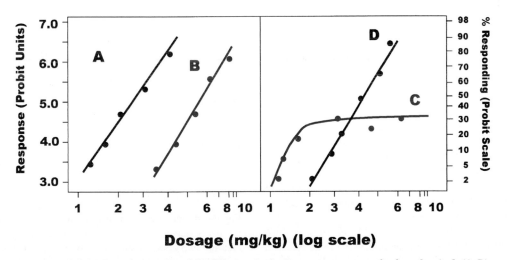

Figure 2-8. Schematic representation of the difference in the dose–response curves for four chemicals (A–D), illustrating the difference between potency and efficacy (see text).

contact. By taking advantage of biological diversity, it is possible to develop agents that are lethal for an undesired species and harmless for other species. Such selective toxicity can be due to differences in distribution (absorption, biotransformation, or excretion) or to differing biochemical processing of the toxicant by different organisms.

Species Differences

Although a basic tenet of toxicology is that "experimental results in animals, when properly qualified, are applicable to humans," it is important to recognize that both quantitative and qualitative differences in the response to toxic substances may occur among different species. Identifying the mechanistic basis for species differences in response to chemicals establishes the relevance of animal data to human response.

Individual Differences in Response

Even within a species, there can be large interindividual differences in response to a chemical because of subtle genetic differences referred to as *genetic polymorphisms.* These differences may be responsible for idiosyncratic reactions to chemicals and interindividual differences in toxic responses.

DESCRIPTIVE ANIMAL TOXICITY TESTS

Two main principles underlie all descriptive animal toxicity testing. The first is that the effects produced by a compound in laboratory animals, when properly qualified, are applicable to humans. The second principle is that exposure of experimental animals to toxic agents in high doses is a necessary and valid method of discovering possible hazards in humans because the incidence of an effect in a population is greater as the dose or exposure increases. Obtaining statistically valid results from the small groups of animals used in toxicity testing requires the use of relatively large doses so that the effect of interest will occur frequently enough to be detected. However, the use of high doses can create problems in interpretation if the response(s) obtained at high doses does not occur at low doses.

Toxicity tests are not designed to demonstrate that a chemical is safe but to characterize the toxic effects a chemical can produce. There are no set toxicology tests that have to be performed on every chemical intended for commerce. Depending on the eventual use of the chem-

ical, the toxic effects produced by structural analogs of the chemical, as well as the toxic effects produced by the chemical itself, contribute to the determination of the toxicology tests that should be performed.

Acute Lethality

The first toxicity test performed on a new chemical is acute toxicity. The LD_{50} and other acute toxic effects are determined after one or more routes of administration (one route being oral or the intended route of exposure) in one or more species, usually the mouse and the rat but sometimes the rabbit and the dog. Daily examination of the animals and tabulation of the number of animals that die in a 14-day period after a single dosage occur. Acute toxicity tests (1) give a quantitative estimate of acute toxicity (LD_{50}), (2) identify target organs and other clinical manifestations of acute toxicity, (3) establish the reversibility of the toxic response, and (4) provide dose-ranging guidance for other studies.

If there is a reasonable likelihood of substantial exposure to the material by dermal or inhalation exposure, acute dermal and acute inhalation studies are performed. When animals are exposed acutely to chemicals in the air they breathe or the water they (fish) live in, the lethal concentration 50 (LC_{50}) usually is determined for a known time of exposure, that is, the concentration of the chemical in the air or water that causes death to 50 percent of the animals. The acute dermal toxicity test usually is performed in rabbits. The site of application is shaved, and the substance is applied and covered for 24 h and then removed. The skin is cleaned, and the animals are observed for 14 days to calculate the LD_{50}. Acute inhalation studies are performed that are similar to other acute toxicity studies except that the route of exposure is inhalation for 4 h.

Acute lethality studies are essential for characterizing the toxic effects of chemicals and their hazard to humans. The most meaningful scientific information derived from acute lethality tests comes from clinical observations and postmortem examination of animals rather than from the specific LD_{50} value.

Skin and Eye Irritations

For the dermal irritation test (Draize test), the skin of rabbits is shaved, and the chemical is applied to one intact and two abraded sites and covered for 4 h. The degree of skin irritation is scored for erythema (redness), eschar (scab) and edema (swelling) formation, and corrosive action. These dermal irritation observations are repeated at various intervals after the covered patch has been removed. To determine the degree of ocular irritation, the chemical is instilled into one eye of each test rabbit. The contralateral eye is used as the control. The eyes of the rabbits are examined at various times after application.

Alternative in vitro models, including epidermal keratinocyte and corneal epithelial cell culture models, have been developed for evaluating the cutaneous and ocular toxicity of substances.

Sensitization

Information about the potential of a chemical to sensitize skin is needed in addition to irritation testing for all materials that may come into contact with the skin repeatedly. In general, the test chemical is administered to the shaved skin of guinea pigs topically, intradermally, or both over a period of 2 to 4 weeks. Some 2 to 3 weeks after the last treatment, the animals are challenged with a nonirritating concentration of the test substance, and the development of erythema is evaluated.

Subacute (Repeated-Dose Study)

Subacute toxicity tests are performed to obtain information on the toxicity of a chemical after repeated administration typically for 14 days and as an aid in establishing doses for subchronic studies.

Subchronic

Subchronic exposure usually lasts for 90 days. The principal goals of a subchronic study are to establish a "lowest observed adverse effect level" (LOAEL), establish a NOAEL, and further identify and characterize the specific organ or organs affected by the test compound after repeated administration.

A subchronic study usually is conducted in two species (rat and dog for the U.S. Food and Drug Administration; mouse and rat for the U.S. Environmental Protection Agency) by the route of intended exposure. At least three doses are employed: a high dose that produces toxicity but less than 10 percent fatalities, a low dose that produces no apparent toxic effects, and an intermediate dose. Animals should be observed once or twice daily for signs of toxicity. All premature deaths should be recorded and necropsied. Severely moribund animals should be terminated immediately to preserve tissues and reduce unnecessary suffering. At the end of the 90-day study, all the remaining animals should be terminated and blood and tissues should be

collected for further analysis. The gross condition and microscopic condition of the organs and tissues are recorded and evaluated. Hematology, blood chemistry, and urinalysis measurements usually are done before, in the middle of, and at the termination of exposure. Hematology measurements usually include hemoglobin concentration, hematocrit, erythrocyte counts, total and differential leukocyte counts, platelet count, clotting time, and prothrombin time. Clinical chemistry determinations commonly include glucose, calcium, potassium, urea nitrogen, alanine aminotransferase (ALT), serum aspartate aminotransferase (AST), gamma-glutamyltranspeptidase (GGT), sorbitol dehydrogenase, lactic dehydrogenase, alkaline phosphatase, creatinine, bilirubin, triglycerides, cholesterol, albumin, globulin, and total protein. Urinalysis includes determination of specific gravity or osmolarity, pH, proteins, glucose, ketones, bilirubin, and urobilinogen as well as microscopic examination of formed elements. If humans are likely to have significant exposure to the chemical through dermal contact or inhalation, subchronic dermal and/or inhalation experiments also may be required.

Chronic

Long-term or chronic exposure studies are performed similarly to subchronic studies except that the period of exposure is usually 6 months to 2 years. Chronic toxicity tests often are designed to assess both the cumulative toxicity and the carcinogenic potential of chemicals. Both gross and microscopic pathologic examinations are made not only on animals that survive the chronic exposure but also on those which die prematurely.

Dose selection is critical to ensure that premature mortality from chronic toxicity does not limit the number of animals that survive to a normal life expectancy. Most regulatory guidelines require that the highest administered dose be the estimated maximum tolerable dose (MTD), that is, the dose that suppresses gain in body weight slightly in a 90-day subchronic study. Generally, one or two additional doses, usually one-half and one-quarter of the MTD, and a control group are tested.

Chronic toxicity assays commonly evaluate the potential oncogenicity of test substances. Both benign and malignant tumors must be reported. Properly designed chronic oncogenicity studies require a concurrent control group matched for variables such as age, diet, and housing conditions.

Other Tests

Mutagenesis is the ability of chemicals to cause changes in the genetic material in the nucleus of cells in ways that allow the changes to be transmitted during cell division. Mutagenicity is discussed in detail in Chap. 9.

Information on methods, concepts, and problems associated with inhalation toxicology is provided in Chaps. 15 and 28. A discussion of behavioral toxicology can be found in Chap. 16.

BIBLIOGRAPHY

Calabrese EJ, Baldwin LA: Chemical hormesis: Its historical foundations as a biological hypothesis. *Toxicol Pathol* 27: 195–216, 1999.

Davila JC, Rodriguez RJ, Melchert RB, et al: Predictive value of in vitro model systems in toxicology. *Annu Rev Pharmacol Toxicol* 38: 63–96, 1998.

Derelanko MJ, Hollinger MA (eds): *CRC Handbook of Toxicology.* New York: CRC Press, 1995.

Hayes AW (ed): *Principles and Methods of Toxicology,* 4th ed. New York: Taylor and Francis, 2001.

Kitchin KT (ed): *Carcinogenicity Testing: Predicting and Interpreting Chemical Effects.* New York: Marcel Dekker, 1999.

Levine RR: *Pharmacology: Drug Actions and Reactions.* New York: Parthenon, 1996.

Tennant RW, Stasiewicz S, Mennear J, et al: Genetically altered mouse models for identifying carcinogens. *IARC Sci Publ* 146:123–150, 1999.

Williams PD, Hottendorf GH (eds): *Toxicological Testing and Evaluation.* Volume 2 in Sipes GI, McQueen CA, Gandolfi AJ (eds): *Comprehensive Toxicology.* New York: Pergamon Press, 1997.

CHAPTER 3

MECHANISMS OF TOXICITY

Zoltán Gregus and Curtis D. Klaassen

KEY POINTS

- Toxicity involves the delivery of toxicant to its target or targets and interactions with endogenous target molecules that may trigger perturbations in cell function and/or structure or initiate repair mechanisms at the molecular, cellular, and/or tissue levels.

- Biotransformation to harmful products is called *toxication* or *metabolic activation.*

- Biotransformations that eliminate the ultimate toxicant or prevent its formation are called *detoxications.*

- Apoptosis, or programmed cell death, is a tightly controlled, organized process by which individual cells break into small fragments that are phagocytosed by adjacent cells or macrophages without producing an inflammatory response.

- Sustained elevation of intracellular Ca^{2+} is harmful because it can result in (1) depletion of energy reserves by inhibiting the ATPase used in oxidative phosphorylation, (2) dysfunction of microfilaments, (3) activation of hydrolytic enzymes, and (4) generation of reactive oxygen species and reactive nitrogen species.

- Cell injury progresses toward cell necrosis (death) if molecular repair mechanisms are inefficient or the molecular damage is not readily reversible.

- Chemical carcinogenesis involves insufficient function of various repair mechanisms, including (1) failure of DNA repair, (2) failure of apoptosis (programmed cell death), and (3) failure to terminate cell proliferation.

An understanding of the mechanisms of toxicity provides a rational basis for interpreting descriptive toxicity data. The cellular mechanisms that contribute to the manifestation of toxicities are considered by relating a series of events that begins with exposure, involves a multitude of interactions between the invading toxicant and the organism, and culminates in a toxic effect.

As a result of the huge number of potential toxicants and the multitude of biological structures and processes that can be impaired, a tremendous number of possible pathways may lead to toxicity (Fig. 3-1). Commonly, a toxicant delivered to its target reacts with it, and the resultant cellular dysfunction manifests itself in toxicity. Sometimes a xenobiotic does not react with a specific target molecule but instead adversely influences the biological environment, causing molecular, organellar, cellular, or organ dysfunction that leads to deleterious effects.

The most complex path to toxicity involves more steps (Fig. 3-1). First, the toxicant is delivered to its target or targets (step 1) and interacts with endogenous target molecules (step 2a), triggering perturbations in cell function and/or structure (step 3), which initiate repair mechanisms at the molecular, cellular, and/or tissue levels (step 4). When the perturbations induced by the toxicant exceed repair capacity or when repair becomes malfunctional, toxicity occurs. Tissue necrosis, cancer, and fibrosis are examples of chemically induced toxicities that follow this four-step course.

STEP 1—DELIVERY: FROM THE SITE OF EXPOSURE TO THE TARGET

Theoretically, the intensity of a toxic effect depends on the concentration and persistence of the ultimate toxicant at its site of action. The ultimate toxicant is the chemical species that reacts with the endogenous target molecule or critically alters the biological environment, initiating structural and/or functional alterations that result in toxicity. The ultimate toxicant can be the original chemical to which the organism is exposed (parent compound), a metabolite or a reactive oxygen or nitrogen species (ROS or RNS) generated during the biotransformation of the toxicant, or an endogenous molecule.

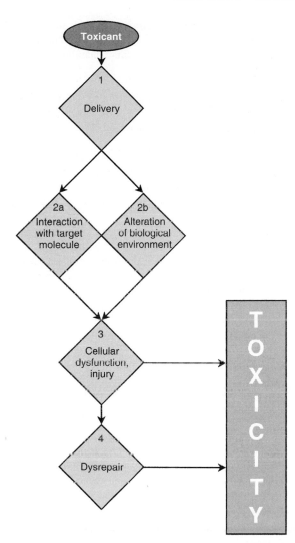

Figure 3-1. Potential stages in the development of toxicity after chemical exposure.

Absorption versus Presystemic Elimination

Absorption Absorption is the transfer of a chemical from the site of exposure, usually an external or internal body surface, into the systemic circulation. Several factors influence absorption (e.g., concentration, surface area of exposure, and characteristics of the epithelial layer through which the toxicant is being absorbed); lipid solubility is usually the most important factor because lipid-soluble molecules are absorbed most easily into cells.

Presystemic Elimination During transfer from the site of exposure to the systemic circulation, toxicants may be eliminated. This is common for chemicals absorbed from the gastrointestinal (GI) tract, because they must pass through the GI mucosal cells, liver, and lung before being distributed to the rest of the body by the systemic circulation. The GI mucosa and the liver may eliminate

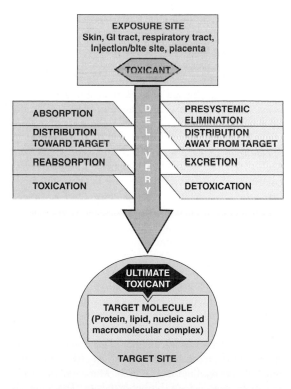

The concentration of the ultimate toxicant at the target molecule depends on the relative effectiveness of the processes that increase or decrease its concentration at the target site (Fig. 3-2). The accumulation of the ultimate toxicant at its target is facilitated by its absorption, distribution to the site of action, reabsorption, and toxication (metabolic activation). Presystemic elimination, distribution away from the site of action, excretion, and detoxication oppose these processes and work against the accumulation of the ultimate toxicant at the target molecule.

Figure 3-2. The process of toxicant delivery is the first step in the development of toxicity. Delivery—that is, movement of the toxicant from the site of exposure to the site of its action in an active form—is promoted by the processes listed on the left and opposed by the events indicated on the right.

a significant fraction of a toxicant during its passage through those tissues. Presystemic or first-pass elimination generally reduces the toxic effects of chemicals that reach their target sites by way of the systemic circulation but may contribute to injury of the digestive mucosa, the liver, and the lungs because these processes promote toxicant delivery to those sites.

Distribution to and Away from the Target

Toxicants exit the blood during the distribution phase, enter the extracellular space, and reach their site or sites of action, usually a macromolecule on either the surface or the interior of a particular type of cell. Chemicals also may be distributed to the site or sites of toxication, usually an intracellular enzyme, where the ultimate toxicant is formed.

Mechanisms Facilitating Distribution to a Target Distribution of toxicants to specific target sites may be enhanced by several factors, as is discussed below.

Porosity of the Capillary Endothelium Endothelial cells in the hepatic sinusoids and the renal peritubular capillaries have large fenestrae (50 to 150 nm in diameter) that permit the passage of even protein-bound xenobiotics. This favors the accumulation of chemicals in the liver and kidneys.

Specialized Transport Across the Plasma Membrane Specialized ion channels and membrane transporters can contribute to the delivery of toxicants to intracellular targets. Na^+, K^+-ATPase, voltage-gated Ca^{2+} channels, carrier-mediated uptake, endocytosis, and membrane recycling facilitate the entry of toxicants into specific cells, rendering those cells targets.

Accumulation in Cell Organelles Amphipathic xenobiotics with a protonatable amine group and a lipophilic character accumulate in lysosomes as well as mitochondria. Lysosomal accumulation occurs by means of pH trapping, that is, diffusion of the amine in an unprotonated form into the acidic interior of the organelle, where the amine is protonated, preventing its efflux, so that it impairs phospholipid degradation. Mitochondrial accumulation takes place electrophoretically. The amine is protonated in the intermembrane space and then sucked into the matrix space by the strong negative potential (-220 mV), where it may impair β-oxidation and oxidative phosphorylation.

Reversible Intracellular Binding Chemicals such as organic and inorganic cations and polycyclic aromatic hydrocarbons accumulate in melanin-containing cells by binding to melanin.

Mechanisms Opposing Distribution to a Target Distribution of toxicants to specific sites may be hindered by several processes, as is discussed below.

Binding to Plasma Proteins Most xenobiotics must dissociate from proteins in order to leave the blood and enter cells. Therefore, strong binding to plasma proteins delays and prolongs the effects and elimination of toxicants.

Specialized Barriers Brain capillaries lack fenestrae and are joined by extremely tight junctions, preventing the access of hydrophilic chemicals to the brain except by active transport. The spermatogenic cells are surrounded by Sertoli cells that are tightly joined to form the blood-testis barrier. Transfer of hydrophilic toxicants across the placenta also is restricted. However, none of these barriers is effective against lipophilic substances.

Distribution to Storage Sites Some chemicals accumulate in tissues (i.e., storage sites) where they do not exert significant effects. Such storage decreases toxicant availability for the target sites.

Association with Intracellular Binding Proteins Binding to nontarget intracellular sites, such as metallothionein, temporarily reduces the concentration of toxicants at the target site.

Export from Cells Intracellular toxicants may be transported back into the extracellular space. An ATP-dependent membrane transporter known as the multidrug-resistance (mdr) protein extrudes chemicals from cells.

Excretion versus Reabsorption

Excretion Excretion is the removal of xenobiotics from the blood and their return to the external environment. Excretion is a physical mechanism, whereas biotransformation is a chemical mechanism for eliminating the toxicant.

The route and speed of excretion depend largely on the physicochemical properties of the toxicant. The major excretory organs—the kidney and the liver—efficiently remove highly hydrophilic chemicals such as organic acids and bases.

There are no efficient elimination mechanisms for nonvolatile, highly lipophilic chemicals. If they are resistant to biotransformation, such chemicals are eliminated very slowly and tend to accumulate in the body after repeated exposure. Three rather inefficient processes are available for the elimination of such chemicals: excretion from the mammary gland in breast milk, excretion in bile, and excretion into the intestinal lumen from blood. Volatile, nonreactive toxicants such as gases and volatile liquids diffuse from pulmonary capillaries into the alveoli and are exhaled.

Reabsorption Toxicants delivered into the renal tubules may diffuse back across the tubular cells and into the peritubular capillaries. This tubular fluid reabsorption increases the intratubular concentration as well as the residence time of the chemical by slowing urine flow. Reabsorption by diffusion is dependent on the lipid solubility of the chemical and inversely related to the extent of ionization.

Toxicants delivered to the GI tract by biliary, gastric, and intestinal excretion and secretion by the salivary glands and the exocrine pancreas may be reabsorbed by diffusion across the intestinal mucosa. Reabsorption of compounds excreted into bile is possible only if the compounds are sufficiently lipophilic or are converted to more lipid-soluble forms in the intestinal lumen.

Toxication versus Detoxication

Toxication Biotransformation to harmful products is called *toxication* or *metabolic activation*. With some xenobiotics, toxication confers physicochemical properties that adversely alter the microenvironment of biological processes or structures. Occasionally, chemicals acquire structural features and reactivity by means of biotransformation that allows a more efficient interaction with specific receptors or enzymes. Most often, however, toxication renders endo- and xenobiotics indiscriminately reactive toward endogenous molecules with susceptible functional groups by conversion into one of several chemical species: (1) electrophiles (positively charged, electron-deficient chemical species that easily react with nucleophiles), (2) free radicals (chemical species with highly reactive unpaired electrons, such as superoxide anion ($O_2^{\cdot-}$) and hydroxyl radical ($HO^{\cdot}$), (3) nucleophiles (negatively charged molecules that react with electrophiles), and (4) redox-active reactants (molecules that can donate and accept electrons). The most reactive metabolites are electron-deficient molecules and molecular fragments such as electrophiles and

neutral or cationic free radicals. Some nucleophiles are reactive (e.g., HCN, CO).

Detoxication Biotransformations that eliminate the ultimate toxicant or prevent its formation are called *detoxications*. In some cases, detoxication may compete with toxication.

Detoxication of Toxicants with No Functional Groups In general, chemicals without functional groups, such as benzene and toluene, are detoxicated in two phases. Initially, a functional group such as hydroxyl or carboxyl is introduced into the molecule, and then an endogenous acid such as glucuronic acid, sulfuric acid, or an amino acid is added to the functional group by a transferase. With some exceptions, the final products are inactive, highly hydrophilic organic acids that are excreted readily.

Detoxication of Nucleophiles Nucleophiles generally are detoxicated by conjugation at the nucleophilic functional group.

Detoxication of Electrophiles Generally, detoxication of electrophilic toxicants involves conjugation with the nucleophile glutathione. This reaction may occur spontaneously or can be facilitated by glutathione *S*-transferases.

Detoxication of Free Radicals Because $O_2^{\cdot-}$ can be converted into much more reactive compounds (Fig. 3-3), its elimination is an important detoxication mechanism. Superoxide dismutases (SOD) located in the cytosol (Cu, Zn-SOD) and the mitochondria (Mn-SOD) convert $O_2^{\cdot-}$ to HOOH (Fig. 3-4). Subsequently, HOOH is reduced to water by cytosolic glutathione peroxidase or peroxisomal catalase (Fig. 3-4).

No enzyme eliminates $HO^{\cdot}$ owing to its extremely short half-life (10^{-9} s). The only effective protection against $HO^{\cdot}$ is to prevent its formation by converting its precursor, HOOH, to water (Fig. 3-4).

Peroxynitrite ($ONOO^{-}$, which is not a free radical oxidant) is significantly more stable than $HO^{\cdot}$ and reacts rapidly with CO_2 to form reactive free radicals (Fig. 3-3). Glutathione peroxidase can reduce $ONOO^{-}$ to nitrite (ONO^{-}). In addition, $ONOO^{-}$ reacts with oxyhemoglobin, heme-containing peroxidases, and albumin, all of which can be important sinks for $ONOO^{-}$. Furthermore, elimination of the two $ONOO^{-}$ precursors—$^{\cdot}NO$ by reaction with oxyhemoglobin and $O_2^{\cdot-}$ by SODs—is a significant mechanism in preventing $ONOO^{-}$ buildup.

Peroxidase-generated free radicals are eliminated by electron transfer from glutathione. This results in the

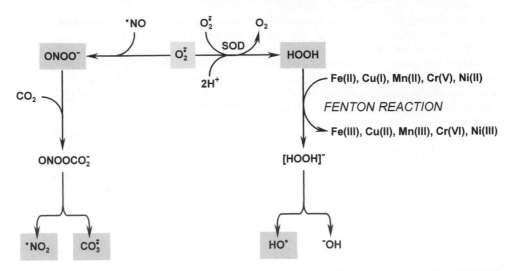

Figure 3-3. Two pathways for toxication of superoxide anion radical ($O_2^{\bar{\cdot}}$) via nonradical products (ONOO⁻ and HOOH) to radical products (•NO₂, CO₃•⁻ and HO•).   In one pathway, conversion of ($O_2^{\bar{\cdot}}$) to HOOH is spontaneous or is catalyzed by superoxide dismutase (SOD). Homolytic cleavage of HOOH to hydroxyl radical and hydroxyl ion is called the Fenton reaction and is catalyzed by the transition metal ions shown. Hydroxyl radical formation is the ultimate toxication for xenobiotics that form $O_2^{\bar{\cdot}}$ or for HOOH, the transition metal ions listed, and some chemicals that form complexes with these transition metal ions. In the other pathway, $O_2^{\bar{\cdot}}$ reacts avidly with nitric oxide (•NO), the product of •NO synthase (NOS), forming peroxynitrite (ONOO⁻). Spontaneous reaction of ONOO⁻ with carbon dioxide (CO₂) yields nitrosoperoxy carbonate (ONOOCO₂⁻) that is homolytically cleaved to nitrogen dioxide (•NO₂) and carbonate anion radical (CO₃•⁻). All three radical products indicated in this figure are oxidants, whereas •NO₂ is also a nitrating agent.

oxidation of glutathione, which is reversed by NADPH-dependent glutathione reductase (Fig. 3-5). Thus, glutathione plays an important role in the detoxication of both electrophiles and free radicals.

Detoxication of Protein Toxins Extra- and intracellular proteases are involved in the inactivation of toxic polypeptides. Venom toxins, such as α- and β-bungarotoxin, erabutoxin, and phospholipase, lose their activity when thioredoxin reduces their essential disulfide bond.

When Detoxication Fails Detoxication may be insufficient because the toxicant overwhelms the detoxication processes, a reactive toxicant inactivates a detoxicating enzyme, the detoxication is reversed after transfer to other tissues, or harmful by-products are produced by the detoxication process.

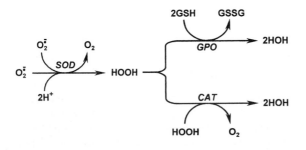

Figure 3-4. Detoxication of superoxide anion radical ($O_2^{\bar{\cdot}}$) by superoxide dismutase (SOD), glutathione peroxidase (GPO), and catalase (CAT).

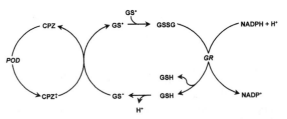

Figure 3-5. Detoxication of peroxidase (POD)–generated free radicals such as chlorpromazine free radical (CPZ⁺•) by glutathione (GSH). The by-products are glutathione thiyl radical (GS•) and glutathione disulfide (GSSG), from which GSH is regenerated by glutathione reductase (GR).

STEP 2—REACTION OF THE ULTIMATE TOXICANT WITH THE TARGET MOLECULE

Toxicity typically is mediated by a reaction of the ultimate toxicant with a target molecule (step 2a in Fig. 3-1). Subsequently, a series of secondary biochemical events occurs, leading to dysfunction or injury that is manifest at various levels of biological organization, such as at the target molecule itself, cell organelles, cells, tissues and organs, and even the whole organism.

Attributes of Target Molecules

Practically all endogenous compounds are potential targets for toxicants. The most prevalent and toxicologically relevant targets are nucleic acids (especially DNA), proteins, and membranes. The first target for reactive metabolites is often the enzyme responsible for their production or the adjacent intracellular structures. Not all targets for chemicals contribute to the harmful effects. Covalent binding to proteins without adverse consequences may represent a form of detoxication by sparing toxicologically relevant targets.

Types of Reactions

The ultimate toxicant may bind to the target molecules noncovalently or covalently and may alter it by hydrogen abstraction, by electron transfer, or enzymatically.

Noncovalent Binding Apolar interactions or the formation of hydrogen and ionic bonds typically is involved in the interaction of toxicants with targets such as membrane receptors, intracellular receptors, ion channels, and some enzymes. Noncovalent binding usually is reversible because of the comparatively low bonding energy.

Covalent Binding Being practically irreversible, covalent binding permanently alters endogenous molecules. Covalent adduct formation is common with electrophilic toxicants such as nonionic and cationic electrophiles and radical cations. These toxicants react with nucleophilic atoms that are abundant in biological macromolecules, such as proteins and nucleic acids. Neutral free radicals such as $HO^{\bullet}$, $^{\bullet}NO_2$, and $Cl_3C^{\bullet}$ also can bind covalently to biomolecules.

Hydrogen Abstraction Neutral free radicals can readily abstract H atoms from endogenous compounds, converting those compounds into radicals. Radicals also can remove hydrogen from CH_2 groups of free amino acids

or from amino acid residues in proteins and convert them to carbonyls, forming cross-links with DNA or other proteins.

Electron Transfer Chemicals can exchange electrons to oxidize or reduce other molecules, leading to the formation of harmful by-products. For example, chemicals can oxidize Fe(II) in hemoglobin to Fe(III) in methemoglobinemia.

Enzymatic Reactions A few toxins act enzymatically on specific target proteins. For example, diphtheria toxin blocks the function of elongation factor 2 in protein synthesis and cholera toxin activates a G protein through such a mechanism.

In summary, most ultimate toxicants act on endogenous molecules on the basis of their chemical reactivity. Those with more than one type of reactivity may react by different mechanisms with various target molecules.

Effects of Toxicants on Target Molecules

Dysfunction of Target Molecules Some toxicants activate protein target molecules, mimicking endogenous ligands. More commonly, chemicals inhibit the function of target molecules by blocking neurotransmitter receptors or ion channels or by inhibiting enzymes.

Protein function is impaired when conformation or structure is altered by interaction with the toxicant. Many proteins possess critical moieties that are essential for catalytic activity or assembly to macromolecular complexes. Covalent and/or oxidative modification of these moieties by xenobiotics can cause aberrant signal transduction and/or impaired maintenance of a cell's energy and metabolic homeostasis. Toxicants also may interfere with the template function of DNA. The covalent binding of chemicals to DNA causes nucleotide mispairing during replication.

Destruction of Target Molecules In addition to adduct formation, toxicants alter the primary structure of endogenous molecules by means of cross-linking and fragmentation. Cross-linking imposes both structural and functional constraints on the linked molecules.

Other target molecules are susceptible to spontaneous degradation after chemical attack. Free radicals such as $Cl_3COO^{\bullet}$ and $HO^{\bullet}$ can initiate peroxidative degradation of lipids by hydrogen abstraction from fatty acids, destroying lipids in cellular membranes and also generating endogenous lipid radicals and electrophiles, which can harm the structure of DNA.

Neoantigen Formation Covalent binding of xenobiotics or their metabolites to protein may evoke an immune response. Some chemicals (e.g., dinitrochlorobenzene, penicillin, nickel) bind to proteins spontaneously. Others may obtain reactivity by autooxidation to quinones (e.g., urushiols, the allergens in poison ivy) or by enzymatic biotransformation.

Toxicity Not Initiated by Reaction with Target Molecules

Some xenobiotics alter the biological microenvironment (see step 2b in Fig. 3-1), leading to a toxic response. Included here are (1) chemicals that alter H^+ ion concentrations in the aqueous biophase, (2) solvents and detergents that physicochemically alter the lipid phase of cell membranes and destroy transmembrane solute gradients, and (3) xenobiotics that cause harm merely by occupying a site or space.

STEP 3—CELLULAR DYSFUNCTION AND RESULTANT TOXICITIES

The reaction of toxicants with a target molecule may result in impaired cellular function as the third step in the development of toxicity (Figs. 3-1 and 3-6). Each cell in a multicellular organism carries out defined processes that are essential to cellular function. Certain programs determine whether cells undergo division, differentiation, or apoptosis. Other programs control the ongoing (momentary) activity of differentiated cells. To regulate these cellular programs, cells possess signaling networks that can be activated and inactivated by external signaling molecules.

As outlined in Fig. 3-6, the nature of the primary cellular dysfunction caused by toxicants, but not necessarily the ultimate outcome, depends on the role of the target molecule affected. If the target molecule is involved in cellular regulation (signaling), dysregulation of gene expression and/or dysregulation of momentary cellular function occurs primarily. However, if the target molecule is involved predominantly in the cell's internal

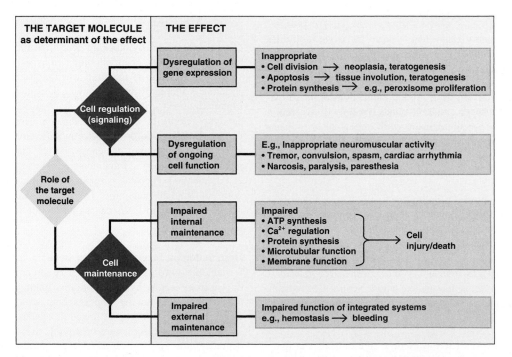

Figure 3-6. The third step in the development of toxicity: alteration of the regulatory or maintenance function of the cell.

maintenance, the resultant dysfunction ultimately can compromise survival of the cell. The reaction of a toxicant with targets serving external functions can influence the operation of other cells and integrated organ systems.

Toxicant-Induced Cellular Dysregulation

Cells are regulated by signaling molecules that activate specific cellular receptors linked to signal transducing networks that transmit the signals to the regulatory regions of genes and/or to functional proteins. Receptor activation ultimately may lead to altered gene expression and/or a chemical modification of specific proteins, typically by phosphorylation. Programs that control the destiny of cells primarily affect gene expression, whereas those which regulate the ongoing activities primarily influence the activity of functional proteins; however, one signal often evokes both responses because of branching and interconnection of signaling networks.

Dysregulation of Gene Expression Dysregulation of gene expression may occur at elements that are directly responsible for transcription, at components of the intracellular signal transduction pathway, and at the synthesis, storage, or release of the extracellular signaling molecules.

Dysregulation of Transcription   Transcription of genetic information from DNA to mRNA is controlled largely by an interplay between transcription factors (TFs) and the regulatory or promoter region of genes. Xenobiotics may interact with the promoter region of the gene, the TFs, or other components of the transcription initiation complex. However, altered activation of TFs appears to be the most common modality.

Many natural compounds, such as hormones and vitamins, influence gene expression by binding to and activating TFs. Natural or xenobiotic ligands may cause toxicity when they are administered at extreme doses or at critical periods during ontogenesis. Other compounds that act on TFs also can change the pattern of cell differentiation by overexpressing various genes.

Dysregulation of Signal Transduction Extracellular signaling molecules, such as growth factors, cytokines, hormones, and neurotransmitters, can ultimately activate TFs by utilizing cell surface receptors and intracellular signal transducing networks. Figure 3-7 depicts such networks and identifies some important signal-activated TFs

that control the transcriptional activity of genes that influence cell cycle progression and thus determine the fate of cells. An example is the c-Myc protein, which, upon dimerizing with Max protein and binding to its cognate nucleotide sequence, transactivates cyclin D and E genes. The cyclins in turn accelerate the cell division cycle by activating cyclin-dependent protein kinases that are involved in regulating the cell cycle. Mitogenic signaling molecules thus induce cellular proliferation.

The signal from the cell surface receptors to the TFs is relayed by successive protein–protein interactions and protein phosphorylations; that is, a signal molecule phosphorylates another protein, such as mitogen-activated kinase (MAPK), which activates that protein to phosphorylate and activate another protein. For example, ligands induce growth factor receptors (item 6 in Fig. 3-7) on the surface of all cells to self-phosphorylate, and these phosphorylated receptors then bind to adapter proteins through which they activate Ras. The active Ras initiates the MAPK cascade, involving serial phosphorylations of protein kinases, which finally reaches the TFs. These signal transducers are typically but not always activated by phosphorylation catalyzed by protein kinases and usually are inactivated by dephosphorylation carried out by protein phosphatases.

Chemicals may cause aberrant signal transduction most often by altering protein phosphorylation and occasionally by interfering with the GTPase activity of G proteins by disrupting normal protein–protein interactions or establishing abnormal ones or by altering the synthesis or degradation of signaling proteins. Such interventions ultimately may influence cell cycle progression.

Chemically Altered Signal Transduction with Proliferative Effect Xenobiotics that facilitate the phosphorylation of signal transducers often promote mitosis and tumor formation. The phorbol esters and fumonisin B activate protein kinase C (PKC), mimicking diacylglycerol (DAG), one of the physiologic activators of PKC (Fig. 3-7). The other physiologic PKC activator, Ca^{2+}, is mimicked by Pb^{2+}. Activated PKC promotes mitogenic signaling by starting a cascade that activates other kinases and allows certain transcription factors to bind to DNA. Protein kinases also may be activated by interacting proteins that have been altered by a xenobiotic.

Aberrant phosphorylation of proteins also may result from decreased dephosphorylation by phosphatases. Inhibition of phosphatases appears to be the underlying mechanism of the mitogenic effect of various chemicals,

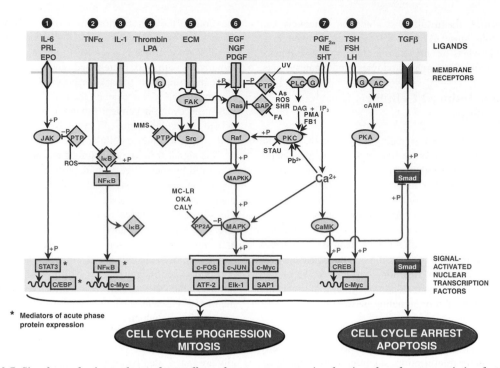

Figure 3-7. Signal transduction pathways from cell membrane receptors to signal-activated nuclear transcription factors that influence transcription of genes involved in cell cycle regulation. The symbols of cell membrane receptors are numbered 1–9, and some of their activating ligands are indicated. Circles represent G proteins, oval symbols protein kinases, rectangles transcription factors, wavy lines genes, and diamond symbols inhibitory proteins, such as protein phosphatases (PTP, PP2A), the GTPase-activating protein GAP, and the inhibitory binding protein IκB. Arrowheads indicate stimulation or formation of second messengers (e.g., DAG, IP$_3$, cAMP, Ca^{2+}), whereas blunt arrows indicate inhibition. Phosphorylation and dephosphorylation are indicated as +P and −P, respectively. Abbreviations for interfering chemicals are printed in black (As = arsenite; CALY = caly-culin A; FA = fatty acids; FB1 = fumonisin B; MC-LR = microcystin-LR; OKA = okadaic acid; MMS = methylmethane sul-fonate; PMA = phorbol miristate acetate; ROS = reactive oxygen species; SHR = SH-reactive chemicals, such as iodoacetamide; STAU = staurosporin).

In the center of the depicted networks is the pathway activated by growth factors, such as EGF, that acts on a tyrosine kinase receptor (#6), which uses adapter proteins (Shc, Grb2, and SOS; not shown) to convert the inactive GDP-bound Ras to the active GTP-bound form, which in turn activates the MAP-kinase phosphorylation cascade (Raf, MAPKK, MAPK). The phosphorylated MAPK moves into the nucleus and phosphorylates transcription factors, thereby enabling them to bind to cognate sequences in the promoter regions of genes to facilitate transcription. There are numerous interconnections between the signal transduction pathways. Some of these connections permit the use of the growth factor receptor (#6)-MAPK "highway" for other receptors (e.g., 4, 5, 7) to send mitogenic signals. For example, receptor (#4) joins in via its G protein β/γ subunits and tyrosine kinase Src; the integrin re-ceptor (#5), whose ligands are constituents of the extracellular matrix (ECM), possibly connects via G-protein Rho (not shown) and focal adhesion kinase (FAK); and the G-protein-coupled receptor (#7) via phospholipase C (PLC)-catalyzed formation of second messengers and activation of protein-kinase C (PKC). The mitogenic stimulus relayed along the growth factor receptor (#6)-MAPK axis can be amplified by, for example, the Raf-catalyzed phosphorylation of IκB, which unleashes NF-κB from this inhibitory pro-tein, and by the MAPK-catalyzed inhibitory phosphorylation of Smad that blocks the cell cycle arrest signal from the TGF-β re-ceptor (#9). Activation of protein kinases (PKC, CaMK, MAPK) by Ca^{2+} also can trigger mitogenic signaling. Several xenobiotics that are indicated in the figure may dysregulate the signaling network. Some may induce cell proliferation either by activating mi-togenic protein kinases (e.g., PKC) or by inhibiting inactivating proteins, such as protein phosphatases (PTP, PP2A), GAP, or IκB. Others, e.g., inhibitors of PKC, oppose mitosis and facilitate apoptosis.

This scheme is oversimplified and tentative in several details. Virtually all components of the signaling network (e.g., G pro-teins, PKCs, MAPKs) are present in multiple, functionally different forms whose distribution may be cell-specific. The pathways depicted are not equally relevant for all cells. In addition, these pathways regulating gene expression not only determine the fate of cells but also control certain aspects of the ongoing cellular activity. For example, NF-κB induces synthesis of acute phase proteins.

oxidative stress, and ultraviolet (UV) irradiation. Soluble protein phosphatase 2A (PP2A) in cells probably is responsible for reversing the growth factor–induced stimulation of MAPK, thus controlling the extent and duration of MAPK activity. PP2A also removes an activating phosphate from a mitosis-triggering protein kinase.

Apart from phosphatases, other inhibitory binding proteins can keep signaling under control. One is IκB, which binds to NF-κB, preventing its transfer into the nucleus and its function as a TF. Upon phosphorylation, IκB becomes degraded and NF-κB is set free. NF-κB is an important contributor to proliferative and prolife signaling as well as inflammation and acute-phase reactions. IκB degradation and NF-κB activation also can be induced by oxidative stress.

Chemically Altered Signal Transduction with Antiproliferative Effect Downturning of increased proliferative signaling after cell injury may compromise the replacement of injured cells (follow the path in Fig. 3-7: inhibition of Raf → diminished degradation of IκB → diminished binding of NF-κB to DNA → diminished expression of c-Myc mRNA. Downregulation of a normal mitogenic signal is a step away from survival and toward apoptosis.

Dysregulation of Extracellular Signal Production Hormones of the anterior pituitary exert mitogenic effects on endocrine glands in the periphery by acting on cell surface receptors. Pituitary hormone production is under negative feedback control by hormones of the peripheral glands. Perturbation of this circuit adversely affects pituitary hormone secretion and, in turn, the peripheral glands. Decreased secretion of pituitary hormone produces apoptosis followed by involution of the peripheral target gland.

Dysregulation of Ongoing Cellular Activity Toxicants can affect ongoing cellular activity in specialized cells adversely by disrupting any step in signal coupling.

Dysregulation of Electrically Excitable Cells Many xenobiotics influence cellular activity in excitable cells, such as neurons and skeletal, cardiac, and smooth muscle cells. Release of neurotransmitters and muscle contraction are controlled by transmitters and modulators synthesized and released by adjacent neurons. Chemicals that interfere with these mechanisms are listed in Table 3-1.

Perturbation of ongoing cellular activity by chemicals may be due to an alteration in (1) the concentration of neurotransmitters, (2) receptor function, (3) intracellular signal transduction, or (4) the signal-terminating processes.

Alteration in Neurotransmitter Levels Chemicals may alter synaptic levels of neurotransmitters by interfering with their synthesis, storage, release, or removal from the vicinity of the receptor.

Toxicant–Neurotransmitter Receptor Interactions Some chemicals interact directly with neurotransmitter receptors, including (1) agonists that associate with the ligand-binding site on the receptor and mimic the natural ligand, (2) antagonists that occupy the ligand-binding site but cannot activate the receptor, (3) activators, and (4) inhibitors that bind to a site on the receptor that is not directly involved in ligand binding. In the absence of other actions, agonists and activators mimic, whereas antagonists and inhibitors block, the physiologic responses characteristic of endogenous ligands.

Toxicant–Signal Transducer Interactions Many chemicals alter neuronal and/or muscle activity by acting on signal-transduction processes. Voltage-gated Na^+ channels, which transduce and amplify excitatory signals generated by ligand-gated cation channels, are activated or inactivated by several toxins (see Table 3-1).

Toxicant–Signal Terminator Interactions The cellular signal generated by cation influx is terminated by removal of the cations through channels or by transporters. Inhibition of cation export may prolong excitation.

Dysregulation of the Activity of Other Cells Whereas many signaling mechanisms operate in nonexcitable cells, such as exocrine secretory cells, Kupffer cells, and pancreatic beta cells, disturbance of these processes is usually less consequential.

Impairment of Internal Cellular Maintenance: Mechanisms of Toxic Cell Death For survival, all cells must synthesize endogenous molecules; assemble macromolecular complexes, membranes, and cell organelles; maintain the intracellular environment; and produce energy for operation. Agents that disrupt these functions jeopardize survival. There are three critical biochemical disorders that chemicals inflicting cell death may initiate: ATP depletion, a sustained rise in intracellular Ca^{2+}, and overproduction of ROS and RNS.

Depletion of ATP ATP plays a central role in cellular maintenance both as a chemical for biosynthesis and as

Table 3-1
Agents Acting on Signaling Systems for Neurotransmitters and Causing Dysregulation of the Momentary Activity of Electrically Excitable Cells Such as Neurons and Muscle Cells*

Receptor/Channel/Pump		Agonist/Activator		Antagonist/Inhibitor	
NAME	**LOCATION**	**AGENT**	**EFFECT**	**AGENT**	**EFFECT**
1. Acetylcholine nicotinic receptor	Skeletal muscle	Nicotine Anatoxin-a Cytisine *Ind:* ChE inhibitors	Muscle fibrillation, then paralysis	Tubocurarine, lophotoxin α-Bungarotoxin α-Cobrotoxin α-Conotoxin Erabutoxin b *Ind:* botulinum toxin	Muscle paralysis
	Neurons	See above	Neuronal activation	Pb^{2+}, general anesthetics	Neuronal inhibition
2. Glutamate receptor	CNS neurons	N-Methyl-D-aspartate Kainate, domoate Quinolinate Quisqualate *Ind:* hypoxia, HCN → glutamate release	Neuronal activation → convulsion, neuronal injury ("excitotoxicity")	Phencyclidine Ketamine General anesthetics	Neuronal inhibition → anesthesia Protection against "excitotoxicity"
3. GABA$_A$ receptor	CNS neurons	Muscimol, avermectins sedatives (barbiturates, benzodiazepines) General anesthetics (halothane) Alcohols (ethanol)	Neuronal inhibition → sedation, general anesthesia, coma, depression of vital centers	Bicuculline Picrotoxin Pentylenetetrazole Cyclodiene insecticides Lindane *Ind:* isoniazid	Neuronal activation → tremor, convulsion
4. Glycine receptor	CNS neurons, motor neurons	Avermectins (?) General anesthetics	Inhibition of motor neurons → paralysis	Strychnine *Ind:* tetanus toxin	Disinhibition of motor neurons → tetanic convulsion
5. Acetylcholine M$_2$ muscarinic receptor	Cardiac muscle	*Ind:* ChE inhibitors	Decreased heart rate and contractility	Belladonna alkaloids (e.g., atropine) atropinelike drugs (e.g., TCAD)	Increased heart rate
6. Opioid receptor	CNS neurons, visceral neurons	Morphine and congeners (e.g., heroin, meperidine)	Neuronal inhibition → analgesia, central respiratory depression, constipation, urine retention	Naloxone	Antidotal effects in opiate intoxication

(continued)

Table 3-1
(Continued)

Receptor/Channel/Pump		Agonist/Activator		Antagonist/Inhibitor	
NAME	**LOCATION**	**AGENT**	**EFFECT**	**AGENT**	**EFFECT**
7. Voltage-gated Na$^+$ channel	Neurons, muscle cells, etc.	Aconitine, veratridine Grayanotoxin Batrachotoxin Scorpion toxins Ciguatoxin DDT, pyrethroids	Neuronal activation → convulsion	Tetrodotoxin, saxitoxin μ-Conotoxin Local anesthetics Phenytoin Quinidine	Neuronal inhibition → paralysis, anesthesia Anticonvulsive action
8. Voltage-gated Ca$^+$ channel	Neurons, muscle cell, etc.	Maitotoxin (?) Atrotoxin (?) Latrotoxin (?)	Neuronal/muscular activation, cell injury	ω-Conotoxin Pb^{2+}	Neuronal inhibition → paralysis
9. Voltage/Ca^{2+}-activated K$^+$ Channel	Neurons, muscle cells	Pb^{2+}	Neuronal/muscular inhibition	Ba^{2+} Apamin (bee venom) Dendrotoxin	Neuronal/muscular activation → convulsion/spasm
10. Na$^+$,K$^+$-ATPase	Universal			Digitalis glycosides Oleandrin Chlordecone	Increased cardiac contractility, excitability Increased neuronal excitability → tremor
11. Acetylcholine M$_3$ muscarinic receptor	Smooth muscle, glands	*Ind:* ChE inhibitors	Smooth muscle spasm Salivation, lacrimation	Belladonna alkaloids (e.g., atropine) Atropine-like drugs (e.g., TCAD)	Smooth muscle relaxation → intestinal paralysis, decreased salivation, decreased perspiration
Acetylcholine M$_1$ muscarinic receptor	CNS neurons	Oxotremorine *Ind:* ChE inhibitors	Neuronal activation → convulsion	See above	
12. Adrenergic alpha$_1$ receptor	Vascular smooth muscle	(Nor)epinephrine *Ind:* cocaine, tyramine amphetamine, TCAD	Vasoconstriction → ischemia, hypertension	Prazosin	Antidotal effects in intoxication with alpha$_1$-receptor agonists
13. 5-HT$_2$ receptor	Smooth muscle	Ergot alkaloids (ergotamine, ergonovine)	Vasoconstriction → ischemia, hypertension	Ketanserine	Antidotal effects in ergot intoxication
14. Adrenergic beta$_1$ receptor	Cardiac muscle	(Nor)epinephrine *Ind:* cocaine, tyramine amphetamine, TCAD	Increased cardiac contractility and excitability	Atenolol, metoprolol	Antidotal effects in intoxication with beta$_1$-receptor agonists

*This tabulation is simplified and incomplete. Virtually all receptors and channels listed occur in multiple forms with different sensitivity to the agents. The reader should consult the pertinent literature for more detailed information. CNS = central nervous system; ChE = cholinesterase; *Ind* = indirectly acting (i.e., by altering neurotransmitter level); TCAD = tricyclic antidepressant.

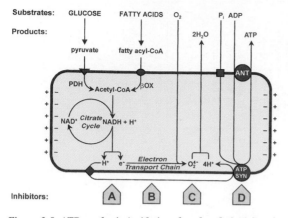

Figure 3-8. ATP synthesis (oxidative phosphorylation) in mitochondria. Arrows with roman numerals point to the ultimate sites of action of four categories of agents that interfere with oxidative phosphorylation (Table 3-2). For simplicity, this scheme does not indicate the outer mitochondrial membrane and show that protons are extruded from the matrix space along the electron transport chain at three sites. βOX = beta-oxidation of fatty acids; e⁻ = electron; P_i = inorganic phosphate; ANT = adenine nucleotide translocator; ATP SYN = ATP synthase (F_0F_1ATPase).

the major source of energy. ATP is utilized in numerous biosynthetic reactions and is incorporated into cofactors as well as nucleic acids. It is required for muscle contraction and polymerization of the cytoskeleton, fueling cellular motility, cell division, vesicular transport, and the maintenance of cell morphology. ATP drives ion transporters that maintain conditions essential for various cell functions.

Chemical energy is released by hydrolysis of ATP to ADP or AMP. The ADP is rephosphorylated in the mitochondria by ATP synthase (Fig. 3-8) through a process that couples oxidation of hydrogen to water and is termed *oxidative phosphorylation*. Oxidative phosphorylation also requires several steps, each of which can be interfered with by toxins, as described in Table 3-2.

Substances in class A interfere with the delivery of hydrogen to the electron transport chain. Class B chemicals inhibit the transfer of electrons along the electron transport chain to oxygen. Class C agents interfere with oxygen delivery to the terminal electron transporter, cytochrome oxidase. Chemicals in class D inhibit the activity of ATP synthase, the key enzyme for oxidative phosphorylation. At this site, the synthesis of ATP may be inhibited in one of four ways: (1) direct inhibition of ATP synthase, (2) interference with ADP delivery, (3) interference with inorganic phosphate delivery, and

(4) deprivation of ATP synthase from its driving force, the controlled influx of protons into the matrix space. Finally, chemicals causing mitochondrial DNA injury, thus impairing the synthesis of specific proteins encoded by the mitochondrial genome, are listed in group E.

Sustained Rise of Intracellular Ca^{2+} Intracellular Ca^{2+} levels are highly regulated and are maintained by the impermeability of the plasma membrane to Ca^{2+} and by transport mechanisms that remove Ca^{2+} from the cytoplasm. Ca^{2+} is pumped actively from the cytosol across the plasma membrane and is sequestered in the endoplasmic reticulum and mitochondria.

Toxicants induce elevation of cytoplasmic Ca^{2+} levels by promoting Ca^{2+} influx into or inhibiting Ca^{2+} efflux from the cytoplasm (Table 3-3). Opening of the ligand- or voltage-gated Ca^{2+} channels or damage to the plasma membrane causes Ca^{2+} to move down its concentration gradient from extracellular fluid to the cytoplasm. Toxicants also may increase cytosolic Ca^{2+}, inducing its leakage from the mitochondria or the endoplasmic reticulum. They also may diminish Ca^{2+} efflux through inhibition of Ca^{2+} transporters or depletion of their driving forces. Sustained elevation of intracellular Ca^{2+} is harmful because it can result in (1) depletion of energy reserves by inhibiting the ATPase used in oxidative phosphorylation, (2) dysfunction of microfilaments, (3) activation of hydrolytic enzymes, and (4) generation of ROS and RNS.

First, high cytoplasmic Ca^{2+} levels cause increased mitochondrial Ca^{2+} uptake by the Ca^{2+} "uniporter," which, like ATP synthase, utilizes the inside negative mitochondrial membrane potential as the driving force. Consequently, mitochondrial Ca^{2+} uptake dissipates the membrane potential and inhibits the synthesis of ATP. Moreover, agents that oxidize mitochondrial NADH activate a transporter that extrudes Ca^{2+} from the matrix space. The ensuing continuous Ca^{2+} uptake and export ("Ca^{2+} cycling") by the mitochondria further compromise oxidative phosphorylation.

Second, an uncontrolled rise in cytoplasmic Ca^{2+} causes cell injury by microfilamental dissociation. An increase of cytoplasmic Ca^{2+} causes dissociation of actin filaments from α-actinin and fodrin, proteins that promote anchoring of the filament to the plasma membrane, predisposing the membrane to rupture.

Third, high Ca^{2+} levels may lead to activation of hydrolytic enzymes that degrade proteins, phospholipids, and nucleic acids. Many integral membrane proteins are targets for Ca^{2+}-activated neutral proteases, or calpains. Indiscriminate activation of phospholipases

Table 3-2
Agents Impairing Mitochondrial ATP Synthesis*

A. Inhibitors of hydrogen delivery to the electron transport chain acting on/as

    1. Glycolysis (critical in neurons): hypoglycemia; iodoacetate and NO^+ at GAPDH

    2. Gluconeogenesis (critical in renal tubular cells): coenzyme A depletors (see below)

    3. Fatty acid oxidation (critical in cardiac muscle): hypoglycin, 4-pentenoic acid

    4. Pyruvate dehydrogenase: arsenite, DCVC, p-benzoquinone

    5. Citrate cycle

       (a) Aconitase: fluoroacetate, $ONOO^-$

       (b) Isocitrate dehydrogenase: DCVC

       (c) Succinate dehydrogenase: malonate, DCVC, PCBD-cys, 2-bromohydroquinone, 3-nitropropionic acid, cis-crotonalide fungicides

    6. Depletors of TPP (inhibit TPP-dependent PDH and α-KGDH): ethanol

    7. Depletors of coenzyme A: 4-(dimethylamino) phenol, p-benzoquinone

    8. Depletors of NADH

       (a) See group A.V.1. in Table 3-3

       (b) Activators of poly (ADP-ribose) polymerase: agents causing DNA damage (e.g., MNNG, hydrogen peroxide, $ONOO^-$)

B. Inhibitors of electron transport acting on/as

    1. Inhibitors of electron transport complexes

       (a) NADH–coenzyme Q reductase (complex I): rotenone, amytal, MPP^+, paraquat

       (b) Cycotochrome Q–cytochrome c reductase (complex III): antimycin-A, myxothiazole

       (c) Cytochrome oxidase (complex IV): cyanide, hydrogen sulfide, azide, formate, $\cdot$NO, phosphine (PH_3)

       (d) Multisite inhibitors: dinitroaniline and diphenylether herbicides, $ONOO^-$

    2. Electron acceptors: CCl_4, doxorubicin, menadione, MPP^+

C. Inhibitors of oxygen delivery to the electron transport chain

    1. Chemicals causing respiratory paralysis: CNS depressants, convulsants

    2. Chemicals causing ischemia: ergot alkaloids, cocaine

    3. Chemicals inhibiting oxygenation of Hb: carbon monoxide, methemoglobin-forming chemicals

D. Inhibitors of ADP phosphorylation acting on/as

    1. ATP synthase: oligomycin, cyhexatin, DDT, chlordecone

    2. Adenine nucleotide translocator: atractyloside, DDT, free fatty acids, lysophospholipids

    3. Phosphate transporter: N-ethylmaleimide, mersalyl, p-benzoquinone

    4. Chemicals dissipating the mitochondrial membrane potential (uncouplers)

       (a) Cationophores: pentachlorophenol, dinitrophenol, benzonitrile, thiadiazole herbicides, salicylate, cationic amphiphilic drugs (amiodarone, perhexiline), valinomycin, gramicidin, calcimycin (A23187)

       (b) Chemicals permeabilizing the mitochondrial inner membrane: PCBD-cys, chlordecone

E. Chemicals causing mitochondrial DNA damage and impaired transcription of key mitochondrial proteins:

    1. Antiviral drugs: zidovudine, zalcitabine, didanosine, fialuridine

    2. Ethanol (when chronically consumed)

*The ultimate sites of action of these agents are indicated in Fig. 3-8. DCVC = dichlorovinyl-cysteine; GAPDH = glyceraldehyde 3-phosphate dehydrogenase; α-KGDH = α-ketoglutarate dehydrogenase; MNNG = N-methyl-N'-nitro-N-nitrosoguanidine; MPP^+ = 1-methyl-4-phenylpyridinium; PCBD-cys = pentachlorobutadienyl-cysteine; PDH = pyruvate dehydrogenase; TPP = thiamine pyrophosphate.

Table 3-3
Agents Causing Sustained Elevation of Cytosolic Ca^{2+}

A. **Chemicals inducing Ca^{2+} influx into the cytoplasm**
  I. Via ligand-gated channels in neurons:
    1. Glutamate receptor agonists ("excitotoxins"): glutamate, kainate, domoate
    2. "Capsaicin receptor" agonists: capsaicin, resiniferatoxin
  II. Via voltage-gated channels: maitotoxin (?), $HO^{\bullet}$
  III. Via "newly formed pores": maitotoxin, amphotericin B, chlordecone, methylmercury, alkyltins
  IV. Across disrupted cell membrane:
    1. Detergents: exogenous detergents, lysophospholipids, free fatty acids
    2. Hydrolytic enzymes: phospholipases in snake venoms, endogenous phospholipase A_2
    3. Lipid peroxidants: carbon tetrachloride
    4. Cytoskeletal toxins (by inducing membrane blebbing): cytochalasins, phalloidin
  V. From mitochondria:
    1. Oxidants of intramitochondrial NADH: alloxan, t-BHP, NAPBQI, divicine, fatty acid hydroperoxides, menadione, MPP^+
    2. Others: phenylarsine oxide, gliotoxin, $^{\bullet}NO$, $ONOO^-$
  VI. From the endoplasmic reticulum:
    1. IP_3 receptor activators: γ-HCH (lindan), IP_3 formed during "excitotoxicity"
    2. Ryanodine receptor activators: δ-HCH

B. **Chemicals inhibiting Ca^{2+} export from the cytoplasm** (inhibitors of Ca^{2+}-ATPase in cell membrane and/or endoplasmic reticulum)
  I. Covalent binders: acetaminophen, bromobenzene, CCl_4, chloroform, DCE
  II. Thiol oxidants: cystamine (mixed disulfide formation), diamide, t-BHP, menadione, diquat
  III. Others: vanadate, Cd^{2+}
  IV. Chemicals impairing mitochondrial ATP synthesis (see Table 3-2)

KEY: DCE = 1,1-dichloroethylene; t-BHP = t-butyl hydroperoxide; HCH = hexachlorocyclohexane; MPP^+ = 1-methyl-4-phenylpyridinium; NAPBQI = N-acetyl-p-benzoquinoneimine.

by Ca^{2+} causes membrane breakdown directly and through the generation of detergents. Activation of a Ca^{2+}-Mg^{2+}-dependent endonuclease causes fragmentation of chromatin.

Overproduction of ROS and RNS A number of xenobiotics can directly generate ROS and RNS, such as the redox cyclers and transition metals (Fig. 3-3). Overproduction of ROS and RNS can be secondary to intracellular hypercalcemia, as Ca^{2+} helps generate ROS and/or RNS by activating dehydrogenases in the citric acid cycle, which lead to increased activity in the electron transport chain, which increases the formation of $O_2^{-\bullet}$ and

HOOH, and by activating nitric oxide synthase, which leads to the formation of $ONOO^-$.

Interplay between the Primary Metabolic Disorders Spells Cellular Disaster The primary derailments in cellular biochemistry discussed above may interact and amplify each other in a number of ways:

1. Depletion of cellular ATP reserves deprives the endoplasmic and plasma membrane Ca^{2+} pumps of fuel, causing elevation of Ca^{2+} in the cytoplasm. With the influx of Ca^{2+} into the mitochondria, the mitochondrial membrane potential $\Delta\Psi m$ declines, hindering ATP synthase.

2. Intracellular hypercalcemia facilitates the formation of ROS and RNS, which oxidatively inactivate the Ca^{2+} pump, aggravating the hypercalcemia.

3. ROS and RNS also can drain the ATP reserves. $^{\bullet}NO$ is a reversible inhibitor of cytochrome oxidase, NO^+ (nitrosonium cation, a product of $^{\bullet}NO$) inactivates glyceraldehyde 3-phosphate dehydrogenase and impairs glycolysis, and $ONOO^-$ irreversibly inactivates several components of the electron transport chain, inhibiting cellular ATP synthesis.

4. Furthermore, $ONOO^-$ can induce DNA single-strand breaks, which activate poly (ADP-ribose) polymerase (PARP). As part of the repair strategy, activated PARP transfers multiple ADP-ribose moieties from NAD^+ to nuclear proteins and to PARP itself. Because consumption of NAD^+ severely compromises ATP synthesis (see Fig. 3-8) and resynthesis of NAD^+ consumes ATP, a cellular energy deficit occurs as a major consequence of DNA damage by $ONOO^-$.

Mitochondrial Permeability Transition (MPT) and the Worst Outcome: Necrosis Mitochrondrial Ca^{2+} uptake, decreased mitochondrial membrane potential, generation of ROS and RNS, depletion of ATP, and consequences of the primary metabolic disorders (e.g., accumulation of inorganic phosphate, free fatty acids, and lysophosphatides) are all considered causative factors in an abrupt increase in the mitochondrial inner-membrane permeability, termed MPT, that is believed to be caused by the opening of a proteinaceous pore that spans mitochondrial membranes and is permeable to solutes of 1500 Da. Opening permits free influx into the matrix space of protons, causing rapid and complete dissipation of the membrane potential, cessation of ATP synthesis, and the osmotic influx of water, resulting in mitochondrial swelling. Ca^{2+} that accumulated in the matrix space effluxes through the pore, flooding the cytoplasm. Such mitochondria not only are incapable of synthesizing ATP but even waste the remaining sources because depolarization of the inner membrane forces the ATP synthase to operate in the reverse mode, as an ATPase, hydrolyzing ATP. Then even glycolysis may be compromised by the insufficient ATP supply to the glycolytic enzymes that require ATP (hexokinase, phosphofructokinase). A complete bioenergetic catastrophe ensues in the cell if the metabolic disorders evoked by the toxic agent (such as the one listed in Tables 3-2 and 3-3) are so extensive that most or all mitochondria in the cell undergo MPT, causing depletion of cellular ATP and culminating in cell lysis or necrosis (see Fig. 3-9).

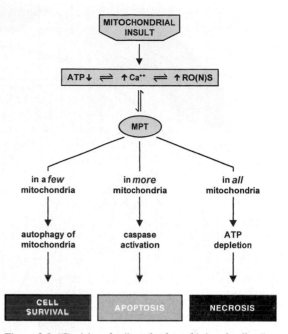

Figure 3-9. "Decision plan" on the fate of injured cell. See the text for details. MPT = mitochondrial permeability transition; RO (N) S = reactive oxygen or nitrogen species.

An Alternative Outcome of MPT: Apoptosis Chemicals that adversely affect cellular energy metabolism, Ca^{2+} homeostasis, and redox state and ultimately cause necrosis also may induce apoptosis. Whereas the necrotic cell swells and lyses, the apoptotic cell shrinks; its nuclear and cytoplasmic materials condense, and then it breaks into membrane-bound fragments (apoptotic bodies) that are phagocytosed.

As was discussed above, the multiple metabolic defects a cell suffers on its way to necrosis are rather random in sequence. In contrast, the routes to apoptosis are ordered, involving cascade-like activation of catabolic processes that finally disassemble the cell. Many details of the apoptotic pathways are presented schematically in Fig. 3-10.

It appears that most if not all cases of chemical-induced cell death involve the mitochondria and that MPT is a crucial event. Another related event is release into the cytoplasm of cytochrome c (cyt c), a small heme-protein that normally resides in the mitochondrial intermembrane space attached to the surface of the inner membrane.

As cyt c is the penultimate link in the mitochondrial electron transport chain, its loss will block ATP synthesis,

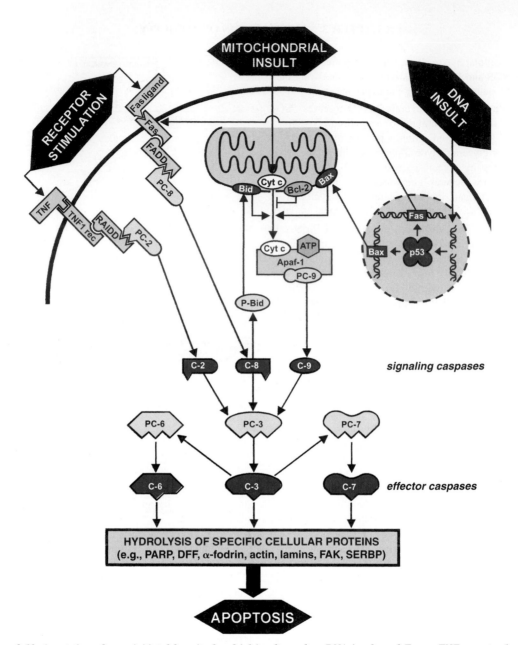

Figure 3-10. Apoptotic pathways initiated by mitochondrial insult, nuclear DNA insult, and Fas or TNF receptor-1 stimulation. The figure is a simplified scheme of three pathways to apoptosis. (1) Mitochondrial insult (see text) ultimately opens the permeability transition pore spanning both mitochondrial membranes and/or causes release of cytochrome *c* (Cyt *c*) from the mitochondria. Cyt *c* release is facilitated by Bax or Bid proteins and opposed by Bcl-2 protein. (2) DNA insult, especially double-strand breaks, activates p53 protein, which increases the expression of Bax (which mediates Cyt *c* release) and the membrane receptor protein Fas. (3) Fas ligand or tumor necrosis factor binds to and activates their respective receptors, the Fas and TNF1 receptors. These ligand-bound receptors and the released Cyt *c* interact with specific adapter proteins (i.e., FADD, RAIDD, and Apaf-1), through which they proteolytically activate procaspases (PC) to active caspases (C). The latter in turn cleave and activate other proteins (e.g., the precursor of Bid, P-Bid) and PC-3, a main effector procaspase. The active effector caspase-3 activates other effector procaspases (PC-6, PC-7). Finally, C-3, C-6, and C-7 clip specific cellular proteins by which apoptosis occurs. These pathways are not equally relevant in all types of cells, and other pathways, such as those employing TGF-β as an extracellular signaling molecule and ceramide as an intracellular signaling molecule, also exist. DFF = DNA fragmentation factor; FAK = focal adhesion kinase; PARP = poly(ADP-ribose) polymerase; SREBP = sterol regulatory element binding protein.

increase the formation of $O_2^{-\bullet}$, and potentially push the cell toward necrosis. Simultaneously, the unleashed cyt c represents a signal or an initial link in the chain of events directing the cell to the apoptotic path (Fig. 3-10). Upon binding, together with ATP, to an adapter protein, cyt c can induce proteolytic cleavage of proteins called caspases or cysteine proteases that cleave cytoplasmic proteins into fragments, beginning apoptosis. Some caspases (e.g., 2, 8, and 9) activate procaspases. These signaling caspases carry the activation wave to the so-called effector caspases (e.g., 3, 6, and 7), which clip specific cellular proteins, activating or inactivating them.

The decisive mitochondrial events of cell death—MPT and release of cyt c—are controlled by the Bcl-2 family of proteins, which includes members that facilitate (e.g., Bax, Bad, Bid) and those that inhibit (e.g., Bcl-2, Bcl-XL) these processes. The relative amount of these antagonistic proteins functions as a regulatory switch between cell survival and death.

The proapoptotic Bax and Bid proteins also represent links by which death programs that are initiated extramitochondrically, for example, by DNA damage in the nucleus or by stimulation of certain receptors called Fas receptors at the cell surface, can engage the mitochondria into the apoptotic process (Fig. 3-10). DNA damage induces stabilization and activation of p53 protein, which increases the expression of Bax protein, a proapoptotic member of the Bcl-2 family. As is discussed below, DNA damage is potentially mutagenic and carcinogenic; therefore, apoptosis of cells with damaged DNA is an important self-defense mechanism of the body against oncogenesis. Stimulation of Fas receptors can directly activate caspases and can engage the mitochondria in the death program through caspase-mediated activation of Bid, another member of the Bcl-2 family (Fig. 3-10).

Thus, apoptosis can be executed through multiple pathways, all involving caspase activation. The route preferred depends on the initial insult as well as on the type and state of the cell.

ATP Availability Determines the Form of Cell Death Many xenobiotics can cause both apoptosis and necrosis. Toxicants tend to induce apoptosis at low exposure levels or early after exposure at high levels, whereas they cause necrosis later at high exposure levels. Recent findings suggest that the availability of ATP is critical in determining the form of cell death. When only a few mitochondria develop MPT, they, and with them the proapoptotic signals (e.g., externalized cyt c), are removed by lysosomal autophagy. When MPT involves more mitochondria, the autophagic mechanism is over-whelmed and the released cyt c initiates caspase activation and apoptosis (Fig. 3-10). When MPT involves virtually all the mitochondria, ATP is severely depleted, preventing execution of the ATP-requiring apoptotic program, and cytolysis occurs.

STEP 4—REPAIR OR DYSREPAIR

The fourth step in the development of toxicity is inappropriate repair (Fig. 3-1). Many toxicants alter macromolecules, which, if not repaired, cause damage at higher levels of the biological hierarchy in the organism and influence the progression of toxicity.

Molecular Repair

Damaged molecules may be repaired in different ways. Some chemical alterations, such as oxidation of protein thiols and methylation of DNA, are simply reversed. Hydrolytic removal of the molecule's damaged unit or units and the insertion of a newly synthesized unit or units often occur with chemically altered DNA and peroxidized lipids. In some instances, the damaged molecule is totally degraded and resynthesized.

Repair of Proteins Thiol groups are essential for the function of numerous proteins. Oxidation of protein thiols can be reversed by enzymatic reduction that is catalyzed by thioredoxin and glutaredoxin. Once they are oxidized, the catalytic thiol groups in these proteins are recycled by reduction with NADPH.

Repair of oxidized hemoglobin (methemoglobin) occurs by means of electron transfer from cytochrome b_5, which then is regenerated by an NADH-dependent cytochrome b_5 reductase. Molecular chaperones such as the heat-shock proteins are synthesized in large quantities in response to protein denaturation and are important in the refolding of altered proteins. Damaged proteins also can be eliminated by proteolytic degradation. Also, the ATP/ubiquitin–dependent proteolytic system is specialized in controlling the level of regulatory proteins (e.g., p53, IκB, cyclins) that eliminate damaged or mutated intracellular proteins.

Repair of Lipids Peroxidized lipids are repaired by a complex process that involves a series of reductants, glutathione peroxidase, and glutathione reductase. NADPH is needed to recycle the reductants that are oxidized in the process.

Repair of DNA Despite its high reactivity with electrophiles and free radicals, nuclear DNA is remarkably stable, in part because it is packaged in chromatin and because several repair mechanisms are available to correct alterations. Mitochondrial DNA, however, lacks histones and efficient repair mechanisms and therefore is more prone to damage.

Direct Repair Certain covalent DNA modifications are directly reversed by enzymes such as DNA photolyase, which cleaves adjacent pyrimidines dimerized by UV light. This chromophore-equipped enzyme functions only in light-exposed cells. Minor adducts, such as methyl groups, attached to the O^6 position of guanine are removed by O^6-alkylguanine-DNA-alkyltransferase.

Excision Repair Base excision and nucleotide excision are two mechanisms for removing damaged bases from DNA (Chaps. 8 and 9). Lesions that do not cause major distortion of the helix typically are removed by base excision, in which the altered base is recognized by a relatively substrate-specific DNA-glycosylase that hydrolyzes the N-glycosidic bond, releasing the modified base and creating an apurinic or apyrimidinic (AP) site in the DNA. The AP site is recognized by the AP endonuclease, which hydrolyzes the phosphodiester bond adjacent to the abasic site. After its removal, the abasic sugar is replaced with the correct nucleotide by a DNA polymerase and is sealed in place by a DNA ligase.

Bulky adducts are removed by nucleotide-excision repair. An ATP-dependent nuclease recognizes the distorted double helix and excises a number of intact nucleotides on both sides of the lesion, together with the one containing the adduct. The excised section of the strand is restored by the insertion of nucleotides into the gap by DNA polymerase and ligase, using the complementary strand as a template.

Poly(ADP-ribose)polymerase (PARP) appears to be an important contributor to excision repair. Upon base damage or a single-strand break, PARP binds to the injured DNA and becomes activated. The active PARP cleaves NAD^+ to use the ADP-ribose moiety of this cofactor to attach long chains of polymeric ADP-ribose to nuclear proteins. Because one ADP-ribose unit contains two negative charges, the poly(ADP-ribosyl)ated proteins accrue negativity and the resultant electrorepulsive force between the negatively charged proteins and DNA causes decondensation of the chromatin structure. It has been hypothesized that PARP-mediated opening of the tightly packed chromatin allows the repair enzymes to access the broken DNA and fix it.

Recombinational (or Postreplication) Repair Recombinational repair occurs when the excision of a bulky adduct or an intrastrand pyrimidine dimer fails to occur before DNA replication begins. At replication, such a lesion prevents DNA polymerase from polymerizing a daughter strand along a sizable stretch of the parent strand that carries the damage. Replication results in two homologous ("sister") yet dissimilar DNA duplexes: one that has a large postreplication gap in its daughter strand and an intact duplex that is synthesized at the opposite leg of the replication fork. This intact sister duplex completes the postreplication gap in the damaged sister duplex by means of recombination ("crossover") of the appropriate strands of the two homologous duplexes. After separation, the sister duplex that originally contained the gap carries in its daughter strand a section originating from the parent strand of the intact sister, which in turn carries in its parent strand a section originating from the daughter strand of the damaged sister—a process of sister chromatid exchange. A combination of excision and recombinational repairs occurs in the restoration of DNA with interstrand cross-links.

Cellular Repair: A Strategy in Peripheral Neurons

Repair of damaged neurons is applied minimally in overcoming cellular injuries, because mature neurons have lost the ability to multiply. In peripheral neurons with axonal damage, repair does occur and requires macrophages and Schwann cells. Macrophages remove debris by phagocytosis and produce cytokines and growth factors, which activate Schwann cells to proliferate and transdifferentiate into a growth-supporting mode. While comigrating with the regrowing axon, Schwann cells physically guide as well as chemically lure the axon to reinnervate the target cell.

In the mammalian central nervous system, axonal regrowth is prevented by growth inhibitory glycoproteins and chondroitin sulfate proteoglycans produced by the oligodendrocytes and by the scar produced by astrocytes. Although damage to central neurons is irreversible, the large number of reserve nerve cells can partly compensate by taking over the functions of lost neurons.

Tissue Repair

In tissues with cells capable of multiplying, damage is reversed by apoptosis or necrosis of the injured cells and regeneration of the tissue by proliferation.

Apoptosis: An Active Deletion of Damaged Cells
Apoptosis initiated by cell injury can be regarded as tissue repair. A cell undergoing apoptosis shrinks as its nuclear and cytoplasmic materials condense, and then it breaks into membrane-bound fragments (apoptotic bodies) that are phagocytosed without inflammation. Also, apoptosis may intercept the process that leads to neoplasia by eliminating cells with potentially mutagenic DNA damage.

Apoptosis of damaged cells has full value as a tissue repair process only for tissues that are made up of constantly renewing cells (e.g., bone marrow, respiratory and gastrointestinal epithelium, and epidermis of the skin) or of conditionally dividing cells (e.g., hepatic and renal parenchymal cells), because the apoptotic cells are replaced readily. The value of apoptosis as a tissue repair strategy is markedly lessened in organs that contain nonreplicating and nonreplaceable cells, such as neurons, cardiac muscle cells, and female germ cells.

Proliferation: Regeneration of Tissue Tissues are composed of various cells and the extracellular matrix. Cadherins allow adjacent cells to adhere to one other, whereas connexins connect neighboring cells internally by association of these proteins into gap junctions. Integrins link cells to the extracellular matrix. Therefore, repair of injured tissues involves both regeneration of lost cells and the extracellular matrix and reintegration of the newly formed elements into tissues and organs.

Replacement of Lost Cells by Mitosis Soon after injury, cells adjacent to the damaged area enter the cell division cycle. Quiescent cells residing in G_0 enter G_1 and progress to mitosis (M).

Sequential changes in gene expression occur in cells that are destined to divide. Early after injury, intracellular signaling turns on, and the expression of numerous genes is increased. Among these so-called immediate-early genes are those which code for transcription factors that amplify the initial gene-activation process by stimulating other genes directly or through cell surface receptors and the coupled transducing networks. A few hours later the so-called delayed-early genes are expressed, whose products regulate the cell-division cycle. Genes for the cell cycle accelerator proteins and genes whose products decelerate the cell cycle are temporarily overexpressed, suggesting that this duality keeps tissue regeneration regulated precisely. Thus, genetic expression is reprogrammed so that DNA synthesis and mitosis gain priority over specialized cellular activities.

The regenerative process probably is initiated by the release of chemical mediators from damaged cells. Nonparenchymal cells, such as resident macrophages and endothelial cells, are receptive to these chemical signals and produce a host of signaling molecules that promote and propagate the regenerative process. The cytokines tumor necrosis factor-α (TNF-α) and interleukin-6 (IL-6) purportedly promote transition of the quiescent cells into cell cycle ("priming"), whereas the growth factors, especially the hepatocyte growth factor (HGF) and transforming growth factor-α (TGF-α), initiate the progression of the "primed" cells in the cycle toward mitosis.

Besides mitosis, cell migration significantly contributes to the restitution of certain tissues. In the mucosa of the GI tract, cells of the residual epithelium rapidly migrate to the site of injury as well as elongate and thin to reestablish the continuity of the surface even before this could be achieved by cell replication. Mucosal repair is dictated by growth factors and cytokines that are operative in tissue repair elsewhere and also by specific peptides associated with the mucous layer of the GI tract that are overexpressed at sites of mucosal injury.

Replacement of the Extracellular Matrix The extracellular matrix is composed of proteins, glycosaminoglycans, and the glycoproteins and proteoglycans. Activation of resting stellate cells is mediated chiefly by two growth factors—platelet-derived growth factor (PDGF) and transforming growth factor-β (TGF-β)—that may be released from platelets accumulating and degranulating at sites of injury and later from the activated stellate cells themselves. Proliferation of stellate cells is induced by the potent mitogen PDGF, whereas TGF-β acts on the stellate cells to stimulate the synthesis of extracellular matrix components, including collagens, fibronectin, tenascin, and proteoglycans.

Side Reactions to Tissue Injury In addition to mediators that aid in the replacement of lost cells and the extracellular matrix, resident macrophages and endothelial cells activated by cell injury produce inflammation, altered production of acute-phase protein, and generalized reactions such as fever.

Inflammation Cells and Mediators Alteration of the microcirculation and accumulation of inflammatory cells are initiated largely by resident macrophages secreting cytokines such as TNF-α and interleukin-1 (IL-1) in response to tissue damage. These cytokines in turn stimulate neighboring stromal cells, such as the endothelial cells and fibroblasts, to release mediators that induce dilation of the local microvasculature and cause permeabilization of capillaries. Activated endothelial cells also facilitate the egress of circulating leukocytes into the injured tissue by releasing chemoattractants and expressing cell-adhesion molecules. Subsequently, a stronger interaction (adhesion) is established between the endothelial cells and leukocytes with participation of intercellular adhesion molecules (e.g., ICAM-1), and leukocytes are able to enter the tissues by crossing the endothelial layer. This process is facilitated by gradients of chemoattractants that induce expression of leukocyte integrins. Chemoattractants originate from various stromal cells and include chemotactic cytokines (or chemokines), as well as lipid-derived compounds, such as platelet-activating factor (PAF) and leukotriene B_4 (LTB_4). Ultimately, all types of cells in the vicinity of injury express ICAM-1, thus promoting leukocyte invasion; the invading leukocytes also synthesize mediators, thus propagating the inflammatory response.

Inflammation Produces Reactive Oxygen and Nitrogen Species Macrophages, as well as leukocytes, recruited to the site of injury undergo a respiratory burst, producing free radicals and activated enzymes. Membrane-bound NAD(P)H oxidase, which is activated in both macrophages and granulocytes, produces superoxide anion radical ($O_2^{-\bullet}$) from molecular oxygen. The $O_2^{-\bullet}$ can give rise to the hydroxyl radical ($HO^\bullet$).

Macrophages generate another cytotoxic free radical, nitric oxide ($^\bullet NO$), from arginine by means of nitric oxide synthase:

$$\text{L-arginine} + O_2 \rightarrow \text{L-citrulline} + {}^\bullet NO$$

Subsequently, $O_2^{-\bullet}$ and $^\bullet NO$, both of which are products of activated macrophages, can react with each other, yielding peroxynitrite anion; upon reaction with carbon dioxide, this decays into two radicals, nitrogen dioxide and carbonate anion radical:

$$O_2^{-\bullet} + {}^\bullet NO \rightarrow ONOO^-$$
$$ONOO^- + CO_2 \rightarrow ONOOCO_2^-$$
$$ONOOCO_2^- \rightarrow {}^\bullet NO_2 + CO_3^{-\bullet}$$

Granulocytes discharge the lysosomal enzyme myeloperoxidase into engulfed extracellular spaces, the phagocytic vacuoles. Myeloperoxidase catalyzes the formation of hypochlorous acid (HOCl) from hydrogen peroxide (HOOH) and chloride ion:

$$HOOH + H^+ + Cl^- \rightarrow HOH + HOCl$$

HOCl can form $HO^\bullet$ as a result of electron transfer from Fe^{2+} or from $O_2^{-\bullet}$ to HOCl:

$$HOCl + O_2^{-\bullet} \rightarrow O_2 + Cl^- + HO^\bullet$$

All these reactive chemicals, as well as the discharged lysosomal proteases, are destructive products of inflammatory cells. Although these chemicals exert antimicrobial activity at the site of microbial invasion, at the site of toxic injury they can damage adjacent healthy tissues and contribute to the propagation of tissue injury.

Altered Protein Synthesis: Acute-Phase Proteins Cytokines released from macrophages and endothelial cells of injured tissues—IL-6, IL-1, and TNF—act on cell surface receptors to increase or decrease the transcriptional activity of genes that encode certain proteins called positive and negative acute-phase proteins.

Positive acute-phase proteins may play a role in minimizing tissue injury and facilitating repair. For example, many of them inhibit lysosomal proteases released from the injured cells and recruited leukocytes.

Negative acute-phase proteins include some plasma proteins, such as albumin, transthyretin, and transferrin, as well as several forms of cytochrome P450 and glutathione *S*-transferase. Because the latter enzymes play important roles in the toxication and detoxication of xenobiotics, the disposition and toxicity of chemicals may be altered markedly during the acute phase of tissue injury.

Generalized Reactions Cytokines released from activated macrophages and endothelial cells at the site of injury also may evoke neurohormonal responses. Thus, IL-1, TNF, and IL-6 alter the temperature set point of the hypothalamus, triggering fever. In addition, IL-1 and IL-6 act on the pituitary to induce the release of ACTH, which in turn stimulates the secretion of cortisol from the adrenals. This represents a negative feedback loop because corticosteroids inhibit cytokine gene expression.

When Repair Fails

Repair mechanisms often fail to protect against injury because the fidelity of the repair mechanisms is not absolute, making it possible for some lesions to be overlooked. Repair fails most typically when the damage overwhelms the repair mechanisms, such as when necessary enzymes or cofactors are consumed. Sometimes the toxicant-induced injury adversely affects the repair process itself. Finally, some types of toxic injuries cannot be repaired effectively, as occurs when xenobiotics are covalently bound to proteins.

It is also possible that repair contributes to toxicity, as occurs when excessive amounts of NAD^+ are cleaved by PARP when this enzyme assists in repairing broken DNA strands or when too much NAD(P)H is consumed for the repair of oxidized proteins and endogenous reductants. Either event can compromise oxidative phosphorylation, which is also dependent on the supply of reduced cofactors (see Fig. 3-8), thus causing or aggravating ATP depletion that contributes to cell injury. However, repair also may play an active role in toxicity. This is observed after chronic tissue injury, when the repair process goes astray and leads to uncontrolled proliferation instead of tissue remodeling. Such proliferation of cells may result in neoplasia, whereas overproduction of extracellular matrix results in fibrosis.

Toxicity Resulting from Dysrepair

Dysrepair occurs at the molecular, cellular, and tissue levels. Some toxicities involve dysrepair at an isolated level, such as a specific enzyme or process, or at different levels, such as tissue necrosis, fibrosis, and chemical carcinogenesis.

Tissue Necrosis Several mechanisms that may lead to cell death may involve molecular damage that is potentially reversible by repair mechanisms. Cell injury progresses toward cell necrosis if molecular repair mechanisms are inefficient or if the molecular damage is not readily reversible.

Progression of cell injury to tissue necrosis can be intercepted by two repair mechanisms working in concert: apoptosis and cell proliferation. Injured cells can initiate apoptosis, which counteracts the progression of the toxic injury by preventing necrosis of injured cells and the consequent inflammatory response.

Another important repair process that can halt the propagation of toxic injury is proliferation of cells adjacent to the injured cells. Initiated soon after cellular injury, this early cell division is thought to be instrumental in the rapid and complete restoration of the injured tissue and the prevention of necrosis. The sensitivity of a tissue to injury and the capacity of the tissue for repair are apparently independent variables, both influencing whether tissue restitution ensues with survival or tissue necrosis occurs with death.

The efficiency of repair is also an important determinant of the dose–response relationship for toxicants that cause tissue necrosis. Tissue necrosis is caused by a cer-

tain dose of a toxicant not only because that dose ensures a sufficient concentration of the ultimate toxicant at the target site to initiate injury but also because that quantity of toxicant causes a degree of damage sufficient to compromise repair, allowing for progression of the injury. Tissue necrosis occurs because the injury overwhelms and disables the repair mechanisms, including (1) repair of damaged molecules, (2) elimination of damaged cells by apoptosis, and (3) replacement of lost cells by cell division.

Fibrosis Fibrosis, a pathologic condition that is characterized by excessive deposition of an extracellular matrix of abnormal composition, is a specific manifestation of dysrepair of injured tissue. As was discussed above, cellular injury initiates a surge in cellular proliferation and extracellular matrix production, which normally ceases when the injured tissue is remodeled. If increased production of extracellular matrix is not halted, fibrosis develops.

TGF-β appears to be a major mediator of fibrogenesis. The increased expression of TGF-β is a common response mediating regeneration of the extracellular matrix after an acute injury. Normally, TGF-β production ceases when repair is complete. Failure to halt TGF-β overproduction, which leads to fibrosis, could be caused by continuous injury or a defect in the regulation of TGF-β.

The fibrotic action of TGF-β is due to (1) stimulation of the synthesis of individual matrix components by specific target cells and (2) inhibition of matrix degradation. Interestingly, TGF-β induces transcription of its own gene in target cells, suggesting that the TGF-β produced by these cells can amplify in an autocrine manner the production of the extracellular matrix. This positive feedback may facilitate fibrogenesis.

Fibrosis involves not only excessive accumulation of the extracellular matrix but also changes in its composition. Basement membrane components, such as collagens and laminin, increase disproportionately during fibrogenesis.

Carcinogenesis Chemical carcinogenesis involves insufficient function of various repair mechanisms, including (1) failure of DNA repair, (2) failure of apoptosis, and (3) failure to terminate cell proliferation.

Failure of DNA Repair: Mutation, the Initiating Event in Carcinogenesis. Chemical and physical insults may induce neoplastic transformation of cells by genotoxic and nongenotoxic mechanisms. Chemicals that react with DNA may cause damage such as adduct formation, oxidative alteration, and strand breakage. If these lesions are not repaired or if injured cells are not eliminated, a lesion in the parental DNA strand may induce a heritable alteration, or mutation, in the daughter strand during replication. The most unfortunate scenario for the organism occurs when the altered genes express mutant proteins that reprogram cells for multiplication. When such cells undergo mitosis, their descendants also have a similar propensity for proliferation. Moreover, because enhanced cell division increases the likelihood of mutations, these cells eventually acquire additional mutations that may further increase their growth advantage over their normal counterparts. The final outcome of this process is a tumor consisting of transformed, rapidly proliferating cells.

Mutation of Proto-Oncogenes Proto-oncogenes are highly conserved genes that encode proteins that stimulate the progression of cells through the cell cycle. The products of proto-oncogenes include (1) growth factors, (2) growth factor receptors, (3) intracellular signal transducers such as G proteins, protein kinases, cyclins, and cyclin-dependent protein kinases, and (4) nuclear transcription factors. Transient increases in the production or activity of proto-oncogene proteins are required for regulated growth, as occurs during embryogenesis, tissue regeneration, and stimulation of cells by growth factors or hormones. In contrast, permanent activation and/or overexpression of these proteins favors neoplastic transformation. One mechanism by which genotoxic carcinogens induce neoplastic cell transformation is the production of an activating mutation of a proto-oncogene. The altered gene (called an *oncogene*) encodes a permanently active protein that forces the cell into the division cycle.

An example of mutational activation of an oncogene protein is that of the Ras proteins. Ras proteins are localized on the inner surface of the plasma membrane and function as crucial mediators in responses initiated by growth factors (see Fig. 3-7). Ras serves as a molecular switch, being active in the GTP-bound form and inactive in the GDP-bound form. Some mutations of the *ras* gene dramatically lower the GTPase activity of the protein, which in turn locks Ras in the permanently active GTP-bound form. Continual rather than signal-dependent activation of Ras can lead eventually to uncontrolled proliferation and transformation.

Mutation of Tumor-Suppressor Genes Tumor-suppressor genes encode proteins that inhibit the progression of cells in the division cycle, which include cyclin-dependent protein kinase inhibitors, transcription factors that transactivate genes encoding cyclin-dependent protein kinase inhibitors, and proteins that block transcription factors involved in DNA synthesis and cell division.

The p53 tumor suppressor gene encodes a 53,000-Da protein with multiple functions. Acting as a transcription factor, the p53 protein transactivates genes whose products arrest the cell cycle or promote apoptosis and represses genes that encode antiapoptotic proteins. DNA damage and illegitimate expression of oncogenes stabilize the p53 protein, causing its accumulation and inducing cell cycle arrest (permitting DNA repair) or even apoptosis of the affected cells.

Cooperation of Proto-Oncogenes and Tumor-Suppressor Genes in Carcinogenesis The accumulation of genetic damage in the form of (1) mutant proto-oncogenes (which encode activated proteins) and (2) mutant tumor-suppressor genes (which encode inactivated proteins) is the main driving force in the transformation of normal cells with controlled proliferative activity to malignant cells with uncontrolled proliferative activity. Because the number of cells in a tissue is regulated by a balance between mitosis and apoptosis, uncontrolled proliferation results from perturbation of this balance.

Failure of Apoptosis: Promotion of Mutation and Clonal Growth Preneoplastic cells, or cells with mutations, have much higher apoptotic activity than do normal cells. Therefore, apoptosis counteracts clonal expansion of the initiated cells and tumor cells. Facilitation of apoptosis can induce tumor regression, whereas inhibition of apoptosis is detrimental because mutations and clonal expansion of preneoplastic cells are facilitated.

Failure to Terminate Proliferation: Promotion of Mutation, Proto-Oncogene Expression, and Clonal Growth Enhanced mitotic activity promotes carcinogenesis for a number of reasons.

1. Enhanced mitotic activity increases the probability of mutations. With activation of the cell-division cycle, a substantial shortening of the G_1 phase occurs, and less time is available for the repair of injured DNA before replication.

2. Overproduced proto-oncogene proteins may cooperate with oncogene proteins to facilitate the neoplastic transformation of cells, allowing less time for DNA methylation, which decreases gene transcription by inhibiting the interaction of transcription factors with the promoter region. Nonexpressed genes are fully methylated.

3. Cell-to-cell communication through gap junctions and intercellular adhesion through cadherins are temporarily disrupted during proliferation, and this contributes to the invasiveness of tumor cells.

Nongenotoxic Carcinogens: Promoters of Mitosis and Inhibitors of Apoptosis Many chemicals do not alter DNA or induce mutations but still induce cancer after chronic administration. Designated *nongenotoxic* or *epigenetic carcinogens,* these chemicals cause cancer by promoting carcinogenesis initiated by genotoxic agents or spontaneous DNA damage. Spontaneous DNA damage commonly occurs in normal human cells at a rate of 1 of 10^8 to 10^{10} base pairs. Nongenotoxic carcinogens increase the frequency of spontaneous mutations through a mitogenic effect and by inhibiting apoptosis, thus increasing the number of cells with DNA damage and mutations.

Cell injury evokes the release of mitogenic growth factors such as HGF and TGF-α from tissue macrophages and endothelial cells. Thus, cells in chronically injured tissues are exposed continuously to endogenous mitogens. Although these growth factors are instrumental in tissue repair after acute cell injury, their continuous presence is potentially harmful because they ultimately may transform the affected cells into neoplastic cells. It is important to realize that even epigenetic carcinogens can exert a genotoxic effect, although indirectly.

CONCLUSIONS

Selective or altered toxicity may be due to different or altered (1) exposure, (2) delivery, thus resulting in a different concentration of the ultimate toxicant at the target site, (3) target molecules, (4) biochemical processes triggered by the reaction of the chemical with the target molecules, (5) repair at the molecular, cellular, or tissue level, or (6) mechanisms such as circulatory and thermoregulatory reflexes by which the affected organism can adapt to some of the toxic effects. Although a simplified scheme can be used to outline the development of toxicity (see Fig. 3-1), the route to toxicity can be considerably more diverse and complicated. An organism has mechanisms that (1) counteract the delivery of toxicants, such as detoxication, (2) reverse the toxic injury, such as repair mechanisms, and (3) offset some dysfunctions, such as adaptive responses. Thus, toxicity is not an inevitable consequence of toxicant exposure because it may be prevented, reversed, or compensated for by such mechanisms. Toxicity develops if the toxicant exhausts or impairs the protective mechanisms and/or overrides the adaptability of biological systems.

BIBLIOGRAPHY

Dalton TP, Shertzer HG, Puga A: Regulation of gene expression by reactive oxygen. *Annu Rev Pharmacol Toxicol* 39:67–101, 1999.

Green DR: Apoptotic pathways: The roads to ruin. *Cell* 94:695–698, 1998.

Hershko A, Ciechanover A: The ubiquitin system. *Annu Rev Biochem* 67:425–479, 1998.

Jäättelä M: Escaping cell death: Survival proteins in cancer. *Exp Cell Res* 248:30–43, 1999.

Johnson DG, Walker CL: Cyclins and cell cycle checkpoints. *Annu Rev Pharmacol Toxicol* 39:295–312, 1999.

Kroemer G, Dallaporta B, Resche-Rigon M: The mitochondrial death/life regulator in apoptosis and necrosis. *Annu Rev Physiol* 60:619–642, 1998.

Lee JI, Burckart GJ: Nuclear factor kappa B: Important transcription factor and therapeutic target. *J Clin Pharmacol* 38:981–993, 1998.

Murphy MP: Nitric oxide and cell death. *Biochim Biophys Acta* 1411:401–414, 1999.

Nicholson DW, Thornberry NA: Caspases: Killer proteases. *Trends Biochem Sci* 22:299–306, 1997.

Podolsky DK: Mucosal immunity and inflammation: V. Innate mechanisms of mucosal defense and repair: The best offense is a good defense. *Am J Physiol* 277:G495–G499, 1999.

Puga A, Wallace KB (eds): *Molecular Biology of the Toxic Response.* Philadelphia: Taylor & Francis, 1999.

Pumford NR, Halmes NC: Protein targets of xenobiotic reactive intermediates. *Annu Rev Pharmacol Toxicol* 37:91–117, 1997.

Reed JC, Jurgensmeier JM, Matsuyama S: Bcl-2 family proteins and mitochondria. *Biochim Biophys Acta* 1366:127–137, 1998.

Toivola DM, Eriksson JE: Toxins affecting cell signalling and alteration of cytoskeletal structure. *Tox In Vitro* 13:521–530, 1999.

Wallace KB, Starkov AA: Mitochondrial targets of drug toxicity. *Annu Rev Pharmacol Toxicol* 40:353–388, 2000.

C H A P T E R   4

RISK ASSESSMENT

Elaine M. Faustman and Gilbert S. Omenn

KEY POINTS

* *Risk assessment* is the systematic scientific characterization of potential adverse health effects resulting from human exposures to hazardous agents or situations.
* *Risk* is defined as the probability of an adverse outcome.
* *Risk management* refers to the process by which policy actions are chosen to control hazards.

INTRODUCTION AND HISTORICAL CONTEXT

Toxicologic research and toxicity testing conducted and interpreted by toxicologists constitute the scientific core of an important activity known as *risk assessment* for chemical exposures. The National Research Council detailed the steps of hazard identification, dose–response assessment, exposure analysis, and characterization of risks in *Risk Assessment in the Federal Government: Managing the Process,* widely known as "The Red Book." The scheme shown in Fig. 4-1 provides a consistent framework for risk assessment across agencies, with bidirectional arrows showing an ideal situation in which mechanistic research feeds directly into risk assessments and critical data uncertainty drives research. Often public policy objectives require extrapolations that go far beyond the observation of actual effects and reflect different tolerances for risks, generating controversy.

The Presidential/Congressional Commission on Risk Assessment and Risk Management formulated a comprehensive framework that applies two crucial concepts: (1) putting each environmental problem or issue into a public health and/or ecological context and (2) proactively engaging the relevant stakeholders—affected or potentially affected community groups—from the very

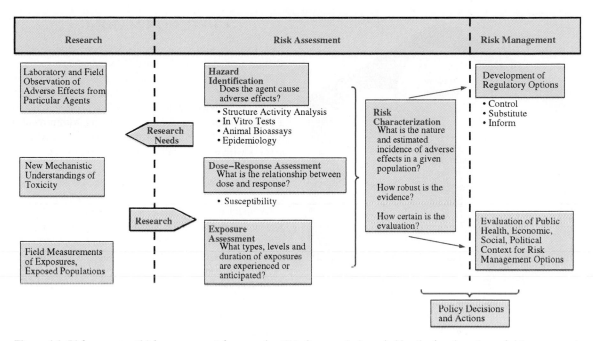

Figure 4-1. Risk assessment/risk management framework.   This framework shows in blue the four key steps of risk assessment: hazard identification, dose–response assessment, exposure assessment, and risk characterization. It shows an interactive, two-way process in which research needs from the risk assessment process drive new research and new research findings modify risk assessment outcomes.

beginning of the six-stage process shown in Fig. 4-2. Particular exposures and potential health effects must be evaluated across sources and exposure pathways and in light of multiple endpoints, as opposed to the current general approach of evaluating one chemical, in one environmental medium (air, water, soil, food, products), for one health effect at a time.

DEFINITIONS

Risk assessment is the systematic scientific characterization of potential adverse health effects resulting from human exposures to hazardous agents or situations. *Risk* is defined as the probability of an adverse outcome. The term *hazard* is used in the United States and Canada to refer to intrinsic toxic properties, whereas internationally this term is defined as the probability of an adverse outcome. Risk assessment requires qualitative information about the strength of the evidence and the nature of the outcomes—as well as quantitative assessment of the exposures, host susceptibility factors, and the potential magnitude of the risk—and then a description of the uncertainties in the estimates and conclusions. The objectives of risk assessment are outlined in Table 4-1.

The phrase *characterization of risk* may better reflect the combination of qualitative analysis and quantitative analysis. Unfortunately, many toxicologists, public health practitioners, environmentalists, and regulators tend to equate risk assessment with quantitative risk assessment, generating a number (or a number with uncertainty bounds) for an overly precise risk estimate and then ignoring crucial information about the mechanism of effect across species, inconsistent findings across studies, multiple variable health effects, and means of avoiding or reversing the effects of exposures.

Risk management refers to the process by which policy actions are chosen to control hazards identified in the risk assessment/risk characterization stage of the six-stage framework (Fig. 4-2). Risk managers consider scientific evidence and risk estimates—along with statutory, engineering, economic, social, and political factors—in evaluating alternative options and choosing among those options.

Risk communication is the challenging process of making information about risk assessment and risk management comprehensible to community groups, lawyers, local elected officials, judges, businesspeople, labor, and environmentalists. A crucial, too often neglected

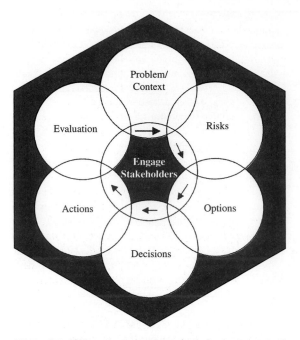

Figure 4-2. Risk management framework for environmental health from the U.S. Commission on Risk Assessment and Risk Management, "Omenn Commission." The framework includes six stages: (1) formulating the problem in a broad public health context, (2) analyzing the risks, (3) defining the options, (4) making risk-reduction decisions, (5) implementing those actions, and (6) evaluating the effectiveness of the actions taken. Interactions with stakeholders are critical and thus have been put at the center of the framework.

requirement for communication is listening to the fears, perceptions, priorities, and proposed remedies of these "stakeholders."

Table 4-1
Objectives of Risk Assessment

1. Balance risks and benefits
   Drugs
   Pesticides
2. Set target levels of risk
   Food contaminants
   Water pollutants
3. Set priorities for program activities
   Regulatory agencies
   Manufacturers
   Environmental/consumer organizations
4. Estimate residual risks and extent of risk reduction after steps are taken to reduce risks

DECISION MAKING

Risk management decisions are reached under diverse statutes in the United States and many other countries. Some statutes specify reliance on risk alone, whereas others require a balancing of the risks and benefits of a product or activity (Table 4-1). Risk assessments provide a valuable framework for priority setting within regulatory and health agencies, in the chemical development process within companies, and in resource allocation by environmental organizations. Currently, there are significant efforts toward the harmonization of testing protocols and the assessment of risks and standards.

A major challenge for risk assessment, risk communication, and risk management is to work across disciplines to demonstrate the biological plausibility and clinical significance of the conclusions from studies of chemicals that are thought to have potential adverse effects. Biomarkers of exposure, effect, or individual susceptibility can link the presence of a chemical in various environmental compartments to specific sites of action in target organs and to host responses. Individual behavioral and social risk factors may be critically important both to the risk and to the reduction of risk. Finally, public and media attitudes toward local polluters, other responsible parties, and relevant government agencies greatly influence the communication process and the choices for risk management.

HAZARD IDENTIFICATION

Assessing Toxicity of Chemicals— Methods

Structure/Activity Relationships Given the cost of $1 to $2 million and the 3 to 5 years required for testing a single chemical in a lifetime rodent carcinogenicity bioassay, initial decisions on whether to continue the development of a chemical, submit a premanufacturing notice (PMN), or require additional testing may be based largely on structure/activity relationships (SARs) and limited short-term assays. A chemical's structure, solubility, stability, pH sensitivity, electrophilicity, volatility, and chemical reactivity can be important information for hazard identification.

Structure/activity relationships have been used for the assessment of complex mixtures. However, it is difficult to predict activity across chemical classes and especially across multiple toxic endpoints by using a single biological response. Computerized SAR methods have provided limited results, whereas three-dimensional (3D) molecular modeling, which utilizes pharmacophore mapping, 3D searching and molecular design, and establishment of 3D quantitative structure/activity relationships, has been more successful.

In Vitro and Short-Term Tests The next approach for hazard identification involves in vitro or short-term tests ranging from bacterial mutation assays performed entirely in vitro to more elaborate short-term tests such as skin-painting studies in mice and altered rat liver-foci assays conducted in vivo (see Chaps. 8 and 9). Other assays evaluate developmental and reproductive toxicity, neurotoxicity, and immunotoxicity (Chap. 12). New assay methods from molecular and developmental biology for developmental toxicity risk assessment should accelerate the use of a broader range of model organisms and assay approaches for noncancer risk assessments.

Animal Bioassays Data from animal bioassays are key components of the hazard identification process. A basic premise of risk assessment is that chemicals that cause tumors in animals can cause tumors in humans. All human carcinogens that have been tested adequately in animals have produced positive results in at least one animal model. Although this association cannot establish that all agents and mixtures that cause cancer in experimental animals also cause cancer in humans, in the absence of adequate data on humans, it is biologically plausible and prudent to regard agents and mixtures for which there is sufficient evidence of carcinogenicity in experimental animals as if they presented a carcinogenic risk to humans—a reflection of the "precautionary principle." In general, the most appropriate rodent bioassays are those which test the exposure pathways of most relevance to predicted or known human exposure pathways. Bioassays for reproductive and developmental toxicity and other noncancer endpoints have a similar rationale.

Consistent features in the design of standard cancer bioassays include testing in two species and both sexes, with 50 animals per dose group and near lifetime exposure. Important choices include the strains of rats and mice, the number of doses, dose levels [typically 90, 50, and 10 to 25 percent of the maximally tolerated dose (MTD)], and the details of the required histopathology (number of organs to be examined, choice of interim sacrifice pathology, etc.). Positive evidence of chemical carcinogenicity can include increases in the number of tumors at a particular organ site, induction of rare tumors, earlier induction (shorter latency) of commonly observed tumors, and/or increases in the total number of observed tumors.

Critical problems exist in using the hazard identification data from rodent bioassays for quantitative risk assessments. This is the case because of the limited dose–response data available from these rodent bioassays and nonexistent response information for environmentally relevant exposures. Results thus traditionally have been extrapolated from a dose–response curve in the 10 to 100 percent biologically observable tumor response range down to 10^{-6} risk estimates (upper confidence limit) or to a benchmark or reference dose-related risk.

The addition of investigations of mechanisms and the assessment of multiple noncancer endpoints into the bioassay design represent important enhancements of lifetime bioassays. It is feasible and desirable to tie these bioassays together with mechanistically oriented short-term tests and biomarker and genetic studies in lower doses than those leading to frank tumor development and address the issues of extrapolation over multiple orders of magnitude to predict response at environmentally relevant doses.

Use of Epidemiologic Data in Risk Assessment The most convincing line of evidence for human risk is a well-conducted epidemiologic study in which a positive association between exposure and disease has been observed. Table 4-2 shows examples of epidemiologic study designs and provides clues on the types of outcomes and exposures evaluated. There are important limitations. When the study is exploratory, hypotheses are often weak. Exposure estimates are often crude and retrospective, especially for conditions with a long latency before clinical manifestations appear. Generally, there are multiple exposures, especially when a full week or a lifetime is considered. There is always a trade-off between detailed information on relatively few persons and very limited information on large numbers of persons. Contributions from lifestyle factors such as smoking and diet are a challenge to sort out. Humans are highly outbred, and so the method must consider variation in susceptibility among those who are exposed.

Nevertheless, human epidemiology studies provide very useful information for hazard identification and sometimes quantitative information for data characterization. Three major types of epidemiology study designs are available: cross-sectional studies, cohort studies, and case-control studies (Table 4-2). Cross-sectional studies survey groups of humans to identify risk factors (exposure) and disease but are not useful for establishing cause and effect. Cohort studies evaluate individuals selected on the basis of their exposure to an agent under study. These prospective studies monitor over time individuals

Table 4-2
Example of Three Types of Epidemiological Study Designs

METHODOLOGICAL ATTRIBUTES	Type of Study		
	COHORT	CASE-CONTROL	CROSS-SECTIONAL
Initial classification	Exposure–nonexposure	Disease–nondisease	Either one
Time sequence	Prospective	Retrospective	Present time
Sample composition	Nondiseased individuals	Cases and controls	Survivors
Comparison	Proportion of exposed with disease	Proportion of cases with exposure	Either one
Rates	Incidence	Fractional (%)	Prevalence
Risk index	Relative risk–attributable risk	Relative odds	Prevalence
Advantages	Lack of bias in exposure; yields incidence and risk rates	Inexpensive, small number of subjects, rapid results, suitable for rare diseases, no attrition	Quick results
Disadvantages	Large number of subjects required, long follow-up, attrition, change in time of criteria and methods, costly, inadequate for rare diseases	Incomplete information, biased recall, problem in selecting control and matching, yields only relative risk—cannot establish causation, population of survivors	Cannot establish causation (antecedent consequence); population of survivors; inadequate for rare diseases

who initially are disease-free to determine the rates at which they develop disease. In case-control studies, subjects are selected on the basis of disease status: disease cases and matched cases of disease-free individuals. Exposure histories of the two groups are compared to determine key consistent features in their exposure histories. All case-control studies are retrospective studies.

Epidemiologic findings are judged by the following criteria: strength of association, consistency of observations (reproducibility in time and space), specificity (uniqueness in quality or quantity of response), appropriateness of temporal relationship (did the exposure precede responses?), dose responsiveness, biological plausibility and coherence, verification, and analogy (biological extrapolation). In addition, epidemiologic study designs should be evaluated for their power of detection, appropriateness of outcomes, verification of exposure assessments, completeness in assessing confounding factors, and general applicability of the outcomes to other populations at risk. The power of detection is calculated by using study size, variability, accepted detection lim-

its for the endpoints under study, and a specified significance level.

Recent advances from the Human Genome Project, increased sophistication and molecular biomarkers, and improved mechanistic bases for epidemiologic hypotheses have allowed epidemiologists to expand our understanding of biological plausibility and clinical relevance. "Molecular epidemiology" is a new focus of human studies in which improved molecular biomarkers of exposure, effect, and susceptibility have allowed investigators to link molecular events in the causative disease pathway more effectively.

RISK CHARACTERIZATION

Quantitative considerations in risk assessment include dose–response assessment, exposure assessment, variation in susceptibility, and characterization of uncertainty. For dose–response assessment, varying approaches have been proposed for threshold versus nonthreshold endpoints. Traditionally, threshold approaches have been applied for assessment of noncancer endpoints and nonthreshold approaches have been used for cancer endpoints.

Dose–Response Assessment

The fundamental basis of the quantitative relationships between exposure to an agent and the incidence of an adverse response is the dose–response assessment. Analysis of dose–response relationships must start with determination of the critical effects that will be evaluated quantitatively. It is customary to choose the data sets with adverse effects occurring at the lowest levels of exposure; the "critical" adverse effect is defined as the significant adverse biological effect that occurs at the lowest exposure level. Approaches for characterizing threshold dose–response relationships include identification of NOAELs or LOAELs, "no or lowest observed adverse effect levels." On the dose–response curve illustrated in Fig. 4-3, the threshold, indicated with a T, represents the dose below which no additional increase in response is observed. The NOAEL is identified as the highest non-statistically significant dose tested; in this example, it is point E, at 2 mg/kg body weight. Point F is the LOAEL (2.5 mg/kg body weight), as it is the lowest dose tested that has a statistically significant effect.

In general, animal bioassays are constructed with sufficient numbers of animals to detect low-level biological responses at the 10 percent response range. *Significance* usually refers to both biological and statistical criteria and is dependent on the number of dose levels tested, the number of animals tested at each dose, and the background incidence of the adverse response in the nonexposed control groups. The NOAEL should not be perceived as risk-free.

As was described in Chap. 2, approaches for characterizing dose–response relationships include identification of effect levels such as LD_{50} (dose producing 50 percent lethality), LC_{50} (concentration producing 50 percent lethality), and ED_{10} (dose producing a 10 percent response), as well as NOAELs.

NOAELs traditionally have served as the basis for risk assessment calculations, such as reference doses and acceptable daily intake values. References doses (RfDs) and reference concentrations (RfCs) are estimates of daily exposure to an agent that is assumed to be without adverse health impact on the human population. Acceptable daily intake (ADI) values may be defined as the daily intake of a chemical during an entire lifetime that appears to be without appreciable risk on the basis of all known facts at that time. Reference doses and ADI values typically are calculated from NOAEL values by dividing by uncertainty (UF) and/or modifying factors (MF):

$$RfD = NOAEL/(UF * MF)$$
$$ADI = NOAEL/(UF * MF)$$

In principle, dividing by these factors allows for interspecies (animal-to-human) and intraspecies (human-to-human) variability with default values of 10 each. An additional uncertainty factor can be used to account for experimental inadequacies; for example, to extrapolate from short-exposure-duration studies to a situation more relevant for chronic study, to account for inadequate numbers of animals, or to describe other experimental limitations. If only a LOAEL value is available, an additional 10-fold factor commonly is used to arrive at a value more comparable to a NOAEL. Traditionally, a safety factor of 100 was used for RfD calculations to extrapolate from a well-conducted animal bioassay

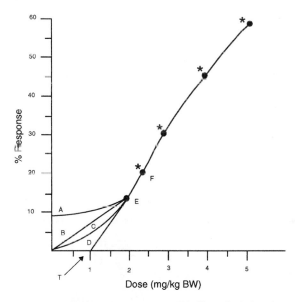

Figure 4-3. Dose–response curve. This figure is designed to illustrate a typical dose–response curve, with "•'s" indicating the biologically determined responses. Statistical significance of these responses is indicated with a * symbol. The threshold dose is shown by T, a dose below which no change in biological response occurs. Point E represents the highest non-statistically significant response point; hence, it is the "no observed adverse effect level" (NOAEL) for this example. Point F is the "lowest observed adverse response level" (LOAEL). Curves A to D show possible options for extrapolating the dose–response relationship below the lowest biologically observed data point, E.

(10-fold factor animal to human) and to account for human variability in response (10-fold factor human-to-human variability).

Modifying factors can be used to adjust the uncertainty factors if data on mechanisms, pharmacokinetics, or the relevance of the animal response to human risk justify such modification.

Recent efforts have focused on using data-derived factors to replace the 10-fold uncertainty factors traditionally used in calculating RfDs and ADIs. Such efforts have included reviewing the human pharmacologic literature from published clinical trials and developing human variability databases for a large range of exposures and clinical conditions. Intra- and interspecies uncertainty factors have two components: toxicokinetic (TK) and toxicodynamic (TD) aspects. Figure 4-4 shows these distinctions. A key advantage of this approach is that it provides a structure for incorporating scientific information on specific aspects of the overall toxicologic process into the reference dose calculations; thus, relevant data can replace a portion of the overall "uncertainty" surrounding these extrapolations.

The NOAEL approach has been criticized on several points, including the following: (1) The NOAEL must, by definition, be one of the experimental doses tested, (2) once this dose is identified, the rest of the dose–response curve is ignored, (3) experiments that test fewer animals result in larger NOAELs and thus larger reference doses, rewarding testing procedures that produce less certain rather than more certain NOAEL values, and (4) the NOAEL approach does not identify the actual responses at the NOAEL and varies with the experimental design, leading to the setting of regulatory limits at varying levels of risk. Because of these limitations, an alternative to the NOAEL approach, the benchmark dose (BMD) method, was proposed. In this approach, the dose–response is modeled and the lower confidence bound for a dose at a specified response level [benchmark response (BMR)] is calculated. The BMR usually is specified at 1, 5, or 10 percent. The BMDx (with "x" representing the percent benchmark response) is used as an alternative to the NOAEL value for reference dose calculations. Thus, the RfD would be

$$RfD = BMDx/UF * MF$$

The proposed values to be used for the uncertainty factors and modifying factors for BMDs can range from the same factors used for the NOAEL to lower values resulting from increased confidence in the response level and increased recognition of experimental variability resulting from the use of a lower confidence bound on the dose.

The advantages of the benchmark dose approach can include (1) the ability to take into account the full dose–response curve, as opposed to focusing on a single test dose, as is done in the NOAEL approach, (2) the inclusion of a measure of variability (confidence limit), (3) the use of responses within the experimental range versus extrapolation of responses to low doses not tested experimentally, and (4) the use of a consistent benchmark response level for RfD calculations across studies. Obviously, limitations in the animal bioassays in regard to minimal test doses for evaluation, shallow dose re-

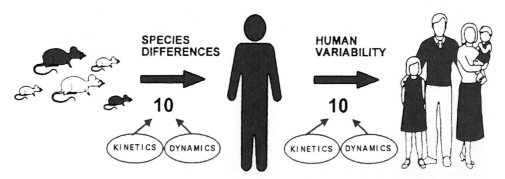

Figure 4-4. Toxicokinetic (TK) and toxicodynamic (TD) considerations inherent in interspecies and interindividual extrapolations. *Toxicokinetics* refers to the processes of absorption, distribution, elimination, and metabolism of a toxicant. *Toxicodynamics* refers to the actions and interactions of the toxicant within the organism and describes processes at the organ, tissue, cellular, and molecular levels. This figure shows how uncertainty in extrapolation both across and within species can be considered as being due to two key factors: a kinetic component and a dynamic component. Refer to the text for detailed explanations.

sponses, and use of study designs with widely spaced test doses will limit the utility of these assays for any type of quantitative assessments, whether NOAEL- or BMD-based approaches.

Nonthreshold Approaches

As Fig. 4-3 shows, numerous dose–response curves can be proposed in the low-dose region of the dose–response curve if a threshold assumption is not made. Because the risk assessor generally needs to extrapolate beyond the region of the dose–response curve for which experimentally observed data are available, the choice of models to generate curves in this region has received a lot of attention. For nonthreshold responses, methods for dose–response assessments also have utilized models for extrapolation to de minimus (10^{-4} to 10^{-6}) risk levels at very low doses, far below the biologically observed response range and far below the effect levels evaluated for threshold responses. Two general types of dose–response models exist: statistical (or probability distribution) models and mechanistic models.

The distribution models are based on the assumption that each individual has a tolerance level for a test agent and that that response level is a variable that follows a specific probability distribution function. These responses can be modeled by using a cumulative dose–response function. However, extrapolation of the experimental data from 50 percent response levels to a "safe," "acceptable," or "de minimus" level of exposure— for example, one in a million risk above background— illustrates the huge gap between scientific observations and highly protective risk limits (sometimes called *virtually safe doses,* or those corresponding to a 95 percent upper confidence limit on adverse response rates).

Models Derived from Mechanistic Assumptions

This modeling approach designs a mathematical equation to describe dose–response relationships that are consistent with postulated biological mechanisms of response. These models are based on the idea that a response (toxic effect) in a particular biological unit (animal or human) is the result of the random occurrence of one or more biological events (stochastic events).

A series of "hit models" for cancer modeling, in which a hit is defined as a critical cellular event that must occur before a toxic effect is produced, assume that (1) an infinitely large number of targets exists, for example, in the DNA, (2) the organism responds with a toxic response

only after a minimum number of targets has been modified, (3) a critical target is altered if a sufficient number of hits occurs, and (4) the probability of a hit in the low dose range of the dose–response curve is proportional to the dose of the toxicant. The simplest mechanistic model is the one-hit (one-stage) linear model, in which only one hit or critical cellular interaction is required for a cell to be altered. As theories of cancer have grown in complexity, multihit models have been developed that can describe hypothesized single-target multihit events as well as multitarget, multihit events in carcinogenesis.

Toxicologic Enhancements of the Models

Three exemplary areas of research that have improved the models used in risk extrapolation are time to tumor information, physiologically based toxicokinetic modeling (described in Chap. 7), and biologically based dose–response modeling. The biologically based dose–response (BBDR) model is intended to make the generalized mechanistic models discussed in the previous section more clearly reflect specific biological processes. Measured rates are incorporated into the mechanistic equations to replace default or computer-generated values.

The development of biologically based dose–response models for endpoints other than cancer has been limited; however, several approaches have been explored in developmental toxicity, that use cell cycle kinetics, enzyme activity, litter effects, and cytotoxicity as critical endpoints. Unfortunately, the lack of specific, quantitative biological information for most toxicants and most endpoints limits the study and utilization of these models.

One key challenge for toxicologists doing risk assessments will be interpretation and linking of observations from highly sensitive molecular and genome-based methods with the overall process of toxicity. The basic need for linkage of observations was highlighted in early biomarker work. Biomarkers of early effects, such as frank clinical pathology, arise as a function of exposure, response, and time. Early, subtle, and possibly reversible effects generally can be distinguished from irreversible disease states.

The challenge for the interpretation of early and highly sensitive responses (biomarkers) is made clear in the analysis of data from gene expression arrays. Because our relatively routine ability to monitor gene responses— up to tens of thousands of them simultaneously—has grown exponentially in the last 5 years, the need for toxicologists to interpret such observations for risk assessment and for the overall process of toxicity has been magnified with equal or greater intensity. For microarray data, each gene response or cluster of genes can have its own pattern of response (peak and overall duration of response).

Microarray analysis for risk assessment requires sophisticated analyses. Because of the vast number of measured responses with gene expression arrays, pattern analysis techniques are being used. The extensive databases across chemical classes, pathologic conditions, and stages of disease progression that are essential for these analyses are being developed.

Exposure Assessment

The primary objectives of exposure assessment are to determine the source, type, magnitude, and duration of contact with the agent of interest. Obviously a key element of the risk assessment process, hazard does not occur in the absence of exposure. However, exposure data frequently are identified as the key area of uncertainty in overall risk determination. The primary goal of using exposure information in quantitative risk assessment is not only to determine the type and amount of total exposure but also to find out specifically how much may be reaching target tissues. A key step in making an exposure assessment is determining which exposure pathways are relevant for the risk scenario under development. The subsequent steps entail quantitating each pathway identified as a potentially relevant exposure and then summarizing these pathway-specific exposures for the calculation of overall exposure.

Additional considerations for exposure assessments include how time and duration of exposures are evaluated in risk assessments. In general, estimates for cancer risk use averages over a lifetime. In a few cases, short-term exposure limits (STELs) are required and characterization of brief but high levels of exposure is required. In these cases, exposures are not averaged over the lifetime. With developmental toxicity, a single exposure can be sufficient to produce an adverse developmental effect; thus, daily doses rather than lifetime weighted averages are used.

Variation in Susceptibility

Toxicology has been slow to recognize the marked variation among humans. Generally, assay results and toxicokinetic modeling utilize means and standard deviations to measure variation, or even standard errors of the mean, to make the range as small as possible. Outliers seldom

are investigated. Thus, it is important to know whether and how one patient might be at higher risk than others. When investigators focus on the most susceptible individuals, there may be a better chance of recognizing and elucidating underlying mechanisms.

Host factors that influence susceptibility to environmental exposures include genetic traits, sex and age, preexisting diseases, behavioral traits (most important, smoking and chronic ethanol consumption), coexisting exposures, medications, vitamins, and protective measures. Genetic studies are of two kinds: (1) investigations of the effects of chemicals and radiation on the genes and chromosomes (Chap. 9) and (2) ecogenetic studies, which identify inherited variation in susceptibility (predisposition and resistance) to specific exposures, ranging across pharmaceuticals ("pharmacogenetics"), pesticides, inhaled pollutants, foods, food additives, sensory stimuli, allergic and sensitizing agents, and infectious agents. Inherited variation in susceptibility has been demonstrated for all these kinds of external agents.

INFORMATION RESOURCES

The Toxicology Data Network (TOXNET) from the National Library of Medicine (http://sis.nlm.nih.gov/sisl/) provides access to databases on toxicology, hazardous chemicals, and related areas. These information sources vary in terms of the included level of assessment, ranging from listings of scientific references without comment to extensive peer-reviewed risk assessment information.

The World Health Organization (http://www.who.int) provides chemical-specific information through the International Programme on Chemical Safety (http://www.who.int/pcs/IPCS/index.htm) criteria documents and health and safety documents. The International Agency for Research on Cancer (IARC) provides data on specific classes of carcinogens as well as individual agents. The National Institutes for Environmental Health Sciences (NIEHS) National Toxicology Program provides technical reports on the compounds tested as a part of this national program and in its reports on carcinogens also provides carcinogen-specific information (http://ehis.niehs.nih.gov/roc/toc9.html).

RISK PERCEPTION AND COMPARATIVE ANALYSES OF RISK

Individuals respond very differently to information about hazardous situations and products, as do communities and whole societies. Understanding these behavioral responses is critical in stimulating constructive risk communication and evaluating potential risk management options. In a classic study, students, League of Women Voters members, active club members, and scientific experts were asked to rank 30 activities or agents in order of their annual contribution to deaths. Club members ranked pesticides, spray cans, and nuclear power as safer than did other laypersons. Students ranked contraceptives and food preservatives as riskier and mountain climbing as safer than did others. Experts ranked electric power, surgery, swimming, and x-rays as more risky and nuclear power and police work as less risky than did laypersons. There are also group differences in perceptions of risk from chemicals among toxicologists, correlated with their employment in industry, academia, or government.

Psychological factors such as dread, perceived uncontrollability, and involuntary exposure interact with factors that represent the extent to which a hazard is familiar, observable, and "essential" for daily living. Figure 4-5 shows a grid on the parameters controllable/uncontrollable and observable/not observable for a large number of risky activities; for each of the two paired main factors, highly correlated factors are described in the boxes.

Public demand for government regulations often focuses on involuntary exposures (especially in the food supply, drinking water, and air) and unfamiliar hazards, such as radioactive waste, electromagnetic fields, asbestos insulation, and genetically modified crops and foods. Many people respond very negatively when they perceive that information about hazards or even about new technologies without reported hazards has been withheld by the manufacturers (genetically modified foods) or government agencies (HIV-contaminated blood transfusions in the 1980s, the extent of hazardous chemical or radioactive wastes).

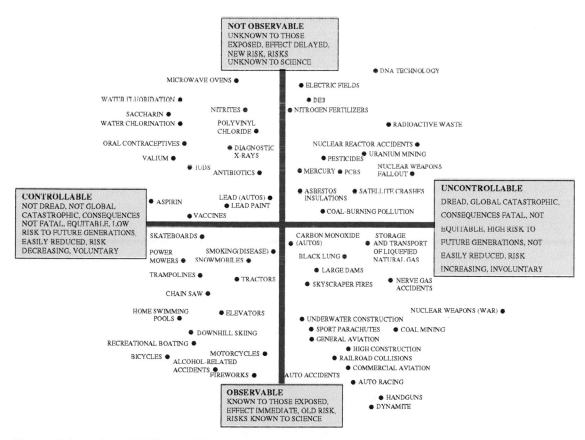

Figure 4-5. Perceptions of risk illustrated by using a "risk space" axis diagram. Risk space has axes that correspond roughly to a hazard's perceived "dreadedness" and to the degree to which it is familiar or observable. Risks in the upper right quadrant of this space are most likely to provoke calls for government regulation.

Most people regularly compare the risks of alternative activities—on the job, in recreational pursuits, in interpersonal interactions, and in investments. Determining how best to conduct comparative risk analyses has proved difficult because of the great variety of health and environmental benefits, the gross uncertainties of dollar estimates of benefits and costs, and the different distributions of benefits and costs across the population.

SUMMARY

The National Research Council and Risk Commission frameworks for risk assessment and risk management provide a consistent databased approach for evaluating risks and taking action to reduce risks. The objectives of risk assessments vary with issues, risk management needs, and statutory requirements. However, the frameworks are sufficiently flexible to address these various objectives and accommodate new knowledge while also providing guidance for priority setting in industry, environmental organizations, and government regulatory and public health agencies. Toxicology, epidemiology, exposure assessment, and clinical observations can be linked with biomarkers, cross-species investigations of mechanisms of effects, and systematic approaches to risk assessment, risk communication, and risk management. Advances in toxicology are certain to improve the quality of risk assessments for a broad array of health endpoints as scientific findings substitute data for assumptions and help describe and model uncertainty more credibly.

BIBLIOGRAPHY

Cullen AC, Frey HC: *Probabilistic Techniques in Exposure Assessment: A Handbook for Dealing with Variability and Uncertainty in Models and Inputs.* New York: Plenum Press, 1999.

EPA: *Health Effects Test Guidelines: 870 Series Final Guidelines.* Washington, DC: Office of Prevention, Pesticides and Toxic Substances, 2000 (*http://www.epa.gov/OPPTS_Harmonized/870_Health_Effects_Test_Guidelines*).

ILSI: *A Framework for Cumulative Risk Assessment.* Washington, DC: International Life Sciences Institute, 1999.

Maines MD, Costa LG, Reed DJ, et al (eds): *Current Protocols in Toxicology.* New York: Wiley, 2000.

NRC: *Scientific Frontiers in Developmental Toxicology and Risk Assessment.* Washington, DC: National Research Council, 2000.

Perera FP, Weinstein IB: Molecular epidemiology: Recent advances and future directions (review). *Carcinogenesis* 21:517–524, 2000.

Wernick IK (ed): *Community Risk Profiles: A Tool to Improve Environment and Community Health.* New York: Rockefeller University, 1995.

WHO: *International Programme on Chemical Safety (IPCS)/OECD Joint Project on Harmonization of Chemical Hazard: Risk Assessment Terminology.* Geneva: WHO, 2000 (http://www.who.int/pes/rsk_term/term_des.htm).

UNIT 2

DISPOSITION OF TOXICANTS

CHAPTER 5

ABSORPTION, DISTRIBUTION, AND EXCRETION OF TOXICANTS

Karl K. Rozman and Curtis D. Klaassen

KEY POINTS

- Absorption is the transfer of a chemical from the site of exposure, usually an external or internal body surface, into the systemic circulation.

- Toxicants are removed from the systemic circulation by biotransformation, excretion, and storage at various sites in the body.

- Excretion is the removal of xenobiotics from the blood and their return to the external environment via urine, feces, or exhalation.

INTRODUCTION

The toxicity of a substance depends on the dose. The concentration of a chemical at the site of action is usually proportional to the dose, but the same dose of two or more chemicals may lead to vastly different concentrations in a particular target organ of toxicity owing to differences in the disposition of the chemicals.

Disposition may be conceptualized as consisting of absorption, distribution, biotransformation, and excretion. Various factors affecting disposition are depicted in Fig. 5-1. For example, (1) if the fraction absorbed or the rate of absorption is low, a chemical may never attain a sufficiently high concentration at a potential site of action to cause toxicity, (2) the distribution of a toxicant may be such that it is concentrated in a tissue other than the target organ, thus decreasing toxicity, (3) biotransformation of a chemical may result in the formation of less toxic or more toxic metabolites at a fast or slow rate, with obvious consequences for the concentration and thus the toxicity at the target site, and (4) the more rap-

idly a chemical is eliminated from an organism, the lower will be its concentration and hence its toxicity in a target tissue or tissues. If a chemical is distributed to and stored in fat, its elimination is likely to be slow because very low plasma levels preclude rapid renal clearance or other clearances.

The quantitation and determination of the time course of absorption, distribution, biotransformation, and excretion of chemicals are referred to as *pharmacokinetics* or *toxicokinetics* (see Chap. 7).

The skin, lungs, and alimentary canal are the main barriers that separate higher organisms from an environment that contains a large number of chemicals. Exceptions are caustic and corrosive agents (acids, bases, salts, oxidizers) that act topically. A chemical absorbed into the bloodstream through any of these three barriers is distributed throughout the body, including the site where it produces damage: the *target organ* or *target tissue*. A chemical may have one or several target organs. Because several factors other than concentration influence the susceptibility of organs to toxicants, the organ or tissue with

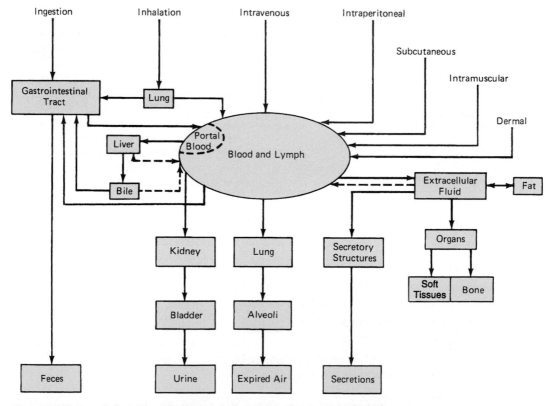

Figure 5-1. Routes of absorption, distribution, and excretion of toxicants in the body.

the highest concentration of a toxicant is not necessarily the site of toxicity.

Toxicants are removed from the systemic circulation by biotransformation, excretion, and storage at various sites in the body. The relative contribution of these processes to total elimination depends on the physical and chemical properties of the chemical. The kidney plays a major role in the elimination of most toxicants, along with the lungs and the liver. The liver is the most active organ in the biotransformation of toxicants. Biotransformation is often a prerequisite for renal excretion, because many toxicants are lipid-soluble and must be transformed into water-soluble forms to be excreted by the kidney.

CELL MEMBRANES

Toxicants usually pass through the membranes of a number of cells, such as the stratified epithelium of skin, the thin cell layers of lungs or the gastrointestinal tract, the capillary endothelium, and the cells of the target organ or tissue. Proteins are inserted in the bilayer, and some proteins even cross it, allowing the formation of aqueous pores. A toxicant may pass through a membrane by either (1) passive transport, in which the cell expends no energy, and (2) specialized transport, in which the cell provides energy to translocate the toxicant across its membrane.

Passive Transport

Simple Diffusion Most toxicants cross membranes by simple diffusion. Small hydrophilic molecules (up to a molecular weight of about 600) permeate membranes through aqueous pores, whereas hydrophobic molecules diffuse across the lipid domain of membranes. The majority of toxicants are larger organic molecules with differing lipid solubility. Their rate of transport across membranes correlates with their lipid solubility.

The ionized form of weak organic acids or bases usually has low lipid solubility and does not permeate readily through the lipid domain of a membrane. In contrast, the nonionized form is more lipid-soluble and diffuses across membranes at a rate that is proportional to its lipid solubility. The pH at which a weak organic acid or base is 50 percent ionized is called its pK_a or pK_b. Like pH, both pK_a and pK_b are defined as the negative logarithm of the ionization constant of a weak organic acid or base. With the equation $pK_a = 14 - pK_b$, pK_a also can be calculated for weak organic bases. An organic acid with a low pK_a is a relatively strong acid, and one with a high pK_a is a weak acid. The opposite is true for bases. Knowl-

edge of the chemical structure is required to distinguish between organic acids and bases.

The degree of ionization of a chemical depends on its pK_a and the pH of the solution. The relationship between pK_a and pH is described by the Henderson-Hasselbalch equations.

$$\text{For acids: } pK_a - pH = \log \frac{[\text{nonionized}]}{[\text{ionized}]}$$

$$\text{For bases: } pK_a - pH = \log \frac{[\text{ionized}]}{[\text{nonionized}]}$$

Filtration When water flows in bulk across a porous membrane, any solute small enough to pass through the pores flows with it. Passage through these channels is called *filtration*. One of the main differences between various membranes is the size of these channels. In the renal glomeruli, these pores allow molecules smaller than albumin (molecular weight of 60,000) to pass through. The channels in most cells are much smaller, permitting substantial passage of molecules with molecular weights of no more than a few hundred.

Special Transport

Active Transport The following properties characterize an active transport system: (1) Chemicals are moved against electrochemical or concentration gradients, (2) the transport system is saturated at high substrate concentrations and thus exhibits a transport maximum (T_m), (3) the transport system is selective for certain structural features of chemicals and has the potential for competitive inhibition between compounds that are transported by the same transporter, and (4) the system requires expenditure of energy, and so metabolic inhibitors block the transport process.

There are a number of distinct active transport systems for endobiotics and xenobiotics. The multidrug-resistant (mdr) proteins or p-glycoproteins exude chemicals out of numerous cells. The multiresistant drug proteins (mrp) also exude chemicals out of cells; however, phase II metabolites (glucuronides and glutathione conjugates) appear to be their preferred substrates. The name *organic-anion transporting peptide (oatp) family* is a misnomer because this transporter family transports not only acids but also bases and neutral compounds and is important in the hepatic uptake of xenobiotics. In contrast, the organic anion transporter (oat) family is especially important in the renal uptake of anions, whereas the organic cation transporter (oct) family is important in both the renal and the hepatic uptake of xenobiotics.

The nucleotide transporter (nt) family, the divalent-metal ion transporter (dmt), and the peptide transporter (pept) aid in gastrointestinal absorption of nucleotides, metals, and di- and tripeptides.

Facilitated Diffusion Facilitated diffusion is carrier-mediated transport that exhibits the properties of active transport except that the substrate is not moved against an electrochemical or concentration gradient and the transport process does not require the input of energy.

Additional Transport Processes Other forms of specialized transport, including phagocytosis and pinocytosis, are proposed mechanisms for cell membranes flowing around and engulfing particles.

ABSORPTION

The process by which toxicants cross body membranes and enter the bloodstream is referred to as *absorption*. The main sites of absorption are the gastrointestinal (GI) tract, lungs, and skin. Enteral administration includes all routes pertaining to the alimentary canal (sublingual, oral, and rectal), whereas parenteral administration involves all other routes (intravenous, intraperitoneal, intramuscular, subcutaneous, etc.).

Absorption of Toxicants by the Gastrointestinal Tract

The GI tract is one of the most important sites of toxicant absorption. Many environmental toxicants enter the food chain and are absorbed together with food from the GI tract.

The GI tract may be viewed as a tube traversing the body. Although it is within the body, its contents can be considered exterior to the body. Therefore, unless a noxious agent has caustic or irritating properties, poisons in the GI tract usually do not produce systemic injury to an individual until they are absorbed.

Absorption of toxicants can take place along the entire GI tract, even in the mouth and rectum. If a toxicant is an organic acid or base, it tends to be absorbed by simple diffusion in the part of the GI tract in which it exists in the most lipid-soluble (nonionized) form. Factors such as the mass action law, surface area, and blood flow rate also influence the absorption of weak organic acids or bases.

The mammalian GI tract has specialized transport systems (carrier-mediated) for the absorption of nutrients and electrolytes (Table 5-1). The GI tract also has at least one active transport system that decreases the absorption

Table 5-1
Site Distribution of Specialized Transport Systems in the Intestine of Humans and Animals

SUBSTRATES	Location of Absorptive Capacity			
	Small Intestine			
	UPPER	MIDDLE	LOWER	COLON
Sugar (glucose, galactose, etc.)	+ +	+ + +	+ +	0
Neutral amino acids	+ +	+ + +	+ +	0
Basic amino acids	+ +	+ +	+ +	?
Gamma globulin (newborn animals)	+	+ +	+ + +	?
Pyrimidines (thymine and uracil)	+	+	?	?
Triglycerides	+ +	+ +	+	?
Fatty acid absorption and conversion to triglyceride	+ + +	+ +	+	0
Bile salts	0	+	+ + +	
Vitamin B_{12}	0	+	+ + +	0
Na^+	+ + +	+ +	+ + +	+ + +
H^+ (and/or HCO_3^- secretion)	0	+	+ +	+ +
Ca^{2+}	+ + +	+ +	+	?
Fe^{2+}	+ + +	+ +	+	?
Cl^-	+ + +	+ +	+	0

SOURCE: Adapted from Wilson TH: *Mechanisms of Absorption*. Philadelphia: Saunders, 1962, pp 40–68.

of xenobiotics. The mdr transporter (also termed p-glycoprotein) is localized in enterocytes. When chemicals that are substrates for mdr enter an enterocyte, they are exuded back into the intestinal lumen.

The number of toxicants actively absorbed by the GI tract is low; most enter the body by simple diffusion. Lipid-soluble substances are absorbed by this process more rapidly and extensively than are water-soluble substances.

The resistance or lack of resistance of chemicals to alteration by the acidic pH of the stomach, the enzymes of the stomach or intestine, or the intestinal flora is of great importance. Simple diffusion is proportional not only to the surface area of villi and microvilli and permeability but also to residency time in various segments of the alimentary canal. Therefore, the rate of absorption of a toxicant remaining for longer periods in the intestine increases, whereas that of a toxicant with a shorter residency time decreases. The residency time of a chemical in the intestine depends on intestinal motility.

Experiments have shown that the oral toxicity of some chemicals is increased when the dose is diluted. This phenomenon may be explained by more rapid stomach emptying induced by increased dosage volume, which in turn leads to more rapid absorption in the duodenum because of the larger surface area there.

The absorption of a toxicant from the GI tract also depends on the physical properties of a compound, such as lipid solubility, and the dissolution rate. An increase in lipid solubility typically increases the absorption of chemicals, and the dissolution rate is inversely proportional to particle size.

The amount of a chemical entering the systemic circulation after oral administration depends on the amount absorbed into the GI cells, biotransformation by the GI cells, and extraction by the liver into bile. This phenomenon of the removal of chemicals before entrance into the systemic circulation is referred to as *presystemic elimination,* or the *first-pass effect.*

Absorptive differences between species may be due to differences in absorptive capabilities among animals, anatomic considerations such as relative surface area of the GI tract, and differences in gastrointestinal flora, since absorption sometimes depends on previous biotransformation by GI bacteria.

Absorption of Toxicants by the Lungs

Toxicants absorbed by the lungs are usually gases, vapors of volatile or volatilizable liquids, and aerosols.

Gases and Vapors The absorption of inhaled gases takes place mainly in the lungs. However, before a gas reaches the lungs, it passes through the nose, with its turbinates, which increase the surface area. Because the mucosa of the nose is covered by a film of fluid, gas molecules can be retained by the nose and not reach the lungs if they are very water-soluble or react with cell surface components. Therefore, the nose acts as a "scrubber" for water-soluble gases and highly reactive gases.

When a gas is inhaled into the lungs, gas molecules diffuse from the alveolar space into the blood and then dissolve until gas molecules in the blood are in equilibrium with gas molecules in the alveolar space. At equilibrium, the ratio of the concentration of chemical in the blood and chemical in the gas phase is constant. This solubility ratio is called the *blood-to-gas partition coefficient.* This constant is unique for each gas. When equilibrium is reached, the rate of transfer of gas molecules from the alveolar space to blood equals the rate of removal by blood from the alveolar space.

The rate of absorption of gases in the lungs is variable and depends on a toxicant's solubility ratio (concentration in blood/concentration in gas phase before or at saturation) at equilibrium. For gases with a very low solubility ratio, the rate of transfer depends mainly on blood flow through the lungs (perfusion-limited), whereas for gases with a high solubility ratio, the rate of transfer is primarily a function of the rate and depth of respiration (ventilation limited).

The blood carries the dissolved gas molecules to the rest of the body. In each tissue, gas molecules are transferred from the blood to the tissue until equilibrium is reached. After releasing part of the gas to tissues, blood returns to the lungs to take up more of the gas. The process continues until a gas reaches equilibrium between the blood and each tissue. At this time, no net absorption of gas takes place as long as the exposure concentration remains constant, because a steady state has been reached. Of course, if biotransformation and excretion occur, alveolar absorption will continue until a corresponding steady state is established.

Aerosols and Particles The major characteristics that affect absorption after exposure to aerosols are the aerosol size and water solubility of a chemical present in the aerosol. The site of deposition of aerosols depends largely on the size of the particles. Particles 5 μm or larger usually are deposited in the nasopharyngeal region (Fig. 5-2) and are removed by nose wiping, blowing, or sneezing. The mucous blanket of the ciliated nasal surface propels insoluble particles by means of the

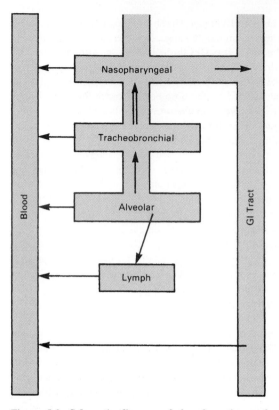

Figure 5-2. Schematic diagram of the absorption and translocation of chemicals by the lungs.

movement of the cilia. These particles and particles inhaled through the mouth are swallowed within minutes. Soluble particles may dissolve in the mucus and be carried to the pharynx or may be absorbed through the nasal epithelium into blood.

Particles 2 to 5 μm are deposited mainly in the tracheobronchiolar regions of the lungs, from which they are cleared by retrograde movement of the mucus layer in the ciliated portions of the respiratory tract. Particles eventually may be swallowed and absorbed from the GI tract.

Particles 1 μm and smaller penetrate to the alveolar sacs of the lungs. They may be absorbed into blood or cleared through the lymphatics after being scavenged by alveolar macrophages.

Removal or absorption of particulate matter from the alveoli appears to occur by three major mechanisms. First, particles may be removed from the alveoli by a physical process. It is thought that particles deposited on the fluid layer of the alveoli are aspirated onto the mucociliary escalator of the tracheobronchial region. From there, they are transported to the mouth and may be swallowed. Second, particles from the alveoli may be removed by phagocytosis by the mononuclear phagocytes, the macrophages. These cells are found in large numbers in normal lungs and contain many phagocytized particles of both exogenous and endogenous origin. They migrate to the distal end of the mucociliary escalator and are cleared and eventually swallowed. Third, removal may occur through the lymphatics, although particulates may remain in lymphatic tissue for long periods.

The overall removal of particles from the alveoli is relatively inefficient; on the first day, only about 20 percent of particles are cleared, and the portion remaining longer than 24 h is cleared very slowly. The rate of clearance by the lungs can be predicted by a compound's solubility in lung fluids. The lower the solubility, the lower the removal rate.

Absorption of Toxicants through the Skin

Human skin comes into contact with many toxic agents. Fortunately, the skin is not very permeable and therefore is a relatively good barrier for separating organisms from their environment. However, some chemicals can be absorbed by the skin in sufficient quantities to produce systemic effects.

To be absorbed through the skin, a toxicant must pass through the epidermis or the appendages (sweat and sebaceous glands and hair follicles). Chemicals that are absorbed through the skin have to pass through several cell layers before entering the blood and lymph capillaries in the dermis (Fig. 5-3). The rate-determining barrier in the dermal absorption of chemicals is the stratum corneum (horny layer), the uppermost layer of the epidermis, with densely packed keratinized cells that have lost their nuclei and thus are biologically inactive.

All toxicants move across the stratum corneum by passive diffusion. Polar substances appear to diffuse through the outer surface of protein filaments of the hydrated stratum corneum, whereas nonpolar molecules dissolve in and diffuse through the lipid matrix between the protein filaments. The permeability of the skin depends on both the diffusivity and the thickness of the stratum corneum. For example, the stratum corneum is much thicker on the palms and soles (400 to 600 μm in callous areas) than it is on the arms, back, legs, and abdomen (8 to 15 μm).

Percutaneous absorption also consists of diffusion of the toxicant through the lower layers of the epidermis (stratum granulosum, spinosum, and germinativum) and

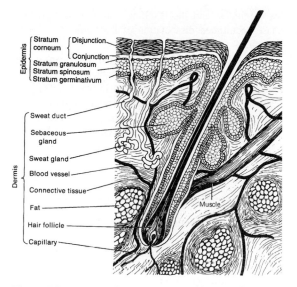

Figure 5-3. Diagram of a cross section of human skin.

the dermis. These cell layers, which are far inferior to the stratum corneum as a barrier, contain a porous, nonselective aqueous diffusion medium. Toxicants pass through this area by diffusion and enter the systemic circulation through the numerous venous and lymphatic capillaries in the dermis.

Absorption of Toxicants after Special Routes of Administration

Besides absorption through the skin, lungs, or GI tract, chemical agents can be administered to laboratory animals by special routes, including the (1) intraperitoneal, (2) subcutaneous, (3) intramuscular, and (4) intravenous routes. The intravenous route introduces the toxicant directly into the bloodstream, eliminating the process of absorption. Intraperitoneal injection results in rapid absorption of xenobiotics because of the rich blood supply and the relatively large surface area of the peritoneal cavity. Intraperitoneally administered compounds are absorbed primarily through the portal circulation and therefore must pass through the liver before reaching other organs. Subcutaneously and intramuscularly administered toxicants usually are absorbed at slower rates but enter directly into the general circulation.

The toxicity of a chemical may or may not depend on the route of administration. If a toxicant is injected intraperitoneally, most of the chemical enters the liver through the portal circulation before reaching the general

circulation. Therefore, an intraperitoneally administered compound may be completely extracted and biotransformed by the liver with subsequent excretion into the bile without gaining access to the systemic circulation. Any toxicant displaying the first-pass effect with selective toxicity for an organ other than the liver and GI tract is expected to be less toxic when administered intraperitoneally than when injected intravenously, intramuscularly, or subcutaneously.

DISTRIBUTION

After entering the blood, a toxicant may undergo distribution (translocation) throughout the body. The rate of distribution to organs or tissues is determined primarily by blood flow and the rate of diffusion out of the capillary bed and into the cells of a particular organ or tissue. The final distribution depends largely on the affinity of a xenobiotic for various tissues.

Volume of Distribution

Total body water may be divided into three distinct compartments. (1) plasma water, (2) interstitial water, and (3) intracellular water. Extracellular water is made up of plasma water plus interstitial water. The concentration of a toxicant in blood depends largely on its volume of distribution. A high concentration will be observed in the plasma if the chemical is distributed into plasma water only, and a much lower concentration will be reached if it is distributed into a large pool, such as total body water.

Distribution of toxicants is usually complex, and binding to and/or dissolution in various storage sites of the body, such as fat, liver, and bone, are critical factors in determining the distribution of chemicals.

Some toxicants do not cross cell membranes readily and therefore have restricted distribution, whereas other toxicants pass rapidly through cell membranes and are distributed throughout the body. Some toxicants accumulate in certain parts of the body as a result of protein binding, active transport, or high solubility in fat. The site of accumulation of a toxicant also may be its site of major toxic action, but more often it is not. If a toxicant accumulates at a site other than the target organ or tissue, the accumulation may be viewed as a protective process in that plasma levels and consequently the concentration of a toxicant at the site of action are diminished. However, because any chemical in a storage depot is in equilibrium with the free fraction of toxicant in plasma, it is released into the circulation as the unbound fraction of the toxicant is eliminated.

Storage of Toxicants in Tissues

Because only the free fraction of a chemical is in equilibrium throughout the body, binding to or dissolving in certain body constituents greatly alters the distribution of a xenobiotic. Toxicants often are concentrated in a specific tissue, which may or may not be their site of toxic action. As a chemical is biotransformed or excreted from the body, more of it is released from the storage site. As a result, the biological half-life of stored compounds can be very long.

Plasma Proteins as Storage Depot Several plasma proteins bind xenobiotics as well as some physiologic constituents of the body. As depicted in Fig. 5-4, albumin, transferrin, globulins, and lipoproteins can bind a large number of different compounds.

Protein-ligand interactions occur primarily as a result of hydrophobic forces, hydrogen bonding, and Van der Waals forces. Because of their high molecular weight, plasma proteins and the toxicants bound to them cannot cross capillary walls. Consequently, the fraction of toxicant bound to plasma proteins is not immediately available for distribution into the extravascular space or filtration by the kidneys. However, the interaction of a chemical with plasma proteins is a reversible process. As unbound chemical diffuses out of capillaries, bound chemical dissociates from the protein until the free fraction reaches equilibrium between the vascular space and the extravascular space. In turn, diffusion in the extravascular space to sites more distant from the capillar-

ies continues, and the resulting concentration gradient causes continued dissociation of the bound fraction in plasma.

Severe toxic reactions can occur if a toxicant is displaced from plasma proteins by another agent, increasing the free fraction of the toxicant in plasma. This will result in an increased equilibrium concentration of the toxicant in the target organ, with the potential for toxicity. Xenobiotics also can compete with and displace endogenous compounds that are bound to plasma proteins.

Liver and Kidney as Storage Depots The liver and the kidneys have a high capacity for binding a multitude of chemicals. These two organs probably concentrate more toxicants than do all the other organs combined. Proteins such as ligandin and metallothionein have a high affinity for many organic compounds and metals, respectively.

Fat as Storage Depot Many highly lipophilic toxicants are distributed and concentrated in body fat. Thus, large amounts of toxicants with a high lipid/water partition coefficient may be stored in body fat. Storage lowers the concentration of a toxicant in the target organ; therefore, the toxicity of such a compound can be expected to be less severe in an obese person than in a lean individual. However, the possibility of a sudden increase in the concentration of a chemical in the blood and thus in the target organ of toxicity when rapid mobilization of fat occurs must be considered.

Bone as Storage Depot Skeletal uptake of xenobiotics is essentially a surface chemistry phenomenon, with exchange taking place between the bone surface of hydroxyapatite crystals and the extracellular fluid that is in contact with it. Deposition and reversible storage of toxicants in bone are dynamic and may or may not be detrimental. Lead is not toxic to bone, but the chronic effects of fluoride deposition (skeletal fluorosis) and radioactive strontium (osteosarcoma and other neoplasms) are well documented.

Blood-Brain Barrier

The blood-brain barrier, though not an absolute barrier to the passage of toxic agents into the central nervous system (CNS), is less permeable than most other areas of the body. There are four major anatomic and physiologic reasons why some toxicants do not enter the CNS readily. First, the capillary endothelial cells of the CNS are tightly joined, leaving few or no pores between the cells. Second, the brain capillary endothelial cells con-

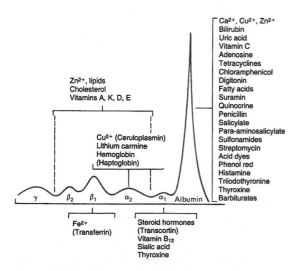

Figure 5-4. Ligand interactions with plasma proteins.

tain an ATP-dependent multidrug-resistant protein that exudes some chemicals back into the blood. Third, the capillaries in the CNS are to a large extent surrounded by glial cell processes (astrocytes). Fourth, the protein concentration in the interstitial fluid of the CNS is much lower than that in other body fluids, limiting the movement of water-insoluble compounds by paracellular transport, which is possible in a largely aqueous medium only when such compounds are bound to proteins.

In general, only the free unbound toxicant equilibrates rapidly with the brain. Lipid solubility and the degree of ionization are important determinants of the rate of entry of a compound into the CNS. Increased lipid solubility enhances the rate of penetration of toxicants into the CNS, whereas ionization greatly diminishes it. Some xenobiotics, although very few, appear to enter the brain through carrier-mediated processes.

Active transport processes decrease the concentration of xenobiotics in the brain. The multidrug-resistant protein in endothelial cells of the brain is responsible for transporting some chemicals from endothelial cells back into the blood.

The blood-brain barrier is not fully developed at birth, and this is one reason why some chemicals are more toxic in newborns than they are in adults.

Passage of Toxicants across the Placenta

Many foreign substances can cross the placenta. In addition to chemicals, viruses (e.g., rubella virus), cellular pathogens (e.g., syphilis spirochetes), globulin antibodies, and erythrocytes can traverse the placenta. Anatomically, the placental barrier consists of a number of cell layers—at most six—interposed between the fetal and maternal circulations. The placenta contains active transport systems and biotransformation enzymes that protect the fetus from some xenobiotics.

Among the substances that cross the placenta by passive diffusion, more lipid-soluble substances more rapidly attain a maternal-fetal equilibrium. Under steady-state conditions, the concentrations of a toxic compound in the plasma of the mother and that of the fetus are usually the same. The concentration in the various tissues of the fetus depends on the ability of fetal tissue to concentrate a toxicant. Differential body composition between mother and fetus may be another reason for an apparent placental barrier. For example, fetuses have very little fat; hence, they do not accumulate highly lipophilic chemicals.

Redistribution of Toxicants

Blood flow to and the affinity of an organ or tissue are the most critical factors that affect the distribution of xenobiotics. Chemicals can have an affinity to a binding site or to a cellular constituent. The initial phase of distribution is determined primarily by blood flow to the various parts of the body. Therefore, a well-perfused organ such as the liver may attain high initial concentrations of a xenobiotic. However, the affinity of less well perfused organs or tissues may be higher for a particular xenobiotic, causing redistribution with time.

EXCRETION

Toxicants are eliminated from the body by several routes. Many xenobiotics, though, have to be biotransformed to more water-soluble products before they can be excreted into urine (Chap. 6). All body secretions appear to have the ability to excrete chemicals; toxicants have been found in sweat, saliva, tears, and milk.

Urinary Excretion

Toxic compounds are excreted into urine by the same mechanisms the kidney uses to remove end products of intermediary metabolism from the body: glomerular filtration, tubular excretion by passive diffusion, and active tubular secretion. Compounds up to a molecular weight of about 60,000 are filtered at the glomeruli. The degree of plasma protein binding affects the rate of filtration, because protein-xenobiotic complexes are too large to pass through the pores of the glomeruli.

A toxicant filtered at the glomeruli may remain in the tubular lumen and be excreted with urine or may be reabsorbed across the tubular cells of the nephron back into the bloodstream. Toxicants with a high lipid/water partition coefficient are reabsorbed efficiently, whereas polar compounds and ions are excreted with urine.

Xenobiotics can also be excreted into urine by active secretion. Figure 5-5 illustrates the various families of transporters in the kidney. The oat family is localized on the basolateral membranes of the proximal tubule. The oct family is responsible for the renal uptake of some cations. Once xenobiotics are in the tubular cell, they are exuded into the lumen by multidrug-resistant (mdr) protein and by multiresistant drug protein (mrp). In contrast, the organic cation transporter (octn2) and peptide transporter (PEP2) reabsorb chemicals from the tubular lumen. Some less polar xenobiotics may diffuse into the lumen. In contrast to filtration, protein-bound toxicants are available for active transport.

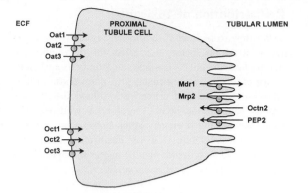

Figure 5-5. Schematic model showing the transport systems in the proximal tubule of the kidney. The families of transporters are organic-anion transporters (oat), organic-cation transporters (oct), multidrug-resistant protein (mdr), multiresistant drug protein (mrp), and peptide transporters (PEP). ECF = extracellular fluid.

Because many functions of the kidney are incompletely developed at birth, some xenobiotics are eliminated more slowly in newborns than they are in adults and therefore may be more toxic to newborns. The development of this organic acid transport system in newborns can be stimulated by the administration of substances normally excreted by this transporter.

The renal proximal tubule reabsorbs small plasma proteins that are filtered at the glomerulus. A toxicant binding those small proteins can be carried into the proximal tubule cells and exert toxicity.

Fecal Excretion

Fecal excretion is the other major pathway for the elimination of xenobiotics from the body.

Nonabsorbed Ingesta In addition to indigestible material, varying proportions of nutrients and xenobiotics that are present in food or are ingested voluntarily (drugs) pass through the alimentary canal unabsorbed, contributing to fecal excretion.

Biliary Excretion The biliary route of elimination is perhaps the most important contributing source to the fecal excretion of xenobiotics and their metabolites. The liver removes toxic agents from blood after absorption from the GI tract, because blood from the GI tract passes through the liver before reaching the general circulation. Thus, the liver can extract compounds from blood and prevent their distribution to other parts of the body. Fur-

thermore, the liver is the main site of the biotransformation of toxicants, and the metabolites thus formed may be excreted directly into bile. Xenobiotics and/or their metabolites entering the intestine with bile may be excreted with feces or undergo an enterohepatic circulation.

Figure 5-6 illustrates the many transporters localized on hepatic parenchymal cells that move foreign substances from plasma into liver and from liver into bile. Sodium-dependent taurocholate peptide (ntcp) present on the sinusoidal side of the parenchymal cell transports bile acids such as taurocholate into the liver, whereas the bile salt excretory protein (bsep) transports bile acids out of liver cells into the bile canaliculi. The sinusoidal membrane of the hepatocyte has a number of transporters, including oatp 1 and 2, liver specific transporter (1st), and organic-cation (oct) transporters that move xenobiotics into the liver. Once inside the hepatocyte, the xenobiotic itself can be transported into the blood or bile or can be biotransformed by phase I and II drug-metabolizing enzymes to more water-soluble products that then are transported into the bile or back into the blood. Multidrug-resistant protein one (mdr1) and multiresistant drug protein two (mrp2) are responsible for transporting xenobiotics into bile, whereas mrp3 and mrp6 transport xenobiotics back into the blood.

Once a compound is excreted into bile and enters the intestine, it can be reabsorbed or eliminated with feces.

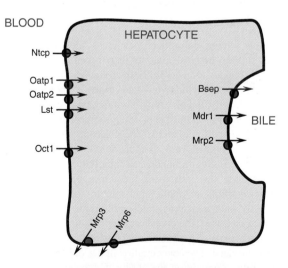

Figure 5-6. Schematic model showing the transport systems in the liver. ntcp = sodium-dependent taurocholate peptide; oatp = organic-anion transporting polypeptide; lst = liver specific transporter; oct = organic-cation transporter; bsep = bile salt excretory protein; mdr = multidrug resistant protein; mrp = multiresistant drug protein.

Many organic compounds are conjugated before excretion into bile. Such polar metabolites are not sufficiently lipid-soluble to be reabsorbed. However, intestinal microflora may hydrolyze glucuronide and sulfate conjugates, making them sufficiently lipophilic for reabsorption and enterohepatic cycling.

Intestinal Excretion Many chemicals in feces directly transfer from blood into the intestinal contents by passive diffusion. In some instances, rapid exfoliation of intestinal cells may contribute to the fecal excretion of some compounds. Intestinal excretion is a relatively slow process that is a major pathway of elimination only for compounds that have low rates of biotransformation and/or low renal or biliary clearance.

Intestinal Wall and Flora Mucosal biotransformation and reexcretion into the intestinal lumen occur with many compounds. It has been estimated that 30 to 42 percent of fecal dry matter originates from bacteria. Moreover, a considerable proportion of fecally excreted xenobiotic is associated with excreted bacteria. However, chemicals may be altered profoundly by bacteria before excretion with feces. It seems that biotransformation by intestinal flora favors reabsorption rather than excretion. Nevertheless, there is evidence that, in many instances, xenobiotics found in feces derive from bacterial biotransformation.

Exhalation

Substances that exist predominantly in the gas phase at body temperature and volatile liquids are eliminated mainly by the lungs. A practical application of this principle is seen in the breath analyzer test for determining the amount of ethanol in the body.

No specialized transport systems have been described for the excretion of toxic substances by the lungs. These substances seem to be eliminated by simple diffusion. Elimination of gases is roughly inversely proportional to the rate of their absorption. The rate of elimination of a gas with low solubility in blood is perfusion-limited, whereas that of a gas with high solubility in blood is ventilation-limited.

Other Routes of Elimination

Cerebrospinal Fluid All compounds can leave the CNS with the bulk flow of cerebrospinal fluid (CSF). In addition, lipid-soluble toxicants can exit at the site of the blood-brain barrier.

Milk The secretion of toxic compounds into milk is extremely important because (1) a toxic material may be passed with milk from the mother to the nursing offspring and (2) compounds can be passed from cows to people in dairy products. Toxic agents are excreted into milk by simple diffusion. Because milk is more acidic (pH $\approx$ 6.5) than plasma, basic compounds may be concentrated in milk, whereas acidic compounds may attain lower concentrations in milk than in plasma. Whereas about 3 to 4 percent of milk consists of lipids and the lipid content of colostrum after parturition is even higher, lipid-soluble xenobiotics diffuse along with fats from plasma into the mammary gland and are excreted with milk during lactation.

Sweat and Saliva The excretion of toxic agents in sweat and saliva is quantitatively of minor importance. Toxic compounds excreted into sweat may produce dermatitis. Substances excreted in saliva enter the mouth, where they usually are swallowed and thus are available for GI absorption.

CONCLUSION

Humans are in continuous contact with toxic agents. Depending on their physical and chemical properties, toxic agents may be absorbed by the GI tract, the lungs, and/or the skin. The body has the ability to biotransform and excrete these compounds into urine, feces, and air. However, when the rate of absorption exceeds the rate of elimination, toxic compounds may accumulate, reaching a critical concentration at a target site, and toxicity may ensue (Fig. 5-7). Whether a chemical elicits toxicity depends not only on its inherent potency and site specificity but also on how an organism can dispose of that toxicant.

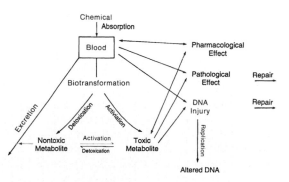

Figure 5-7. Schematic representation of the disposition and toxic effects of chemicals.

Many chemicals have very low inherent toxicity but have to be activated by biotransformation into toxic metabolites, and the toxic response depends on the rate of production of toxic metabolites. Alternatively, a very potent toxicant may be detoxified rapidly by biotransformation. Toxic effects are related to the concentration of "toxic chemical" at the site of action (in the target organ), whether a chemical is administered or generated by biotransformation in the target tissue or at a distant site. Thus, the toxic response exerted by chemicals is critically influenced by the rates of absorption, distribution, biotransformation, and excretion.

BIBLIOGRAPHY

Friedman G, Jacobson ED: *Gastrointestinal Pharmacology and Therapeutics.* Philadelphia: Lippincott-Raven, 1997.

Goodman LS, Hardman JG, Limbird LL, Gilman AG: *Goodman and Gilman's the Pharmacological Basis of Therapeutics,* 10th ed. New York: McGraw-Hill, 2002.

Maibach HI (eds): *Toxicology of the Skin,* New York: Taylor & Francis, 2000.

C H A P T E R   6

BIOTRANSFORMATION OF XENOBIOTICS

Andrew Parkinson

KEY POINTS

- *Biotransformation* is the metabolic conversion of endogenous and xenobiotic chemicals to more water-soluble compounds.

- Xenobiotic biotransformation is accomplished by a limited number of enzymes with broad substrate specificities.

- Phase I reactions involve hydrolysis, reduction, and oxidation. These reactions expose or introduce a functional group ($-OH$, $-NH_2$, $-SH$, or $-COOH$) and usually result in only a small increase in hydrophilicity.

- Phase II biotransformation reactions include glucuronidation, sulfonation (more commonly called sulfation), acetylation, methylation, and conjugation with glutathione (mercapturic acid synthesis), which usually results in increased hydrophilicity and elimination.

Biotransformation is the metabolic conversion of endogenous and xenobiotic chemicals to more water-soluble compounds. Generally, the physical properties of a xenobiotic are changed from those favoring absorption (lipophilicity) to those favoring excretion in urine or feces (hydrophilicity). An exception to this general rule is the elimination of volatile compounds by exhalation.

Chemical modification of a xenobiotic by biotransformation may alter its biological effects. Some drugs undergo biotransformation to active metabolites that exert their pharmacodynamic or toxic effect. In most cases, however, biotransformation terminates the pharmacologic effects of a drug and lessens the toxicity of xenobiotics. Enzymes catalyzing biotransformation reactions often determine the intensity and duration of action of drugs and play a key role in chemical toxicity and chemical tumorigenesis.

GENERAL PRINCIPLES

Basic Properties of Xenobiotic Biotransforming Enzymes

Xenobiotic biotransformation is accomplished by a limited number of enzymes with broad substrate specificities. The synthesis of some of these enzymes is triggered by the xenobiotic (through the process of enzyme induction), but in most cases the enzymes are expressed constitutively (i.e., synthesized in the absence of a discernible external stimulus). Although the synthesis of steroid hormones is catalyzed by cytochrome P450 enzymes in steroidogenic tissues, this family of enzymes in the liver converts steroid hormones into water-soluble metabolites to be excreted.

The structure (i.e., amino acid sequence) of a biotransforming enzyme may differ among individuals, and this can give rise to differences in rates of xenobiotic biotransformation. The study of the causes, prevalence, and impact of heritable differences in xenobiotic biotransforming enzymes is known as *pharmacogenetics.*

Biotransformation versus Metabolism

The terms *biotransformation* and *metabolism* often are used synonymously, particularly when applied to drugs. The term *metabolism* often is used to describe the total fate of a xenobiotic, which includes absorption, distribution, biotransformation, and elimination. However, *metabolism* commonly is used to mean biotransformation, which is understandable from the standpoint that the products of xenobiotic biotransformation are known as *metabolites.* Furthermore, individuals with a genetic enzyme deficiency that results in impaired xenobiotic biotransformation are described as *poor metabolizers* rather than poor biotransformers.

Stereochemical Aspects of Biotransformation

Many xenobiotics, especially drugs, contain one or more chiral centers and can exist in two mirror-image stereoisomers or enantiomers. The biotransformation of some chiral xenobiotics occurs stereoselectively, which means that one enantiomer (stereoisomer) is biotransformed faster than is its antipode.

Table 6-1
General Pathways of Xenobiotic Biotransformation and Their Major Subcellular Location

REACTION	ENZYME	LOCALIZATION
Phase I		
Hydrolysis	Esterase	Microsomes, cytosol, lysosomes, blood
	Peptidase	Blood, lysosomes
	Epoxide hydrolase	Microsomes, cytosol
Reduction	Azo- and nitro-reduction	Microflora, microsomes, cytosol
	Carbonyl reduction	Cytosol, blood, microsomes
	Disulfide reduction	Cytosol
	Sulfoxide reduction	Cytosol
	Quinone reduction	Cytosol, microsomes
	Reductive dehalogenation	Microsomes
Oxidation	Alcohol dehydrogenase	Cytosol
	Aldehyde dehydrogenase	Mitochondria, cytosol
	Aldehyde oxidase	Cytosol
	Xanthine oxidase	Cytosol
	Monoamine oxidase	Mitochondria
	Diamine oxidase	Cytosol
	Prostaglandin H synthase	Microsomes
	Flavin-monooxygenases	Microsomes
	Cytochrome P450	Microsomes
Phase II		
	Glucuronide conjugation	Microsomes
	Sulfate conjugation	Cytosol
	Glutathione conjugation	Cytosol, microsomes
	Amino acid conjugation	Mitochondria, microsomes
	Acetylation	Mitochondria, cytosol
	Methylation	Cytosol, microsomes, blood

Phase I and Phase II Biotransformation

The reactions catalyzed by xenobiotic biotransforming enzymes generally are divided into two groups, called phase I and phase II, as shown in Table 6-1. Phase I reactions involve hydrolysis, reduction, and oxidation. These reactions expose or introduce a functional group (—OH, —NH$_2$, —SH, or —COOH) and usually result in only a small increase in hydrophilicity. Phase II biotransformation reactions include glucuronidation, sulfonation (more commonly called sulfation), acetylation, methylation, conjugation with glutathione (mercapturic acid synthesis), and conjugation with amino acids such as glycine, taurine, and glutamic acid. Most phase II biotransformation reactions result in a large increase in

xenobiotic hydrophilicity; hence, they greatly promote the excretion of foreign chemicals.

Distribution of Xenobiotic Biotransforming Enzymes

Xenobiotic biotransforming enzymes are distributed widely throughout the body and are present in several subcellular compartments. In vertebrates, the liver is the richest source of enzymes that catalyze biotransformation reactions. These enzymes also are located in the skin, lung, nasal mucosa, kidney, eye, and gastrointestinal tract as well as numerous other tissues. Intestinal microflora play an important role in the biotransformation of certain xenobiotics. Biotransformation enzymes are located primarily in the endoplasmic reticulum (microsomes) and the soluble fraction of the cytoplasm (cytosol), with lesser amounts in mitochondria, nuclei, and lysosomes (see Table 6-1).

XENOBIOTIC BIOTRANSFORMATION BY PHASE I ENZYMES

Hydrolysis

Carboxylesterases, Pseudocholinesterase, and Paraoxonase The hydrolysis of carboxylic acid esters, amides, and thioesters is catalyzed largely by carboxylesterases and by two esterases: true acetylcholinesterase in erythrocyte membranes and pseudocholinesterase, which also is known as butyrylcholinesterase and is located in serum. Phosphoric acid esters are hydrolyzed by paraoxonase, a serum enzyme also known as aryldialkylphosphatase. Phosphoric acid anhydrides are hydrolyzed by a related organophosphatase.

Carboxylesterases in serum and tissues and serum cholinesterase collectively determine the duration and site of action of certain drugs. In general, enzymatic hydrolysis of amides occurs more slowly than does that of esters.

Esterases play an important role in limiting the toxicity of organophosphates, which inhibit acetylcholinesterase and thus the termination of the action of the neurotransmitter acetylcholine. Factors that decrease esterase activity potentiate the toxic effects of organophosphates.

Carboxylesterases are glycoproteins that are present in serum and most tissues. Carboxylesterases hydrolyze numerous endogenous lipid compounds and generate pharmacologically active metabolites from several ester or amide prodrugs. In addition, carboxylesterases may convert xenobiotics to toxic and tumorigenic metabolites.

Peptidases Numerous human peptides and several recombinant peptide hormones, growth factors, cytokines, soluble receptors, and monoclonal antibodies are used therapeutically. These peptides are hydrolyzed in the blood and tissues by a variety of peptidases, which cleave the amide linkage between adjacent amino acids.

Epoxide Hydrolase Epoxide hydrolase catalyzes the *trans*-addition of water to alkene epoxides and arene oxides and is present in virtually all tissues. There are five distinct forms of epoxide hydrolase in mammals: microsomal epoxide hydrolase (mEH), soluble epoxide hydrolase (sEH), cholesterol epoxide hydrolase, LTA4 hydrolase, and hepoxilin hydrolase. The last three enzymes appear to hydrolyze endogenous epoxides

exclusively and have virtually no capacity to detoxify xenobiotic oxides.

In contrast to the high degree of substrate specificity displayed by the cholesterol, LTA4, and hepoxilin epoxide hydrolases, the microsomal and soluble epoxide hydrolases (mEH and sEH) hydrolyze many alkene epoxides and arene oxides. Generally, these two forms of epoxide hydrolases and cytochrome P450 enzymes, which are often responsible for producing the toxic epoxides, have a similar cellular localization that presumably ensures the rapid detoxication of the alkene epoxides and arene oxides generated during the oxidative biotransformation of xenobiotics.

Epoxide hydrolase is one of several inducible enzymes in liver microsomes. Induction of epoxide hydrolase invariably is associated with the induction of cytochrome P450.

Reduction

Certain metals and xenobiotics containing an aldehyde, ketone, disulfide, sulfoxide, quinone, *N*-oxide, alkene, azo, or nitro group often are reduced in vivo. The reaction may proceed enzymatically or nonenzymatically by means of interaction with reducing agents, such as the reduced forms of glutathione, FAD, FMN, and NADP.

Azo- and Nitro-Reduction Azo-reduction and nitro-reduction are catalyzed by intestinal microflora and by two liver enzymes: cytochrome P450 and NADPH-quinone oxidoreductase (also known as DT-diaphorase). These reactions require NADPH and are inhibited by oxygen. The anaerobic environment of the lower gastrointestinal tract is well suited for azo- and nitro-reduction.

Carbonyl Reduction The reduction of certain aldehydes to primary alcohols and of ketones to secondary alcohols is catalyzed by alcohol dehydrogenase and by a family of carbonyl reductases. Carbonyl reductases are monomeric, NADPH-dependent enzymes that are present in blood and the cytosolic fraction of various tissues. Hepatic carbonyl reductase activity is present mainly in the cytosolic fraction, with a different carbonyl reductase being present in the microsomes.

Disulfide Reduction Disulfide reduction by glutathione is a three-step process, the last step of which is catalyzed by glutathione reductase. The first steps can be catalyzed by glutathione *S*-transferase or can occur nonenzymatically.

Sulfoxide and *N*-Oxide Reduction Thioredoxin-dependent enzymes in liver and kidney cytosol can reduce sulfoxides, which were formed by cytochrome P450. Under reduced oxygen tension, the NADPH-dependent reduction of *N*-oxides in liver microsomes may be catalyzed by cytochrome P450 or NADPH-cytochrome P450 reductase.

Quinone Reduction Quinones can be reduced to hydroquinones by NADPH-quinone oxidoreductase (DT-diaphorase), a cytosolic flavoprotein, *without* oxygen consumption. The two-electron reduction of quinones also can be catalyzed by carbonyl reductase. This pathway of quinone reduction is essentially nontoxic and is not associated with oxidative stress.

The second pathway of quinone reduction catalyzed by microsomal NADPH-cytochrome P450 reductase results in the formation of a semiquinone free radical by a one-electron reduction of the quinone. The oxidative stress associated with the autooxidation of a semiquinone free radical, which produces superoxide anion, hydrogen peroxide, and other active oxygen species, can be extremely cytotoxic.

Dehalogenation There are three major mechanisms for removing halogens (F, Cl, Br, and I) from aliphatic xeno-biotics: (1) *Reductive dehalogenation* involves the replacement of a halogen with hydrogen, (2) *oxidative dehalogenation* replaces a halogen and hydrogen on the same carbon atom with oxygen, and (3) *double dehalogenation* involves the elimination of two halogens on adjacent carbon atoms to form a carbon–carbon double bond. A variation on the third mechanism is *dehydrohalogenation,* in which a halogen and hydrogen on adjacent carbon atoms are eliminated to form a carbon–carbon double bond.

Oxidation

Alcohol Dehydrogenase Alcohol dehydrogenase (ADH) is a cytosolic enzyme that is present in several tissues, including the liver, which has the highest levels, the kidney, the lung, and the gastric mucosa. There are four major classes of ADH. The class I ADH isozymes (α-ADH, β-ADH, and γ-ADH) are responsible for the oxidation of ethanol and other small aliphatic alcohols (Fig. 6-1). Class II ADH (π-ADH) is expressed primarily in liver, where it preferentially oxidizes larger aliphatic and aromatic alcohols. Long-chain alcohols (pentanol and larger) and aromatic alcohols are preferred substrates for class III

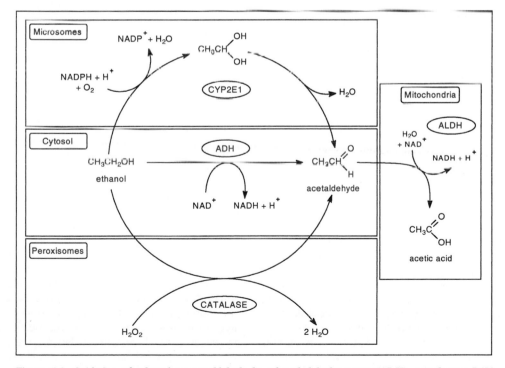

Figure 6-1. Oxidation of ethanol to acetaldehyde by ethanol dehydrogenase (ADH), cytochrome P450 (CYP2E1), and catalase. Note that the oxidation of ethanol to acetic acid involves multiple organelles.

ADH (χ-ADH). Class IV ADH (σ- or μ-ADH), which is not expressed in the liver, is the most active of the medium-chain ADHs in oxidizing retinol.

Aldehyde Dehydrogenase Aldehyde dehydrogenase (ALDH) oxidizes aldehydes to carboxylic acids with NAD^+ as the cofactor. These enzymes also have esterase activity. The ALDHs differ in their primary amino acid sequences and in the quaternary structure. In contrast to ALDH1 and ALDH2, which specifically reduce NAD^+, ALDH3 reduces both NAD^+ and $NADP^+$.

As shown in Fig. 6-1, ALDH2 is a mitochondrial enzyme that, by virtue of its high affinity, is primarily responsible for oxidizing simple aldehydes, such as acetaldehyde. Genetic deficiencies in other ALDHs impair the metabolism of other aldehydes.

Dihydrodiol Dehydrogenase The aldo-keto reductase (AKR) superfamily includes several forms of dihydrodiol dehydrogenases, which are cytosolic, NADPH-requiring oxidoreductases that oxidize various polycyclic aromatic hydrocarbons.

Molybdenum Hydroxylases Two major molybdenum hydroxylases or molybdozymes participate in the biotransformation of xenobiotics: aldehyde oxidase and xanthine dehydrogenase/xanthine oxidase (XD/XO). Sulfite oxidase, a third molybdozyme, oxidizes sulfite, an irritating air pollutant, to sulfate, which is relatively innocuous. All three molybdozymes are flavoprotein enzymes. During substrate oxidation, aldehyde oxidase and xanthine oxidase are reduced and then reoxidized by molecular oxygen. The oxygen incorporated into the xenobiotic is derived from water rather than oxygen, and this distinguishes the oxidases from oxygenases.

Xanthine Dehydrogenase–Xanthine Oxidase Xanthine dehydrogenase (XD) and xanthine oxidase (XO) are two forms of the same enzyme that differ in regard to the electron acceptor used in the final step of catalysis. In the case of XD, the final electron acceptor is NAD^+, whereas in the case of XO, the final electron acceptor is oxygen. XD is converted to XO by oxidation of cysteine residues and/or proteolytic cleavage. The conversion of XD to XO in vivo may be important in ischemia-reperfusion injury, lipopolysaccharide-mediated tissue injury, and alcohol-induced hepatotoxicity. XO contributes to oxidative stress and lipid peroxidation because the oxidase activity of XO involves reduction of molecular oxygen, which can lead to the formation of reactive oxygen species.

Aldehyde Oxidase The molybdozyme aldehyde oxidase exists only in the oxidase form. Cytosolic aldehyde oxidase transfers electrons to molecular oxygen, which can generate reactive oxygen species and lead to lipid peroxidation. Aldehyde oxidase plays an important role in the catabolism of biogenic amines and catecholamines.

Monoamine Oxidase Monoamine oxidases (MAOs) are involved in the oxidative deamination of primary, secondary, and tertiary amines, including serotonin, and a number of xenobiotics. Oxidative deamination of a primary amine produces ammonia and an aldehyde, whereas oxidative deamination of a secondary amine produces a primary amine and an aldehyde. The aldehydes formed by MAO usually are oxidized further by other enzymes to the corresponding carboxylic acids. Monoamine oxidase is located throughout the brain and in the outer membrane of mitochondria in the liver, kidney, intestine, and blood platelets. The substrate is oxidized by monamine oxidase, which itself is reduced using FAD. The oxygen incorporated into the substrate is derived from water, not molecular oxygen. The catalytic cycle is completed by reoxidation of the reduced enzyme (FADH$_2$ → FAD) by oxygen, which generates hydrogen peroxide.

Peroxidase-Dependent Cooxidation Oxidative biotransformation of xenobiotics by peroxidases couples the reduction of hydrogen peroxide and lipid hydroperoxides to the oxidation of other substrates through a process known as *cooxidation*. An important peroxidase is prostaglandin H synthetase (PHS), which possesses two catalytic activities: a *cyclooxygenase* that converts arachidonic acid to prostaglandins and a *peroxidase* that converts the hydroperoxide to the corresponding alcohol PGH$_2$. Peroxidases are important in the activation of xenobiotics to toxic or tumorigenic metabolites, particularly in extrahepatic tissues that contain low levels of cytochrome P450.

In certain cases, the oxidation of xenobiotics by peroxidases involves direct transfer of the peroxide oxygen to the xenobiotic, as shown in Fig. 6-2 for the conversion of substrate X to product XO. Xenobiotics that can serve as electron donors, such as amines and phenols, also can be oxidized to free radicals during the reduction of a hydroperoxide by peroxidases. In this case, the hydroperoxide is still converted to the corresponding alcohol, but the peroxide oxygen is reduced to water instead of being incorporated into the xenobiotic. For each molecule of hydroperoxide reduced (this is a two-electron process), two molecules of xenobiotic can be oxidized

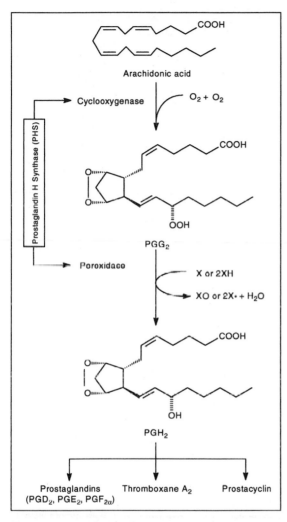

Figure 6-2. Cooxidation of xenobiotics (X) during the conversion of arachidonic acid to PGH$_2$ by prostaglandin H synthase.

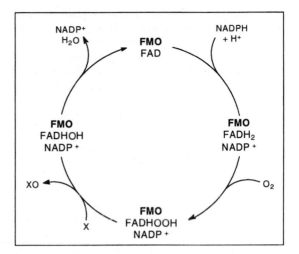

Figure 6-3. Catalytic cycle of flavin monooxygenase (FMO). X and XO are the xenobiotic substrate and the oxygenated product, respectively. The 4a-hydroperoxyflavin and 4a-hydroxyflavin of FAD are depicted as FADHOOH and FADHOH, respectively.

(each by a one-electron process). Many of the metabolites produced are reactive electrophiles that can cause tissue damage.

Cyclooxygenase may play at least two distinct roles in tumor formation: It may convert certain xenobiotics to DNA-reactive metabolites and *initiate* tumor formation, and it may *promote* subsequent tumor growth, perhaps through the formation of growth-promoting eicosanoids.

PHS is unique among peroxidases because it can both generate hydroperoxides and catalyze peroxidase-dependent reactions, as is shown in Fig. 6-2. Xenobiotic biotransformation by PHS is controlled by the availabil-

ity of arachidonic acid, whereas conversion by other peroxidases is controlled by the availability of hydroperoxide substrates.

Flavin Monooxygenases Liver, kidney, and lung contain one or more FAD-containing monooxygenases (FMOs) that oxidize the nucleophilic nitrogen, sulfur, and phosphorus heteroatom of various xenobiotics. The mammalian FMO gene family includes five microsomal enzymes that require NADPH and O$_2$, and many of the reactions catalyzed by FMO also can be catalyzed by cytochrome P450.

The mechanism of catalysis by FMO is depicted in Fig. 6-3. After the FAD moiety is reduced to FADH$_2$ by NADPH, the oxidized cofactor NADP$^+$ remains bound to the enzyme. FADH$_2$ then binds oxygen to produce a peroxide that is relatively stable. During the oxygenation of xenobiotics, the flavin peroxide oxygen is transferred to the substrate (depicted as X $\rightarrow$ XO in Fig. 6-3). The final step in the catalytic cycle involves restoration of FAD to its oxidized state and release of NADP$^+$. This final step is rate-limiting, and it occurs after substrate oxygenation.

Cytochrome P450 Among the phase I biotransforming enzymes, the cytochrome P450 system ranks first in terms of catalytic versatility and the number of xenobiotics it detoxifies or activates. The highest concentration of P450 enzymes involved in xenobiotic biotransformation is found in hepatic endoplasmic reticulum (microsomes), but P450 enzymes are present in virtually all tissues. All P450 enzymes are heme-containing proteins. The basic reaction catalyzed by cytochrome P450 is the monooxygenation of one atom of oxygen into a substrate; the other oxygen atom is reduced to water with reducing equivalents derived from NADPH.

During catalysis, cytochrome P450 does not interact directly with NADPH or NADH. In the endoplasmic reticulum, where most of the P450 enzymes involved in xenobiotic biotransformation are localized, electrons are relayed from NADPH to cytochrome P450 through a flavoprotein called NADPH–cytochrome P450 reductase. In mitochondria, electrons are transferred from NADPH to cytochrome P450 through two proteins: ferredoxin and ferredoxin reductase.

There are some notable exceptions to the general rule that cytochrome P450 requires a second enzyme (i.e., a flavoprotein) for catalytic activity. One exception applies to two P450 enzymes involved in the conversion of arachidonic acid to eicosanoids: thromboxane synthase and prostacyclin synthase. In both cases, cytochrome P450 functions as an isomerase and catalyzes a rearrangement of the oxygen atoms that are introduced into arachidonic acid by cyclooxygenase. The second exception involves two cytochrome P450 enzymes expressed in the bacterium *Bacillus megaterium.* These P450 enzymes are considerably larger than most P450 enzymes because the P450 moiety and flavoprotein are expressed in a single protein that is encoded by a single gene.

Cytochrome P450 and NADPH–cytochrome P450 reductase are embedded in the phospholipid bilayer of the endoplasmic reticulum, which facilitates their interaction. The catalytic cycle of cytochrome P450 is shown in Fig. 6-4. The first part of the cycle involves the activation of oxygen, and the final part involves substrate oxidation, which entails the abstraction of a hydrogen atom or an electron from the substrate followed by oxygen rebound (radical recombination). After the binding of substrate to the P450 enzyme, the heme iron is reduced from the ferric (Fe^{3+}) state to the ferrous (Fe^{2+}) state by the addition of a single electron from NADPH–cytochrome P450 reductase. Release of the oxidized substrate returns cytochrome P450 to its initial state. If the catalytic cycle is interrupted, oxygen is released as superoxide anion ($O_2^{\bullet -}$) or hydrogen peroxide (H_2O_2).

Cytochrome P450 catalyzes the following types of oxidation reactions:

1. Hydroxylation of an aliphatic or aromatic carbon
2. Epoxidation of a double bond

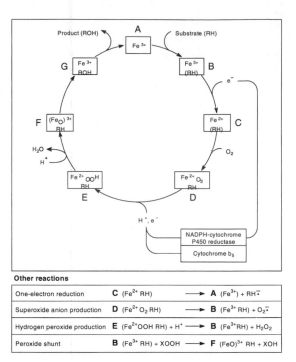

Other reactions

One-electron reduction	**C** (Fe^{2+} RH)	⟶	**A** (Fe^{3+}) + RH⁻
Superoxide anion production	**D** (Fe^{2+} O_2 RH)	⟶	**B** (Fe^{3+} RH) + $O_2^{\bullet -}$
Hydrogen peroxide production	**E** (Fe^{2+}OOH RH) + H^+	⟶	**B** (Fe^{3+}RH) + H_2O_2
Peroxide shunt	**B** (Fe^{3+} RH) + XOOH	⟶	**F** $(FeO)^{3+}$ RH + XOH

Figure 6-4. Catalytic cycle of cytochrome P450.

3. Heteroatom (*S*-, *N*-, and *I*-) oxygenation and *N*-hydroxylation
4. Heteroatom (*O*-, *S*-, *N*- and *Si*-) dealkylation
5. Oxidative group transfer
6. Cleavage of esters
7. Dehydrogenation

Liver microsomes from all mammalian species contain numerous P450 enzymes, each with the potential to catalyze the various reactions shown in Figs. 6-5 through 6-12. In general, P450 enzymes are classified into subfamilies on the basis of amino acid sequence identity. Human liver microsomes can contain 15 or more distinct P450 enzymes.

The function and regulation of CYP1A1, CYP1A2, CYP1B1, and CYP2E1 are highly conserved among mammalian species, and these proteins have the same names in all mammalian species. In all other cases, the P450 enzymes are named in a species-specific manner. The levels and activity of each P450 enzyme vary from one individual to the next because of environmental and/or genetic factors. Decreased P450 enzyme activity can result from (1) a genetic mutation that either blocks the synthesis of a P450 enzyme or leads to the synthesis of a catalytically compromised or inactive enzyme, (2) exposure to an

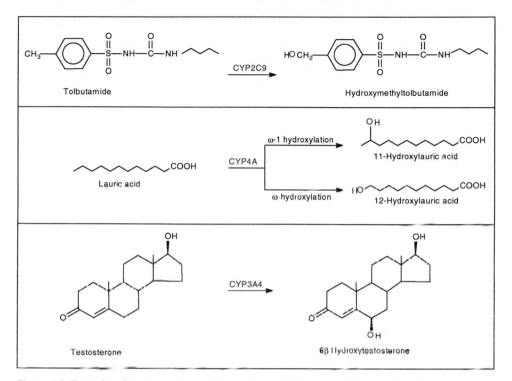

Figure 6-5. Examples of reactions catalyzed by cytochrome P450: hydroxylation of aliphatic carbon.

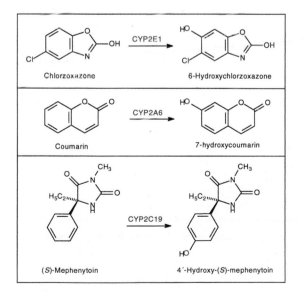

Figure 6-6. Examples of reactions catalyzed by cytochrome
P450: hydroxylation of aromatic carbon.

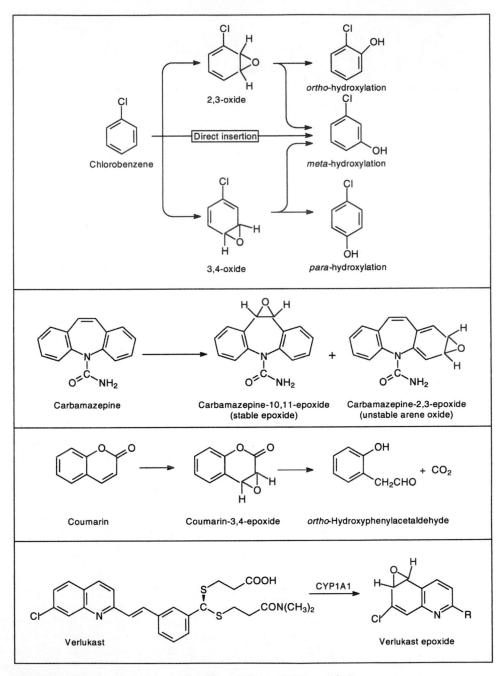

Figure 6-7. Examples of reactions catalyzed by cytochrome P450: epoxidation.

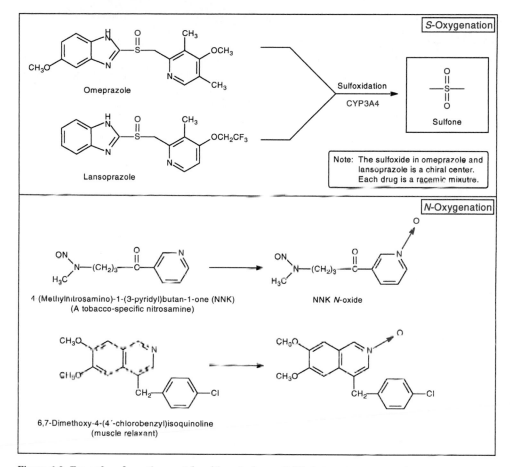

Figure 6-8. Examples of reactions catalyzed by cytochrome P450: heteroatom oxygenation.

environmental factor (such as an infectious disease or a xenobiotic) that suppresses P450 enzyme expression, or (3) exposure to a xenobiotic that inhibits or inactivates a preexisting P450 enzyme. By inhibiting cytochrome P450, one drug can impair the biotransformation of another, and this may lead to an exaggerated pharmacologic or toxicologic response to the second drug. Increased P450 enzyme activity can result from (1) gene duplication leading to overexpression of a P450 enzyme, (2) exposure to environmental factors, such as xenobiotics, that induce the synthesis of cytochrome P450, or (3) stimulation of a preexisting enzyme by a xenobiotic.

Induction of cytochrome P450 by xenobiotics increases P450 enzyme activity. By inducing cytochrome P450, one drug can stimulate the metabolism of a second drug and thus decrease or ameliorate its therapeutic effect. Allelic variants, which arise from point mutations in the wild-type gene, are another source of interindividual variation in

P450 activity. Environmental factors that are known to affect P450 levels include medications, foods, social habits (e.g., alcohol consumption, cigarette smoking), and disease status (diabetes, inflammation, viral and bacterial infection, hyperthyroidism, and hypothyroidism). When environmental factors influence P450 enzyme levels, considerable variation may be observed during repeated measures of xenobiotic biotransformation (e.g., drug metabolism) in the same individual. As a result of their broad substrate specificity, two or more P450 enzymes can contribute to the metabolism of a single compound.

The pharmacologic or toxic effects of certain drugs are exaggerated in a significant percentage of the population because of a heritable deficiency in a P450 enzyme. Inasmuch as the biotransformation of a xenobiotic in humans frequently is dominated by a single P450 enzyme, considerable attention has been paid to defining the substrate specificity of the P450 enzymes expressed in human liver

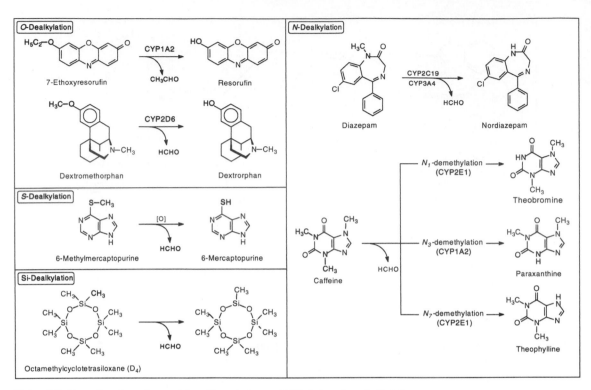

Figure 6-9. Examples of reactions catalyzed by cytochrome P450: heteroatom dealkylation.

microsomes through a process commonly referred to as *reaction phenotyping* or *enzyme mapping*. Three approaches to reaction phenotyping are as follows:

1. *Correlation analysis* involves measuring the rate of xenobiotic metabolism by several samples of human liver microsomes and correlating reaction rates with the variation in the level or activity of the individual P450 enzymes in the same microsomal samples.

2. *Chemical and antibody inhibition* evaluates the effects of known P450 enzyme inhibitors or inhibitory antibodies on the metabolism of a xenobiotic by human liver microsomes. Chemical inhibitors of cytochrome P450 must be used cautiously because most of them can inhibit more than one P450 enzyme.

3. *Biotransformation by purified or recombinant human P450 enzymes* establishes whether a particular P450 enzyme can or cannot biotransform a xenobiotic, but it does not address whether that P450 enzyme contributes substantially to reactions catalyzed by human liver microsomes.

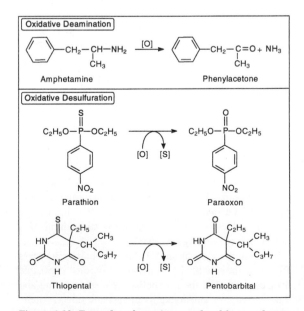

Figure 6-10. Examples of reactions catalyzed by cytochrome P450: oxidative group transfer.

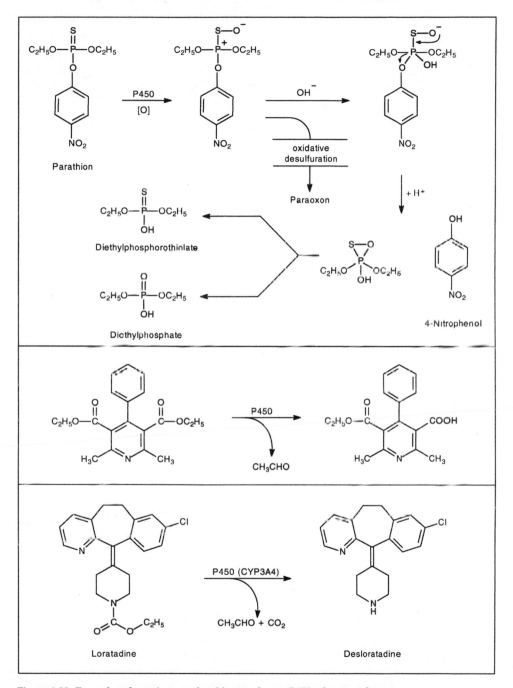

Figure 6-11. Examples of reactions catalyzed by cytochrome P450: cleavage of esters.

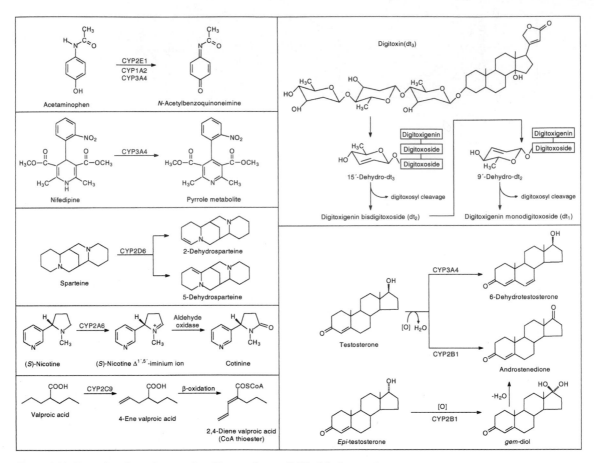

Figure 6-12. Examples of reactions catalyzed by cytochrome P450: dehydrogenation.

Examples of substrates, inhibitors, and inducers for each P450 enzyme in human liver microsomes are given in Table 6-2. Because reaction phenotyping in vitro is not always carried out with toxicologically relevant substrate concentrations, the P450 enzyme that appears to be responsible for biotransforming the drug in vitro may not be the P450 enzyme responsible for biotransforming the drug in vivo.

Activation of Xenobiotics by Cytochrome P450

The role of human P450 enzymes in the activation of procarcinogens and protoxicants and some cytochrome P450-dependent reactions are summarized in Table 6-3. Many of the chemicals listed in Table 6-3 also are detoxified by cytochrome P450 by biotransformation to less toxic metabolites. In some cases, the same P450 enzyme

catalyzes both activation and detoxication reactions. For example, CYP3A4 activates aflatoxin B_1 to the hepatotoxic and tumorigenic 8,9-epoxide, but it also detoxifies aflatoxin B_1 by 3-hydroxylation to aflatoxin Q_1. This shows that complex factors determine the balance between xenobiotic activation and detoxication.

P450 Knockout Mice

Transgenic mice that lack one or more P450 enzymes may be used to evaluate the role of specific P450 enzymes in xenobiotic activation. Studies in knockout mice are relevant to humans because their counterpart can be found in individuals who lack certain P450 enzymes or other xenobiotic biotransforming enzymes. Experiments in knockout mice underscore how genetic polymorphisms in the human population are risk modifiers for the development of chemically induced disease.

Table 6-2

Examples of Substrates, Inhibitors, and Inducers of the Major Human Liver Microsomal P450 Enzymes Involved in Xenobiotic Biotransformation

	CYP2A6	CYP2B6	CYP2C8	CYP2C9	CYP2C19	CYP2E1
Substrates	Coumarin Butadiene Nicotine	Benzphetamine 7-Benzyloxyresorufin Bupropion Cyclophosphamide 7-Ethoxy-4-trifluoro-methylcoumarin Ifosphamide S-Mephenytoin	Arachidonic acid Carbamazepine Paclitaxel (Taxol)	Celecoxib Diclofenac Phenacetin Phenobarbital Phenytoin Piroxicam Tenoxicam Tetrahydrocannabinol Tienilic acid Tolbutamide Torsemide S-Warfarin	Citalopram Diazepam Diphenylhydantoin Hexobarbital Imipramine Lansoprazole S-Mephenytoin Mephobarbital Omeprazole Pentamidine Phenobarbital Proguanil Propranolol	Acetaminophen Alcohols Aniline Benzene Caffeine Chlorzoxazone Dapsone Enflurane Halogenated alkanes Isoflurane Methylformamide 4-Nitrophenol Nitrosamines Styrene Theophylline
Inhibitors	Diethyldithiocarbamate Letrozole 8-Methoxypsoralen* Pilocarpine Tranylcypromine	9-Ethynylphenanthrene Methoxychlor Orphenadrine*	Etoposide Nicardipine Quercetin Tamoxifen R-Verapamil	Sulfaphenazole Sulfinpyrazone	Fluconazole Teniposide Tranylcypromine	3-Amino-1,2,4-triazole* Diethyldithiocarbamate Dihydrocapsaicin Dimethyl sulfoxide Disulfiram 4-Methylpyrazole Phenethylisothiocyanate*
Inducers	Barbiturates?	Phenobarbital Phenytoin Rifampin Troglitazone	Not known	Rifampin	Artemisinin? Rifampin	Ethanol Isoniazid

*Metabolism-dependent (mechanism-based) inhibitor.

(continued)

Table 6-2
Examples of Substrates, Inhibitors, and Inducers of the Major Human Liver Microsomal P450 Enzymes Involved in Xenobiotic Biotransformation (*continued*)

	CYP1A2	CYP2D6			CYP3A4		
Substrates	Acetaminophen	Amiflamine	Dolasetron	Miniaprine	Acetaminophen	Erythromycin	Rapamycin
	Acetanilide	Amitriptyline	Encainide	Nortriptyline	Aldrin	Ethinylestradiol	Retinoic acid
	Aminopyrine	Aprindine	Flecainide	Ondansetron	Alfentanil	Etoposide	Saquinavir
	Antipyrine	Brofaromine	Fluoxetine	Paroxetine	Amiodarone	Flutamide	Steroids (e.g., cortisol)
	Aromatic amines	Bufurolol	Flunarizine	Perhexiline	Aminopyrine	Hydroxyarginine	Tacrolimus (FK 506)
	Caffeine	Captopril	Fluphenazine	Perphenazine	Amprenavir	Ifosphamide	Tamoxifen
	Estradiol	Chlorpromazine	Guanoxan	Propafenone	Antipyrine	Imipramine	Taxol
	Ethoxyresorufin	Cinnarizine	Haloperidol (reduced)	Propranolol	Astemizole	Indinavir	Teniposide
	Imipramine	Citalopram		*N*-Propylajmaline	Benzphetamine	Lansoprazole	Terfenadine
	Methoxyresorufin	Clonipramine	Hydrocodone	Remoxipride	Budesonide	Lidocaine	Tetrahydrocannabinol
	Phenacetin	Clozapine	Imipramine	Sparteine	Carbamazepine	Loratadine	Theophylline
	Tacrine	Codeine	Indoramin	Tamoxifen	Celecoxib	Losartan	Toremifene
	Theophylline	Debrisoquine	Methoxyamphetamine	Thioridazine	Cisapride	Lovastatin	Triazolam
	Trimethadone	Deprenyl	Methoxyphenamine	Timolol	Cyclophosphamide	Midazolam	Trimethadone
	Warfarin	Desmethylcitalopram	Metoprolol	Tomoxetine	Cyclosporine	Nelfinavir	Troleandomycin
		Despiramine	Mexiletine	Trifluperidol	Dapsone	Nicardipine	Verapamil
		Dextromethorphan	Mianserin	Tropisetron	Delavirdine	Nifedipine	Warfarin
					Diazepam	Omeprazole	Zatosetron
					Digitoxin	Quinidine	Zonisamide
					Diltiazem		
Inhibitors	Ciprofloxacin	Ajmalicine	Fluoxetine	Quinidine	Amprenavir	Indinavir	Ritonavir
	Fluvoxamine	Celecoxib	Lobelin	Trifluperidol	Clotrimazole	Itraconazole	Saquinavir
	Furafylline*	Chinidin	Propidin	Yohimbine	Delavirdine	Ketoconazole	Troleandomycin*
	α-Naphthoflavone	Corynanthine			Ethinylestradiol*	Miconazole	Verapamil
					Fluoxetine	Nelfinavir	*Activator:*
					Gestodene*	Nicardipine	α-Naphthoflavone
Inducers	Charcoal-broiled beef	None known			Carbamazepine	Phenytoin	Sulfadimidine
	Cigarette smoke				Dexamethasone	Rifabutin	Sulfinpyrazone
	Cruciferous vegetables				Glutethimide	Rifampin	Troglitazone
	Omeprazole				Nevirapine	Ritonavir?	Troleandomycin
					Phenobarbital	St. John's wort	

*Metabolism-dependent (mechanism-based) inhibitor.

Table 6-3
Examples of Xenobiotics Activated by Human P450 Enzymes

CYP1A1	**CYP2E1**
Benzo[a]pyrene and other polycyclic	Acetaminophen
aromatic hydrocarbons	Acrylonitrile
CYP1A2	Benzene
Acetaminophen	Carbon tetrachloride
2-Acetylaminofluorene	Chloroform
4-Aminobiphenyl	Dichloromethane
2-Aminofluorene	1,2-Dichloropropane
2-Naphthylamine	Ethylene dibromide
NNK*	Ethylene dichloride
Amino acid pyrrolysis products	Ethyl carbamate
(DiMeQx, MeIQ, MeIQx, Glu P-1,	Halothane
Glu P-2, IQ, PhIP, Trp P-1, Trp P-2)	N-Nitrosodimethylamine
Tacrine	Styrene
CYP2A6	Trichloroethylene
N-Nitrosodiethylamine	Vinyl chloride
NNK*	**CYP3A4**
CYP2B6	Acetaminophen
6-Aminochrysene	Aflatoxin B_1 and G_1
Cyclophosphamide	6-Aminochrysene
Ifosphamide	Benzo[a]pyrene 7,8-dihydrodiol
CYP2C8, 9, 18, 19	Cyclophosphamide
Tienilic acid	Ifosphamide
Valproic acid	1-Nitropyrene
CYP2D6	Sterigmatocystin
NNK*	Senecionine
	Tris(2,3-dibromopropyl) phosphate
	CYP4A9/11
	None known

*NNK, 4-(methylnitrosamino)-1-(3-pyridyl)-1-butanone, a tobacco-specific nitrosamine.

Inhibition of Cytochrome P450

In addition to predicting the likelihood of some individuals being poor metabolizers as a result of a genetic deficiency in P450 expression, information about which human P450 enzyme metabolizes a drug can help predict or explain drug interactions. Inhibitory drug interactions generally fall into three categories. The first involves competition between two drugs that are metabolized by the same P450 enzyme. The second is also competitive in nature, but the inhibitor is not a substrate for the affected P450 enzyme. The third type of drug interaction results from noncompetitive inhibition of cytochrome P450 by covalent binding to P450.

Induction of Cytochrome P450

Inducers of cytochrome P450 increase the rate of xenobiotic biotransformation. Some of the P450 enzymes in human liver microsomes are inducible (Table 6-2). As an underlying cause of serious adverse effects, P450 induction lowers blood levels; this compromises the therapeutic goal of drug therapy but does not cause an exaggerated response to the drug.

Induction of cytochrome P450 may increase the activation of procarcinogens to DNA-reactive metabolites, leading to increased tumor formation. There is little evidence from either human epidemiologic studies or animal experiments that P450 induction enhances the incidence or multiplicity of tumors caused by known chemical carcinogens. In fact, most evidence points to a protective role of enzyme induction against chemical-induced neoplasia. Cytochrome P450 induction can cause pharmacokinetic tolerance by which larger drug doses must be administered to achieve therapeutic blood levels because of increased drug biotransformation.

PHASE II ENZYME REACTIONS

Phase II biotransformation reactions include glucuronidation, sulfonation (more commonly called sulfa- tion), acetylation, methylation, conjugation with glutathione (mercapturic acid synthesis), and conjugation with amino acids such as glycine, taurine, and glutamic acid. The cosubstrates for these reactions, which are shown in Fig. 6-13, react with functional groups that either are present on the xenobiotic or are introduced/exposed during phase I biotransformation. With the exception of methylation and acetylation, phase II biotransformation reactions result in a large increase in xenobiotic hydrophilicity, which greatly promotes the excretion of foreign chemicals. Glucuronidation, sulfation, acetylation, and methylation involve reactions with acti-

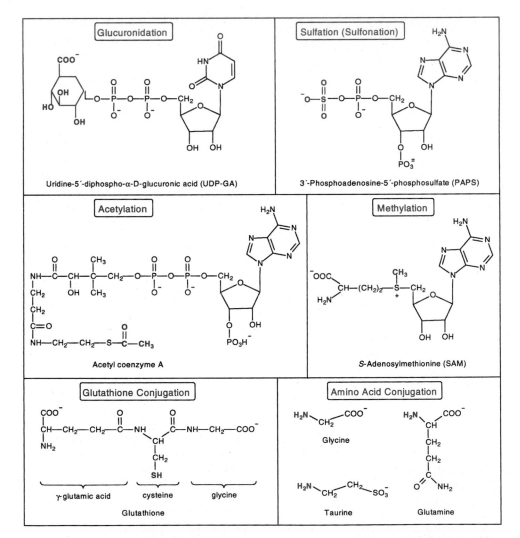

Figure 6-13. Structures of cofactors for phase II biotransformation. The functional group that reacts with or is transferred to the xenobiotic is shown in blue.

vated or "high-energy" cosubstrates, whereas conjugation with amino acids or glutathione involves reactions with activated xenobiotics. Most phase II biotransforming enzymes are located mainly in the cytosol (Table 6-1). Phase II reactions generally proceed much faster than do phase I reactions. Therefore, the rate of elimination of xenobiotics whose excretion depends on biotransformation by cytochrome P450 followed by phase II conjugation generally is determined by the first reaction.

Glucuronidation

Glucuronidation requires the cosubstrate uridine diphosphate-glucuronic acid (UDP-glucuronic acid), and the reaction is catalyzed by UDP-glucuronosyltransferases (UGTs). Examples of xenobiotics that are glucuronidated are shown in Fig. 6-14. The site of glucuronidation is generally an electron-rich nucleophilic heteroatom (O, N, or S), as found in aliphatic alcohols and phenols, carboxylic acids, primary and secondary aromatic and aliphatic amines, and free sulfhydryl groups. Endogenous substrates for glucuronidation include bilirubin, steroid hormones, and thyroid hormones.

Glucuronide conjugates of xenobiotics and endogenous compounds are polar, water-soluble conjugates. Whether glucuronides are excreted from the body in bile or urine depends on the size of the aglycone (parent compound or phase I metabolite). The carboxylic acid moiety of glucuronic acid, which is ionized at physiologic pH, promotes excretion because it (1) increases the aqueous solubility of the xenobiotic and (2) is recognized by the biliary and renal organic anion transport systems, enabling glucuronides to be secreted into urine and bile. Glucuronides of xenobiotics are substrates for β-glucuronidase present in the intestinal microflora. The intestinal enzyme can release the aglycone, which undergoes *enterohepatic circulation* and delays the elimination of the xenobiotic.

Cofactor availability can limit the rate of glucuronidation of drugs that are administered in high doses and are conjugated extensively, such as aspirin and acetaminophen.

UDP-glucuronosyltransferases expressed in rat liver microsomes belong to two gene families, UGT1 and UGT2, each of which contains several subfamilies with many similar members. Members of gene family 2 are all distinct gene products (i.e., each member is encoded by a separate gene). In contrast, members of family 1 are formed from a single gene with multiple copies of the first exon, each of which can be connected in cassette fashion with a common set of exons.

Sulfation

Many xenobiotics and endogenous substrates are conjugated with sulfate. Sulfate conjugation is catalyzed by sulfotransferases, a multigene family of cytosolic enzymes, and generally produces a highly water-soluble sulfuric acid ester. The cosubstrate for the reaction is 3′-phosphoadenosine-5′-phosphosulfate (PAPS) (see Fig. 6-13).

Sulfate conjugation involves the transfer of sulfonate, not sulfate (i.e., SO_3^-, not SO_4^-), from PAPS to the xenobiotic. (The commonly used terms *sulfation* and *sulfate conjugation* are used here even though *sulfonation* and *sulfonate conjugation* are more appropriate descriptors.) Table 6-4 lists examples of xenobiotics and endogenous compounds that are sulfated without prior biotransformation by phase I enzymes. An even greater number of xenobiotics are sulfated after a hydroxyl group is exposed or introduced during phase I biotransformation.

Sulfate conjugates of xenobiotics are excreted mainly in urine. Sulfatases are also present in the endoplasmic reticulum and lysosomes, where they primarily hydrolyze sulfates of endogenous compounds. Some sulfate conjugates are substrates for further biotransformation.

The sulfate donor PAPS is synthesized from inorganic sulfate (SO_4^{2-}) and ATP in a two-step reaction. The major source of sulfate required for the synthesis of PAPS appears to be derived from cysteine through a complex oxidation sequence. The cellular concentrations of PAPS ($\sim75~\mu$M) are considerably lower than those of UDP-glucuronic acid ($\sim350~\mu$M) and glutathione (~10 mM). The relatively low concentration of PAPS limits the capacity for xenobiotic sulfation.

Multiple sulfotransferases have been identified in all mammalian species that have been examined. The sulfotransferases are arranged into gene families (SULT1–SULT5) that share less than 40 percent amino acid sequence identity and are further subdivided into several subfamilies. Each family appears to work on a specific functional group (i.e., phenols, alcohols, amines).

In general, sulfation is an effective means of decreasing the pharmacologic and toxicologic activity of xenobiotics. However, as shown in Fig. 6-15, sulfation plays a role in the activation of aromatic amines, methyl-substituted polycyclic aromatic hydrocarbons, and safrole to tumorigenic metabolites.

Methylation

Methylation, a minor pathway of biotransformation, generally decreases the water solubility of xenobiotics and masks functional groups that might otherwise be

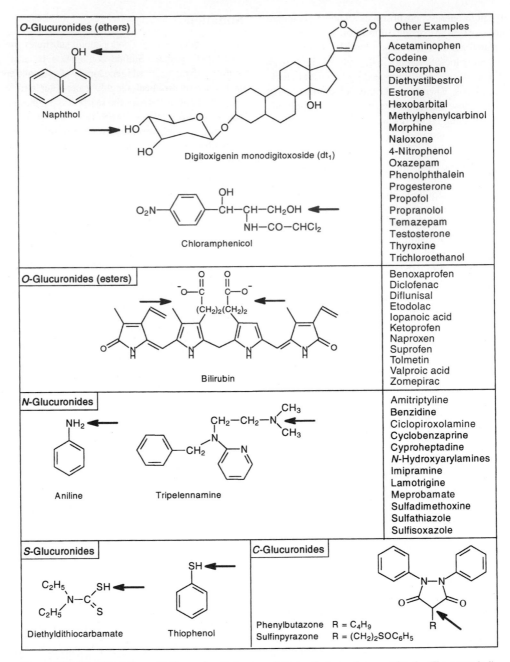

Figure 6-14. Examples of xenobiotics and endogenous substrates that are glucuronidated. The arrow indicates the site of glucuronidation.

Table 6-4
Examples of Xenobiotics and Endogenous Compounds That Undergo Sulfate Conjugation

FUNCTIONAL GROUP	EXAMPLE
Primary alcohol	Chloramphenicol, ethanol, hydroxymethyl polycyclic aromatic hydrocarbons, polyethylene glycols
Secondary alcohol	Bile acids, 2-butanol, cholesterol, dehydroepiandrosterone, doxaminol
Phenol	Acetaminophen, estrone, ethinylestradiol, naphthol, pentachlorophenol, phenol, picenadol, salicylamide, trimetrexate
Catechol	Dopamine, ellagic acid, α-methyl-DOPA
N-oxide	Minoxidil
Aliphatic amine	2-Amino-3,8-dimethylimidazo[4,5,-f]-quinoxaline (MeIQx)*
	2-Amino-3-methylinidazo-[4,5-f]-quinoline (IQ)*
	2-Cyanoethyl-N-hydroxythioacetamide, despramine
Aromatic amine	2-Aminonaphthalene, aniline
Aromatic hydroxylamine	N-hydroxy-2-aminonaphthalene
Aromatic hydroxyamide	N-hydroxy-2-acetylaminofluorene

*Amino acid pyrolysis products.

conjugated by other phase II enzymes. The structure of the consubstrate for methylation, S-adenosylmethionine (SAM), is shown in Fig. 6-13. The methyl group bound to the sulfonium ion in SAM is transferred to xenobiotics and endogenous substrates by nucleophilic attack from an electron-rich heteroatom (O, N, or S). Examples of xenobiotics and endogenous substrates that undergo O-, N-, or S-methylation are shown in Fig. 6-16. During these methylation reactions, SAM is converted to S-adenosylhomocysteine.

The O-methylation of phenols and catechols is catalyzed by two different enzymes known as phenol O-methyltransferase (POMT) in microsomes and catechol-O-methyltransferase (COMT) in cytosol and microsomes. In rats and humans, COMT is encoded by a single gene with two different transcription initiation sites. Transcription at one site produces a cytosolic form of COMT, whereas transcription from the other site produces a membrane-bound form by adding a 50–amino acid segment that targets COMT to the endoplasmic reticulum. Substrates for COMT include several catecholamine neurotransmitters and catechol drugs, such as L-dopa and methyldopa.

Several N-methyltransferases have been described in humans and other mammals. Phenylethanolamine N-methyltransferase catalyzes the N-methylation of the neurotransmitter norepinephrine to form epinephrine. This enzyme is expressed in the adrenal medulla and in certain regions of the brain and has minimal significance in xenobiotic biotransformation. However, histamine and nicotine N-methyltransferases expressed in liver, intestine, and/or kidney methylate xenobiotics.

S-Methylation is an important pathway in the biotransformation of sulfhydryl-containing xenobiotics. In humans, S-methylation is catalyzed by two enzymes: thiopurine methyltransferase in cytosol and thiol methyltransferase in microsomes.

Acetylation

N-Acetylation is a major route of biotransformation for xenobiotics that contain an aromatic amine (R–NH$_2$) or a hydrazine group (R–NH–NH$_2$), which are converted to aromatic amides (R–NH–COCH$_3$) and hydrazides (R–NH–NH–COCH$_3$), respectively. Like methylation, N-acetylation masks an amine with a nonionizable group so that many N-acetylated metabolites are less water-soluble than is the parent compound. Nevertheless, N-acetylation of certain xenobiotics, such as isoniazid, facilitates their urinary excretion.

The N-acetylation of xenobiotics is catalyzed by cytosolic N-acetyltransferases and requires the cosubstrate acetyl-coenzyme A (acetyl-CoA), which is shown in Fig. 6-13. The reaction occurs in two sequential steps: (1) The acetyl group from acetyl-CoA is transferred to an active site cysteine residue within an N-acetyltransferase with release of coenzyme A, and (2) the acetyl group is transferred from the acylated enzyme to the amino group of the substrate with regeneration of the enzyme.

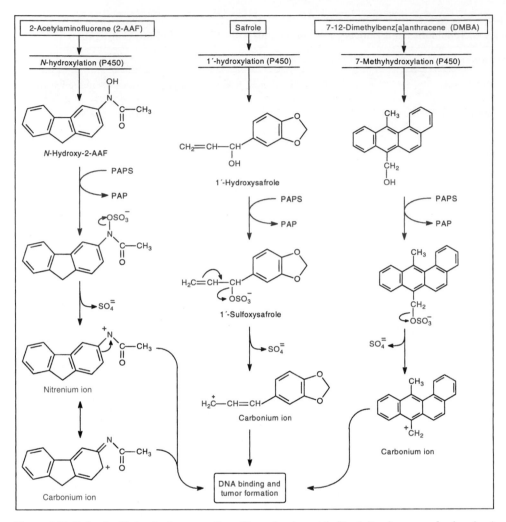

Figure 6-15. Role of sulfation in the generation of tumorigenic metabolites (nitrenium or carbonium ions) of 2-acetylaminofluorene, safrole, and 7,12-dimethylbenz[a]anthracene (DMBA).

NAT1 and NAT2, the two acetyltransferases that exist in humans, are closely related proteins (79 to 95 percent identical in amino acid sequence) with an active site cysteine residue in the N-terminal region. Although encoded by genes on the same chromosome, NAT1 and NAT2 are independently regulated proteins: NAT1 is expressed in most tissues of the body, whereas NAT2 is expressed mainly in the liver and the intestine. However, most (but not all) of the tissues that express NAT1 also appear to express low levels of NAT2, at least at the level of mRNA. NAT1 and NAT2 also have different but overlapping substrate specificities. Examples of drugs that are N-acetylated by NAT1 and NAT2 are shown in Fig. 6-17.

Genetic polymorphisms for N-acetylation have been documented in humans, hamsters, rabbits, and mice. Genetic polymorphisms in *NAT2* have a number of pharmacologic and toxicologic consequences: Slow NAT2 acetylators are predisposed to several drug toxicities, including an excessive response from the antihypertensive agent hydralazine, peripheral neuropathy from isoniazid and dapsone, systemic lupus erythematosus from hydralazine and procainamide, and the toxic effects of coadministration of the anticonvulsant phenytoin with isoniazid.

The N-acetyltransferases generally detoxify aromatic amines by converting them to the corresponding amides

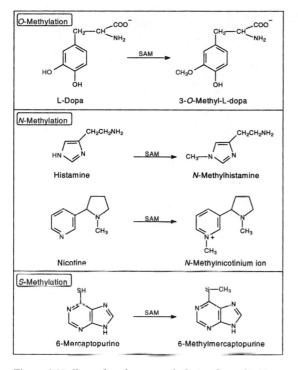

Figure 6-16. *Examples of compounds that undergo O-, N-, or S-methylation.*

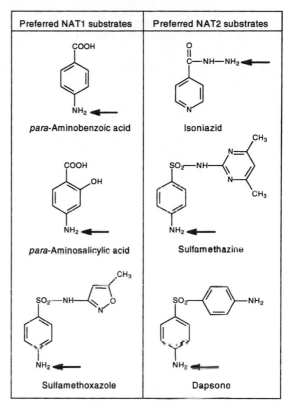

Figure 6-17. *Examples of substrates for the human N-acetyltransferases, NAT1, and the highly polymorphic NAT2.*

that are less likely to be activated to DNA-reactive metabolites. However, *N* acetyltransferases can activate aromatic amines if they are first *N*-hydroxylated by cytochrome P450. The acetoxy esters of *N*-hydroxyaromatic amines, like the corresponding sulfate esters (Fig. 6-15), can break down to form highly reactive nitrenium and carbonium ions that bind to DNA. Whether fast acetylators are protected from or predisposed to the cancer-causing effects of aromatic amines depends on the nature of the aromatic amine and other risk modifiers.

Amino Acid Conjugation

Two principal pathways by which xenobiotics are conjugated with amino acids are illustrated in Fig. 6-18. The first pathway involves conjugation of xenobiotics containing a carboxylic acid group with the amino group of amino acids such as glycine, glutamine, and taurine (see Fig. 6-13). After activation of the xenobiotic by conjugation with CoA, the acyl-CoA thioether reacts with the *amino group* of an amino acid to form an amide linkage. The second pathway involves conjugation of xenobiotics containing an aromatic hydroxylamine with the *car-boxylic acid group* of amino acids such as serine and proline. This pathway involves the activation of an amino acid by aminoacyl-tRNA-synthetase, which reacts with an aromatic hydroxylamine to form a reactive *N*-ester.

Substrates for amino acid conjugation are restricted to certain aliphatic, aromatic, heteroaromatic, cinnamic, and arylacetic acids. The ability of xenobiotics to undergo amino acid conjugation depends on steric hindrance around the carboxylic acid group and by substituents on the aromatic ring or aliphatic side chain. Amino acid conjugates of xenobiotics are eliminated primarily in urine. The acceptor amino acid used for conjugation is both species- and xenobiotic-dependent.

Amino acid conjugation of *N*-hydroxy aromatic amines (hydroxylamines) is an activation reaction because it produces *N*-esters that can degrade to form electrophilic nitrenium and carbonium ions. Conjugation of hydroxylamines with amino acids is catalyzed by cytosolic aminoacyl-tRNA synthetases and requires ATP (Fig. 6-18).

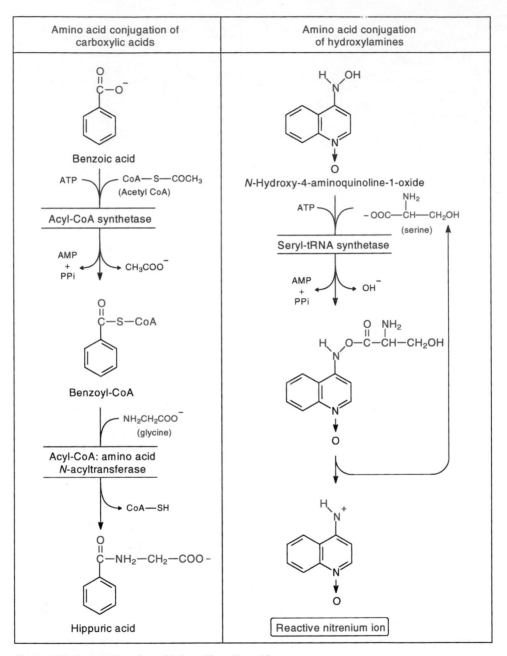

Figure 6-18. Conjugation of xenobiotics with amino acids.

Glutathione Conjugation

Conjugation of xenobiotics with glutathione includes an enormous array of electrophilic xenobiotics, or xenobiotics that can be biotransformed to electrophiles. The tripeptide glutathione is composed of glycine, cysteine, and glutamic acid (Fig. 6-13). Glutathione conjugates are thioethers, which form by nucleophilic attack of glutathione thiolate anion (GS⁻) with an electrophilic carbon, oxygen, nitrogen, or sulfur atom in the xenobiotic.

This conjugation reaction is catalyzed by a family of glutathione S-transferases that are present in most tissues, where they are localized in the cytoplasm (>95 percent) and the endoplasmic reticulum (<5 percent).

Substrates for glutathione S-transferase share three common features: They are hydrophobic, they contain an electrophilic atom, and they react nonenzymatically with glutathione at a measurable rate. The mechanism by which glutathione S-transferase increases the rate of glutathione conjugation involves deprotonation of GSH to GS⁻. The concentration of glutathione in liver is extremely high (~10 mM); hence, the nonenzymatic conjugation of certain xenobiotics with glutathione can be significant. However, some xenobiotics are conjugated with glutathione stereoselectively, indicating that the reaction is catalyzed largely by glutathione S-transferase. Like glutathione, the glutathione S-transferases are abundant cellular components, accounting for up to 10 percent of the total cellular protein. These enzymes bind, store, and/or transport a number of compounds that are not substrates for glutathione conjugation. The cytoplasmic protein formerly known as ligandin, which binds heme, bilirubin, steroids, azo-dyes, and polycyclic aromatic hydrocarbons, is one of the glutathione S-transferases.

As shown in Fig. 6-19, substrates for glutathione conjugation can be divided into two groups: those sufficiently

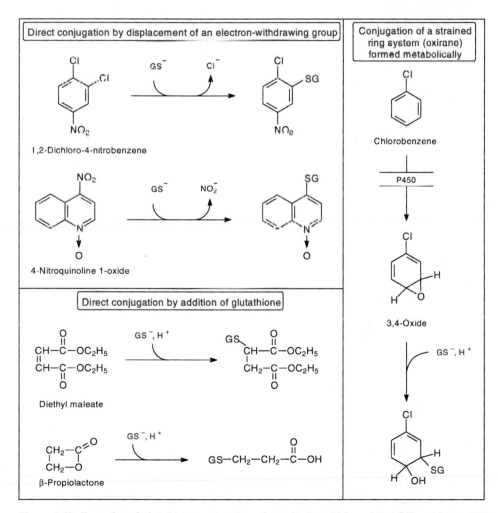

Figure 6-19. Examples of glutathione conjugation of xenobiotics with an electrophilic carbon. GS⁻ represents the anionic form of glutathione.

electrophilic to be conjugated directly, and those which must be biotransformed to an electrophilic metabolite before conjugation. The conjugation reactions can be divided into two types: *displacement reactions,* in which glutathione displaces an electron-withdrawing group, and *addition reactions,* in which glutathione is added to an activated double bond or strained ring system.

The displacement of an electron-withdrawing group by glutathione typically occurs when the substrate contains halide, sulfate, sulfonate, phosphate, or a nitro group (i.e., good *leaving groups*) attached to an allylic or benzylic carbon atom.

The addition of glutathione to a carbon–carbon double bond also is facilitated by the presence of a nearby electron-withdrawing group; hence, substrates for this reaction typically contain a double bond attached to —CN, —CHO, —COOR, or —COR.

Glutathione also can conjugate xenobiotics with an electrophilic heteroatom (O, N, and S). In each of the examples shown in Fig. 6-20, the initial conjugate formed

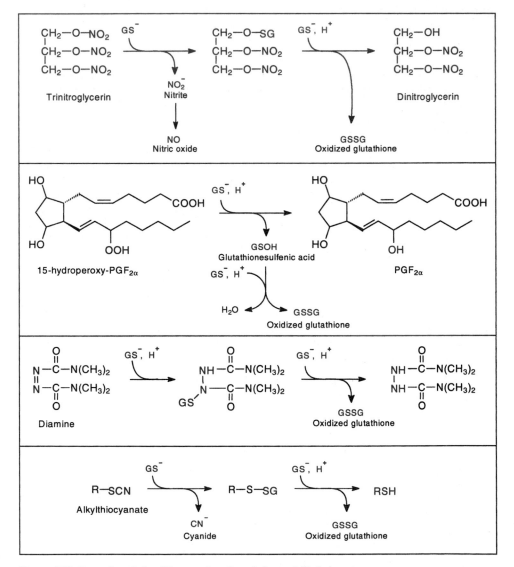

Figure 6-20. Examples of glutathione conjugation of electrophilic heteroatoms.

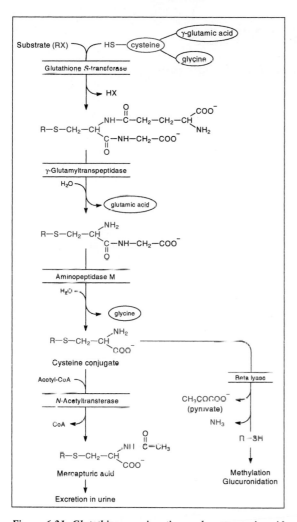

Figure 6-21. Glutathione conjugation and mercapturic acid biosynthesis.

between glutathione and the heteroatom is cleaved by a second molecule of glutathione to form oxidized glutathione (GSSG). The initial reactions are catalyzed by glutathione *S*-transferase, whereas the second reaction (which leads to GSSG formation) generally occurs nonenzymatically.

Glutathione conjugates formed in the liver can be excreted intact in bile or can be converted to mercapturic acids in the kidney and excreted in urine. As is shown in Fig. 6-21, the conversion of glutathione conjugates to mercapturic acids involves the sequential cleavage of glutamic acid and glycine from the glutathione moiety, followed by *N*-acetylation of the resulting cysteine conjugate.

Glutathione *S*-transferases are dimers that are composed of identical subunits, although some forms are heterodimers. Each subunit contains 200 to 240 amino acids and one catalytic site. Numerous subunits have been cloned and sequenced and differ in substrate specificity, tissue location, and cellular location.

Conjugation with glutathione represents an important detoxication reaction because electrophiles are potentially toxic species that can bind to critical nucleophiles, such as proteins and nucleic acids, and cause cellular damage and genetic mutations. Glutathione is also a cofactor for glutathione peroxidase, which plays an important role in protecting cells against lipid peroxidation.

In some cases, conjugation with glutathione enhances the toxicity of a xenobiotic. Glutathione conjugates of various compounds can activate xenobiotics to become toxic by releasing a toxic metabolite, by being inherently toxic, or by being degraded to a toxic metabolite.

BIBLIOGRAPHY

Gibson GG, Skett P: *Introduction to Drug Metabolism,* 3d ed. Cheltenham, UK: Nelson Thornes, 2001.

Guengerich FP: *Human Cytochromes P450 (Human CYPs): Human Cytochrome P450 Enzymes, Status Report Summarizing Their Reactions, Substrates, Inducers and Inhibitors—1st Update.* New York: Marcel Dekker, 2002.

Ryder W (ed): *Metabolic Polymorphisms and Susceptibility to Cancer.* IARC Sci. Pub. No. 148. Lyon, France: International Agency for Research on Cancer, 1999.

Williams G, Aruoma OI: *Molecular Drug Metabolism and Toxicology.* London: OICA, 2000.

Woolf TF (ed): *Handbook of Drug Metabolism.* New York: Marcel Dekker, 1999.

C H A P T E R   7

TOXICOKINETICS

Michele A. Medinsky and John L. Valentine

KEY POINTS

- *Toxicokinetics* is the study of the modeling and mathematical description of the time course of disposition (absorption, distribution, biotransformation, and excretion) of xenobiotics in the whole organism.

- The apparent volume of distribution (V_d) is the apparent space into which an amount of chemical is distributed in the body to result in a given plasma concentration.

- Clearance describes the rate of chemical elimination from the body in terms of the volume of fluid containing chemical that is cleared per unit of time.

- The half-life of elimination ($T_{1/2}$) is the time required for the blood or plasma chemical concentration to decrease by one-half.

INTRODUCTION

Toxicokinetics is the study of the modeling and mathematical description of the time course of disposition (absorption, distribution, biotransformation, and excretion) of xenobiotics in the whole organism. In the *classic model,* chemicals are said to move throughout the body as if there were one or two compartments that might have no apparent physiologic or anatomic reality. In physiologically based toxicokinetic models, the body is represented as a series of mass balance equations that describe each organ or tissue on the basis of physiologic considerations. There is no inherent contradiction between the classic and physiologically based approaches, yet certain assumptions differ between the two models. Ideally, physiologic models can predict tissue concentrations, whereas classic models cannot.

CLASSIC TOXICOKINETICS

The least invasive and simplest method for gathering information on the absorption, distribution, metabolism, and elimination of a compound is sampling blood or plasma over time. If one assumes that the concentration of a compound in blood or plasma is in equilibrium with concentrations in tissues, changes in plasma chemical concentrations reflect changes in tissue chemical concentrations. Compartmental pharmacokinetic models consist of a central compartment representing plasma and tissues that equilibrate rapidly with chemical, connected to one or more peripheral compartments that represent tissues that equilibrate more slowly with chemical (Fig. 7-1). Chemical is administered into the central compartment and is distributed between central and peripheral compartments. Chemical elimination occurs from

One-compartment model

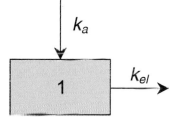

Two-compartment model

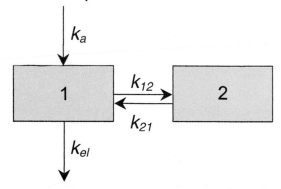

Figure 7-1. Compartmental pharmacokinetic models where k_a is the first-order extravascular absorption rate constant into the central compartment (1), k_{el} is the first-order elimination rate constant from the central compartment (1), and k_{12} and k_{21} are the first-order rate constants for distribution of chemical into and out of the peripheral compartment (2) in a two-compartment model.

the central compartment, which is assumed to contain rapidly perfused tissues that are capable of eliminating chemical (e.g., kidneys and liver). Compartmental pharmacokinetic models require no information on tissue physiology or anatomic structure, and they are valuable in predicting plasma chemical concentrations at different doses, establishing the time course of chemical in plasma and tissues and the extent of chemical accumulation with multiple doses, and determining effective doses and dose regimens in toxicity studies.

One-Compartment Model

The simplest toxicokinetic analysis entails measurement of the plasma concentrations of a xenobiotic at several time points after the administration of a bolus intravenous injection. If the data obtained yield a straight line when they are plotted as the logarithms of plasma concentrations versus time, the kinetics of the xenobiotic can be described with a one-compartment model (Fig. 7-2). Compounds whose toxicokinetics can be described with a one-compartment model equilibrate rapidly, or mix uniformly, between blood and the various tissues relative to the rate of elimination. The one-compartment model depicts the body as a homogeneous unit. This does not mean that the concentration of a compound is the same throughout the body, but it does assume that the changes that occur in the plasma concentration reflect proportional changes in tissue chemical concentrations.

In the simplest case, a curve of this type can be described by the expression

$$C = C_0 \times e^{-k_{el} \times t}$$

where C is the blood or plasma chemical concentration over time t, C_0 is the initial blood concentration at time $t = 0$, and k_{el} is the first-order elimination rate constant with dimensions of reciprocal time (e.g., t^{-1}).

Two-Compartment Model

After the rapid intravenous administration of some chemicals, the semilogarithmic plot of plasma concentration versus time yields a curve rather than a straight line, and this implies that there is more than one dispositional phase. In these instances, the chemical requires a longer time for tissue concentrations to reach equilibrium with the concentration in plasma, and a multicompartmental analysis of the results is necessary (Fig. 7-2). A multiexponential mathematical equation then best characterizes the elimination of the xenobiotic from the plasma.

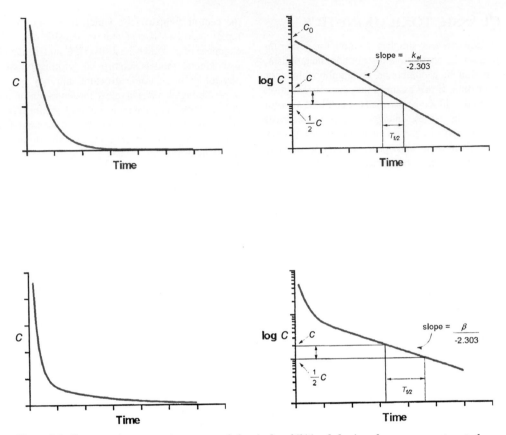

Figure 7-2. Concentration versus time curves of chemicals exhibiting behavior of a one-compartment phar-
macokinetic model **(top)** *and a two-compartment pharmacokinetic model* **(bottom)** *on a linear scale* **(left)**
and a semilogarithmic scale **(right).**   Elimination rate constants, k_{el} and β are determined from the slope of
the log-linear concentration versus time curve. Half-life ($T_{1/2}$) is the time required for blood or plasma chemical concentration to decrease by one-half. C_0 is the concentration of the chemical at t = 0 determined by
extrapolating the log-linear concentration time curve to the Y-axis (t = 0).

Generally, a curve of this type can be resolved into
two monoexponential terms (a two-compartment model)
and is described by

$$C = A \times e^{-\alpha \times t} + B \times e^{-\beta \times t}$$

where A and B are proportionality constants and α and
β are the first-order distribution and elimination rate constants, respectively (Fig. 7-2). During the distribution (α)
phase, concentrations of the chemical in the plasma
decrease more rapidly than they do in the postdistribu-
tional elimination (β) phase. The distribution phase may
last for only a few minutes or for hours or days. The
equivalent of k_{el} in a one-compartment model is β in a
two-compartment model.

Elimination

Elimination includes biotransformation, exhalation, and
excretion. The elimination of a chemical from the body
whose disposition is described by a one-compartment
model usually occurs through a first-order process; that
is, the rate of elimination at any time is proportional to
the amount of the chemical in the body at that time. First-
order reactions occur at chemical concentrations that are
not sufficiently high to saturate elimination processes.

The equation for a monoexponential model, $C = C_0$
$\times e^{-k_{el} \times t}$, can be transformed to a logarithmic equation
that has the general form of a straight line, $y = mx + b$:

$$\log C = (k_{el}/2.303) \times t + \log C_0$$

where $\log C_0$ represents the y-intercept or initial concentration and $(k_{el}/2.303)$ represents the slope of the line. The first-order elimination rate constant (k_{el}) can be determined from the slope of the log C versus time plot (i.e., $k_{el} = 2.303 \times slope$). The first-order elimination rate constants, k_{el} and β, have units of reciprocal time (e.g., min^{-1} and h^{-1}) and are independent of dose.

Mathematically, the fraction of dose remaining in the body over time (C/C_0) is calculated by using the elimination rate constant by rearranging the equation for the monoexponential function and taking the antilog to yield

$$C/C_0 = antilog \left[(-k_{el}/2.303) \times t \right]$$

Apparent Volume of Distribution

In a one-compartment model, all chemical is assumed to distribute into plasma and tissues instantaneously. The apparent volume of distribution (V_d) is a proportionality constant that relates the total amount of chemical in the body to the concentration of a xenobiotic in plasma and typically is described in units of liters or liters per kilogram of body weight. V_d is the apparent space into which an amount of chemical is distributed in the body to result in a given plasma concentration. For example, the apparent volume of distribution of a chemical in the body is determined after intravenous bolus administration and is defined mathematically as the quotient of the amount of chemical in the body and its plasma concentration. V_d is calculated as

$$V_d = Dose_{iv}/(\beta \times AUC_0^\infty)$$

where $Dose_{iv}$ is the intravenous dose or known amount of chemical in body at time zero, β is the elimination rate constant, and AUC_0^∞ is the area under the chemical concentration versus time curve from time zero to infinity. The product, $\beta \times AUC_0^\infty$, is the concentration of xenobiotic in plasma.

For a one-compartment model, V_d can be simplified by the equation $V_d = Dose_{iv}/C_0$, where C_0 is the concentration of chemical in plasma at time zero. C_0 is determined by extrapolating the plasma disappearance curve after intravenous injection to the zero time point (Fig. 7-2). V_d is called the *apparent volume of distribution*. The magnitude of the V_d term is chemical-specific and represents the extent of distribution of chemical out of plasma and into other body tissues. Thus, a chemical with high affinity for tissues also will have a large volume of distribution. Conversely, a chemical that predominantly remains in the plasma will have a low V_d that

approximates the volume of plasma. Once the V_d for a chemical is known, it can be used to estimate the amount of chemical remaining in the body at any time if the plasma concentration at that time also is known by the relationship $X_c = V_d \times C_p$, *where X_c is the amount of* chemical in the body and C_p is the plasma chemical concentration.

Clearance

Clearance describes the rate of chemical elimination from the body in terms of the volume of fluid containing chemical that is cleared per unit of time. Thus, clearance has the units of flow (milliliters per minute). A clearance of 100 mL/min means that 100 mL of blood or plasma containing xenobiotic is cleared completely each minute.

The overall efficiency of the removal of a chemical from the body can be characterized by clearance. High values of clearance indicate efficient and generally rapid removal, whereas low clearance values indicate slow and less efficient removal of a xenobiotic from the body. *Total body clearance* is defined as the sum of clearances by individual eliminating organs:

$$Cl = Cl_r + Cl_h + Cl_i + \ldots$$

where Cl_r depicts renal, Cl_h hepatic, and Cl_i intestinal clearance. After bolus intravenous administration, total body clearance is defined as

$$Cl = Dose_{iv}/AUC_0^\infty$$

Clearance also can be calculated if the volume of distribution and elimination rate constants are known and can be defined as $Cl = V_d \times k_{el}$ for a one-compartment model and $Cl = V_d \times \beta$ for a two-compartment model.

Half-Life

The half-life of elimination $(T_{1/2})$ is the time required for the blood or plasma chemical concentration to decrease by one-half and is dependent on both volume of distribution and clearance. $T_{1/2}$ can be calculated if V_d and Cl are known:

$$T_{1/2} = (0.693 \times V_d)/Cl$$

Because of the relationship $T_{1/2} = 0.693 \times k_{el}$, the half-life of a compound can be calculated after k_{el} (or β) has been determined from the slope of the line that designates the elimination phase on the log C versus time plot. The $T_{1/2}$ also can be determined by means of visual inspection of the log C versus time plot, as is shown in Fig. 7-2. For compounds eliminated by first-order kinetics, the time required for the plasma concentration to decrease by one-half is constant. After seven half-lives, 99.2 percent of a chemical is eliminated, and this can be practically viewed as complete elimination. The half-life of a chemical obeying first-order elimination kinetics is independent of the dose and does not change with increasing dose.

Saturation Toxicokinetics

As the dose of a compound increases, its volume of distribution or its rate of elimination may change owing to saturation kinetics. Biotransformation, active transport processes, and protein binding have finite capacities and can be saturated. When the concentration of a chemical in the body is higher than the K_M (chemical concentration at one-half V_{max}, the maximum metabolic capacity), the rate of elimination is no longer proportional to the dose. The transition from first-order kinetics to saturation kinetics is important in toxicology because it can lead to prolonged residency time of a compound in the body or increased concentration at the target site of action, which may result in increased toxicity.

Nonlinear toxicokinetics are indicated by the following: (1) The decline in the levels of the chemical in the body is not exponential, (2) AUC_0^∞ is not proportional to the dose, (3) V_d, Cl, k_{el} (or β), or $T_{1/2}$ changes with increasing dose, (4) the composition of excretory products changes quantitatively or qualitatively with the dose, (5) competitive inhibition by other chemicals that are biotransformed or actively transported by the same enzyme system occurs, and (6) dose–response curves show a nonproportional change in response with an increasing dose, starting at the dose level at which saturation effects become evident.

The elimination of some chemicals from the body is readily saturated. Important characteristics of zero-order processes are as follows: (1) An arithmetic plot of plasma concentration versus time yields a straight line, (2) the rate or amount of chemical eliminated at any time is constant and is independent of the amount of chemical in the body, and (3) a true $T_{1/2}$ or k_{el} does not exist but differs depending on the dose.

By comparison, the important characteristics of first-order elimination are as follows: (1) The rate at which a chemical is eliminated at any time is directly proportional to the amount of that chemical in the body at that time. (2) A semilogarithmic plot of plasma concentration versus time yields a single straight line. (3) The elimination rate constant (k_{el} or β), apparent volume of distribution (V_d), clearance (Cl), and half-life ($T_{1/2}$) are independent of dose. (4) The concentration of the chemical in plasma and other tissues decreases similarly by some constant fraction per unit of time, the elimination rate constant (k_{el} or β).

Bioavailability

The extent of absorption of a xenobiotic can be determined experimentally by comparing the plasma AUC_0^∞ after intravenous and extravascular dosing. The resulting index quantifies the fraction of the dose absorbed systemically and is called *bioavailability* (F). Bioavailability can be determined by using different doses provided that the compound does not display dose-dependent or saturable kinetics. Pharmacokinetic data after intravenous administration are used as the reference from which to compare extravascular absorption because all chemical is delivered (or is 100 percent bioavailable) to the systemic circulation. For example, bioavailability after an oral exposure can be determined as follows:

$$F = (AUC_{po}/Dose_{po}) \times (Dose_{iv}/AUC_{iv})$$

where AUC_{po}, AUC_{iv}, $Dose_{po}$, and $Dose_{iv}$ are the respective areas under the plasma concentration versus time curves and doses for oral and intravenous administration. Bioavailabilities for various chemicals range in value between 0 and 1. Complete absorption of chemical is demonstrated when $F = 1$. When $F < 1$, incomplete absorption of chemical is indicated. The fraction of a chemical that reaches the systemic circulation is of critical importance in determining toxicity. Several factors can alter this systemic availability greatly, including (1) limited absorption after oral dosing, (2) intestinal first-pass effect, (3) hepatic first-pass effect, and (4) mode of formulation, which affects, for example, dissolution rate or incorporation into micelles (for lipid-soluble compounds).

PHYSIOLOGIC TOXICOKINETICS

In classic kinetics, the rate constants are defined by the data, and these models often are referred to as *data-based*. In *physiologically based* models, the rate constants represent known or hypothesized biological processes. The advantages of physiologically based models are that (1) these models can provide the time course of distribution of xenobiotics to any organ or tissue, (2) they allow estimation of the effects of changing physiologic parameters on tissue concentrations, (3) the same model can predict the toxicokinetics of chemicals across species by means of allometric scaling, and (4) complex dosing regimes and saturable processes such as metabolism and binding are accommodated easily.

Basic Model Structure

Physiologic models often look like a number of classic one-compartment models that are linked together. The actual model *structure,* or *how* the compartments are linked together, depends on both the chemical and the organism being studied. It is important to realize that there is no generic physiologic model. Models are simplifications of reality and ideally should contain elements that are believed to be important in describing a chemical's disposition.

Physiologic modeling has enormous potential predictive power. Because the kinetic constants in physiologic models represent measurable biological or chemical processes, the resultant physiologic models have the potential for extrapolation from observed data to predicted situations.

One of the best illustrations of the predictive power of physiologic models is their ability to extrapolate kinetic behavior from laboratory animals to humans. *Simulations* are the outcomes or results (such as a chemical's concentration in blood or tissue) of numerically integrating model equations over a simulated time period, using a set of initial conditions (such as intravenous dose) and parameter values (such as organ weights). Whereas the model structures for the kinetics of chemicals in rodents and humans may be identical, the parameter values, such as organ weight, heart beat rate, and respiration rate, for rodents and humans are different. Other parameters, such as solubility in tissues, are similar in rodents and human models because the composition of tissues in different species is similar. Because the parameters underlying the model structure represent measurable biological and chemical determinants, the appropriate values for those parameters can be chosen for each species, forming the basis for successful interspecies extrapolation.

Compartments

The basic unit of the physiologic model is the lumped *compartment* (Fig. 7-3), which is a single region of the body with a *uniform* xenobiotic concentration. A compartment may be a particular functional or anatomic portion of an organ, a single blood vessel with the sur-

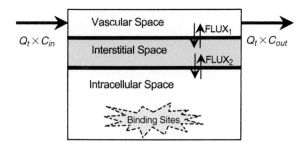

Figure 7-3. Schematic representation of a lumped compartment in a physiologic model. The blood capillary and cell membranes separating the vascular, interstitial, and intracellular subcompartments are depicted in black. The vascular and interstitial subcompartments often are combined into a single extracellular subcompartment. Q_t is blood flow, C_{in} is chemical concentration into the compartment, and C_{out} is chemical concentration out of the compartment.

rounding tissue, an entire discrete organ such as the liver or kidney, or a widely distributed tissue type such as fat or skin. Compartments consist of three individual well-mixed phases, or *subcompartments.* These subcompartments are (1) the *vascular* space through which the compartment is perfused with blood, (2) the *interstitial* space that forms the matrix for the cells, and (3) the *intracellular* space consisting of the cells in the tissue.

As shown in Fig. 7-3, the xenobiotic enters the vascular subcompartment at a certain rate in mass per unit of time (e.g., milligrams per hour). The rate of entry is a product of the blood flow rate to the tissue (Q_t, in liters per hour) and the concentration of the xenobiotic in the blood entering the tissue (C_{in}, in milligrams per liter). Within the compartment, the xenobiotic moves from the vascular space to the interstitial space at a certain net rate (*Flux$_1$*) and from the interstitial space to the intracellular space at different net rate (*Flux$_2$*). Some xenobiotics can bind to cell components; thus, within a compartment there may be both free and bound xenobiotics. The xenobiotic leaves the vascular space at a certain venous concentration (C_{out}). C_{out} is equal to the concentration of the xenobiotic in the vascular space.

Parameters

The most common types of parameters, or information required, in physiologic models are *anatomic, physiologic, thermodynamic,* and *transport.*

Anatomic   Anatomic parameters are used to describe the various compartments physically. The *size* of each of the compartments in the physiologic model must be known. The size generally is specified as a volume (milliliters or liters) because a unit density is assumed even though weights most frequently are obtained experimentally. If a compartment contains subcompartments such as those shown in Fig. 7-3, those volumes also must be known. Volumes of compartments often can be obtained from the literature or from specific toxicokinetic experiments.

Physiologic Physiologic parameters encompass various processes, including blood flow, ventilation, and elimination. The blood flow rate (Q_t, in volume per unit time, such as mL/min or L/h) to individual compartments must be known. Additionally, information on the total blood flow rate or *cardiac output* (Q_c) is necessary. If inhalation is the route for exposure to the xenobiotic or is a route of elimination, the alveolar ventilation rate (Q_p) also must be known. Blood flow rates and ventilation rates can be taken from the literature or can be obtained experimentally. Renal clearance rates and parameters to describe rates of biotransformation are required if these processes are important in describing the elimination of a xenobiotic.

Thermodynamic Thermodynamic parameters relate the *total* concentration of a xenobiotic in a tissue (C) to the concentration of *free* xenobiotic in that tissue (C_f). Two important assumptions are that (1) total and free concentrations are in equilibrium with each other and (2) only free xenobiotic can enter and leave the tissue. Whereas total concentration is measured experimentally, it is the free concentration that is available for binding, metabolism, or removal from the tissue by blood. The extent to which a xenobiotic partitions into a tissue is directly dependent on the composition of the tissue and independent of the concentration of the xenobiotic. Thus, the relationship between free and total concentration becomes one of proportionality: total = free × partition coefficient, or $C = C_f \times P$. Knowledge of the value of P, a *partition* or *distribution* coefficient, permits an indirect calculation of the free concentration of xenobiotic or $C_f \cdot C_f = C/P$.

A more complex relationship between the free concentration and the total concentration of a chemical in tissues occurs when the chemical may bind to saturable binding sites on tissue components. In these cases, nonlinear functions relating the free concentration in the tissue to the total concentration are necessary.

Transport The passage of a xenobiotic across a biological membrane is complex and may occur by passive diffusion, carrier-mediated transport, facilitated transport, or a combination of processes. The simplest of these processes—passive diffusion—is a first-order process. Diffusion of xenobiotics can occur across the blood capillary membrane ($Flux_1$ in Fig. 7-3) or across the cell membrane ($Flux_2$ in Fig. 7-3). *Flux* refers to the rate of transfer of a xenobiotic across a boundary. For simple diffusion, the net flux (milligrams per hour) from one side of a membrane to the other is described as Flux = permeability coefficient × driving force, or

$$Flux = [PA] \times (C_1 - C_2) = [PA] \times C_1 - [PA] \times C_2$$

The permeability coefficient [PA] often is called the *permeability-area cross-product* for the membrane (in units of liters per hour) and is a product of the cell membrane permeability constant (P, in micrometers per hour) for the xenobiotic and the total membrane area (A, in square micrometers). The cell membrane permeability constant takes into account the rate of diffusion of the specific xenobiotic and the thickness of the cell membrane. C_1 and C_2 are the *free* concentrations of xenobiotic on each side of the membrane. For any given xenobiotic, thin membranes, large surface areas, and large concentration differences enhance diffusion.

There are two *limiting conditions* for the transport of a xenobiotic across membranes: *perfusion-limited* and *diffusion-limited*.

Perfusion-Limited Compartments

A perfusion-limited compartment also is referred to as *blood flow–limited* or simply *flow-limited*. A flow-limited compartment can be developed if the cell membrane permeability coefficient [PA] for a particular xenobiotic is much greater than the blood flow rate to the tissue (Q_t). In this case, the rate of xenobiotic uptake by tissue subcompartments is limited by the rate at which the blood containing a xenobiotic arrives at the tissue, not by the rate at which the xenobiotic crosses the cell membranes. In most tissues, transport across vascular cell membranes is perfusion-limited. In the generalized tissue compartment shown in Fig. 7-3, this means that transport of the xenobiotic through the loosely knit blood capillary walls of most tissues is rapid compared with delivery of the xenobiotic to the tissue by the blood. As a result, the vascular blood is in equilibrium with the interstitial subcompartment and the two subcompartments usually are lumped together as a single compartment that often is called the *extracellular space*.

As is indicated in Fig. 7-3, the cell membrane separates the extracellular compartment from the intracellular compartment. The cell membrane is the most important diffusional barrier in a tissue. Nonetheless, for molecules that are very small (molecular weight <100) or lipophilic, cellular permeability generally does not limit the rate at which a molecule moves across cell membranes. For these molecules, flux across the cell membrane is fast compared with the tissue perfusion rate ($[PA]\,Q_t$), the intracellular compartment is in equilibrium with the extracellular compartment, and these tissue subcompartments usually are lumped as a single compartment. This flow-limited tissue compartment is shown in Fig. 7-4. Movement into and out of the entire tissue compartment can be described by a single equation:

$$V_t \times dC/dt = Q_t \times (C_{in} - C_{out})$$

where V_t is the volume of the tissue compartment, C is the concentration of free xenobiotic in the compartment ($V_t \times C$ equals the amount of xenobiotic in the compartment), $V_t \times dC/dt$ is the change in the amount of xenobiotic in the compartment with time expressed as mass per unit of time, Q_t is blood flow to the tissue, C_{in} is xenobiotic concentration entering the compartment, and C_{out} is xenobiotic concentration leaving the compartment. These mass balance *differential* equations require that input into one equation be balanced by outflow from another equation in the physiologic model.

In the perfusion-limited case, C_{out}, or the venous concentration of xenobiotic leaving the tissue, is equal to the free concentration of xenobiotic in the tissue, C_f. As was noted above, C_f (or C_{out}) can be related to the total concentration of xenobiotic in the tissue through a simple linear partition coefficient, $C_{out} = C_f = C/P$. In this case, the differential equation describing the rate of change in the amount of a xenobiotic in a tissue becomes $V_t \times dC/dt = Q_t \times (C_{in} - C/P)$

In a flow-limited compartment, the assumption is that the concentrations of a xenobiotic in all parts of the tissue are in equilibrium. Additionally, estimates of flux are not required to develop the mass balance differential equation for the compartment. Given the information required to estimate flux, this simplifying assumption significantly reduces the number of parameters required in the physiologic model.

Diffusion-Limited Compartments

When uptake into a compartment is governed by cell membrane permeability and total membrane area, the model is said to be *diffusion-limited*, or *membrane-limited*. Diffusion-limited transport occurs when the flux, or the transport of a xenobiotic across cell membranes, is slow compared with blood flow to the tissue. In this case, the permeability-area cross-product $[PA]$ is small compared with blood flow, Q_t, or $PA << Q_t$. Figure 7-5 shows the structure of a compartment of this type. The xenobiotic concentrations in the interstitial and vascular spaces are in equilibrium and make up the extracellular subcompartment where uptake from the incoming blood is flow-limited. The rate of xenobiotic uptake across the cell membrane (into the intracellular space from the extracellular space) is limited by cell membrane permeability and thus is diffusion-limited. Two mass balance differential equations are necessary to describe this compartment:

$$\text{Extracellular space: } V_{t1} \times dC_1/dt = Q_t \times (C_{in} - C_{out}) - [PA] \times C_1 + [PA] \times C_2$$
$$\text{Intracellular space: } V_{t2} \times dC_2/dt = [PA] \times C_1 - [PA] \times C_2$$

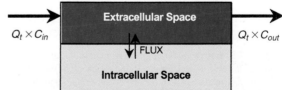

Figure 7-5. Schematic representation of a compartment that is membrane-limited.

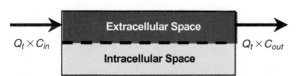

Figure 7-4. Schematic representation of a compartment that is blood flow–limited.

Q_t is blood flow, and C is *free* xenobiotic concentration in entering blood (in), exiting blood (out), extracellular space (1), or intracellular space (2). Both equations contain terms for flux, or transfer across the cell membrane, $[PA] \times (C_1 - C_2)$.

Specialized Compartments

Lung The inclusion of a lung compartment in a physiologic model is an important consideration because inhalation is a common route of exposure to many toxic chemicals. The assumptions inherent in lung compartment description are as follows: (1) Ventilation is continuous, not cyclic, (2) conducting airways function as inert tubes, carrying the vapor to the gas exchange region, (3) diffusion of vapor across the lung cell and capillary walls is perfusion-limited, (4) all xenobiotic disappearing from inspired air appears in arterial blood (i.e., there is no storage of xenobiotic in the lung tissue and insignificant lung mass), and (5) vapor in the alveolar air and arterial blood within the lung compartment are in rapid equilibrium.

In the lung compartment depicted in Fig. 7-6, the rate of inhalation of xenobiotic is controlled by the ventilation rate (Q_p) and the inhaled concentration (C_{inh}). The rate of exhalation of a xenobiotic is a product of the ventilation rate and the xenobiotic concentration in the alveoli (C_{alv}). Xenobiotic also can enter the lung compartment in venous blood returning from the heart, represented by the product of cardiac output (Q_c) and the concentration of xenobiotic in venous blood (C_{ven}). Xenobiotic leaving the lungs in the blood is a function of both cardiac output and the concentration of xenobiotic in arterial blood (C_{art}). Putting these four processes together, a mass balance differential equation can be written for the rate of change in the amount of xenobiotic in the lung compartment (L):

$$dL/dt = Q_p \times (C_{inh} - C_{alv}) + Q_c \times (C_{ven} - C_{art})$$

Because of some of these assumptions, the rate of change in the amount of xenobiotic in the lung compartment becomes equal to zero ($dL/dt = 0$). C_{alv} can be replaced by C_{art}/P_b, and the differential equation can be solved for the arterial blood concentration:

$$C_{art} = (Q_p \times C_{inh} + Q_c \times C_{ven})/(Q_c + Q_p/P_b)$$

The lung is viewed here as a portal of entry and not as a target organ, and the concentration of a xenobiotic delivered to other organs by the blood, or the arterial concentration of that xenobiotic, is of primary interest.

Liver The liver often is represented as a compartment in physiologic models because hepatic biotransformation is an important aspect of the toxicokinetics of many xenobiotics. A simple compartmental structure for the liver is assumed to be flow-limited, and this compartment is similar to the general tissue compartment shown in Fig. 7-4, except that the liver compartment contains an additional process for metabolic elimination. One of the simplest expressions for this process is first-order elimination:

$$R = C_f \times V_l \times K_f$$

where R is the rate of metabolism (milligrams per hour), C_f is the free concentration of xenobiotic in the liver (milligrams per liter), V_l is the liver volume (liters), and K_f is the first-order rate constant for metabolism in units of h^{-1}.

In physiologic models, the Michaelis-Menten expression for *saturable metabolism*, which employs two parameters, V_{max} and K_M, is written as follows:

$$R = (V_{max} \times C_f)/(K_M + C_f)$$

where V_{max} is the maximum rate of metabolism (in milligrams per hour) and K_M is the Michaelis constant, or xenobiotic concentration at one-half the maximum rate of metabolism (in milligrams per liter). Because many xenobiotics are metabolized by enzymes that display saturable metabolism, this equation is a key factor in the success of physiologic models for the simulation of chemical disposition across a range of doses.

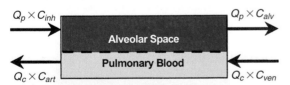

Figure 7-6. Simple model of gas exchange in the alveolar region of the respiratory tract.   Rapid exchange in the lumped lung compartment between the alveolar gas (*blue*) and the pulmonary blood (*light blue*) maintains the equilibrium between them as symbolized by the dashed line. Q_p is alveolar ventilation (L/h), Q_c is cardiac output (L/h), C_{inh} is inhaled vapor concentration (mg/L), C_{art} is concentration of vapor in the arterial blood, and C_{ven} is concentration of vapor in the mixed venous blood. The equilibrium relationship between the chemical in the alveolar air (C_{alv}) and the chemical in the arterial blood (C_{art}) is determined by the blood/air partition coefficient P_b, e.g., $C_{alv} = C_{art}/P_b$.

Other, more complex expressions for metabolism also can be incorporated into physiologic models. Bisubstrate second-order reactions—reactions involving the destruction of enzymes, the inhibition of enzymes, or the depletion of cofactors—have been simulated by using physiologic models. Metabolism also can be included in other compartments in much the same way as was described for the liver.

CONCLUSION

This chapter has overviewed the simpler elements of physiologic models and the important and often neglected assumptions that underlie model structures. The field of physiologic modeling is expanding rapidly. Physiologic models of a parent chemical linked in series with one or more active metabolites, models describing biochemical interactions among xenobiotics, and more biologically realistic descriptions of tissues previously viewed as simple lumped compartments are just a few of the most recent applications. Finally, physiologically based *toxicokinetic* models are beginning to be linked to biologically based *toxicodynamic* models to simulate the entire exposure → dose → response paradigm that is basic to the science of toxicology.

BIBLIOGRAPHY

Brown RP, Delp MD, Lindstedt SL, et al: Physiological parameter values for physiologically based pharmacokinetic models. *Toxicol Ind Health* 13(4):407–484, 1997.

Collins AS, Sumner SCJ, Borghoff SJ, et al: A physiological model for *tert*-amyl alcohol: Hypothesis testing of model structures. *Toxicol Sci* 49:15–28, 1999.

Shargel L, Yu ABC: *Applied Biopharmaceutics and Pharmacokinetics,* 3d ed. Norwalk, CT: Appleton & Lange, 1993.

UNIT 3

NONORGAN-DIRECTED TOXICITY

CHEMICAL CARCINOGENESIS

Henry C. Pitot III and Yvonne P. Dragan

EVALUATION OF CARCINOGENIC
  POTENTIAL
    The Problem of Extrapolation
    The Dose–Response Problem
    The Problem of the Potency of Carcinogenic
      Agents

RELATION (EXTRAPOLATION) OF
  BIOASSAY DATA TO HUMAN RISK

STATISTICAL ESTIMATES OF HUMAN RISK
  FROM BIOASSAY DATA BY USING
  MATHEMATICAL MODELS

RISK–BENEFIT CONSIDERATIONS IN THE
  REGULATION OF ACTUAL AND
  POTENTIAL CARCINOGENIC
  ENVIRONMENTAL HAZARDS

KEY POINTS

- The term *cancer* describes a subset of neoplastic lesions.
- A *neoplasm* is defined as a heritably altered, relatively autonomous growth of tissue with abnormal regulation of gene expression.
- *Metastases* are secondary growths of cells from the primary neoplasm.
- A *carcinogen* is an agent whose administration to previously untreated animals leads to a statistically significant increased incidence of neoplasms of one or more histogenetic types compared with the incidence in appropriate untreated animals.
- Initiation requires one or more rounds of cell division for the "fixation" of DNA damage.
- *Promotion* results from the selective functional enhancement of the initiated cell and its progeny by continuous exposure to the promoting agent.
- *Progression* is the transition from early progeny of initiated cells to the biologically malignant cell population of the neoplasm.

Cancer resulting from exposure to chemicals in the environment has taken on new importance. Knowledge about the mechanisms and natural history of cancer development as well as the epidemiology of human cancer is critical in the control and prevention of human neoplastic disease.

DEFINITIONS

The term *cancer* describes a subset of neoplastic lesions. A *neoplasm* is defined as a heritably altered, relatively autonomous growth of tissue with abnormal regulation of gene expression. Neoplasms may be either *benign* or *malignant*. The critical distinction between these classes is related to *metastatic* growth of malignant but not benign neoplasms. *Metastases* are secondary growths of cells from the primary neoplasm. Cancers are malignant neoplasms, whereas the term *tumor* describes space-occupying lesions that may or may not be neoplastic.

The nomenclature of neoplasia depends primarily on whether a neoplasm is benign or malignant and, in the latter case, whether it is derived from epithelial or mesenchymal tissue. For most benign neoplasms, the tissue of origin is followed by the suffix *-oma:* fibroma, lipoma, adenoma, and so on. For malignant neoplasms derived from tissues of mesenchymal origin, the term *sarcoma* is added to the tissue descriptor: fibrosarcoma, osteosarcoma, liposarcoma, and so on. Malignant neoplasms derived from tissues of ectodermal or endodermal (epithelial) origin are termed *carcinomas* with an antecedent tissue descriptor: epidermoid carcinoma (skin), hepatocellular carcinoma, gastric adenocarcinoma, and so on.

In general, a *carcinogen* is an agent that causes or induces neoplasia. A more appropriate definition is as follows: A *carcinogen* is an agent whose administration to previously untreated animals leads to a statistically significant increased incidence of neoplasms of one or more histogenetic types compared with the incidence in appropriate untreated animals.

CARCINOGENESIS BY CHEMICALS

Organic Chemical Carcinogens

Several organic compounds can cause cancer: polycyclic aromatic hydrocarbons (PAHs), dialkylnitrosamines, nitrite (which is metabolized into carcinogenic nitrosamines or nitrosamides), and aflatoxin B_1.

Inorganic Chemical Carcinogens

A number of inorganic elements and their compounds, including compounds of cadmium, chromium, nickel, lead, beryllium, and arsenic, have been shown to be carcinogenic.

Hormonal Carcinogenesis

Some cancers may result from abnormal internal production of specific hormones. Alternatively, excessive production or the derangement of the homeostatic mechanisms of an organism may result in neoplastic transformation. Theoretically, neoplasms of any of the end organs, including testes, ovary, adrenal gland, mammary gland, and uterus, may be produced by a manipulation that breaks the feedback loop between the pituitary and the target organ.

Chemical Carcinogenesis by Mixtures: Defined and Undefined

Relatively few detailed studies on mixtures of carcinogenic chemicals have been carried out experimentally. The most common environmental mixtures are those seen in tobacco smoke and other combustion products, including engine exhaust and air pollution. Interactions between the chemicals in mixtures may be additive, synergistic, or inhibitory.

Studies of the carcinogenic action of defined mixtures of chemicals usually are done with a knowledge of the carcinogenic effect of the chemicals involved. Common mixtures of carcinogens important for human disease are tobacco smoke, diesel exhaust, and diet.

Chemical Carcinogenesis by Diet Substantial evidence in humans indicates that many dietary components, including excessive caloric intake, excessive alcohol intake, and a variety of chemical contaminants of the diet, including aflatoxin B_1, are carcinogenic.

MECHANISMS OF CHEMICAL CARCINOGENESIS

Metabolism of Chemical Carcinogens in Relation to Carcinogenesis

A critical step in the induction of cancer by chemicals is the covalent interaction of some form of the chemical with macromolecules. Some parent compounds require metabolic alteration to a metabolite that is capable of covalent binding directly with macromolecules. Chemical carcinogens that require metabolism for their carcinogenic effect are termed procarcinogens, whereas their highly reactive metabolites are termed ultimate carcinogens. A number of metabolic reactions are involved in the "activation" of chemicals to their ultimate carcinogenic forms (see Chap. 6).

Free Radicals and the Metabolism of Chemical Carcinogens

Free radical reactions also are involved in the formation of ultimate carcinogens. Free radicals are chemical elements or their compounds that possess a single unpaired electron. Although biological reduction of molecular oxygen is the prime generative pathway for the development of free radicals, free radical intermediates sometimes are formed during the metabolism of chemical carcinogens. Free radicals may react directly with DNA to produce a variety of structural changes in bases.

Mutagenesis and Carcinogenesis

The process of mutagenesis consists of structural DNA alteration, cell proliferation that fixes the DNA damage, and DNA repair that either directly repairs the alkylated base or bases or results in the removal of larger segments of the DNA. The reaction of electrophiles with DNA results in alkylation products that are covalent derivatives of the reactive chemical species with DNA. Direct-acting alkylation agents induce preferential binding to highly nucleophilic centers such as the N^7 position of guanine. The position of an adduct in DNA and its chemical and physical properties in that context dictate the types of mutations induced. Different adducts can induce a distinct spectrum of mutations, and any adduct can result in a multitude of different DNA lesions. Mutagenesis can be the result of several different alterations in the physical and chemical nature of DNA. Methylating and ethylating agents result in mutations as a result of base mispairing. The active metabolites of numerous compounds, such as PAHs and aromatic amines, can form bulky DNA adducts that block DNA synthesis, resulting in a noncoding lesion. The synthetic machinery employs bypass synthesis to avoid the lethal impact of these unrepaired lesions. The role of DNA repair in protection of the genome and in the induction of mutations is an essential component in mutagenesis.

Macromolecular Adducts Resulting from Reaction with Ultimate Carcinogens

The most nucleophilic site in DNA is the N^7 position of guanine, and many carcinogens form covalent adducts at that site. Another common structural change in DNA is the hydroxylation of DNA bases, which have been found in the DNA of target organs in animals administered chemical carcinogens but are also present in the DNA of organisms not subjected to any known carcinogenic agent, probably as a result of endogenous oxidative stress from normal metabolism. Such oxidative reactions, occurring either as a result of an endogenous oxidative phenomenon or from the administration of exogenous chemical and radiation carcinogens, presumably are repaired rapidly by the mechanisms discussed below.

The methylation of deoxycytidine residues results in the heritable expression or repression of specific genes in eukaryotic cells. Genes that are transcribed actively are hypomethylated, whereas those which are hypermethylated rarely tend to be transcribed. Chemical carcinogens may inhibit DNA methylation through several mechanisms. Therefore, the inhibition of DNA methylation by chemical carcinogens may represent a further potential mechanism for carcinogenesis induced by chemicals.

Structural changes in DNA of largely unknown character also have been reported. The exact role of structural adducts of DNA in carcinogenesis is not a simple one to characterize with adduct = mutation = carcinogenesis. Adducts of known carcinogens may play a significant role in carcinogenesis induced by their procarcinogenic forms, but the function of structurally undefined, endogenously produced adducts in the carcinogenic process is not as clear.

DNA REPAIR AND CHEMICAL CARCINOGENESIS

Persistence of DNA Adducts and DNA Repair

The extent to which DNA adducts occur after the administration of chemical carcinogens depends on the overall metabolism of the chemical agent as well as the chemical reactivity of the ultimate metabolite. Once an adduct is formed, its continued presence in the DNA of the cell depends primarily on the ability of the cellular machinery to repair the structural alteration in the DNA. On the basis of such considerations as well as the presumed critical nature of the adduct in the carcinogenic process, it has been postulated that the extent of formation of DNA adducts and their persistence in the DNA should correlate with the biological effect of the agent.

Various adducts are found in both normal individuals and those potentially exposed to specific carcinogenic agents. In addition to DNA adducts, specific carcinogens covalently bind to serum proteins. Thus, the persistence of macromolecular adducts of the ultimate forms of chemical carcinogens may be very important in the carcinogenic mechanism of such agents.

Mechanisms of DNA Repair

The persistence of DNA adducts is predominantly a result of the failure of DNA repair. The types of structural alterations that may occur in the DNA molecule as a result of interaction with reactive chemical species or directly with radiation are considerable. The reaction of DNA with reactive chemical species produces adducts on bases, sugars, and the phosphate backbone. In addition, bifunctional reactive chemicals may cause the cross-linking of DNA strands through reaction with two opposing bases. Other structural changes, such as pyrimidine dimer formation, are specific for ultraviolet radiation, while double-strand DNA breaks are seen most commonly with ionizing radiation.

Two types of damage response pathways exist: repair pathways and the tolerance mechanism. In repair mechanisms the DNA damage is removed, whereas tolerance mechanisms circumvent the damage without fixing it. Certain repair mechanisms reverse the DNA damage, for example, removal of adducts from bases and insertion of new bases into apurinic/apyrimidinic (AP) sites, and direct reversal of the premutational lesions restores normal base pairing specificity.

The excisional repair of DNA may involve the removal of a single altered base having a relatively low-molecular-weight adduct, such as an ethyl or methyl group, and is termed *base excision repair,* or the repair may involve a base with a very large bulky group adducted to it, such as the dimerization of pyrimidines, which is termed *nucleotide excision repair.* This nucleotide excision pathway is represented in Fig. 8-1. The series of reactions includes recognition of the damage, unwinding of the DNA, 3′ and 5′ sequential dual incisions of the damaged strand, repair synthesis of the eliminated patch, and final ligation.

Whereas animal cell DNA polymerases are not absolutely faithful in their replication of the template strand, there is the potential for a mutation to occur in the form of one or more mispaired bases during the process outlined above. This possibility is greater in the case of nucleotide excision repair compared with simple base excision, because a much longer base sequence is removed and resynthesized during the nucleotide excision mechanism.

Whereas the repair of adducts involves several possible pathways, the repair of double DNA strand breaks is more prone to error than is either the excisional or the direct reversal pathway. Double-strand breaks in DNA are largely the result of ionizing radiation, high doses of alkylating carcinogens such as nitrogen mustards and polycyclic hydrocarbons, and even the normal function of topoisomerases involved in the winding and unwinding of DNA. Double-strand breaks also may occur at sites of single-strand DNA resulting from adduction of bulky molecules, preventing further polymerase action and subsequent endonuclease cleavage and resulting in double-strand breaks and potential chromosomal aberrations.

Mismatch repair can be distinguished from nucleotide excision repair and base excision repair by several characteristics. Nucleotide and base excision repair generally involves the recognition of nucleotides and bases that have been modified chemically or fused to an adjacent nucleotide. In contrast, mismatch repair recognizes normal nucleotides that are unpaired or paired with a noncomplementary nucleotide.

DNA Repair, Cell Replication, and Chemical Carcinogenesis

The persistence of DNA adducts in relation to the development of neoplasia in specific tissues and differences in the repair of the adducts are critical factors in chemical carcinogenesis. Some adducts are extremely difficult, if not impossible, for the cell to repair. Of equal

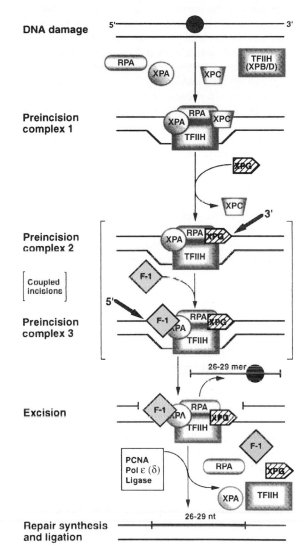

Figure 8-1. Model for transcription-independent nucleotide excision repair of DNA in humans. 1. The damage is recognized by XPA · RPA, which recruits XPC and TFIIH, to form the preincision complex 1 (PIC1). 2. XPG binds PIC1 and XPC dissociates, leading to PIC2 complex. 3. PIC2 recruits XPF · ERCC1 (F-1) to form PIC3. XPG makes the 3′ incision and F-1 makes the 5′ incision a fraction of a second later. 4. The excised damaged fragment is released, leaving in place a postincision complex. The proliferating cell nuclear antigen (PCNA) forms a torus around the DNA molecule associating with DNA polymerase δ and/or ε [Pol ε (δ)] and a DNA ligase replacing the postincision complex with these repair synthesis proteins. 5. The gap is filled and the repair patch is ligated. (From Petit C, Sancar A: Nucleotide excision repair: From *E. coli* to man. *Biochimie* 81:15–25, 1999, with permission of authors and publisher.)

importance is the continuous damage to DNA that occurs within cells as a result of ambient mutagens, radiation, and endogenous processes, including oxidation, methylation, deamination, and depurination. DNA damage induced by oxidative stress is probably the source of most endogenous DNA damage.

Because the formation of a mutation occurs during the synthesis of a new DNA strand through the use of the damaged template, cell replication becomes an important factor in the "fixation" of a mutation. Many DNA repair mechanisms may not be abnormal in neoplastic cells compared with their normal counterparts; a high rate of cell division tends to enhance both the spontaneous level and the induced level of mutation through the chance inability of a cell to repair damage before DNA synthesis.

Enhanced mitogenesis also may trigger more dramatic genetic alterations, including mitotic recombination, gene conversion, and nondisjunction. These genetic changes result in further progressive genetic alterations with a high likelihood of cancer.

CHEMICAL CARCINOGENS AND THE NATURAL HISTORY OF NEOPLASTIC DEVELOPMENT

Numerous chemicals can alter the structure of the genome and/or the expression of genetic information, with the subsequent appearance of cancer. However, cancer as a disease usually develops slowly, with a long latent period between the first exposure to the chemical carcinogen and the ultimate development of malignant neoplasia. Thus, carcinogenesis involves various biological changes that to a great extent reflect the structural and functional alterations in the genome of the affected cell.

The Pathogenesis of Neoplasia: Biology

The pathogenesis of neoplasia is felt to consist of at least three operationally defined stages, beginning with initiation, followed by an intermediate stage of promotion, from which evolves the stage of progression (see Table 8-1). It is in the first and last stages of neoplastic development—initiation and progression—that structural changes in the genome (DNA) can be observed. The intermediate stage of promotion does not appear to involve direct structural changes in the genome of the cell but instead depends on altered expression of genes.

Initiation Initiation requires one or more rounds of cell division for the "fixation" of the process. Initiation is irreversible in that the genotype/phenotype of the initiated cell is established at the time of initiation. Spontaneous initiation of cells in a variety of tissues is a very common occurrence. However, not all initiated cells survive over the life span of the organism or the period of an experiment owing to the normal process of programmed cell death, or apoptosis.

Promotion Unlike chemicals that induce the stage of initiation, promoting agents and their metabolites generally do not interact directly with DNA. Some promoting agents are polypeptide hormones, halogenated hydrocarbons, a high intake of dietary calories, and xenobiotics such as saccharin, phorbol acetate, phenobarbital, butylated hydroxytoluene, estradiol, and naphenopin.

The reversible nature of this stage is a distinctive characteristic of promotion in contrast to initiation or progression. The regression of preneoplastic lesions upon withdrawal of the promoting agents may be due to apoptosis or to "redifferentiation," or remodeling. Thus, cells in the stage of promotion are dependent on continued administration of the promoting agent.

Promotion is susceptible to modulation by physiologic factors, including the aging process and dietary and hormonal factors. The relative potency of promoting agents may be determined as a function of their ability to induce the clonal growth of initiated cells.

Progression The transition from the early progeny of initiated cells to the biologically malignant cell population constitutes the major part of the natural history of neoplastic development. Malignant progression is characterized by a high growth rate, invasiveness, metastatic frequency, hormonal responsiveness, and morphologic characteristics that vary independently as the disease develops.

Cell and Molecular Mechanisms of the Stages of Carcinogenesis

Table 8-2 lists a number of the molecular mechanistic characteristics of the stages of initiation, promotion, and progression.

Initiation At least three processes are important in initiation: metabolism, DNA repair, and cell proliferation. Individual variability, species differences, and organotropism of the stage of initiation represent a balance of carcinogen metabolism, cell proliferation, and DNA repair.

Table 8-1
Morphologic and Biologic Characteristics of the Stages of Initiation, Promotion, and Progression during Carcinogenesis

INITIATION	PROMOTION	PROGRESSION
Irreversible in viable cells Initiated "stem cell" not morphologically identifiable	Operationally reversible both at the level of gene expression and at the cell level	Irreversible Morphologically discernible alteration in cellular genomic structure resulting from karyotypic instability
Efficiency sensitive to xenobiotic and other chemical factors	Promoted cell population existence dependent on continued administration of the promoting agent	
Spontaneous (endogenous) occurrence of initiated cells	Efficiency sensitive to aging and dietary and hormonal factors Endogenous promoting agents may effect "spontaneous" promotion	Growth of altered cells sensitive to environmental factors during early phase of this stage
Requires cell division for "fixation"		
Dose response does not exhibit a readily measurable threshold	Dose response exhibits measurable threshold and maximal effect	Benign or malignant neoplasms observed in this stage
Relative potency of initiators depends on quantitation of preneoplastic lesions after a defined period of promotion	Relative potency of promoters is measured by their effectiveness in causing an expansion of the cell progeny of the initiated population	"Progressor" agents act to advance promoted cells into this stage

Molecular Genetic Targets of DNA-Damaging Carcinogenic Agents Although many genes are affected by the mutagenic action of certain chemical carcinogens, mutations in a relatively few specific genes—proto-oncogenes, oncogenes, and tumor suppressor genes—may be most critical to neoplastic transformation (Table 8-3). Oncogenes are involved primarily in cellular growth, signal transduction, and nuclear transcription. Similar functions are attributed to known tumor suppressor genes as well as being involved in regulation of the cell cycle.

Promotion The regulation of genetic information is mediated through recognition of the environmental effector, hormone, promoting agent, drug, and so on, and its specific molecular interaction with either a surface receptor or a cytosolic receptor. The ligand receptor complex then travels to the nucleus before interacting directly with specific DNA sequences known as response elements.

Binding to cell surface receptors usually causes the initiation of a kinase cascade that ultimately results in the phosphorylation and activation of transcription factors that include Jun, Fos, Myc, CREB, E2F, and Rb, the retinoblastoma tumor suppressor gene.

In addition to the plasma membrane receptors, gene expression can be regulated through the interaction of cytoplasmic receptors with their ligands, as was discussed previously. As is the case with membrane receptors, the pathways of the cytoplasmic receptors involve multiple, interactions with proteins, phosphorylation, and ultimate alteration of transcription through the interaction of a transcription factor with DNA. Many promoting agents exert their effects on gene expression through perturbation of one of the signal transduction pathways.

Table 8-2
Some Cell and Molecular Mechanisms in Multistage Carcinogenesis

INITIATION	PROMOTION	PROGRESSION
Simple mutations (transitions, transversions, small deletions, etc.) involving the cellular genome.	Reversible enhancement or repression of gene expression mediated via receptors specific for the individual promoting agent.	Complex genetic alterations (chromosomal translocations, deletions, gene amplification, recombination, etc.) resulting from evolving karyotypic instability.
In some species and tissues, point mutations occur in proto-oncogenes and/or potential cellular oncogenes.	Inhibition of apoptosis by promoting agent.	Irreversible changes in gene expression, including fetal gene expression, altered MHC gene expression, and ectopic hormone production.
Mutations in genes of signal transduction pathways may result in altered phenotype.	No direct structural alteration in DNA results from action or metabolism of promoting agent.	Selection of neoplastic cells for optimal growth genotype/phenotype in response to the cellular environment and including the evolution of karyotypic instability.

The Molecular Basis of the Reversibility of the Stage of Tumor Promotion

The basic assumption of the ligand-receptor interaction is that the effect of the agent is directly proportional to the number of receptors occupied by that chemical ligand and that a maximum response of the target is obtained only when all receptors are occupied. The dose response of the receptor-ligand interaction takes the shape of a sigmoidal curve. Withdrawal of the ligand returns the system to its original state. The regulation of genetic expression that occurs through the ligand-receptor mechanism predicts a threshold and reversible effect. Furthermore, at very low doses of some carcinogenic agents, an apparent "protective" effect of the agent actually can be demonstrated. This phenomenon has been termed *hormesis*. Thus, the stage of tumor promotion, unlike that of initiation and progression, does not involve mutational or structural events in the genome but instead involves the reversible

Table 8-3
Characteristics of Proto-Oncogenes, Cellular Oncogenes, and Tumor Suppressor Genes

PROTO-ONCOGENES	CELLULAR ONCOGENES	TUMOR SUPPRESSOR GENES
Dominant	Dominant	Recessive
Broad tissue specificity for cancer development	Broad tissue specificity for cancer development	Considerable tissue specificity for cancer development
Germline inheritance rarely involved in cancer development	Germline inheritance rarely involved in cancer development	Germline inheritance frequently involved in cancer development
Analogous to certain viral oncogenes	No known analogs in oncogenic viruses	No known analogs in oncogenic viruses
Somatic mutations activate during all stages of neoplastic development	Somatic mutations activate during all stages of neoplastic development	Germline mutations may initiate, but mutation to neoplasia occurs only during the stage of progression

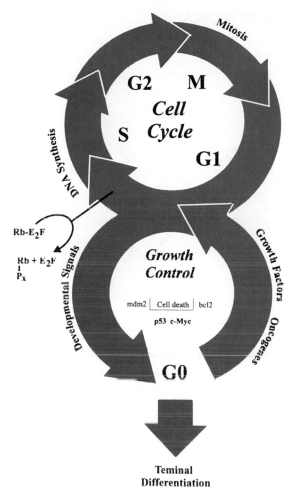

Figure 8-2. Diagram of the cell cycle and its associated cycle to apoptosis or terminal differentiation with the potential to return to the active cycle under the influence of growth factors and related components. Signal transduction may regulate the cell cycle through kinase activation involving the E_2F-Rb interaction or other kinases and related molecules involved in the cell cycle.

alteration of the expression of genetic information. The characteristic of promoting agents at the cellular and molecular levels to increase cell proliferation of preneoplastic cell populations selectively more than that of their normal counterparts may be the result of altered mechanisms of cell cycle control in the preneoplastic cell.

Cell Cycle Regulation Although the exact mechanism(s) by which promoting agents selectively enhance cell replication in preneoplastic cells is unknown, Figure 8-2 diagrams an integration of the cell cycle and apop-

tosis with the signal transduction pathways. Phosphorylation of the mitogen-activated protein kinase (MAPK) through the signal transduction pathway activates this kinase (Fig. 8-2), which then activates various transcription factors. *Rb* is made throughout the cell cycle. It becomes highly phosphorylated at the beginning of DNA synthesis (G_1/S). This releases a transcription factor, E2F. E2F then is available to stimulate the transcription of a variety of genes needed for the transition from G1 and the initiation of DNA synthesis. This involves a variety of protein kinases and proteins, known as *cyclins.* Another tumor suppressor gene, the *p53* gene, also plays a role as a transcription factor, preventing continuance of the cell cycle on the occasion of DNA damage. This pause allows the cells to repair such damage or, if the damage is excessive, to undergo apoptosis (Fig. 8-2). If the *p53* gene is mutated or absent, the pause does not occur, and the cell cycle continues replicating despite the presence of damage resulting in mutations and clastogenesis.

Progression As is noted in Tables 8-1 and 8-2, the major hallmark of the stage of progression is evolving karyotypic instability that potentially leads to multiple "stages" or changes in malignant cells. Cells in the stage of progression may evolve in such a way that the characteristics of invasion, metastatic growth, and anaplasia, as well as the rate of growth and responses to hormonal influences, change toward higher and higher degrees of malignancy, permitting the expression of fetal genes or the major histocompatibility complex (MHC) class I and II surface proteins and the ectopic production of hormones by cells derived from non-hormone-producing tissues.

The Bases for the Stages of Initiation, Promotion, and Progression

The bases for the cell and molecular biology of the stages of neoplastic development may be considered simply as follows (see Fig. 8-3):

Initiation results from a simple mutation in one or more cellular genes that control key regulatory pathways of the cell.

Promotion results from the selective functional enhancement of signal transduction pathways induced in the initiated cell and its progeny by continuous exposure to the promoting agent.

Progression results from continuing change of a basically unstable karyotype.

THE NATURAL HISTORY OF NEOPLASIA

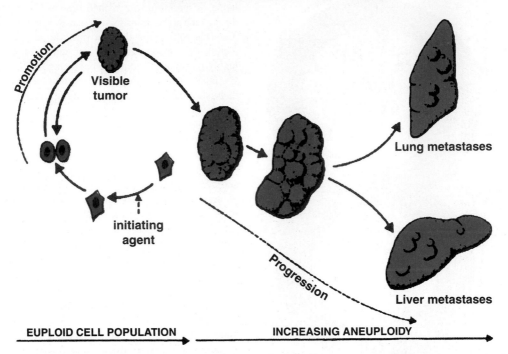

Figure 8-3. The natural history of neoplasia, beginning with the initiated cell after application of an initiating agent (carcinogen), followed by the potentially reversible stage of promotion to a visible tumor, with subsequent progression of this tumor to malignancy. The relation to karyotype is presented as a generalization on the lower arrows. The reader is cautioned that not all neoplastic cells undergo this entire natural history. It is theoretically possible, although this has not been shown definitively, that some neoplasms, such as those induced in animals by radiation or high doses of chemical carcinogens, may enter this sequence in the stage of progression, exhibiting aneuploidy, and thus bypass the early euploid cell stages.

These seminal characteristics of the three stages of carcinogenesis readily distinguish one from the others and also form a basis for the molecular action of chemicals acting at each of these stages (Table 8-4).

Genetic and Nongenetic Mechanisms of Chemical Carcinogenesis in Relation to the Natural History of Cancer Development

Some initiating and progressor agents have the ability to alter the structure of DNA and/or chromosomes. Such "genotoxic" effects have been linked directly to the induction of neoplasia. However, when administered chronically to animals, a number of chemicals induce the development of neoplasia without evidence of a direct "genotoxic" action on target cells. One may classify such agents as promoting agents that act to expand clones of spontaneously initiated cells. The consequent selective enhancement of cell replication in such initiated cell clones sets the stage for the spontaneous transition of an occasional cell into the stage of progression.

Agents that are not mutagenic or genotoxic may induce direct toxicity with sustained tissue damage and subsequent cell proliferation. Both direct DNA toxicity and increased cell proliferation may lead to clastogenesis or may damage genetic DNA indirectly through oxidative mechanisms. Finally, the cell proliferation resulting from toxicity may selectively induce enhanced replication of an already damaged genome in the initi-

Table 8-4
Classification of Chemical Carcinogens in Relation to Their Action on One or More Stages of Carcinogenesis

Initiating agent (incomplete carcinogen): a chemical capable only of initiating cells
Promoting agent: a chemical capable of causing the expansion of initiated cell clones
Progressor agent: a chemical capable of converting an initiated cell or a cell in the stage of promotion to a potentially malignant cell
Complete carcinogen: a chemical possessing the capability of inducing cancer from normal cells, usually possessing properties of initiating, promoting, and progressor agents

ated cell population. Thus, the neoplastic development observed with a test compound may result from the toxicity and cell proliferation associated with the chronic high doses utilized rather than from a direct carcinogenic effect of the agent.

CHEMICAL CARCINOGENESIS IN HUMANS

Epidemiology has been defined as the study of the distribution and determinants of disease from observation rather than through controlled experimentation. Epidemiologic observations may include the following:

1. *Episodic observations.* Observations of isolated cases of cancer in relation to a specific environmental factor(s) have yielded information about cause-and-effect relationships.

2. *Retrospective studies.* Retrospective investigations of the histories and habits of groups of individuals who have developed a disease have been common sources of epidemiologic data.

3. *Prospective studies.* Prospective investigations involve analyses of the continuing and future development of cancers in individuals with specific social habits, occupational exposures, and so on.

Epidemiologic studies may involve a single factor or multiple factors potentially causative of specific human cancers. However, it rarely is possible to identify a single chemical as the sole causative factor in the development of a specific type of human cancer because of the numerous other environmental variables to which the human population or cohort (group under study) is exposed.

Epidemiologic studies can identify only factors that are different between two populations and that are suffi-

ciently important in the etiology of the condition under study to play a determining role under the conditions of exposure. Furthermore, on the basis of epidemiologic studies alone, it is usually very difficult to determine whether a specific chemical is or is not carcinogenic to humans because of the long time interval between exposure and development of neoplasm and because of the imprecise knowledge of the nature of exposure or its cause-and-effect nature. In view of the fact that epidemiologic studies in themselves are often insufficient to establish the carcinogenicity of an agent for humans, laboratory studies with laboratory animals in vivo and cells in vitro have been employed to complement or in some cases supplant epidemiologic observations where they exist.

The International Agency for Research on Cancer (IARC) has devised a system of definitions of relative carcinogenicity:

1. *Sufficient evidence* of carcinogenicity, which indicates that there is a causal relationship between the agent(s) and human cancer.

2. *Limited evidence* of carcinogenicity, which indicates that a causal interpretation is credible but that alternative explanations, such as chance, bias, or confounding variables, cannot be completely excluded.

3. *Inadequate evidence* indicates that (a) there were few pertinent data, (b) the available studies, while showing evidence of association, did not exclude chance, bias, or confounding variables, (c) studies were available that did not show evidence of carcinogenicity.

Lifestyle Carcinogenesis

Chemical factors involved in the development of cancer from lifestyle practices may be related to complex

Table 8-5
Carcinogenic Factors Associated with Lifestyle

CHEMICAL(S), PHYSIOLOGIC CONDITION, OR NATURAL PROCESS	ASSOCIATED NEOPLASM(S)	EVIDENCE FOR CARCINOGENICITY
Alcoholic beverages	Esophagus, liver, oropharynx, and larynx	Sufficient
Aflatoxins	Liver	Sufficient
Betel chewing	Mouth	Sufficient
Dietary intake (fat, protein, calories)	Breast, colon, endometrium, gallbladder	Sufficient
Reproductive history		
1. Late age at 1st pregnancy	Breast	Sufficient
2. Zero or low parity	Ovary	Sufficient
Tobacco smoking	Mouth, pharynx, larynx, lung, esophagus, bladder	Sufficient

chemical mixtures or, in some instances, to specific external or internal environmental chemicals. Table 8-5 lists chemical carcinogenic agents associated with lifestyle. Among the agents listed, three—alcoholic beverages, aflatoxins, and dietary intake—are related to the nutritional status of the individual. While aflatoxin has been shown to be a complete carcinogen in experimental animals, the carcinogenic effect of alcoholic beverages and dietary intake is not readily apparent. As is noted in the table, elevated risks of several neoplasms in the human result from excessive intake of alcoholic beverages because ethanol is metabolized into acetaldehyde, an incomplete carcinogen that can contribute to the progression of cancer that already has been initiated or can act as a cocarcinogen when administered with another carcinogen. For example, cancer of the oral cavity and pharynx is markedly increased when an individual smokes tobacco as well as abuses alcoholic beverages.

Aflatoxins, especially aflatoxin B_1, which are produced by some strains of the ubiquitous mold *Aspergillus flavus,* are potent hepatocarcinogens. Other dietary contaminants—produced directly by organisms such as molds, substances naturally occurring in plants such as the pyrrolizidine alkaloids, and products of the metabolism of dietary components by contaminating molds—have been demonstrated as carcinogenic in experimental systems.

The most common mechanism of diet-associated carcinogenesis in the human is the action of major dietary constituents (fat, carbohydrate, and protein) as promoting agents. Considerable experimental evidence has demonstrated that carbohydrate and lipid are effective promoting agents in the development of several tissue types of neoplasms.

There is substantial epidemiologic evidence that being overweight may increase the incidence of a variety of human cancers. The fact that overnutrition in experimental animals is carcinogenic has been described for decades. Relatively high levels of dietary fat are associated with increased death rates from cancer of the prostate, colon, and breast in humans.

Endogenous hormone production probably also is related to the phenomenon of the enhanced risk of breast cancer in patients who wait until the fourth decade or more to have the first child. In addition to late first full-term pregnancy, early menarche and late menopause appear to increase the risk of breast cancer in humans.

Perhaps the most common exogenous cause of human cancer is tobacco smoking and other forms of tobacco abuse. The chewing of tobacco leads to cancer of the mouth. It has been estimated that about 30 percent of all cancer deaths in the United States result from this habit. Smoking cessation decreases the incidence of lung cancer because the stage of tumor promotion occupies the longest time interval and poses the greatest risk in the development of cancer in smokers.

Although mechanisms of cancer induction by lifestyle factors are poorly understood, cancers resulting from lifestyle account for two-thirds or more of the chemical induction of this human disease (Fig. 8-4). The stage involved in lifestyle-induced human cancer is primarily that of promotion.

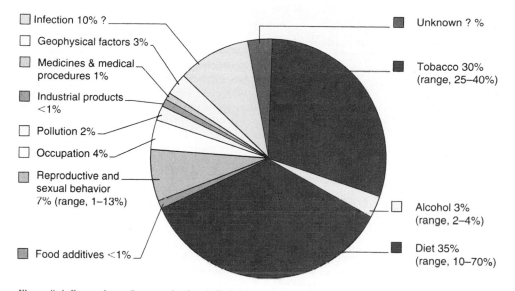

Figure 8-4. *Proportions of cancer deaths attributed to various environmental factors.*   (After Doll R, Peto R: *The Causes of Cancer.* New York: Oxford University Press, 1981.)

Chemical Carcinogens Associated with Occupations

Table 8-6 lists a number of chemical processes for which there is sufficient data to implicate these agents as carcinogenic to humans or animals.

Chemical Carcinogenesis Resulting from Medical Therapy and Diagnosis

There are risk–benefit considerations in the use of a number of drugs and hormones in humans, and the most striking is the utilization of known carcinogenic agents in chemotherapy for neoplasia, as is noted in Table 8-7. Immunosuppression as a result of genetic abnormalities, therapeutic immunosuppression (as in transplants), and immunosuppression resulting from diseases such as advanced cancer or the acquired immune deficiency syndrome (AIDS) are associated with increased incidences of a variety of different cancers.

THE PREVENTION OF HUMAN CANCER INDUCED BY CHEMICALS

Definitive epidemiologic observations and investigations are the surest way to relate a specific etiologic agent—chemical, physical, or biological—causally with human neoplasms, but epidemiologic studies are relatively insensitive in identifying causative factors in human cancer because of the extended lag between exposure and the clinical occurrence of a neoplasm, the high background incidence of many cancers in the general population, the relatively imprecise knowledge of the nature of the exposure in most instances, and a number of other confounding variables. Such studies can identify only factors that are different between two populations and that are sufficiently important to play a determining role under the conditions of exposure. The ultimate goal of such epidemiologic and basic studies is the prevention of human cancer.

Cancer prevention in humans in general may be grouped into two approaches: active and passive. Table 8-8 depicts an outline of various methods of cancer prevention with an indication of the stage of carcinogenesis toward which the preventive measure is directed. The passive prevention of cancer involves the cessation of smoking, dietary restrictions, and modification of other personal habits. Active prevention of cancer development usually is accomplished by the administration of an agent to prevent infection by carcinogenic viruses and other organisms or by the intake of chemicals, nutrients, or other factors that may modify or prevent the action of carcinogenic agents.

In reviewing Table 8-8, one can see that most methods of cancer prevention are linked to action at the stage of promotion, because this is the reversible stage of

Table 8-6
Exposures to Chemical Carcinogens in the Workplace

AGENT	INDUSTRIES AND TRADES WITH PROVED EXCESS CANCERS AND EXPOSURE	PRIMARY AFFECTED SITE
Established		
Para-aminodiphenyl	Chemical manufacturing	Urinary bladder
Asbestos	Construction, asbestos mining and milling, production of friction products and cement	Pleura, peritoneum, bronchus
Arsenic	Copper mining and smelting	Skin, bronchus, liver
Alkylating agents (mechloro-ethamine hydrochloride and bis[chloromethyl]ether)	Chemical manufacturing	Bronchus
Benzene	Chemical and rubber manufacturing, petroleum refining	Bone marrow
Benzidine, beta-naphthylamine, and derived dyes	Dye and textile production	Urinary bladder
Chromium and chromates	Tanning, pigment making	Nasal sinus, bronchus
Isopropyl alcohol manufacture	Chemical manufacturing	Cancer of paranasal sinuses
Nickel	Nickel refining	Nasal sinus, bronchus
Polynuclear aromatic hydrocarbons (from coke, coal tar, shale, mineral oils, and creosote)	Steel making, roofing, chimney cleaning	Skin, scrotum, bronchus
Vinyl chloride monomer	Chemical manufacturing	Liver
Wood dust	Cabinetmaking, carpentry	Nasal sinus

AGENT	INDUSTRIES AND TRADES	SUSPECTED HUMAN SITES
Suspected		
Acrylonitrile	Chemical and plastics	Lung, colon, prostate
Beryllium	Beryllium processing, aircraft manufacturing, electronics, secondary smelting	Bronchus
Cadmium	Smelting, battery making, welding	Bronchus
Ethylene oxide	Hospitals, production of hospital supplies	Bone marrow
Formaldehyde	Plastic, textile, and chemical production; health care	Nasal sinus, bronchus
Synthetic mineral fibers (e.g., fibrous glass)	Manufacturing, insulation	Bronchus
Phenoxyacetic acid	Farming, herbicide application	Soft tissue sarcoma
Polychlorinated biphenyls	Electrical-equipment production and maintenance	Liver
Organochlorine pesticides (e.g., chlordane, dieldrin)	Pesticide manufacture and application, agriculture	Bone marrow
Silica	Casting, mining, refracting	Bronchus

Table 8-7
Carcinogenic Risks of Chemical Agents Associated with Medical Therapy and Diagnosis

CHEMICAL OR DRUG	ASSOCIATED NEOPLASMS	EVIDENCE FOR CARCINOGENICITY
Alkylating agents (cyclophosphamide, melphalan)	Bladder, leukemia	Sufficient
Inorganic arsenicals	Skin, liver	Sufficient
Azathioprine (immunosuppressive drugs)	Lymphoma, reticulum cell sarcoma, skin, Kaposi's sarcoma (?)	Sufficient
Chlornaphazine	Bladder	Sufficient
Chloramphenicol	Leukemia	Limited
Diethylstilbestrol	Vagina (clear cell carcinoma)	Sufficient
Estrogens		
Premenopausal	Liver cell adenoma	Sufficient
Postmenopausal	Endometrium	Limited
Methoxypsoralen with ultraviolet light	Skin	Sufficient
Oxymetholone	Liver	Limited
Phenacetin	Renal pelvis (carcinoma)	Sufficient
Phenytoin (diphenylhydantoin)	Lymphoma, neuroblastoma	Limited
Thorotrast	Liver (angiosarcoma)	Sufficient

neoplastic development. As knowledge of the mechanisms of carcinogenesis has increased, so has the development of methods for the identification of potentially carcinogenic agents in the environment by a variety of different systems, from bacteria to whole animals.

IDENTIFICATION OF POTENTIAL CARCINOGENIC AGENTS

The various tests that have been applied to identifying agents with carcinogenic potential may be classified into several general areas on the basis of the time involved in the assay: short, medium, and long.

Short-Term Tests

Short-term tests for mutagenicity were developed to identify potential carcinogenic agents on the basis of their capacity for inducing mutations in DNA in cells in vitro or in vivo. In the Ames test, *Salmonella typhimurium* cells that are deficient in DNA repair and lack the ability to grow in the absence of histidine are treated with several

dose levels of the test compound, after which reversion to the histidine-positive phenotype is ascertained.

In addition to the bacterial mutational assay, several in vitro mammalian cell mutation assays exist. These mammalian mutagenicity assays use either the hypoxanthine-guanine phosphoribosyltransferase (HG-PRT) or the thymidine kinase (TK) gene as the endpoint. Because these short-term tests are based on the premise that carcinogens damage DNA, their concordance with the chronic bioassay in vivo (see below) is only between 30 and 80 percent.

Gene Mutation Assays in Vivo One of the more popular assays utilized in this area was the dominant lethal assay, in which male mice are exposed to a potential genotoxic stimulus and mated with untreated female mice, after which the percentage of pregnancies or the number of implants is determined.

In recent years, genetically engineered cells and animals have been developed that have found use in short-term mutagenesis assays. The LacZ⁻ mouse, the LacI mouse, and the LacI rat contain transgenes within which are components of the *lac* operon of *Escherichia coli* that

Table 8-8
Modes of the Prevention of Cancer

MODE	STAGE
Passive	
Smoking cessation	Pr, Pg
Dietary restriction	Pr
Moderation of alcohol intake	Pr
Modification of sexual and reproductive habits	I, Pr
Avoidance of excessive ultraviolet exposure	I, Pr
Active	
Dietary modification and supplements	Pr
Vaccination against oncogenic viruses	I, Pr
Application of ultraviolet blocking agents in appropriate situations	I, Pr
Selective screening for certain preneoplastic lesions	I, Pr
Determination of genetic background in relation to neoplastic disease	I, Pr
Administration of antihormones	Pr

KEY: I, initiation; Pr, promotion; Pg, progression.

are involved in lactose metabolism. Basically, the *lacI* and *lacZ* genes are the ones utilized in the mutational assays. By using genetically engineered cells, one may obtain both the number of mutations per unit DNA from the mouse and, more important, the actual sequence changes induced by the mutagenic action of the original agent.

Chromosomal Alterations Chromosomal alterations are extremely common, if not ubiquitous, in all malignant neoplasms. Theoretically, short-term assays for the induction of clastogenicity and related abnormalities allow the rapid identification of potential progressor agents.

Analysis of chromosomal alterations in vivo involves the administration of an agent to male mice shortly before breeding and subsequent examination of male offspring for sterility and/or chromosomal abnormalities in both germ and somatic cells. The micronucleus test measures induced clastogenesis in rodent bone marrow in vivo by means of morphologic evaluation of micronuclei that contain chromosome fragments in cell preparations from bone marrow.

Another short-term test involving changes in chromosomal structure by mechanisms that are not entirely understood is the technique of "sister chromatid exchange" (SCE). During metaphase, sister chromatids, each of which is a complete copy of the chromosome, are bound together by mechanisms that involve specific proteins. SCE reflects an interchange between DNA molecules within different chromatids at homologous loci within a replicating chromosome.

Primary DNA Damage The measurement of DNA damage and repair induced by exogenous chemicals, both in vivo and in vitro, has been used in short-term tests for potential carcinogenicity. The most widely utilized technology involves the analysis of nonreplicative DNA synthesis with appropriately labeled precursor nucleotides.

Transformation and Cell Culture Cell lines that exhibit aneuploidy, such as primary Syrian hamster embryo (SHE) cells, are used extensively in primary culture for predicting the carcinogenic potential of a variety of chemicals.

Chronic Bioassays for Carcinogenicity—Medium- and Long-Term

Chronic 2-Year Bioassay Today the "gold standard" for determining the potential carcinogenic activity of a chemical is the use of the chronic 2-year bioassay for carcinogenicity in rodents. This assay involves test groups of 50 rats and mice of both sexes and at two or three dose levels of the test agent. The animals should be susceptible but not hypersensitive to the tested effect. Animals at about 8 weeks of age are placed on the test agent at the various doses for another 96 weeks of their life span. Various pretest analyses are carried out, such as those for acute toxicity, route of administration, and determination of the maximum tolerated dose (MTD).

The underlying basis for risk extrapolation from animals to human is that the animal is a good model for human cancer development.

Medium-Term Bioassays At least two assays have been designated specifically as having reduced the time for the development of an endpoint. One that is used intensively today takes only 8 weeks, and the endpoint is nodules and focal lesions in the liver of rats that stain for glutathione S-transferase pi (GST-P). There is a significant degree of correlation between long- and medium-term results, indicating the usefulness of this assay as a potential surrogate for the chronic bioassay.

The newborn mouse model of chemical carcinogenesis determines the endpoint of neoplasms in a variety of different tissues, including lung, liver, lymphoid, and hematopoietic tissues, within a 1-year period. The assay is relatively inexpensive, using small amounts of the test materials.

Multistage Models of Neoplastic Development

A number of models of multistage carcinogenesis were developed in the rat liver. Initiation was performed with a nonnecrogenic dose of the initiating agent, followed by the chronic administration of a promoting agent. The endpoint of these systems is the quantitative analysis of altered hepatic foci measured by one of several enzymatic markers, with the most sensitive being the expression of GST-P. However, all such assays utilizing preneoplastic endpoints have not been useful in the identification of potential carcinogenic agents.

Transgenic and Knockout Mice as Models of Carcinogenesis

Recent efforts have been directed toward the development of animal models with specific genetic alterations that make them more susceptible to carcinogenesis by external agents. As noted in Table 8-9, the most popular of these models are mice that exhibit one defective allele of the $p53$ tumor suppressor gene and a transgenic mouse line (TG · AC). $p53$-deficient mice develop a high frequency of a variety of spontaneous neoplasms. The incidence of such tumors varies, but in general, all homozygous $p53$-defective mice develop neoplasms by 10 months of age, whereas heterozygous mice have a

Table 8-9
Animal Models of Neoplastic Development

	ENDPOINT
Chronic 2-year bioassay	Tumors in all organs
Tissue specific bioassays	
Liver, mouse	Hepatomas
Lung, mouse	Pulmonary adenomas
Brain, rat	Gliomas
Mammary gland, rat/mouse	Adenomas and carcinomas
Medium-term bioassays	
Ito model	Hepatic adenomas and carcinomas
Newborn mouse	Neoplasms in liver, lung, lymphoid organs
Multistage models of neoplastic development	
Bladder, rat	Papillomas/carcinomas
Colon, rat	Aberrant crypt polyp
Epidermis, mouse	Papillomas
Liver, rat	Altered hepatic foci
Transgenic mice	
Knockout of $p53$ tumor suppressor gene ($p53^{\text{def}}$)	Tumors in heterozygous animals having normal phenotype
v-Ha-ras with zetaglobin promoter; tandem insertion on chromosome 11 (TG · AC)	Induced transgene expression in skin leads to papilloma development

50 percent incidence by 18 months, with over a 90 percent incidence by 2 years of age.

The TG · AC transgenic mouse, carrying a v-Ha-*ras* oncogene, develops a high incidence of various spontaneous neoplasms and is one of many transgenic mice and rats that may be considered for the study of the development of neoplasia in response to test agents. However, in most cases, the expression of the transgene is targeted to a specific tissue, and thus one deals with a tissue-specific development of neoplasia. The TG · AC transgenic mouse is very effective in the identification of potential promoting agents for the skin.

EVALUATION OF CARCINOGENIC POTENTIAL

The multiple in vivo and in vitro tests present the experimentalist or regulator with an extensive amount of data from which to draw conclusions about the carcinogenic potential of a test agent. In addition, epidemiologic studies provide perhaps the most definitive means of estimating the carcinogenic potential to humans from exposure to a specific agent. If they are definitively positive, epidemiologic studies provide the best evidence for the carcinogenic potential of an agent in humans. The results of in vitro and in vivo tests clearly offer qualitative information with respect to the identification of agents that exhibit some potential hazard with respect to one or more aspects of the process of carcinogenesis. Major difficulties remain in attempting to extrapolate in a scientific and meaningful way information obtained from in vitro and in vivo tests to an estimation of the potential risk of such agents to the human population as inducers of disease, especially neoplasia.

The Problem of Extrapolation

Bacterial mutagenicity is the most widely and extensively utilized test for estimating the qualitative carcinogenic potential of an agent. Several issues are relevant to cross-species extrapolation, including differences in the metabolism of chemical agents between species.

The Dose–Response Problem

Another important component in the analysis of assays for carcinogenic potential is the dose–response to a particular test agent. The effectiveness of the induction of neoplasia by a chemical agent is dependent on the dose of that agent administered to the test animal. The differences in the shapes of the dose–response curves for initiation and promotion are of considerable significance in assessing carcinogenic potential and risk. Other factors that may influence a dose–response curve include the toxicity of the agent, the bioavailability of the agent, and the metabolic or pharmacokinetic characteristics of the agent in the living organism.

The Problem of the Potency of Carcinogenic Agents

It should be apparent by this point that not all carcinogenic agents are equally effective in inducing neoplasia; that is, they exhibit differing carcinogenic potencies. The potency of an agent to induce neoplasia has been simply defined as the slope of the dose–response curve for the induction of neoplasms.

RELATION (EXTRAPOLATION) OF BIOASSAY DATA TO HUMAN RISK

The risk (R) of an agent or event can be estimated as a function of the product of the probability (P) of the event and the severity of the harmfulness of the event or agent (H):

$$R = P \times H$$

From the simplest viewpoint, the risk taker may accept harm of greater severity (high value of H) only if the probability of occurrence (P) is very low. From this argument, safety may be taken as a measure of the acceptability of some degree of risk. As for the risk of cancer, harm (H) is considered by most laypersons to be extremely great.

The gold standard chronic 2-year bioassay that is utilized as the mainstay in the regulation of both industrial and pharmaceutical chemicals does not distinguish between initiating, promoting, and progressor agents. Scientific risk estimation should be carried out with full knowledge of the action of the carcinogenic agent as a complete carcinogen or as having a major action at one or more of the stages of carcinogenesis.

The extrapolation of bioassay data to human risk estimation is one of the most difficult problems that has faced society as numerous new chemicals have entered the environment. Qualitative risk estimation is much easier to develop, based on qualitative analyses of the variety of bioassay procedures utilized. However, quantitative risk analysis is much more difficult. In fact, many epidemiologists have refused to establish such quantitative relationships on the basis of animal data and use only data in the human to carry out such estimates. Still, as we have seen from the utilization of various "safe" doses of carcinogenic agents and a variety of other factors, quantitative risk assessment has been and is being applied to human risk situations involving specific chemicals and mixtures.

STATISTICAL ESTIMATES OF HUMAN RISK FROM BIOASSAY DATA BY USING MATHEMATICAL MODELS

The statistical analyses of whole-animal bioassay data have employed over the years a number of mathematical models in an attempt to relate experimental data to the human situation, especially for the purposes of quantitating human risk insofar as that is possible. Most of these mathematical models have as a basic tenet the assumption that carcinogenic agents lack a threshold, act irreversibly, and have effects that are additive. None of these models can prove or disprove the existence of a threshold of response, and none can be verified completely on the basis of biological argument.

The linear multistage model incorporates the idea of multiple steps into a statistical approach for risk analysis, but cell cycle–dependent processes, the dynamics of cell kinetics, birth rate, and death rate are not considered. Furthermore, the transition from one stage to the next is considered irreversible. Despite these deficiencies, the linearized multistage model is one of the most commonly used models at the present time. Pharmacokinetic and pharmacodynamic models provide information that can help bridge the gap between the high-dose and low-dose scenarios. A second problem is associated with extrapolation of lifetime exposure of animals to the MTD of a compound to the less than lifetime exposure common in humans. More recently, biomathematical modeling of cancer risk assessment has been used in an attempt to relate such models more closely to the biological characteristics of the pathogenesis of neoplasia. These biologically based models reproduce quite well the multistage characteristics of neoplastic development, including the rate at which normal cells are converted to "intermediate" or initiated cells and the rate at which intermediate cells are converted to neoplastic cells. These rates model the rates of initiation and progression in multistage carcinogenesis, and the stage of promotion represents the expansion of the intermediate cell population.

RISK–BENEFIT CONSIDERATIONS IN THE REGULATION OF ACTUAL AND POTENTIAL CARCINOGENIC ENVIRONMENTAL HAZARDS

We have reviewed briefly the methods for determining the actual and potential carcinogenic agents in our environment and methods for the estimation of risk to the human population from such agents. An equally important consideration includes somewhat undefined concepts such as benefit–risk analysis, cost-effectiveness, and risk–cost analysis in the regulation of hazardous agents in our environment. These concepts are concerned with such traditional regulatory terms as *safe, lowest feasible,* and *best practicable technology.*

Attempts have been made to quantitate and characterize risks versus benefits. One way to do this is to consider risks to the environment and to health as opposed to risks to society and to general aspects of health. It is evident that reduction in risk from direct exposure to an environmental factor will, at some level of additional cost of control, create new risks to society in terms of increased costs of products, availability of services, personal freedoms, employment, and so on. In controlling risks to the environment and to health, there is a point beyond which the benefits to society and the individual begin to decrease because of the cost, financial and other, incurred in reducing risk toward actual zero. However, the concept of *necessary risk,* especially in relation to occupational and industrial hazards, points to the importance of making every effort to eliminate hazardous agents in our environment that are important to society by replacing them with equally useful but less hazardous or nonhazardous components. If this cannot be done and a necessary risk is present, this consideration must be balanced against the benefits.

BIBLIOGRAPHY

Arcos JC, Argus MF, Woo YT (eds): *Chemical Induction of Cancer.* Basel: Birkhauser, 1995.

Gold LS, Slone TH, Ames BN: What do animal cancer tests tell us about human cancer risk? Overview of analyses of the carcinogenic potency database. *Drug Metab Rev* 30:359–404, 1998.

Gold LS, Zeiger E (eds): *Handbook of Carcinogenic Potency and Genotoxicity Databases.* Boca Raton, FL: CRC Press, 1997.

Hanahan D, Weinberg RA: The hallmarks of cancer. *Cell* 100:57–70, 2000.

Jacobs MN (ed): *Exercise, Calories, Fat, and Cancer.* New York: Plenum Press, 1992.

Mendelsohn J: *The Molecular Basis of Cancer.* Phildelphia: Saunders, 2001.

Rosenberg MP: Gene knockout and transgenic technologies in risk assessment: The next generation. *Mol Carcinog* 20:262–274, 1997.

Warshawsky D, Landolph JR (eds): *Molecular Carcinogenesis.* Boca Raton, FL: CRC Press, 2002.

GENETIC TOXICOLOGY

R. Julian Preston and George R. Hoffmann

KEY POINTS

- Genetic toxicology assesses the effects of chemical and physical agents on the hereditary material (DNA) and the genetic processes of living cells.
- *Oncogenes* are genes that stimulate the transformation of normal cells into cancer cells.
- Genetic toxicology assays identify mutagens for purposes of hazard identification and characterize dose–response relationships and mutagenic mechanisms.
- A broad range of short-term assays for genetic toxicology identify many mutagens and address the relationship between mutagens and cancer-causing agents.

Genetic toxicology assesses the effects of agents on both DNA and the genetic processes of living cells and organisms. This chapter describes the assays for qualitative and quantitative assessment of cellular changes induced by exposure to chemicals or radiation, the underlying molecular mechanisms for these changes, and how such information is incorporated in risk assessment.

HEALTH IMPACT OF GENETIC ALTERATIONS

Somatic Cells

Oncogenes are genes that stimulate the transformation of normal cells into cancer cells. They originate when genes called proto-oncogenes, which are involved in normal cellular growth and development, are genetically altered. Mutational alteration of proto-oncogenes can lead to overexpression of their growth-stimulating activity, whereas mutations that inactivate tumor suppressor genes, which normally restrain cellular proliferation, free cells from their inhibitory influence.

The action of oncogenes is genetically dominant in that a single active oncogene is expressed even though its normal allele is present in the same cell. Among chromosomal alterations that activate proto-oncogenes, translocations are especially prevalent. A translocation can activate a proto-oncogene by moving it to a new chromosomal location with a more active promoter, where its expression is enhanced.

Unlike oncogenes, the cancer-causing alleles that arise from tumor suppressor genes are typically recessive in that they are not expressed when they are heterozygous. Gene mutations in a tumor suppressor gene on chromosome 17 called *p53* occur in many different human cancers, and molecular characterization of *p53* mutations has linked specific human cancers to mutagen exposures.

Gene mutations, chromosome aberrations (morphologic abnormality), and aneuploidy (an abnormal number of chromosomes) are all implicated in the development of cancer. Many mutagens and clastogens contribute to carcinogenesis as initiators; however, mutagens, clastogens, and aneugens also may contribute to multiple genetic alterations.

Germ Cells

The relevance of gene mutations to health is evident from the many disorders that often are caused by base-pair substitutions or small deletions that are inherited as simple Mendelian characteristics. Many genetic disorders (e.g., cystic fibrosis, phenylketonuria, Tay-Sachs disease) are caused by the expression of recessive mutations. These mutations generally are inherited from previous generations and are expressed when an individual inherits the mutant gene from both parents.

Besides causing diseases that exhibit Mendelian inheritance, gene mutations undoubtedly contribute to human disease through the genetic component of disorders with a complex etiology, such as heart disease, hypertension, and diabetes. Refined cytogenetic methods have led to the discovery of minor variations in chromosome structure that have no apparent effect. Nevertheless, other chromosome aberrations cause fetal death or serious abnormalities. Aneuploidy (the gain or loss of one or more chromosomes) also contributes to fetal deaths and causes disorders such as Down's syndrome. Much of the effect of chromosomal abnormalities occurs prenatally. Among these abnormalities, aneuploidy is the most common, followed by polyploidy. Structural aberrations constitute about 5 percent of the total. Most chromosomal anomalies detected in newborns arise de novo in the germ cells of the parents.

CANCER AND GENETIC RISK ASSESSMENTS

Cancer Risk Assessment

Cancer risk assessment involves investigation of the sensitivity of different species and subpopulations to tumor induction by a chemical and the development of a dose–response curve of mutations to a chemical.

Genetic Risk Assessment

To investigate genetic risk, the frequency of genetic alteration in human germ cells is estimated by extrapolation from data from rodent germ cells and somatic cells. For a complete estimate of genetic risk, it is necessary to obtain an estimate of the frequency of genetic alterations transmitted to the offspring (Fig. 9-1).

MECHANISMS OF INDUCTION OF GENETIC ALTERATIONS

DNA Damage

Types of DNA damage range from single- and double-strand breaks in the DNA backbone to cross-links between DNA bases and between DNA bases and proteins and chemical addition to the DNA bases (adducts) (Fig. 9-2).

Ionizing Radiations   Ionizing radiations produce DNA single- and double-strand breaks and a broad range of base damages. The relative proportions of these different classes of DNA damage vary with the type of radiation.

Ultraviolet Light   Ultraviolet (UV) light, a nonionizing radiation, induces two predominant lesions: cyclobutane pyrimidine dimers and 6,4-photoproducts. These lesions can be quantitated by chemical and immunologic methods.

Chemicals   Chemicals can produce base alterations either directly as adducts or indirectly through the

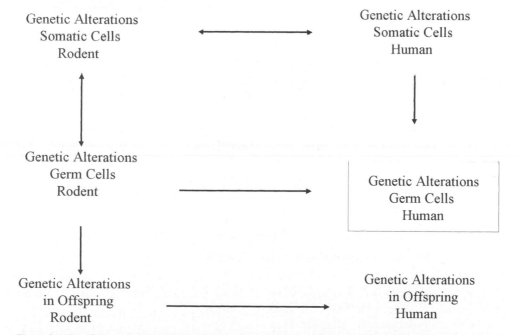

Figure 9-1. Parallelogram approach for genetic risk assessment.   Data obtained for genetic alterations in rodent somatic and germ cells and human somatic cells are used to estimate the frequency of the same genetic alterations in human germ cells. The final step is to estimate the frequency of these genetic alterations that are transmitted to offspring.

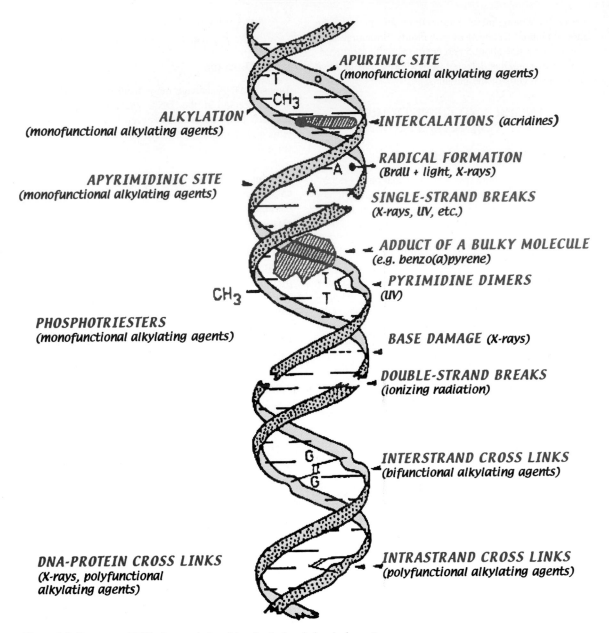

Figure 9-2. Spectrum of DNA damage induced by physical and chemical agents.

intercalation of a chemical between the base pairs. Many electrophilic chemicals react with DNA, forming covalent addition products (adducts). Alkylated bases also can lead to base loss. Base loss from DNA leaves an apurinic or apyrimidinic site that is commonly called an AP site. The insertion of incorrect bases into AP sites causes mutations. Bulky DNA adducts are recognized by

the cell in a similar way to UV damages and are repaired similarly.

Endogenous Agents Endogenous agents are responsible for several hundred DNA damages per cell per day, predominately altered DNA bases (e.g., 8-oxoguanine and thymine glycol) and AP sites. The cellular processes that can lead to DNA damage are the formation of reactive active oxygen species and deamination of cytosines and S-methylcytosines leading to uracils and thymines, respectively. The process of DNA replication is error-prone, and an incorrect base can be added by the polymerase.

DNA Repair

Two processes enable a cell to cope with the extensive DNA damage it sustains. If the damage is extensive, the cell can undergo apoptosis. If the damage is less severe, cells have developed a range of repair processes that return the DNA to its undamaged state (error-free repair) or to an improved but still altered state (error-prone repair). The basic principles underlying most repair processes are damage recognition, removal of damage (except for strand breaks or cleavage of pyrimidine dimers), repair DNA synthesis, and ligation.

Base Excision Repair The major pathways by which DNA base damages are repaired involves removal of the damaged base. The resulting gap can be filled by a DNA polymerase, followed by ligation to the parental DNA. Oxidative damages, either background or induced, are important substrates for base excision repair.

Nucleotide Excision Repair The nucleotide excision repair (NER) system provides a cell's ability to remove bulky lesions from DNA. NER removes a damage-containing oligonucleotide from DNA by means of damage recognition, incision, excision, repair synthesis, and ligation (see Fig. 8-1). The DNA damage in actively transcribing genes, specifically the transcribed strand, is preferentially and thus more rapidly repaired than is the DNA damage in the rest of the genome. Thus, the cell protects the integrity of the transcription process.

Double-Strand Break Repair Cell survival is compromised seriously by the presence of broken chromosomes. Unrepaired double-strand breaks trigger one or more DNA damage response systems to either check cell cycle progression or induce apoptosis. There are two general pathways for repair of DNA double-strand breaks: homologous recombination and nonhomologous end-joining.

Homologous Recombination The repair of double-strand breaks (and single-strand gaps) basically involves the following basic steps. The initial step is the production of a 3'-ended single-stranded tail by exonucleases or helicase activity. Through strand invasion, by which the single-stranded tail invades an undamaged homologous DNA molecule, together with DNA synthesis, a so-called Holliday junction DNA complex is formed. Through cleavage of this junction, two DNA molecules are produced (with or without a structural crossover), neither of which now contains a strand break.

Nonhomologous End-Joining (NHEJ) This type of recombination requires the production of double-strand breaks, recombination of DNA pieces, and subsequent religation. A major component of the NHEJ repair complex is a DNA-dependent protein kinase (DNA-PK). This protein probably functions to align the broken DNA ends to facilitate their ligation or to serve as a signal molecule for recruiting other repair proteins.

Mismatch Repair DNA mismatch repair systems operate to repair mismatched bases. The principal steps are damage recognition by a specific protein that binds to the mismatch, stabilizing of the binding by the addition of one or more proteins, cutting of the DNA at a distance from the mismatch, excision past the mismatch, resynthesis, and ligation.

0^6-Methylguanine-DNA Methyltransferase Repair The enzyme 0^6-methylguanine-DNA methyltransferase (MGMT) protects cells against the toxic effects of simple alkylating agents by transferring the methyl group from 0^6-methylguanine in DNA to a cysteine residue in MGMT.

Formation of Gene Mutations

Somatic Cells Gene mutations, which are considered to be small DNA-sequence changes that are confined to a single gene, are substitutions, small additions, and small deletions. Base substitutions are the replacement of the correct nucleotide by an incorrect one; they can be further subdivided as transitions in which the change is purine for purine or pyrimidine for pyrimidine and transversions in which the change is purine for pyrimidine and vice versa. Frameshift mutations are the addition or deletion of one or a few base pairs (not in multiples of three) in protein coding regions.

The great majority of so-called spontaneous (background) mutations arise from *replication* of an altered template. These DNA alterations either are the result of oxidative damage or are produced from the deamination of 5-methyl cytosine to thymine at CpG sites, resulting in G:C $\rightarrow$ A:T transitions.

Gene mutations produced by a majority of chemicals and nonionizing radiations are base substitutions, frameshifts, and small deletions. Among these mutations, a very high proportion are produced by errors of DNA *replication* on a damaged template. The relative mutation frequency is the outcome of the race between repair and replication; that is, the more repair that takes place before replication, the lower the mutation frequency for a given amount of induced DNA damage. Significant regulators of this race are cell cycle checkpoint genes (e.g., *p53*), since if the cell is checked from entering the S phase at a G_1/S checkpoint, more repair can take place before the cell starts to replicate its DNA.

Germ Cells   The mechanism of production of gene mutations in germ cells is basically the same as that in somatic cells. Ionizing radiations produce mainly deletions through errors of DNA repair; the majority of chemicals induce base substitutions, frameshifts, and small deletions through errors of DNA replication.

An important consideration in assessing gene mutations induced by chemicals in germ cells is the relationship between exposure and the timing of DNA replication (i.e., if there is damage, can it be repaired before replication?). The spermatogonial stem cell is the major contributor to genetic risk assessment, since it generally is present throughout the reproductive lifetime of an individual. Each time a spermatogonial stem cell divides, it produces a differentiating spermatogonium and a stem cell. This stem cell can accumulate genetic damage from chronic exposures.

In oogenesis, the primary oocyte arrests before birth, and there is no further S phase until the zygote. For this reason, the oocyte is resistant to the induction of gene mutations by most chemicals.

Formation of Chromosomal Alterations

Somatic Cells *Structural Chromosome Aberrations*
Sister chromatid exchanges (the apparently reciprocal exchange between the sister chromatids of a single chromosome) and gene mutations are common. In particular, damaged DNA serves as the substrate that leads to chromosomal aberrations. The DNA repair errors that lead to the formation of chromosome aberrations after exposure to ionizing radiation arise from misligation of double-strand breaks or interaction of coincidentally repairing regions during nucleotide excision repair of damaged bases. The broad outcomes of misrepair are that incorrect rejoining of chromosomal pieces during repair leads

to chromosomal exchanges within and between chromosomes. Failure to rejoin double-strand breaks or to complete the repair of other types of DNA damage leads to terminal deletions.

The failure to incorporate an acentric fragment into a daughter nucleus at anaphase/telophase or the failure of a whole chromosome to segregate at anaphase to the cellular poles can result in the formation of a micronucleus that resides in the cytoplasm. Errors of DNA replication on a damaged template can lead to a variety of chromosomal alterations. The majority of these alterations involve deletion or exchanges of individual chromatids, but some can involve both chromatids.

Numerical Chromosome Changes   Numerical changes (e.g., monosomics, trisomics, and ploidy changes) can arise from errors in chromosomal segregation resulting from any of the many possible impairments of mitotic control processes. Alteration of various cellular components can result in failure to segregate the sister chromatids to separate daughter cells or failure to segregate a chromosome to either pole.

Sister Chromatid Exchange   Sister chromatid exchanges (SCEs) are produced during S phase and are assumed to be a consequence of errors in the replication process.

Germ Cells   The formation of chromosomal alterations in germ cells is basically the same as that for somatic cells: through misrepair for ionizing radiations and radiomimetic chemicals for treatments in G_1 and G_2 and through errors of replication for all radiations and chemicals for DNA damage that is present during the S phase.

The types of aberrations formed in germ cells are the same as those formed in somatic cells. The specific segregation of chromosomes during meiosis influences the probability of recovery of an aberration, particularly a reciprocal translocation, in the offspring of a treated parent.

ASSAYS FOR DETECTING GENETIC ALTERATIONS

Introduction to Assay Design

Genetic toxicology assays serve two interrelated but distinct purposes in the toxicologic evaluation of chemicals: (1) identifying mutagens for purposes of hazard identification and (2) characterizing dose–response relationships and mutagenic mechanisms. Table 9-1 lists many of the assays one may encounter in the genetic toxicology

Table 9-1
Overview of Genetic Toxicology Assays

ASSAYS

I. DNA damage and repair assays
    A. Direct detection of DNA damage
        Alkaline elution assays for DNA strand breakage
        Comet assay for DNA strand breakage
        Assays for chemical adducts in DNA
    B. Bacterial assays for DNA damage
        Differential killing of repair-deficient and wild-type strains
        Induction of the SOS system by DNA damage in *E. coli*
    C. Assays for repairable DNA damage in mammalian cells
        Unscheduled DNA synthesis (UDS) in rat hepatocytes
        UDS in rodent hepatocytes in vivo

II. Prokaryote gene mutation assays
    A. Bacterial reverse mutation assays
        Salmonella/mammalian microsome assay (Ames test)
        E. coli WP2 tryptophan reversion assay
        Salmonella-specific base-pair substitution assay (Ames-II assay)
        E. coli lacZ–specific reversion assay
    B. Bacterial forward mutation assays
        E. coli lacI assay
        Arabinose resistance in *Salmonella*

III. Assays in nonmammalian eukaryotes
    A. Fungal assays for gene mutations
        Reversion of auxotrophs in *Neurospora* or yeast
        Forward mutations and deletions in red adenine mutants
    B. Fungal assays for aneuploidy
        Genetic detection of mitotic chromosome loss and gain in yeast
        Meiotic nondisjunction in yeast or *Neurospora*
    C. Fungal assays for induced recombination
        Mitotic crossing over and gene conversion assays in yeast
    D. Plant assays
        Gene mutations affecting chlorophyll in seedlings or waxy in pollen
        Tradescantia stamen hair-color mutations
        Chromosome aberrations or micronuclei in mitotic or meiotic cells
        Aneuploidy detected by pigmentation or cytogenetics
    E. Drosophila assays
        Sex-linked recessive lethal (SLRL) test in germ cells
        Heritable translocation assays
        Sex chromosome loss tests for aneuploidy
        Induction of mitotic recombination in eyes or wings

IV. Mammalian gene mutation assays
    A. In vitro assays for forward mutations
        TK mutations in mouse lymphoma or human cells
        HPRT mutations in Chinese hamster or human cells
        XPRT mutations in Chinese hamster AS52 cells

(continued)

Table 9-1
Overview of Genetic Toxicology Assays *(continued)*

ASSAYS

    B. In vivo assays for gene mutations in somatic cells
        Mouse spot test (somatic cell specific locus test)
        HPRT mutations (6-thioguanine-resistance) in rodent lymphocytes
    C. Transgenic assays
        Gene mutations in the bacterial *lacI* gene in mice and rats
        Gene mutations in the bacterial *lacZ* gene in mice
        Gene mutations in the phage cII gene in *lacI* or *lacZ* transgenic mice
  V. Mammalian cytogenetic assays
    A. Chromosome aberrations
        Metaphase analysis in cultured Chinese hamster or human cells
        Metaphase analysis of rodent bone marrow or lymphocytes in vivo
    B. Micronuclei
        Cytokinesis-block micronucleus assay in human lymphocytes
        Micronucleus assay in mammalian cell lines
        In vivo micronucleus assay in erythrocytes
    C. Sister chromatid exchange
        SCE in human cells or Chinese hamster cells
        SCE in rodent tissues, especially bone marrow
    D. Aneuploidy in mitotic cells
        Mitotic disturbance seen by staining spindles and chromosomes
        Hyperploidy detected by chromosome counting
        Chromosome gain or loss in cells with intact cytoplasm
        Micronucleus assay with centromere labeling
        Hyperploid cells in vivo in mouse bone marrow
        Mouse bone marrow micronucleus assay with centromere labeling
 VI. Germ cell mutagenesis
    A. Measurement of DNA damage
        Molecular dosimetry based on mutagen adducts
        UDS in rodent germ cells
        Alkaline elution assays for DNA strand breaks in rodent testes
    B. Gene mutations
        Mouse-specific locus test for gene mutations and deletions
        Mouse electrophoretic specific locus test
        Dominant mutations causing mouse skeletal defects or cataracts
    C. Chromosomal aberrations
        Cytogenetic analysis in oocytes, spermatogonia, or spermatocytes
        Micronuclei in mouse spermatids
        Mouse heritable translocation test
    D. Dominant lethal mutations
        Mouse or rat dominant lethal assay
    E. Aneuploidy
        Cytogenetic analysis for aneuploidy arising by nondisjunction
        Sex chromosome loss test for nondisjunction or breakage
        Micronucleus assay in spermatids with centromere labeling

literature. Some assays for gene mutations detect forward mutations, whereas others detect reversions. Forward mutations are genetic alterations in a wild-type gene and are detected by a change in phenotype caused by the alteration or loss of gene function. In contrast, a back mutation or reversion is a mutation that restores gene function in a mutant and thus brings about a return to the wild-type phenotype. The simplest gene mutation assays rely on selection techniques to detect mutations. By imposing experimental conditions under which only cells or organisms that have undergone mutation can grow, selection techniques greatly facilitate the identification of the rare cells that have experienced mutation among the many cells that have not.

Studying mutagenesis in intact animals requires more complex assays, which range from inexpensive short-term tests that can be performed in a few days to complicated assays for mutations in mammalian germ cells. Typically, there remains a gradation in which an increase in relevance for human risk entails more elaborate and costly tests.

Many compounds that are not themselves mutagenic or carcinogenic can be activated into mutagens and carcinogens by mammalian metabolism. Such compounds are called promutagens and procarcinogens. The most widely used metabolic activation system in microbial and cell culture assays is a postmitochondrial supernatant from a rat liver homogenate, along with appropriate buffers and cofactors. Most of the short-term assays listed in Table 9-1 require exogenous metabolic activation to detect promutagens. Exceptions are assays in intact mammals.

Despite their usefulness, in vitro metabolic activation systems cannot mimic mammalian metabolism perfectly. There are differences among tissues in the reactions that activate or inactivate foreign compounds, and organisms of the normal flora of the gut can contribute to metabolism in intact mammals.

DNA Damage and Repair Assays

Some assays measure DNA damage itself rather than the mutational consequences of DNA damage. They may do this directly, through such indicators as chemical adducts and strand breaks in DNA, or indirectly, through measurement of biological repair processes. Adducts in DNA can be detected by ^{32}P-postlabeling, immunologic methods that use antibodies against specific adducts, and fluorometric methods in the case of such fluorescent compounds.

A rapid method of measuring DNA damage is the comet assay. In this assay, cells are incorporated into agarose on slides, lysed to liberate their DNA, and subjected to electrophoresis. The DNA is stained with a fluorescent dye for observation and image analysis. Because broken DNA fragments migrate more quickly than do larger pieces of DNA, a blur of fragments (a "comet") is observed when the DNA is damaged extensively. The extent of DNA damage can be estimated from the length and other attributes of the comet tail.

The occurrence of DNA repair can serve as a readily measured indicator of DNA damage. The most common repair assay in mammalian cells is an assay for unscheduled DNA synthesis (UDS), which is a measure of excision repair. The occurrence of UDS indicates that the DNA had been damaged.

Gene Mutations in Prokaryotes

The most common means of detecting mutations in microorganisms is selecting for reversion in strains that have a specific nutritional requirement differing from that of wild-type members of the species; such strains are called auxotrophs. In the Ames assay, one measures the frequency of histidine-independent bacteria that arise in a histidine-requiring strain in the presence or absence of the chemical being tested. Auxotrophic (nutrient-deficient) bacteria are treated with the chemical of interest and plated on a medium that is deficient in histidine; if the colony survives, it must have a reversion mutation that allows it to survive without exogenous histidine.

The development of specific reversion assays of histidine mutations in *Salmonella* strains and of *lacZ* mutations in *Escherichia coli* has made the identification of specific base-pair substitutions more straightforward.

Gene Mutations in Nonmammalian Eukaryotes

The fruit fly, *Drosophila,* has long occupied a prominent place in genetic research because of the sex-linked recessive lethal (SLRL) test. This test permits the detection of recessive lethal mutations at 600 to 800 different loci on the X chromosome by screening for the presence or absence of wild-type males in the offspring of specifically designed crosses. A significant increase over the frequency of spontaneous SLRLs in the lineages derived from treated males indicates mutagenesis. The SLRL test yields information about mutagenesis in germ cells, which is lacking in all microbial and cell culture systems.

Genetic and cytogenetic assays in plants continue to be used in special applications, such as in situ monitoring for mutagens and exploration of the metabolism of pro-mutagens by agricultural plants. In in situ monitoring, one looks for evidence of mutagenic effects in organisms that are grown in the environment of interest.

Assays in nonmammalian eukaryotes continue to be important in the study of induced recombination. Recombinagenic effects in yeast have long been used as a general indicator of genetic damage. The best characterized assays for recombinagens are those which detect mitotic crossing over and mitotic gene conversion in the yeast *Saccharomyces cerevisiae.*

Gene Mutations in Mammals

Gene Mutations in Vitro Mutagenicity assays in cultured mammalian cells have some of the same advantages as microbial assays with respect to speed and cost, and they follow similar approaches. The most widely used assays for gene mutations in mammalian cells detect forward mutations that confer resistance to a toxic chemical.

Gene Mutations in Vivo In vivo assays involve treating intact animals and analyzing genetic effects in appropriate tissues. Mutations may be detected either in somatic cells or in germ cells.

The mouse spot test is a traditional genetic assay for gene mutations in somatic cells. Visible spots of altered phenotype in mice that are heterozygous for coat color genes indicate mutations in the progenitor cells of the altered regions.

Mutation assays also provide information on mechanisms of mutagenesis. Base substitutions and large deletions can be differentiated through the use of probes for the target gene and Southern blotting in that base substitutions are too subtle to be detectable on the blots. Gene mutations have been characterized at the molecular level by DNA sequence analysis both in transgenic rodents and in endogenous mammalian genes.

Transgenic Assays Transgenic animals are products of DNA technology in which the animal contains foreign DNA sequences that have been added to the genome and are transmitted through the germ line. The foreign DNA therefore is represented in all the somatic cells of the animal.

Mice that carry *lac* genes from *E. coli* use *lacI* or *lacZ* as a target for mutagenesis. After mutagenic treatment of the transgenic animals, the *lac* genes are recovered from the animal, packaged into phage λ, and transferred to *E. coli* for mutational analysis. Mutant plaques are identi-fied on the basis of phenotype, and mutant frequencies can be calculated for different tissues of the treated animals.

Mammalian Cytogenetic Assays

Chromosome Aberrations Genetic assays without DNA sequencing are indirect in that one observes a phenotype and reaches conclusions about genes. In contrast, cytogenetic assays use microscopy for direct observation of the effect of interest. In conventional cytogenetics, metaphase analysis is used to detect chromosomal anomalies. Cells should be treated during a sensitive period of the cell cycle (typically S), and aberrations should be analyzed at the first mitotic division after treatment. Examples of chromosome aberrations are shown in Fig. 9-3.

It is essential that a sufficient number of cells be analyzed because a negative result in a small sample is equivocal and inconclusive. The results should be recorded for specific classes of aberrations, not just as an overall index of aberrations per cell.

In interpreting results on the induction of chromosome aberrations in cell cultures, questionable positive results have been found at highly cytotoxic doses, high osmolality, and pH extremes. Although excessively high doses may lead to artifactual positive responses, failure to test to sufficiently high doses also undermines the utility of a test; therefore, testing should be conducted at an intermediate dose and extended to a dose at which some cytotoxicity is observed.

In vivo assays for chromosome aberrations involve treating intact animals and later collecting cells for cytogenetic analysis. The main advantage of in vivo assays is that they include mammalian metabolism, DNA repair, and pharmacodynamics. The target is a tissue from which large numbers of dividing cells are easily prepared for analysis, such as bone marrow.

In interphase cell analysis by fluorescent in situ hybridization (FISH), a nucleic acid probe is hybridized to complementary sequences in chromosomal DNA. The probe is labeled with a fluorescent dye so that the chromosomal location to which it binds is visible on fluorescence microscopy; often probes are used that cover the whole chromosome; this is called "chromosome painting."

Chromosome painting facilitates cytogenetic analysis, because aberrations are detected easily by the number of fluorescent regions in a painted metaphase. FISH permits the scoring of stable aberrations, such as translo-

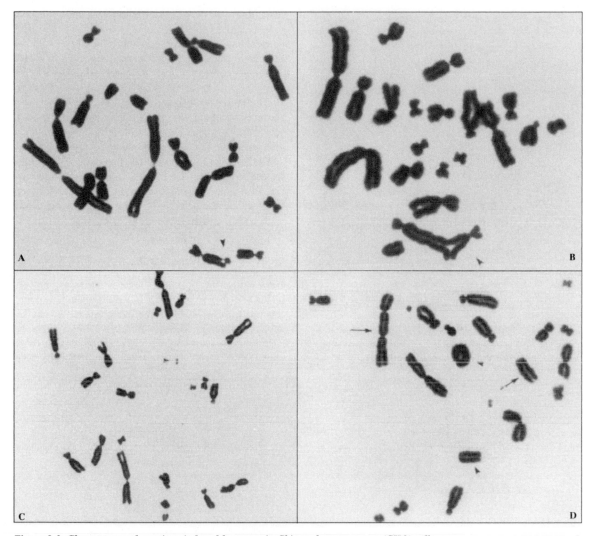

Figure 9-3. Chromosome aberrations induced by x-rays in Chinese hamster ovary (CHO) cells.
A. A chromatid deletion (➤). *B*. A chromatid exchange called a triradial (➤). *C*. A small interstitial deletion
(➤) that resulted from chromosome breakage. *D*. A metaphase with more than one aberration: a centric ring
plus an acentric fragment (➤) and a dicentric chromosome plus an acentric fragment (→).

cations and insertions, that are not readily detected in traditional metaphase analysis of unbanded chromosomes.

Micronuclei Micronuclei are chromatin-containing
bodies that represent chromosomal fragments or sometimes whole chromosomes that were not incorporated
into a daughter nucleus at mitosis. Micronuclei usually
represent acentric chromosomal fragments, and they
commonly are used as simple indicators of chromosomal

damage. Micronuclei in a binucleate human lymphocyte
are shown in Fig. 9-4.

Sister Chromatid Exchange SCE, in which apparently
reciprocal segments have been exchanged between the
two chromatids of a chromosome, is visible cytologically
through differential staining of chromatids (Fig. 9-5).
SCE assays are general indicators of mutagen exposure
rather than measures of a mutagenic effect.

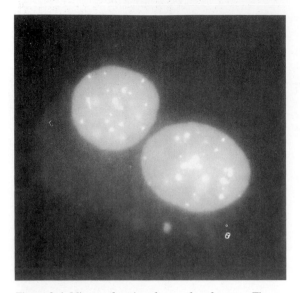

Figure 9-4. Micronucleus in a human lymphocyte.   The cytochalasin B method was used to inhibit cytokinesis that resulted in a binucleate nucleus. The micronucleus resulted from failure of an acentric chromosome fragment or a whole chromosome being included in a daughter nucleus after cell division. (Kindly provided by James Allen, Jill Barnes, and Barbara Collins.)

Aneuploidy Assays for aneuploidy include chromosome counting, the detection of micronuclei that contain kinetochores, and the observation of abnormal spindles or spindle-chromosome associations in cells in which spindles and chromosomes have been stained differentially.

The presence of the spindle attachment region of a chromosome (kinetochore) in a micronucleus can indicate that it contains a whole chromosome. Aneuploidy therefore may be detected by means of antikinetochore antibodies with a fluorescent label or FISH with a probe for centromere-specific DNA. Frequencies of micronuclei ascribable to aneuploidy and to clastogenic effects therefore may be determined concurrently by tabulating micronuclei with and without kinetochores.

Germ Cell Mutagenesis

Gene Mutations Mammalian germ cell assays provide the best basis for assessing risks to human germ cells. Mammalian assays permit the measurement of mutagenesis at different germ cell stages. Late stages of spermatogenesis often are found to be sensitive to mutagenesis, but spermatocytes, spermatids, and sper-

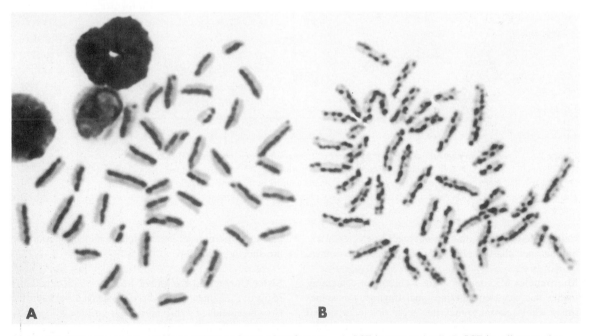

Figure 9-5. Sister chromatid exchanges (SCEs) in human lymphocytes.   *A.* SCE in untreated cell. *B.* SCE in cell exposed to ethyl carbamate. The treatment results in a very large increase in the number of SCEs. (Kindly provided by James Allen and Barbara Collins.)

matozoa are transitory. Mutagenesis in stem cell spermatogonia and resting oocytes is of special interest in genetic risk assessment because of the persistence of these stages throughout reproductive life.

Chromosomal Alterations Knowledge of the induction of chromosome aberrations in germ cells is important in assessing risks to future generations. A germ cell micronucleus assay, in which chromosomal damage induced in meiosis is measured by observation of rodent spermatids, has been developed. Aneuploidy originating in mammalian germ cells may be detected cytologically through chromosome counting for hyperploidy or genetically in the mouse sex-chromosome loss test.

Besides cytologic observation, indirect evidence for chromosome aberrations is obtained in the mouse heritable translocation assay, which measures reduced fertility in the offspring of treated males. This presumptive evidence of chromosomal rearrangements can be confirmed through cytogenetic analysis.

Dominant Lethal Mutations The mouse or rat dominant lethal assay offers an extensive database on the induction of genetic damage in mammalian germ cells. Commonly, males are treated on an acute or subchronic basis with the agent of interest and then mated with virgin females. The females are killed and necropsied during pregnancy so that embryonic mortality that is assumed to be due to chromosomal anomalies can be characterized and quantified.

Development of Testing Strategies

Concern about the adverse effects of mutation on human health, principally carcinogenesis and the induction of transmissible damage in germ cells, has provided the impetus to identify environmental mutagens. The most obvious use of genetic toxicology assays is in screening chemicals to detect mutagens, but these assays also are used to obtain information on mutagenic mechanisms and dose responses that contribute to an evaluation of hazards. Besides the testing of pure chemicals, environmental samples are tested because many mutagens exist in complex mixtures.

The first indication that a chemical is a mutagen often lies in its chemical structure. Potential electrophilic sites in a molecule serve as an alert to possible mutagenicity and carcinogenicity, because such sites confer reactivity with nucleophilic sites in DNA.

Assessment of a chemical's genotoxicity requires data from well-characterized genetic assays. Sensitivity

refers to the proportion of carcinogens that are positive in an assay, whereas specificity is the proportion of noncarcinogens that are negative. Sensitivity and specificity both contribute to the predictive reliability of an assay.

Rather than trying to assemble batteries of complementary assays, it is prudent to emphasize mechanistic considerations in choosing assays. This approach makes a sensitive assay for gene mutations (e.g., the Ames assay) and an assay for clastogenic effects in mammals pivotal in the evaluation of genotoxicity. Beyond gene mutations, one should evaluate damage at the chromosomal level with a mammalian in vitro or in vivo cytogenetic assay. Other assays offer an extensive database on chemical mutagenesis (*Drosophila* SLRL), a unique genetic endpoint (i.e., aneuploidy, mitotic recombination), applicability to diverse organisms and tissues (i.e., DNA damage assays such as the comet assay), or special importance in the assessment of genetic risk (i.e., germ cell assays).

HUMAN POPULATION MONITORING

For considerations of cancer risk assessment, the human data utilized most frequently, absent epidemiologic data, are those collected from genotoxicity assessment in human populations. The studies conducted most frequently are for chromosome aberrations, micronuclei, and sister chromatid exchanges in peripheral lymphocytes.

Each study group should be sufficiently large to prevent any confounder from having undue influence. Certain characteristics should be matched among exposed and unexposed groups. These characteristics include age, sex, smoking status, and general dietary features. Study groups of 20 or more individuals can be used as a reasonable substitute for exact matching because confounders are less influential on chromosome alteration or mutation frequency in larger groups, as was mentioned above. In some instances, it may be informative to compare exposed groups with a historical control as well as to a concurrent control.

Reciprocal translocations are transmissible from cell generation to generation, and frequency can be representative of an accumulation over time of exposure. The importance of this is that stable chromosome aberrations observed in peripheral lymphocytes exposed in vivo, but assessed after in vitro culture, are produced in vivo in hematopoietic stem cells or other precursor cells of the peripheral lymphocyte pool.

NEW APPROACHES FOR GENETIC TOXICOLOGY

As the field of genetic toxicology has moved into the molecular era, the advances in our understanding of basic cellular processes and how they can be perturbed have been enormous. The ability to manipulate and characterize DNA, RNA, and proteins has been the basis of this advance in knowledge. However, the development of sophisticated molecular biology does not in itself imply a corresponding advance in the utility of genetic toxicology and its application to risk assessment. Knowing the types of studies to conduct and knowing how to interpret the data remain fundamental. There is a need for genetic toxicology to avoid the temptation to use more and more sophisticated techniques to address the same questions and in the end make the same mistakes that were made previously.

Advances in Cytogenetics

Conventional chromosome staining with DNA stains such as Giemsa and the process of chromosome banding require a considerable expenditure of time and a high level of expertise. Chromosome banding does allow for the assessment of transmissible aberrations such as reciprocal translocations and inversions with a fairly high degree of accuracy. Stable aberrations are transmissible from parent cell to daughter cell and represent effects of chronic exposures. The more readily analyzed but cell-lethal nontransmissible aberrations, such as dicentrics and deletions, reflect only recent exposures, and only when analyzed at the first division after exposure.

Specific chromosomes, specific genes, and chromosome alterations can be detected readily since the development of FISH. In principle, the technique relies on amplification of DNA from particular genomic regions such as whole chromosomes or gene regions and the hybridization of those amplified DNAs to metaphase chromosome preparations or interphase nuclei. Regions of hybridization can be determined through the use of fluorescent antibodies that detect modified DNA bases incorporated during amplification or by incorporating fluorescent bases during amplification. The fluorescently labeled, hybridized regions are detected by fluorescence microscopy. Alterations in tumors also can be detected on a whole-genome basis. Comparative genomic hybridization (CGH) has allowed an accurate and sensitive assessment of the chromosomal alterations present in tumors. The CGH method is being adapted for automated screening approaches, using biochips.

The types of FISH methodologies available undoubtedly indicate the direction in which cytogenetic analysis will proceed. The types of data collected will affect our understanding of how tumors develop. Data on the dose–response characteristics for a specific chromosomal alteration as a proximate marker of cancer can enhance the cancer risk assessment process by describing the effects of low exposures that are below those for which tumor incidence can be assessed reliably. Cytogenetic data of the types described above also can improve extrapolation from data generated in laboratory animals to humans.

Molecular Analysis of Mutations and Gene Expression

With molecular biology techniques, the exact basis of a mutation at the level of the DNA sequence can be established. With hybridization of test DNAs to oligonucleotide arrays, specific genetic alterations or their cellular consequences can be determined rapidly and automatically. Recent advances using cDNA microarray technologies have allowed the measurement of changes in the expression of hundreds or even thousands of genes at one time. The level of expression at the mRNA level is measured by the amount of hybridization of isolated cDNAs to oligonucleotide fragments from known genes or expressed sequence tags (ESTs) on a specifically laid out grid. This technique holds great promise for establishing a cell's response to exposure to chemical or physical agents in the context of normal cellular patterns of gene expression.

CONCLUSIONS

Genetic toxicology began as basic research demonstrating that ionizing radiations and chemicals could induce mutations and chromosome alterations in plant, insect, and mammalian cells. The development of a broad range of short-term assays for genetic toxicology identified many mutagens and addressed the relationship between mutagens and cancer-causing agents, or carcinogens. The inevitable failure of those assays to be completely predictive resulted in the identification of nongenotoxic carcinogens. Genetic toxicology has begun to take advantage of the knowledge that cancer is a genetic disease with multiple steps, many of which require a mutation. The identification of the chromosome alterations involved in tumor formation has been facilitated greatly by the use of FISH. The ability to distinguish between background and induced mutations can be achieved in some cases by the use of mutation analysis at the level of DNA sequence. Key cellular processes related to mutagenesis have been identified, including multiple pathways of DNA repair, cell cycle controls, and the role of checkpoints in ensuring that the cell cycle does not proceed until the DNA and specific cellular structures are checked for fidelity. Recent developments in genetic toxicology have greatly improved our understanding of basic cellular processes and alterations that can affect the integrity of the genetic material and its functions. The ability to detect and analyze mutations in mammalian germ cells continues to improve and can contribute to a better appreciation of the long-term consequences of mutagenesis in human populations.

BIBLIOGRAPHY

Benhamou S, Sarasin A: Variability in nucleotide excision repair and cancer risk: A review. *Mutat Res* 462:149–158, 2000.

Choy WN: *Genetic Toxicology and Cancer Risk Assessment.* New York: Marcel Dekker, 2001.

Friedberg EC, Walker GC, Siede W: *DNA Repair and Mutagenesis.* Washington, DC: ASM Press, 1995.

Hanahan D, Weinberg RA: The hallmarks of cancer. *Cell* 100:57–70, 2000.

Harrington CA, Rosenow C, Retief J: Monitoring gene expression using DNA microarrays. *Curr Opin Microbiol* 3:285–291, 2000.

Li AP, Heflich RH (eds): *Genetic Toxicology: A Treatise.* Boca Raton, FL: CRC Press, 1991.

McCullough AK, Dodson ML, Lloyd RS: Initiation of base excision repair: Glycosylase mechanisms and structures. *Annu Rev Biochem* 68:255–285, 1999.

McGregor DB, Rice JM, Venitt S (eds): *The Use of Short- and Medium-Term Tests for Carcinogens and Data on Genetic Effects in Carcinogenic Hazard Evaluation.* IARC Sci. Pub. No. 146, Lyon, France: IARC, 1999.

Phillips DH, Farmer PB, Beland FA, et al: Methods of DNA adduct determination and their application to testing compounds for genotoxicity. *Environ Mol Mutagen* 35:222–233, 2000.

Tice RR, Agurell E, Anderson D, et al: Single cell gel/comet assay: Guidelines for in vitro and in vivo genetic toxicology testing. *Environ Mol Mutagen* 35:206–221, 2000.

C H A P T E R   1 0

DEVELOPMENTAL TOXICOLOGY

John M. Rogers and Robert J. Kavlock

KEY POINTS

- Developmental toxicology encompasses the study of pharmacokinetics, mechanisms, pathogenesis, and outcome after exposure to agents or conditions that lead to abnormal development.
- Developmental toxicology includes teratology, or the study of structural birth defects.
- *Gametogenesis* is the process of forming the haploid germ cells: the egg and the sperm.
- *Organogenesis* is the period during which most bodily structures are established. This period of heightened susceptibility to malformations extends from the third week to the eighth week of gestation in humans.

Developmental toxicology describes the biologic outcomes subsequent to exposure to agents or conditions that lead to abnormal progression in the formation of germ cells, as well as maturation from embryonic stages to adulthood.

SCOPE OF PROBLEM: THE HUMAN EXPERIENCE

Successful pregnancy outcome in the general population occurs at a surprisingly low frequency. Estimates of adverse outcomes include postimplantation pregnancy loss, 31 percent; major birth defects, 2 to 3 percent at birth, increasing to 6 to 7 percent at age 1 year as more manifestations are diagnosed; minor birth defects, 14 percent; low birth weight, 7 percent; infant mortality (before 1 year of age), 1.4 percent; and abnormal neurologic function, 16 to 17 percent. Thus, less than half of all human conceptions result in the birth of a completely normal, healthy infant. Many hundreds of chemicals are teratogens; most of them produce birth defects by an unknown mechanism. Table 10-1 lists chemicals, chemical classes, and conditions known to alter prenatal development in humans.

Table 10-1
Human Developmental Toxicants

Radiation	Drugs/Chemicals
Therapeutic	Androgenic chemicals
Radioiodine	Angiotensin converting enzyme inhibitors
Atomic fallout	Captopril, enalapril
	Antibiotics
	Tetracylines
	Anticancer drugs
	Aminopterin, methylaminopterin,
	cyclophosphamide, busulfan
Infections	Anticonvulsants
Rubella virus	Diphenylhydantoin, trimethadione, valproic
Cytomegalovirus (CMV)	acid
Herpes simplex virus I and II	Antithyroid drugs
Toxoplasmosis	Methimazole
Venezuelan equine encephalitis virus	Chelators
Syphilis	Penicillamine
Parvovirus B-19 (erythema infectiosum)	Chlorobiphenyls
Varicella virus	Cigarette smoke
	Cocaine
	Coumarin anticoagulants (warfarin)
	Ethanol
Maternal Trauma and Metabolic Imbalances	Ethylene oxide
Alcoholism	Fluconazole, high dosage
Amniocentesis, early	Diethylstilbestrol
Chorionic villus sampling	Iodides
(before day 60)	Lithium
Cretinism, endemic	Metals
Diabetes	Mercury (organic), lead
Folic acid deficiency	Methylene blue via intraamniotic injection
Hyperthermia	Misoprostol
Phenylketonuria	Retinoids
Rheumatic disease and congenital heart block	13-*cis*-retinoic acid, etretinate
Sjögren's syndrome	Thalidomide
Virilizing tumors	Toluene abuse

Thalidomide

In 1960, a large increase in newborns with rare limb malformations of amelia (absence of the limbs) or various degrees of phocomelia (reduction of the long bones of the limbs) was recorded in West Germany. Congenital heart disease; ocular, intestinal, and renal anomalies; and malformations of the external and inner ears also were found. Thalidomide, which was identified as the causative agent, was used throughout much of the world as a sleep aid and to ameliorate nausea and vomiting in pregnant women. It had no apparent toxicity or addictive properties in adult humans or animals at therapeutic exposure levels.

As a result of this catastrophe, regulatory agencies developed requirements for evaluating the effects of drugs on pregnancy outcomes.

Diethylstilbestrol

Diethylstilbestrol (DES) is a synthetic nonsteroidal estrogen that was used widely from the 1940s to the 1970s in the United States to prevent threatened miscarriage. Maternal use of DES before the eighteenth week of gestation appeared to be necessary for induction of the genital tract anomalies in offspring; the overall incidence of noncancerous alterations in the vagina and cervix was estimated to be as high as 75 percent. In male offspring of exposed pregnancies, a high incidence of reproductive tract anomalies along with low ejaculated semen volume and poor semen quality were observed. The realization of the latent and devastating manifestations of prenatal DES exposure has broadened the magnitude and scope of potential adverse outcomes of intrauterine exposures.

Ethanol

Although the developmental toxicity of ethanol can be traced to biblical times (e.g., Judges 13:3–4), only since the description of the fetal alcohol syndrome (FAS) in 1971 has there been a clear acceptance of alcohol's developmental toxicity. FAS includes craniofacial dysmorphism, intrauterine and postnatal growth retardation, retarded psychomotor and intellectual development, and other nonspecific major and minor abnormalities.

In utero exposure to lower levels of ethanol than those which produce full-blown FAS has been associated with a wide range of effects, including isolated components of FAS and milder forms of neurologic and behavioral disorders. These more subtle expressions of the toxicity of prenatal ethanol exposure have been termed fetal alcohol effects (FAE). Alcohol consumption can affect birth weight in a dose-related fashion.

Tobacco Smoke

Prenatal and early postnatal exposure to tobacco smoke or its constituents may represent the leading cause of environmentally induced developmental disease and morbidity today. The consequences of developmental exposure to tobacco smoke include spontaneous abortions; perinatal deaths; increased risk of sudden infant death syndrome (SIDS); increased risk of learning, behavioral, and attention disorders; and lower birth weight. One component of tobacco smoke, nicotine, is a known neuroteratogen in experimental animals and can by itself produce many of the adverse developmental outcomes associated with tobacco smoke. Perinatal exposure to tobacco smoke also can affect branching morphogenesis and maturation of the lung, leading to altered physiologic function. Environmental (passive) tobacco smoke also represents a significant risk to pregnant nonsmokers.

Cocaine

Cocaine is a local anesthetic with vasoconstrictor properties. Its effects on the fetus are complicated and controversial and demonstrate the difficulty of monitoring the human population for adverse reproductive outcomes. Accurate exposure ascertainment is difficult, as many confounding factors, including socioeconomic status and concurrent use of cigarettes, alcohol, and other drugs of abuse, may be involved. In addition, reported effects on the fetus and infant (neurologic and behavioral changes) are difficult to identify and quantify. Nevertheless, adverse effects reliably associated with cocaine exposure in humans include abruptio placentae; premature labor and delivery; microcephaly; altered prosencephalic development; decreased birth weight; a neonatal neurologic syndrome of abnormal sleep, tremor, poor feeding, irritability, and occasional seizures; and SIDS.

Retinoids

Vitamin A (retinol) exposure can cause malformations of the face, limbs, heart, central nervous system, and skeleton. Spontaneous abortion, live-born infants having at least one major malformation, and numerous exposed children with full-scale IQ scores below 85 at age 5 have been documented.

PRINCIPLES OF DEVELOPMENTAL TOXICOLOGY

Some basic principles of teratology put forth by Jim Wilson in 1959 and listed in Table 10-2 are still important today.

Critical Periods of Susceptibility and Endpoints of Toxicity

Development is characterized by various changes that are orchestrated by a cascade of factors that regulate gene transcription throughout development. Intercellular and intracellular signaling pathways that are essential for normal development rely on transcriptional, translational, and posttranslational controls. The rapid changes that occur during development alter the nature of the embryo/fetus as a target for toxicity. The timing of some key developmental events in humans and experimental animal species is presented in Table 10-3.

Gametogenesis is the process of forming the haploid germ cells: the egg and the sperm. These gametes fuse in the process of *fertilization* to form the diploid *zygote,* or one-celled embryo. Gametogenesis and fertilization are vulnerable to toxicants.

After fertilization, the embryo moves down the fallopian tube and implants in the wall of the uterus. The *preimplantation* period involves mainly an increase in cell number through a rapid series of cell divisions with little growth in size (*cleavage* of the zygote) and cavitation of the embryo to form a fluid-filled blastocoele. This stage, termed the *blastocyst,* contains cells destined to give rise to the embryo proper, and other cells give rise to extraembryonic membranes and support structures.

Toxicity during preimplantation generally is thought to result in no effect or a slight effect on growth (because of regulative growth) or in death (through overwhelming damage or failure to implant). Patterning of the limbs and lower body may begin at this time. Because of the rapid mitoses that occur during the preimplantation period, chemicals affecting DNA synthesis or integrity and those affecting microtubule assembly would be expected to be particularly toxic if given access to the embryo.

After implantation, the embryo undergoes *gastrulation,* the process of the formation of the three primary germ layers: the *ectoderm, mesoderm,* and *endoderm.* As it is a prelude to organogenesis, the period of gastrulation is quite susceptible to teratogenesis.

The formation of the neural plate in the ectoderm marks the onset of *organogenesis,* during which the rudiments of most bodily structures are established. This is a period of heightened susceptibility to malformations and extends from approximately the third week to the eighth week of gestation in humans. The rapid changes of organogenesis require cell proliferation, cell migration, cell–cell interactions, and morphogenetic tissue remodeling. Within organogenesis, there are periods of peak susceptibility for each forming structure. The peak incidence of each malformation coincides with the timing of key developmental events in the affected structure.

The end of organogenesis marks the beginning of the *fetal period,* which is characterized primarily by tissue differentiation, growth, and physiologic maturation. All organs are present and grossly recognizable, although they are not yet completely developed.

Table 10-2
Wilson's General Principles of Teratology

I. Susceptibility to teratogenesis depends on the genotype of the conceptus and the manner in which this interacts with adverse environmental factors.
II. Susceptibility to teratogenesis varies with the developmental stage at the time of exposure to an adverse influence.
III. Teratogenic agents act in specific ways (mechanisms) on developing cells and tissues to initiate sequences of abnormal developmental events (pathogenesis).
IV. The access of adverse influences to developing tissues depends on the nature of the influence (agent).
V. The four manifestations of deviant development are death, malformation, growth retardation, and functional deficit.
VI. Manifestations of deviant development increase in frequency and degree as dosage increases, from the no effect to the totally lethal level.

Table 10-3
Timing of Key Developmental Events in Some Mammalian Species

	RAT	RABBIT	MONKEY	HUMAN
Blastocyst formation	3–5	2.6–6	4–9	4–6
Implantation	5–6	6	9	6–7
Organogenesis	6–17	6–18	20–45	21–56
Primitive streak	9	6.5	18–20	16–18
Neural plate	9.5	—	19–21	18–20
First somite	10	—	—	20–21
First branchial arch	10	—	—	20
First heartbeat	10.2	—	—	22
10 somites	10–11	9	23–24	25–26
Upper limb buds	10.5	10.5	25–26	29–30
Lower limb buds	11.2	11	26–27	31–32
Testes differentiation	14.5	20	—	43
Heart septation	15.5	—	—	46–47
Palate closure	16–17	19–20	45–47	56–58
Urethral groove closed in male	—	—	—	90
Length of gestation	21–22	31–34	166	267

NOTE: Developmental ages are days of gestation.

Exposure during the fetal period is most likely to result in effects on growth and functional maturation. Functional anomalies of the central nervous system and reproductive organs—including behavioral, mental, and motor deficits as well as decreases in fertility—are among the possible adverse outcomes.

Dose–Response Patterns and the Threshold Concept

The major effects of prenatal exposure, observed at the time of birth in developmental toxicity studies, are embryo lethality, malformations, and growth retardation. For some agents, these endpoints may represent a continuum of increasing toxicity, with low dosages producing growth retardation and increasing dosages producing malformations and then lethality.

Another key element of the dose–response relationship is the shape of the dose–response curve at low exposure levels. Because of the high restorative growth potential of the mammalian embryo, cellular homeostatic mechanisms, and maternal metabolic defenses, mammalian developmental toxicity generally has been considered a threshold phenomenon. The assumption of a threshold means that there is a maternal dosage below

which an adverse response is not elicited because some repair or defense system is able to combat the exposure.

MECHANISMS AND PATHOGENESIS OF DEVELOPMENTAL TOXICITY

The term *mechanisms* is used here to refer to cellular-level events that initiate the process leading to abnormal development. *Pathogenesis* includes the cell-, tissue-, and organ-level sequelae that ultimately are manifest in abnormality. Mechanisms of teratogenesis include mutations, chromosomal breaks, altered mitosis, altered nucleic acid integrity or function, diminished supplies of precursors or substrates, decreased energy supplies, altered membrane characteristics, osmolar imbalance, and enzyme inhibition. Although these cellular insults are not unique to development, they may trigger unique pathogenetic responses in the embryo, such as reduced cell proliferation, cell death, altered cell–cell interactions, reduced biosynthesis, inhibition of morphogenetic movements, and mechanical disruption of developing structures.

Cell death plays a critical role in normal morphogenesis. The term *programmed cell death* (pcd) refers to a specific type of cell death, *apoptosis,* under genetic control in the embryo. Cell proliferation rates change both spatially and temporally during ontogenesis. There is a delicate balance between cell proliferation, cell differentiation, and apoptosis in the embryo. Thus, DNA damage may lead to cell cycle perturbations and cell death.

Damage to DNA can inhibit cell cycle progression at the G_1-S transition, through the S phase, and at the G_2-M transition. If DNA damage is repaired, the cell cycle can return to normal, but if the damage is too extensive or the cell cycle arrest is too long, apoptosis may be triggered. The relationship between DNA damage and repair, cell cycle progression, and apoptosis is depicted in Fig. 10-1. From the multiple checkpoints and factors that are present to regulate the cell cycle and apoptosis, it is clear that different cell populations may respond differ-

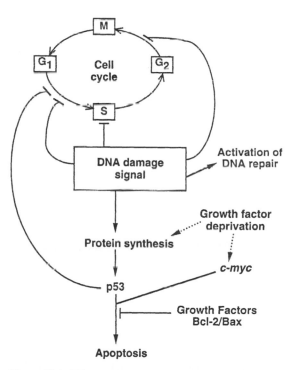

Figure 10-1. Relationships between DNA damage and the induction of cell cycle arrest or apoptosis. DNA damage can signal inhibition of the cell cycle between G_1 and S, in S phase, or between G_2 and mitosis. The signal(s) also can activate DNA repair mechanisms and the synthesis of proteins, including p53, that can initiate apoptosis. Growth factors and products of the proto-oncogene *c-myc* and the Bcl-2/Bax gene family, as well as differentiation state and cell cycle phase, are important determinants of the ultimate outcome of embryonal DNA damage.

ently to a similar stimulus, in part because cellular predisposition to apoptosis can vary.

In addition to affecting proliferation and cell viability, molecular and cellular insults can affect essential processes such as cell migration, cell–cell interactions, differentiation, morphogenesis, and energy metabolism. Although the embryo has compensatory mechanisms that offset such effects, the production of a normal or malformed offspring depends on the balance between damage and repair at each step in the pathogenetic pathway.

Advances in the Molecular Basis of Dysmorphogenesis

Rapid technological advances are bringing a new understanding of the mechanisms of normal and abnormal development. Targeted gene disruption by homologous recombination (gene "knockout") has been used to study the function of members of the retinoic acid receptor (RAR) family of nuclear ligand-inducible transcription factors.

The use of synthetic antisense oligonucleotides allows temporal and spatial restriction of gene ablation by hybridizing to mRNA in the cell, thus inactivating it. In this way, gene function can be turned off at specific times.

Gain of gene function also can be studied by engineering genetic constructs with an inducible promoter attached to the gene of interest. Ectopic gene expression can be made ubiquitous or site-specific, depending on the choice of promoter to drive expression. Transient overexpression of specific genes can be accomplished by adding extra copies by using adenoviral transduction.

PHARMACOKINETICS AND METABOLISM IN PREGNANCY

The extent to which chemicals reach the conceptus are important determinants of whether an agent can affect development. The maternal, placental, and embryonic compartments are independent yet interacting systems that undergo profound changes throughout the course of pregnancy. Alterations in placental physiology can have a significant impact on the uptake, distribution, metabolism, and elimination of xenobiotics. For example, decreases in intestinal motility and increases in gastric emptying time result in longer retention time of ingested chemicals in the upper gastrointestinal tract in the mother. Cardiac output increases by 50 percent during the first trimester in humans and remains elevated throughout pregnancy, whereas blood volume increases and plasma proteins and peripheral vascular resistance decrease. The relative increase in blood volume over red cell volume leads to borderline anemia and a generalized edema with a 70 percent elevation of extracellular space. Thus, the volume of distribution of a chemical and the amount bound by plasma proteins may change considerably during pregnancy. Other changes occur in the renal, hepatic, and pulmonary systems. Clearly, maternal handling of a chemical influences the extent of embryotoxicity.

The placenta also influences embryonic exposure by helping to regulate blood flow, offering a transport barrier, and metabolizing chemicals. The placenta permits bidirectional transfer of substances between the maternal and fetal compartments. It is important to note that virtually any substance present in the maternal plasma will be transported to some extent by the placenta. The passage of most drugs across the placenta seems to occur by simple passive diffusion. Important modifying factors to the rate and extent of transfer include lipid solubility, molecular weight, protein binding, the type of transfer (passive diffusion, facilitated or active transport), the degree of ionization, and placental metabolism. Blood flow probably constitutes the major rate-limiting step for more lipid-soluble compounds.

Maternal metabolism of xenobiotics is an important and variable determinant of developmental toxicity. In regard to other health endpoints, the developing field of pharmacogenomics offers hope for increasing our ability to predict susceptible subpopulations based on empirical relationships between maternal genotype and fetal phenotype.

RELATIONSHIPS BETWEEN MATERNAL AND DEVELOPMENTAL TOXICITY

Although all developmental toxicity ultimately must result from an insult to the conceptus at the cellular level, the insult may occur through a direct effect on the embryo/fetus, indirectly through toxicity of the agent to the mother and/or the placenta, or a combination of direct and indirect effects. Some conditions that may affect the fetus adversely are depicted in Fig. 10-2.

The distinction between direct and indirect developmental toxicity is important for interpreting safety assessment tests in pregnant animals, as the highest dosage level in these experiments is chosen on the basis of its ability to produce some maternal toxicity (e.g., decreased food or water intake, weight loss, clinical signs). However, maternal toxicity defined only by such manifestations provides little insight into the toxic actions of a xenobiotic. When developmental toxicity is observed only in the presence of maternal toxicity, the developmental effects may be indirect (i.e., caused by an inappropriate growing condition resulting from an altered maternal environment rather than by a direct interaction of the fetus with the toxin). Greater understanding of the physiologic changes underlying the observed maternal toxicity and elucidation of the association with developmental effects are needed before one can begin to address the relevance of the observations to human safety assessment.

Maternal Factors Affecting Development

Genetics The genetic makeup of the pregnant female has been well documented as a determinant of developmental outcome. The incidence of cleft lip and/or palate [CL(P)], which occurs more frequently in whites than in blacks, has been investigated in the offspring of interracial couples in the United States. Offspring of white mothers had a higher incidence of CL(P) than did offspring of black mothers after correcting for paternal race, whereas offspring of white fathers did not have a higher incidence of CL(P) than did offspring of black fathers after correcting for maternal race.

Disease Chronic hypertension in the mother, uncontrolled maternal diabetes mellitus, and certain infections in the mother (e.g., cytomegalovirus and *Toxoplasma gondii*) are leading causes of several types of defects in the fetus. Exposure to hyperthermia (such as febrile illness in the mother) also is implicated in neural defects in the fetus.

Nutrition A wide spectrum of dietary insufficiencies ranging from protein-calorie malnutrition to deficiencies of vitamins, trace elements, and/or enzyme cofactors is known to affect pregnancy adversely. In fact, folate supplementation reduces the incidence of pregnant women having infants with neural tube defects.

Stress Diverse forms of maternal toxicity may have in common the induction of a physiologic stress response. Various forms of physical stress have been applied to pregnant animals in attempts to isolate the developmental effects of stress. Noise stress in pregnant rats or mice throughout gestation can produce developmental toxicity. Restraint stress produces increased fetal death in rats and malformations of cleft palate, fused and supernumerary ribs, and encephaloceles in mice. There is a positive correlation in humans between stress and adverse

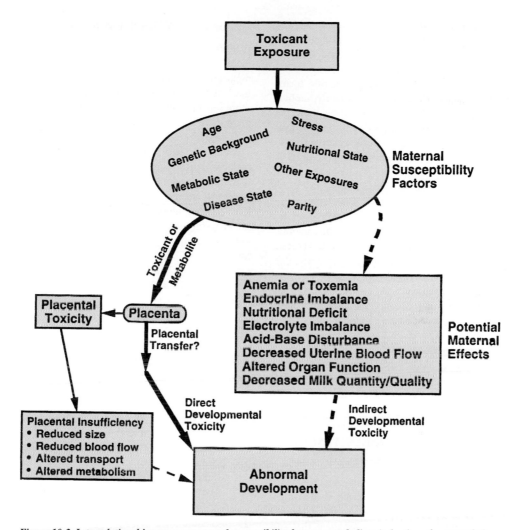

Figure 10-2. Interrelationships among maternal susceptibility factors, metabolism, induction of maternal physiologic or functional alterations, placental transfer and toxicity, and developmental toxicity.   A developmental toxicant can cause abnormal development through any one or a combination of these pathways. Maternal susceptibility factors determine the predisposition of the mother to respond to a toxic insult, and the maternal effects listed can affect the developing conceptus adversely. Most chemicals traverse the placenta in some form, and the placenta also can be a target for toxicity. In most cases, developmental toxicity probably is mediated by a combination of these pathways.

developmental effects, including low birth weight and congenital malformations.

Placental Toxicity   The placenta is the interface between the mother and the conceptus, providing attachment, nutrition, gas exchange, and waste removal. The placenta also produces hormones critical to the maintenance of pregnancy and can metabolize and/or store xenobiotics. Placental toxicity may compromise these

functions. Toxicants that are known to be toxic to the placenta include cadmium (Cd), arsenic and mercury, cigarette smoke, ethanol, cocaine, endotoxin, and sodium salicylate.

Maternal Toxicity   A retrospective analysis of relationships between maternal toxicity and specific types of prenatal effects found species-specific associations between maternal toxicity and specific adverse developmental effects. Various adverse developmental outcomes include increased intrauterine death, decreased fetal weight, supernumerary ribs, and enlarged renal pelves.

A number of studies directly relate specific forms of maternal toxicity to developmental toxicity, including those in which the test chemical causes maternal effects that exacerbate the agent's developmental toxicity. However, clear delineation of the relative role(s) of indirect maternal and direct embryo/fetal toxicity is difficult.

Diflunisal, an analgesic and anti-inflammatory drug, causes axial skeletal defects in rabbits. Developmentally toxic dosages resulted in severe maternal anemia and depletion of erythrocyte ATP levels. Teratogenicity, anemia, and ATP depletion were unique to the rabbit. The teratogenicity of diflunisal in the rabbit probably was due to hypoxia resulting from maternal anemia.

Phenytoin, an anticonvulsant, can affect maternal folate metabolism in experimental animals, and these alterations may play a role in the teratogenicity of this drug. A mechanism of teratogenesis was proposed that relates depressed maternal heart rate and embryonic hypoxia. Supporting studies have demonstrated that hyperoxia reduces the teratogenicity of phenytoin in mice.

DEVELOPMENTAL TOXICITY OF ENDOCRINE-DISRUPTING CHEMICALS

There has been growing concern that exposure to chemicals that can interact with the endocrine system may pose a serious health hazard. An *endocrine disruptor* has been broadly defined as an exogenous agent that interferes with the production, release, transport, metabolism, binding, action, or elimination of natural hormones that are responsible for the maintenance of homeostasis and the regulation of developmental processes. Because of the critical role of hormones in directing differentiation in many tissues, the developing organism is particularly vulnerable to fluctuations in the timing or intensity of exposure to chemicals with hormonal (or antihormonal) activity. Chemicals from a wide variety of chemical classes induce developmental toxicity through at least four modes of action involving the endocrine system: (1) by serving as steroid receptor ligands, (2) by modifying steroid hormone metabolizing enzymes, (3) by perturbing hypothalamic-pituitary release of trophic hormones, and (4) by uncharacterized proximate modes of action.

Laboratory Animal Evidence

Estrogenic (or antiestrogenic) developmental toxicants include DES, estradiol, antiestrogenic drugs such as tamoxifen and clomiphene citrate, and some pesticides and industrial chemicals. Female offspring are generally more sensitive than males, and altered pubertal development, reduced fertility, and reproductive tract anomalies are common findings.

Antiandrogens represent another major class of endocrine-disrupting chemicals. The principal manifestations of developmental exposure to an antiandrogen generally are restricted to males and include hypospadias, retained nipples, reduced testes and accessory sex gland weights, and decreased sperm production. Polychlorinated biphenyls (PCBs) may act at several sites to lower thyroid hormone levels during development and cause body weight and auditory deficits. PCBs also cause learning deficits and alter locomotor activity patterns in rodents and monkeys.

Human Evidence

It is not clear whether human health is being affected adversely by exposures to endocrine disruptors present in the environment. Reports are of two types:

1. Observations of adverse effects on reproductive system development and function after exposure to chemicals with known endocrine activities that are present in medicines, contaminated food, or the workplace. These observations have tended to involve relatively higher exposure to chemicals with known endocrine effects.

2. Epidemiologic evidence of increasing trends in reproductive and developmental adverse outcomes that have an endocrine basis. For example, secular trends have been reported for cryptorchidism, hypospadias, semen quality, and testicular cancer, but because of the lack of exposure assessment, such studies provide limited evidence of a cause-and-effect relationship.

Impact on Screening and Testing Programs

The findings of altered reproductive development after early life stage exposures to endocrine-disrupting chemicals helped prompt revision of traditional safety evaluation tests. These tests now include assessments of female estrous cyclicity, sperm motility and sperm morphology in both the parental and F1 generations, the age at puberty in the F1s, histopathology of target organs, anogenital distance in the F2s, and primordial follicular counts in the parental and F1 generations. For the new prenatal developmental toxicity test guidelines, one important modification aimed at improved detection of endocrine disruptors was the expansion of the period of dosing from the end of organogenesis (i.e., palatal closure) to the end of pregnancy in order to include the developmental period of urogenital differentiation.

MODERN SAFETY ASSESSMENT

Experience with chemicals that have the potential to induce developmental toxicity indicates that both laboratory animal testing and surveillance of the human population (i.e., epidemiologic studies) are necessary to provide adequate public health protection.

Regulatory Guidelines for in Vivo Testing

New and internationally accepted testing protocols rely on the investigator to meet the primary goal of detecting and bringing to light any indication of toxicity to reproduction. Key elements of various tests are provided in Table 10-4. The general goal of these studies is to identify the no observed adverse effect level (NOAEL), which is the highest dosage level that does not produce a significant increase in adverse effects in the offspring.

Multigeneration Tests

Information pertaining to developmental toxicity also can be obtained from studies in which animals are exposed to the test substance continuously over one or more generations. For additional information on this approach, see Chap. 20.

Children's Health

Children have diets different from those of adults and also have activity patterns that change their exposure profile compared with adults, such as crawling on the floor or ground, putting their hands and foreign objects in their mouths, and raising dust and dirt during play. Even the level of their activity (i.e., closer to the ground) can affect their exposure to some toxicants. In addition to exposure differences, children are growing and developing, and

this makes them more susceptible to some types of insults. The effects of early childhood exposure, including neurobehavioral effects and cancer, may not be apparent until later in life. Debate continues over the approach that should be used in risk assessment in infants and children.

Alternative Testing Strategies

A variety of alternative test systems have been proposed to refine, reduce, or replace reliance on the standard regulatory mammalian tests for assessing prenatal toxicity (Table 10-5). These tests can be grouped into assays based on cell cultures, cultures of embryos in vitro (including submammalian species), and short-term in vivo tests. It initially was hoped that the alternative approaches would become generally applicable to all chemicals and help prioritize full-scale testing. Indeed, given the complexity of embryogenesis and the multiple mechanisms and target sites of potential teratogens, it was perhaps unrealistic to have expected a single test or even a small battery to accurately prescreen the activity of chemicals in general.

An exception to the poor acceptance of alternative tests for prescreening for developmental toxicity is the Chernoff/Kavlock in vivo test. In this test, pregnant females are exposed during the period of major organogenesis to a limited number of dosage levels near those inducing maternal toxicity, and then the offspring are evaluated over a brief neonatal period for external malformations, growth, and viability. This test has proved reliable over a large number of chemical agents and classes.

Epidemiology

Reproductive epidemiology is the study of the possible statistical associations between specific exposures of the father or pregnant woman and her conceptus and the outcome of pregnancy. The plausibility of linking a particular exposure with a series of case reports increases with the rarity of the defect, the rarity of the exposure in the population, a small source population, a short time span for study, and biological plausibility for the association. In other situations, such as those which occurred with ethanol and valproic acid, associations are sought through either a case-control or a cohort approach. Both approaches require accurate ascertainment of abnormal outcomes and exposures and a sufficiently large effect and study population to detect an elevated risk. Another challenge to epidemiologists is the high percentage of human pregnancy failures related to a particular exposure

Table 10-4
Summary of in Vivo Regulatory Protocol Guidelines for Evaluation of Developmental Toxicity

STUDY	EXPOSURE	ENDPOINTS COVERED	COMMENTS
Segment I: Fertility and general reproduction study	Males: 10 weeks before mating; Females: 2 weeks before mating	Gamete development, fertility, pre- and postimplantation viability, parturition, lactation	Assesses reproductive capabilities of male and female after exposure over one complete spermatogenic cycle or several estrous cycles.
Segment II: Teratogenicity test	Implantation (or mating) through end of organogenesis (or term)	Viability and morphology (external, visceral, and skeletal) of conceptuses just before birth	Shorter exposure to prevent maternal metabolic adaptation and to provide high exposure to the embryo during gastrulation and organogenesis. Earlier dosing option for bioaccumulative agents or those affecting maternal nutrition. Later dosing option covers male reproductive tract development and fetal growth and maturation.
Segment III: Perinatal study	Last trimester of pregnancy through lactation	Postnatal survival, growth, and external morphology	Intended to observe effects on development of major organ functional competence during the perinatal period; thus, may be relatively more sensitive to adverse effects at this time.
ICH 4.1.1: Fertility protocol	Males: 4 weeks before mating; Females: 2 weeks before mating	Males: reproductive organ weights and histology, sperm counts and motility. Females: Viability of conceptuses at mid-pregnancy or later	Improved assessment of male reproductive endpoints; shorter treatment duration than Segment I.
ICH 4.1.2: Effects on prenatal and postnatal development, including maternal function	Implantation through end of lactation	Relative toxicity to pregnant versus nonpregnant female; postnatal viability, growth, development and functional deficits (including behavior, maturation, and reproduction)	Similar to Segment I study.
ICH 4.1.3: Effects on embryo/fetal development	Implantation through end of organogenesis	Viability and morphology (external, visceral, and skeletal) of fetuses just before birth	Similar to Segment II study. Usually conducted in two species (rodent and nonrodent).
OECD 414 Prenatal developmental toxicity study	Implantation (or mating) through day before cesarean section	Viability and morphology (external, visceral, and skeletal) of fetuses just before birth	Similar to Segment II study. Usually conducted in two species (rodent and nonrodent).

Table 10-5
Brief Survey of Alternative Test Methodologies for Developmental Toxicity

ASSAY	BRIEF DESCRIPTION AND ENDPOINTS EVALUATED
Mouse ovarian tumor	Labeled mouse ovarian tumor cells added to culture dishes with concanavalin A coated disks for 20 min. Endpoint is inhibition of attachment of cells to disks.
Human embryonic palatal mesenchyme	Human embryonic palatal mesenchyme cell line grown in attached culture. Cell number assessed after 3 days.
Micromass culture	Midbrain and limb bud cells dissociated from rat embryos and grown in micromass culture for 5 days. Cell proliferation and biochemical markers of differentiation assessed.
Mouse embryonic stem cell (EST) test	(1) Mouse ESTs in 96-well plates assessed for differentiation and cytotoxicity after 7 days. (2) Mouse ESTs and 3T3 cells in 96-well plates assessed for viability after 3 and 5 days. ESTs grown for 3 days in hanging drops form embryoid bodies that are plated and examined after 10 days for differentiation into cardiocytes.
Chick embryo neural retina cell culture	Neural retinas of day 6.5 chick embryos dissociated and grown in rotating suspension culture for 7 days. Endpoints include cellular aggregation, growth, differentiation, and biochemical markers.
Drosophila	Fly larvae grown from egg disposition through hatching of adults. Adult flies examined for specific structural defects (bent bristles and notched wing).
Hydra	Hydra attenuata cells are aggregated to form an "artificial embryo" and allowed to regenerate. Dose response compared to that for adult Hydra toxicity.
FETAX	Midblastula stage Xenopus embryos exposed for 96 h and evaluated for viability, growth, morphology.
Rodent whole embryo culture	Postimplantation rodent embryos grown in vitro for up to 2 days and evaluated for growth and development.
Chernoff/Kavlock assay	Pregnant mice or rats exposed during organogenesis and allowed to deliver. Postnatal growth, viability, and gross morphology of litters assessed.

that may go undetected in the general population. Furthermore, with the availability of prenatal diagnostic procedures, additional pregnancies of malformed embryos (particularly those with neural tube defects) are electively aborted. Thus, the incidence of abnormal outcomes at birth may not reflect the true rate of abnormalities, and the term *prevalence,* rather than *incidence,* is preferred when the denominator is the number of live births rather than total pregnancies.

Other issues particularly relevant to reproductive epidemiology include homogeneity, recording proficiency, and confounding. Homogeneity refers to the fact that a particular outcome may be described differently by various recording units and that even given a specific outcome, there can be multiple pathogenetic origins (e.g., cleft palate can arise by means of a variety of mechanisms). Recording difficulties relate to inconsistencies of definitions and nomenclature and to difficulties in ascertaining or recalling outcomes as well as exposures. For example, birth weights usually are determined and recalled accurately, but spontaneous abortions and certain malformations may not be. Finally, confounding by factors such as maternal age and parity, dietary factors, diseases and drug use, and social characteristics must be accounted for to control for variables that affect both exposure and outcome.

Epidemiologic studies of abnormal reproductive outcomes usually are undertaken with three objectives in mind: The first is scientific research into the causes of abnormal birth outcomes and usually involves analysis of case reports or clusters; the second is prevention and is targeted at broader surveillance of trends by birth defect registries around the world; and the third is informing the public and providing assurance. Cohort studies, with their prospective exposure assessment and ability to monitor both adverse and beneficial outcomes, may be the most methodologically robust approach to identifying human developmental toxicants.

Information on differential genetic susceptibility to birth defects will continue to accrue. This new knowledge promises to elucidate links between genetics and disease susceptibility at a pace that was not possible previously. Understanding the genetic basis of susceptibility to environmentally induced birth defects will allow more inclusive risk assessments and a better understanding of the mechanisms of action of developmental toxicants.

Concordance of Data

Studies of the similarity of responses of laboratory animals and humans for developmental toxicants support the assumption that the results from laboratory tests are predictive of potential human effects. Concordance is strongest when there are positive data from more than one test species. Humans tend to be more sensitive to developmental toxicants than is the most sensitive test species.

Elements of Risk Assessment

The extrapolation of animal test data for developmental toxicity follows two basic directions: one for drugs for which exposure is voluntary and usually to high dosages and the other for environmental agents for which exposure is generally involuntary and to low levels. For drugs, a use-in-pregnancy rating is utilized in which the letters A, B, C, D, and X are used to classify the evidence that a chemical poses a risk to the human conceptus. For example, drugs are placed in category A if adequate, well-controlled studies in pregnant humans have failed to demonstrate a risk and are placed in category X (contraindicated for pregnancy) if studies in animals or humans or investigational or postmarketing reports have shown fetal risk that clearly outweighs any possible benefit to the patient. The default category C (risks cannot be ruled out) is assigned when there is a lack of human studies and animal studies are lacking or positive for fetal risk but the benefits may justify the potential risk. Categories B and D represent areas of relatively lesser or greater concern for risk, respectively.

For environmental agents, the purpose of the risk assessment process for developmental toxicity is generally to define the dose, route, timing, and duration of exposure that induce effects at the lowest level in the most relevant laboratory animal model. The exposure associated with this "critical effect" then is subjected to a variety of safety or uncertainty factors to derive an exposure level for humans that is assumed to be relatively safe. In the absence of definitive animal test data, certain default assumptions generally are made. They include the following: (1) An agent that produces an adverse developmental effect in experimental animals will potentially pose a hazard to humans after sufficient exposure during development, (2) all four manifestations of developmental toxicity (death, structural abnormalities, growth alterations, and functional deficits) are of concern, (3) the specific types of developmental effects seen in animal studies are not necessarily the same as those which may be produced in humans, (4) the most appropriate species is used to estimate human risk when data are available (in the absence of such data, the most sensitive species is appropriate), and (5) in general, a threshold is assumed for the dose–response curve for agents that produce developmental toxicity.

One troubling and subjective aspect of risk assessment for developmental toxicants is distinguishing between adverse effects that are detrimental to health and lesser effects that are considered not significant for human health. The interpretation of reduced fetal growth in developmental toxicity studies illustrates most of the issues. Although we have accepted definitions of low birth weight in humans and understand how intrauterine growth retardation translates to an elevated risk of infant mortality and mental retardation, similar knowledge in rodents is lacking. Further concerns arise from recent epidemiologic evidence suggesting that birth weight in humans is a predictor of adult-onset diseases, including hypertension, cardiovascular disease, and diabetes.

PATHWAYS TO THE FUTURE

There are several mechanisms of normal development that are conserved in diverse animals, including the fruit fly, roundworm, zebrafish, frog, chick, and mouse. Seventeen conserved intercellular signaling pathways have been described that are used repeatedly at different times and locations during the development of these and other animal species, as well as in humans (Table 10-6). The conserved nature of these key pathways provides a strong scientific rationale for using these animal models to advantage in developmental toxicology. These organisms have well-known genetics and embryology and rapid generation times, and they are also amenable to genetic manipulation to enhance the sensitivity of specific developmental pathways or to incorporate human genes to answer questions of interspecies extrapolation.

Increased understanding of human genetic polymorphisms and their contribution to susceptibility to birth defects, use of sensitized animal models for high-dose to low dose extrapolation, use of stress/checkpoint pathways as indicators of developmental toxicity, implementation of bioinformatic systems to improve data archiving and retrieval, and increased multidisciplinary education and research on the causes of birth defects will aid assessment of the developmental risk of toxicants.

Table 10-6
The 17 Intercellular Signaling Pathways Used in Development by Most Metazoans

PERIOD DURING DEVELOPMENT	SIGNALING PATHWAY
Before organogenesis; later for growth and tissue renewal	1. Wingless-Int pathway 2. Transforming growth factor β pathway 3. Hedgehog pathway 4. Receptor tyrosine kinase pathway 5. Notch-Delta pathway 6. Cytokine pathway (STAT pathway)
Organogenesis and cytodifferentiation; later for growth and tissue renewal	7. Interleukin-1-toll nuclear factor-kappa B pathway 8. Nuclear hormone receptor pathway 9. Apoptosis pathway 10. Receptor phosphotyrosine phosphatase pathway
Larval and adult physiology	11. Receptor guanylate cyclase pathway 12. Nitric oxide receptor pathway 13. G-protein coupled receptor (large G proteins) pathway 14. Integrin pathway 15. Cadherin pathway 16. Gap junction pathway 17. Ligand-gated cation channel pathway

BIBLIOGRAPHY

Fort DJ, Stover EL, Farmer DR, Lemen JK: Assessing the predictive validity of frog embryo teratogenesis assay—*Xenopus* (FETAX). *Teratogenesis Carcinog Mutagen* 20:87–98, 2000.

Kavlock RJ, Daston GP (eds): *Drug Toxicity in Embryonic Development, II*. Berlin: Springer-Verlag, 1997.

Khoury MJ: Genetic susceptibility to birth defects in humans: From gene discovery to public health action. *Teratology* 61:17–20, 2000.

Korach KS (ed): *Reproductive and Developmental Toxicology.* New York: Marcel Dekker, 1998.

Mazo J del (ed): *Reproductive Toxicology: In Vitro Germ Cell Developmental Toxicology from Science to Social Industrial Demand.* New York: Plenum Press, 1998.

Pagon RA, Covington M, Tarczy-Hornoch P: Helix: A directory of medical genetics laboratories, http://www.genetests.org, 1998.

Schardein JL: *Chemically Induced Birth Defects,* 3d ed. New York: Marcel Dekker, 2000.

UNIT 4

TARGET ORGAN
TOXICITY

C H A P T E R   1 1

TOXIC RESPONSES OF THE BLOOD

John C. Bloom and John T. Brandt

KEY POINTS

- Hematotoxicology is the study of the adverse effects of exogenous chemicals on blood and blood-forming tissues.
- Direct or indirect damage to blood cells and their precursors includes tissue hypoxia, hemorrhage, and infection.
- Xenobiotic-induced *aplastic anemia* is a life-threatening disorder characterized by peripheral blood pancytopenia, reticulocytopenia, and bone marrow hypoplasia.
- Idiosyncratic xenobiotic-induced agranulocytosis may involve a sudden depletion of circulating neutrophils concomitant with exposure that persists as long as the agent or its metabolites are in the circulation.
- Leukemias are proliferative disorders of hematopoietic tissue that originate from individual bone marrow cells.
- Xenobiotic-induced thrombocytopenia may result from increased platelet destruction or decreased platelet production, which leads to decreased platelet aggregation and bleeding disorders.
- Blood coagulation is a complex process that involves a number of proteins whose synthesis and function can be altered by many xenobiotics.

BLOOD AS A TARGET ORGAN

Hematotoxicology is the study of the adverse effects of exogenous chemicals on blood and blood-forming tissues. The delivery of oxygen to tissues throughout the body, which maintains vascular integrity and provides the many affector and effector immune functions necessary for host defense, requires a prodigious proliferative and regenerative capacity. The various blood cells (erythrocytes, granulocytes, and platelets) are each produced at a rate of approximately 1 million to 3 million per second in a healthy adult; this characteristic makes hematopoietic tissue a particularly sensitive target for cytoreductive or antimitotic agents, such as those used to treat cancer, infection, and immune-mediated disorders. This tissue is also susceptible to secondary effects of toxic agents that affect the supply of nutrients such as iron, the clearance of toxins and metabolites such as urea, and the production of vital growth factors such as erythropoietin. The consequences of direct or indirect damage to blood cells and their precursors are predictable and potentially life-

threatening. They include hypoxia, hemorrhage, and infection.

Hematotoxicity may be regarded as *primary,* in which one or more blood components are affected directly, or *secondary,* in which the toxic effect is a consequence of other tissue injury or systemic disturbances. Primary toxicity is regarded as among the serious effects of xenobiotics, particularly drugs. Secondary toxicity is exceedingly common because of the propensity of blood cells to reflect various local and systemic effects of toxicants on other tissues.

HEMATOPOIESIS

The production of blood cells, or hematopoiesis, is a highly regulated sequence of events by which blood cell precursors proliferate and differentiate. The bone marrow in the axial skeleton and proximal limbs is the principal site of hematopoiesis.

Whereas the central function of bone marrow is hematopoiesis and lymphopoiesis, bone marrow is also one of the sites of the mononuclear phagocyte system

(MPS), contributing monocytes that differentiate into phagocytic cells in other tissues. A complex interplay of developing cells with stromal cells, extracellular matrix components, and cytokines makes up the *hematopoietic inductive microenvironment.*

TOXICOLOGY OF THE ERYTHRON

The Erythrocyte

Erythrocytes [red blood cells (RBCs)] serve as the principal vehicle for transportating oxygen from the lungs to the peripheral tissues and carbon dioxide from tissues to the lung. Erythrocytes also are involved as a carrier and/or reservoir for drugs and toxins. Xenobiotics may affect the production, function, and/or survival of erythrocytes. These effects most frequently manifest as a change in the circulating red cell mass, usually resulting in a decrease (anemia). Occasionally, agents that affect the oxygen affinity of hemoglobin lead to an increase in the red cell mass (erythrocytosis). Shifts in plasma volume can alter the relative concentration of erythrocytes (and hemoglobin concentration) and can be confused easily with true anemia or erythrocytosis.

Two general mechanisms that lead to true anemia are decreased production and increased destruction of erythrocytes. The usual parameters of a complete blood count (CBC), including the RBC count, hemoglobin concentration, and hematocrit, can establish the presence of anemia. Two additional parameters that are helpful in classifying an anemia are the mean corpuscular volume (MCV) and the reticulocyte count. Increased destruction usually is accompanied by an increase in reticulocytes (young erythrocytes containing residual RNA). Two related processes contribute to the increased number of reticulocytes in humans. First, increased destruction is accompanied by a compensatory increase in bone marrow production, with an increase in the number of cells being released from the marrow and into the circulation. Second, during compensatory erythroid hyperplasia, the marrow releases reticulocytes earlier in their life span; thus, the reticulocytes persist for a longer period in the peripheral blood.

Alterations in Red Cell Production

Erythrocyte production is a continuous process that is dependent on frequent cell division and a high rate of hemoglobin synthesis. Adult hemoglobin (hemoglobin A)

is a tetramer composed of two α-globin and two β-globin chains, each with a heme residue. Abnormalities that lead to decreased hemoglobin synthesis are relatively common (e.g., iron deficiency). Xenobiotics can affect globin-chain synthesis and alter the composition of hemoglobin within erythrocytes.

The synthesis of heme requires the incorporation of iron into a porphyrin ring (Fig. 11-1). Iron deficiency usually results from dietary deficiency or increased blood loss. Any drug that contributes to blood loss may potentiate the risk of developing *iron deficiency anemia.* Defects in the synthesis of the porphyrin ring of heme can lead to *sideroblastic anemia,* with its characteristic accumulation of iron in bone marrow erythroblasts. The accumulated iron precipitates within mitochondria, causing the intracellular injury. A number of xenobiotics (Table 11-1) interfere with one or more steps in erythroblast heme synthesis and result in sideroblastic anemia.

All hematopoietic elements of the marrow continuously proliferate to replace circulating cells. This requires active DNA synthesis and frequent mitoses. Folate and vitamin B_{12} are necessary to maintain the synthesis of thymidine for incorporation into DNA. Deficiency of folate and/or vitamin B_{12} causes *megaloblastic anemia,* which is a result of improper cell division. Xenobiotics that may contribute to a deficiency of vitamin B_{12} and/or folate are listed in Table 11-2.

Many antiproliferative agents used in the treatment of malignancy predictably inhibit hematopoiesis, including erythropoiesis. The resulting bone marrow toxicity may be dose-limiting.

Drug-induced *aplastic anemia* may represent either a predictable or an idiosyncratic reaction to a xenobiotic. This life-threatening disorder is characterized by peripheral blood pancytopenia, reticulocytopenia, and bone marrow hypoplasia; the mechanism is unknown. Agents associated with the development of aplastic anemia are listed in Table 11-3. *Pure red cell aplasia* is a syndrome in which the decrease in marrow production is limited to the erythroid lineage. The drugs most clearly implicated in this idiosyncratic reaction include isoniazid, phenytoin, and azathioprine.

Alterations in the Respiratory Function of Hemoglobin

Hemoglobin transports oxygen and carbon dioxide between the lungs and tissues. The individual globin units show cooperativity in the binding of oxygen, resulting in

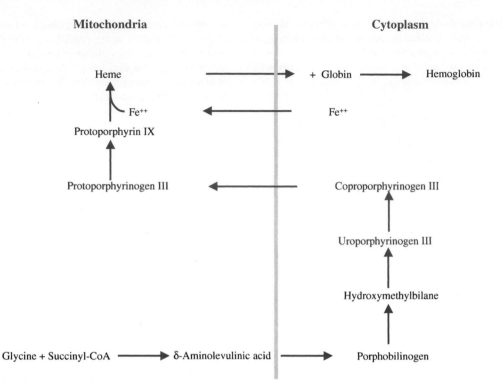

Figure 11-1. Heme and hemoglobin synthesis.   The synthesis of heme involves a series of reactions that occur in the cytoplasm and mitochondria of erythroblasts. The initial step in the pathway is the mitochondria synthesis of δ-aminolevulinic acid, a step that commonly is affected by xenobiotics, including lead. Ferrochelatase catalyzes the incorporation of ferrous iron into the tetrapyrrole protoporphyrin IX. Inhibition of the synthetic pathway leading to protoporphyrin IX, as occurs in the sideroblastic anemias, can cause an imbalance between iron concentration and ferrochelatase activity, resulting in iron deposition within mitochondria. Mitochondrial accumulation of iron is the hallmark lesion of the sideroblastic anemias.

the familiar sigmoid shape to the oxygen dissociation curve (Fig. 11-2).

Homotropic Effects Perhaps one of the most important homotropic (intrinsic) properties of oxyhemoglobin is the slow but consistent oxidation of heme iron to the fer-

Table 11-1
Xenobiotics Associated with Sideroblastic Anemia

Ethanol	Chloramphenicol
Isoniazid	Copper chelation/deficiency
Pyrazinamide	Zinc intoxication
Cycloserine	Lead intoxication

Table 11-2
Xenobiotics Associated with Megaloblastic Anemia

VITAMIN B_{12} DEFICIENCY	FOLATE DEFICIENCY
Paraminosalicylic acid	Phenytoin
Colchicine	Primidone
Neomycin	Carbamazepine
Ethanol	Phenobarbital
Omeprazole	Sulfasalazine
Hemodialysis	Cholestyramine
Zidovudine	Triamterine
Fish tapeworm	Malabsorption
	syndromes
	Antimetabolites

Table 11-3
Drugs and Chemicals Associated with the Development of Aplastic Anemia

Chloramphenicol	Organic arsenicals	Quinacrine
Methylphenylethylhydantoin	Trimethadione	Phenylbutazone
Gold	Streptomycin	Benzene
Penicillin	Allopurinol	Tetracycline
Methicillin	Sulfonamides	Chlortetracycline
Sulfisoxazole	Sulfamethoxypyridazine	Amphotericin B
Mefloquine	Ethosuximide	Felbamate
Carbimazole	Methylmercaptoimidazole	Potassium perchlorate
Propylthiouracil	Tolbutamide	Pyrimethamine
Chlorpropamide	Carbutamide	Tripelennamine
Indomethacin	Carbamazepine	Diclofenac
Meprobamate	Chlorpromazine	Chlordiazepoxide
Mepazine	Chlorphenothane	Parathion
Thiocyanate	Methazolamide	Dinitrophenol
Bismuth	Mercury	Chlordane
Carbon tetrachloride	Cimetidine	Metolazone
Azidothymidine	Ticlopidine	Isoniazid
Trifluoperazine	D-Penicillamine	

ric state to form methemoglobin, which is not capable of binding and transporting oxygen. The presence of methemoglobin in a hemoglobin tetramer results in a leftward shift of the oxygen dissociation curve (Fig. 11-2). The combination of decreased oxygen content and increased affinity may impair the delivery of oxygen to tissues significantly.

The normal erythrocyte has metabolic mechanisms for reducing heme iron back to the ferrous state. Failure of these control mechanisms leads to increased levels of methemoglobin, or *methemoglobinemia*. The large number of chemicals that cause methemoglobinemia are shown in Table 11-4. Most patients tolerate low levels (<10 percent) of methemoglobin without clinical symptoms. Higher levels lead to tissue hypoxemia that eventually is fatal.

Heterotropic Effects   There are three major heterotropic (extrinsic) effectors of hemoglobin function: pH, erythrocyte 2,3-bisphosphoglycerate (2,3-BPG, formerly designated 2,3-diphosphoglycerate) concentration, and temperature. A decrease in pH (e.g., lactic acid, carbon dioxide) lowers the affinity of hemoglobin for oxygen; that is, it causes a right shift in the oxygen dissociation curve, facilitating the delivery of oxygen to tissues. As bicarbonate and carbon dioxide equilibrate in the lung, the hydrogen ion concentration decreases, increasing the

affinity of hemoglobin for oxygen and facilitating oxygen uptake.

Binding of 2,3-BPG to deoxyhemoglobin results in reduced oxygen affinity (a shift to the right of the oxygen dissociation curve). The conformational change induced by the binding of oxygen alters the binding site for 2,3-BPG and results in the release of 2,3-BPG from hemoglobin. This facilitates the uptake of more oxygen for delivery to tissues. The concentration of 2,3-BPG increases whenever there is tissue hypoxemia but may decrease in the presence of acidosis.

The oxygen affinity of hemoglobin decreases as body temperature increases. This facilitates the delivery of oxygen to tissues during periods of extreme exercise and febrile illnesses associated with increased temperature. Correspondingly, oxygen affinity increases and delivery decreases during hypothermia.

The respiratory function of hemoglobin also may be impaired by blocking the ligand-binding site with other substances. Carbon monoxide has a relatively low rate of association with deoxyhemoglobin but shows high affinity once it is bound and causes a left shift in the oxygen dissociation curve, further compromising oxygen delivery to the tissues.

Nitric oxide, an important vasodilator that modulates vascular tone, binds avidly to heme iron. Erythrocytes can influence the availability of nitric oxide in parts of

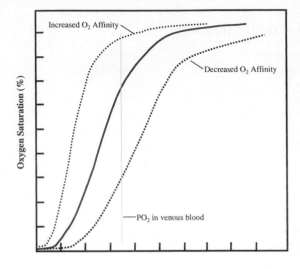

Figure 11-2. Hemoglobin-oxygen dissociation curves. The normal oxygen dissociation curve (solid line) has a sigmoid shape as a result of the cooperative interaction between the four globin chains in the hemoglobin molecule. Fully deoxygenated hemoglobin has a relatively low affinity for oxygen. Interaction of oxygen with one heme-iron moiety induces a conformational change in that globin chain. Through surface interactions, that conformational change affects the other globin chains, causing a conformational change in all the globin chains that increases their affinity for oxygen. Homotropic and heterotropic parameters also affect the affinity of hemoglobin for oxygen. An increase in oxygen affinity results in a shift to the left in the oxygen dissociation curve. Such a shift may decrease oxygen delivery to the tissues. A decrease in oxygen affinity results in a shift to the right in the oxygen dissociation curve, facilitating oxygen delivery to the tissues.

the circulation because the nitric oxide is bound to erythrocyte hemoglobin.

Alterations in Erythrocyte Survival

Erythrocytes normally circulate in blood for about 120 days. Very little protein synthesis occurs during this time, as erythrocytes are anucleate when they enter the circulation and residual mRNA is lost rapidly over the first 1 or 2 days in the circulation. Consequently, senescence occurs over time until the aged erythrocytes are removed by the spleen, where the iron is recovered for reutilization in heme synthesis.

Table 11-4
Xenobiotics Associated with Methemoglobinemia

THERAPEUTIC AGENTS	ENVIRONMENTAL AGENTS
Benzocaine	Nitrites
Lidocaine	Nitrates
Prilocaine	Nitrobenzencs
Dapsone	Aniline dyes
Amyl nitrate	Butyl nitrite
Isobutyl nitrite	Potassium chlorate
Nitroglycerine	Gasoline additives
Primaquine	Aminobenzenes
Sulfonamide	Nitrotoluenes
Phenacetin	Trinitrotoluene
Nitric oxide	Nitroethane
Phenazopyridine	
Metoclopramide	
Flutamide	
Silver nitrate	
Quinones	
Methylene blue	

Nonimmune Hemolytic Anemia

Microangiopathic Anemias Intravascular fragmentation of erythrocytes gives rise to the *microangiopathic hemolytic anemias*. The hallmark of this process is the presence of schistocytes (fragmented RBCs) in the peripheral blood. The formation of fibrin strands in the microcirculation is a common mechanism for RBC fragmentation. The erythrocytes essentially are sliced into fragments by the fibrin strands that extend across the vascular lumen and impede the flow of erythrocytes through the vasculature. Excessive fragmentation also can be seen in the presence of abnormal vasculature.

Infectious Diseases Infectious diseases may be associated with significant hemolysis by a direct effect on the erythrocyte or an immune-mediated hemolytic process. Erythrocytes are parasitized in malaria and babesiosis, leading to their destruction. Clostridial infections are associated with the release of hemolytic toxins that enter the circulation and lyse erythrocytes.

Oxidative Hemolysis Molecular oxygen is a reactive and potentially toxic chemical species; consequently, the normal respiratory function of erythrocytes generates oxidative stress on a continuous basis. Several mechanisms protect against oxidative injury in erythrocytes,

Table 11-5
Xenobiotics Associated with Oxidative Injury

Acetanilide	Phenylhydrazine
Naphthalene	Nitrobenzene
Nitrofurantoin	Phenacetin
Sulfamethoxypyridazine	Phenol
Aminosalicylic acid	Hydroxylamine
Sodium sulfoxone	Methylene blue
Dapsone	Toluidine blue
Phenazopyridine	Furazolidone
Primaquine	Nalidixic acid
Chlorates	Sulfanilamide
Sulfasalazine	

including NADH-diaphorase, superoxide dismutase, catalase, and the glutathione pathway.

Xenobiotics capable of inducing oxidative injury in erythrocytes are listed in Table 11-5. These agents appear to potentiate the normal redox reactions and are capable of overwhelming the usual protective mechanisms. The interaction between these xenobiotics and hemoglobin leads to the formation of free radicals that denature critical proteins, including hemoglobin, thiol-dependent enzymes, and components of the erythrocyte membrane. Significant oxidative injury usually occurs when the concentration of a xenobiotic is high enough to overcome the normal protective mechanisms or, more commonly, when there is an underlying defect in the protective mechanisms.

The most common enzyme defect associated with oxidative hemolysis is glucose-6-phosphate dehydrogenase (G-6-PD) deficiency, a sex-linked disorder characterized by diminished G-6-PD activity. It is often clinically asymptomatic until the erythrocytes are exposed to oxidative stress from the host response to infection or exposure to xenobiotics.

Nonoxidative Chemical-Induced Hemolysis Exposure to some xenobiotics is associated with hemolysis without significant oxidative injury. For example, inhalation of gaseous arsenic hydride (arsine) can result in severe hemolysis, with anemia, jaundice, and hemoglobinuria. Lead poisoning is associated with defects in heme synthesis, a shortening of erythrocyte survival, and hemolysis.

Immune Hemolytic Anemia Immunologic destruction of erythrocytes is mediated by the interaction of IgG or IgM antibodies with antigens expressed on the surface of the erythrocyte. In the case of autoimmune hemolytic anemia, the antigens are intrinsic components of the patient's own erythrocytes. A number of mechanisms have been implicated in xenobiotic-mediated antibody binding to erythrocytes. Some drugs, of which penicillin is a prototype, appear to bind to the surface of the cell, with the "foreign" drug acting as a *hapten* and eliciting an immune response. The antibodies that arise in this type of response bind only to drug-coated erythrocytes. Other drugs, of which quinidine is a prototype, bind to components of the erythrocyte surface and induce a conformational change in one or more components of the membrane. A third mechanism, for which α-methyldopa is a prototype, results in the production of a *drug-induced autoantibody* that cannot be distinguished from the antibodies arising in idiopathic autoimmune hemolytic anemia.

TOXICOLOGY OF THE LEUKON

Components of Blood Leukocytes

The leukon consists of leukocytes, or white blood cells, including granulocytes, which may be subdivided into neutrophils, eosinophils, and basophils; monocytes; and lymphocytes. Granulocytes and monocytes are nucleated ameboid cells that are phagocytic. They play a central role in the inflammatory response and host defense. Unlike RBCs, which reside exclusively within blood, granulocytes and monocytes merely pass through the blood on their way to the extravascular tissues, where they reside in large numbers.

Granulocytes are defined by the characteristics of their cytoplasmic granules as they appear on a blood smear. Neutrophils, the largest component of blood leukocytes, are highly specialized in the mediation of inflammation and the ingestion and destruction of pathogenic microorganisms. Eosinophils and basophils modulate inflammation through the release of various mediators.

Evaluation of Granulocytes

In the blood, neutrophils are distributed between *circulating* and *marginated* pools, which are of equal size and are in constant equilibrium. A blood neutrophil count assesses only the circulating pool, which remains remarkably constant (1800 to 7500 μL^{-1}) in a healthy adult human. During inflammation, an increased number of immature (nonsegmented) granulocytes may be seen in peripheral blood. In certain conditions, neutrophils may show morphologic changes that are indicative of toxicity.

Toxic Effects on Granulocytes

Effects on Proliferation The high rate of proliferation of neutrophils makes their progenitor and precursor granulocyte pool particularly susceptible to inhibitors of mitosis. Agents that affect both neutrophils and monocytes pose a greater risk for toxic sequelae, such as infection. Such effects tend to be dose-related, with mononuclear phagocyte recovery preceding neutrophil recovery.

Methotrexate, cytosine arabinoside, daunorubicin, cyclophosphamide, cisplatin, and the nitrosureas are toxic to resting and actively dividing cells, in which maximum effects usually are seen 7 to 14 days after exposure. Cytokines may enhance these effects. Methylmethacrylate monomer, which is used in orthopedic surgical procedures, is cytotoxic to both neutrophils and monocytes at clinically relevant concentrations.

Effects on Function Ethanol and glucocorticoids impair phagocytosis and microbe ingestion. Iohexol and ioxaglate, which are components of radiographic contrast media, also have been reported to inhibit phagocytosis. Superoxide production, which is required for microbial killing and chemotaxis, reportedly is reduced in patients who use parenteral heroin as well as in former opiate abusers on long-term methadone maintenance. Chemotaxis also is impaired after treatment with zinc salts in antiacne preparations.

Idiosyncratic Toxic Neutropenia Of greater concern are agents that unexpectedly damage neutrophils and granulocyte precursors and induce *agranulocytosis,* which is characterized by a profound depletion in blood neutrophils to less than 500 μL^{-1}. This type of injury occurs in specifically conditioned individuals and therefore is termed idiosyncratic.

Idiosyncratic xenobiotic-induced agranulocytosis may involve a sudden depletion of circulating neutrophils concomitant with exposure, which may persist as long as the agent or its metabolites persist in the circulation. Hematopoietic function usually is restored when the agent is detoxified or excreted. Toxicants that affect uncommitted stem cells induce total marrow failure, as is seen in aplastic anemia. After exposure to agents that affect more differentiated precursors, surviving uncommitted stem cells eventually produce recovery provided that the risk of infection is managed successfully during the leukopenic episodes.

Mechanisms of Toxic Neutropenia In *immune-mediated neutropenia,* antigen-antibody reactions lead to the destruction of peripheral neutrophils, granulocyte precursors, or both. As with RBCs, an immunogenic xenobiotic can act as a hapten, in which case the agent must be physically present to cause cell damage, or, alternatively, may induce immunogenic cells to produce antineutrophil antibodies that do not require the drug to be present.

Nonimmune-mediated toxic neutropenia often shows a genetic predisposition. Direct damage may cause inhibition of granulopoiesis or neutrophil function. Some studies suggest that a buildup of toxic oxidants generated by leukocytes can result in neutrophil damage.

Examples of agents associated with immune and nonimmune neutropenia/agranulocytosis are listed in Table 11-6.

Table 11-6
Examples of Toxicants That Cause Immune and Nonimmune Idiopathic Neutropenia

DRUGS ASSOCIATED WITH WBC ANTIBODIES	DRUGS NOT ASSOCIATED WITH WBC ANTIBODIES
Aminopyrine	Isoniazid
Propylthiouracil	Rifampicin
Ampicillin	Ethambutol
Metiamide	Allopurinol
Dicloxacillin	Phenothiazines
Phenytoin	Flurazepam
Aprindine	Hydrochlorothiazide
Azulfidine	
Chlorpropamide	
Phenothiazines	
Procainamide	
Nafcillin	
Tolbutamide	
Lidocaine	
Methimazole	
Levamisole	
Gold	
Quinidine	
Clozapine	

LEUKEMOGENESIS AS A TOXIC RESPONSE

Human Leukemias

Leukemias are proliferative disorders of hematopoietic tissue that oiginate from individual bone marrow cells. Historically, they have been classified as myeloid or lymphoid, referring to the major lineages for erythrocytes/granulocytes/thrombocytes and lymphocytes, respectively. Poorly differentiated phenotypes have been designated as "acute," including acute lymphoblastic leukemia (ALL) and acute myelogenous leukemia (AML), whereas well-differentiated ones are referred to as "chronic" leukemias, which include chronic lymphocytic leukemia (CLL), chronic myelogenous leukemia (CML), and the myelodysplastic syndromes (MDS).

Mechanisms of Toxic Leukemogenesis

AML is the dominant leukemia associated with drug or chemical exposure, followed by MDS. This represents a continuum of one toxic response that has been linked to cytogenetic abnormalities, particularly the loss of all or part of chromosomes 5 and 7. Remarkably, the frequency of these deletions in patients who develop MDS and/or AML after treatment with alkylating or other antineoplastic agents ranges from 67 to 95 percent, depending on the study. Some of the same changes have been observed in AML patients who have been occupationally exposed to benzene, who also show aneuploidy with a high frequency of involvement of chromosome 7. The relatively low frequency of deletions in chromosomes 5 and 7 in de novo compared with secondary AML suggests that these cytogenetic markers can be useful in discriminating between toxic exposures and other etiologies of this leukemia.

Leukemogenic Agents

Most *alkylating agents* used in cancer chemotherapy can cause MDS and/or AML. Among the *aromatic hydrocarbons,* only benzene has been proven to be leukemogenic. Treatment with the *topoisomerase II inhibitors* etoposide and teniposide can induce AML.

Exposure to *high-dose γ- or x-ray radiation* has long been associated with ALL, AML, and CML, as has been demonstrated in survivors of the atomic bombings of Nagasaki and Hiroshima. Less clear is the association of these diseases with low-dose radiation secondary to fallout or diagnostic radiographs. Other *controversial agents* include 1,3-butadiene, nonionizing radiation (electromagnetic, microwave, infrared, visible, and the high end of the ultraviolet spectrum), and cigarette smoking.

TOXICOLOGY OF PLATELETS AND HEMOSTASIS

Hemostasis is a multicomponent system that is responsible for preventing the loss of blood from sites of vascular injury and maintaining circulating blood in a fluid state. Loss of blood is prevented by the formation of stable hemostatic plugs. The major constituents of the hemostatic system include circulating platelets, a variety of plasma proteins, and vascular endothelial cells. Alterations in these components or systemic activation of this system can lead to the clinical manifestations of deranged hemostasis, including excessive bleeding and thrombosis. The hemostatic system is a common target of therapeutic intervention as well as inadvertent expression of the toxic effect of a variety of xenobiotics.

Toxic Effects on Platelets

The Thrombocyte Platelets are essential for the formation of a stable hemostatic plug in response to vascular injury. Platelets initially adhere to the damaged wall. Activation of a pathway of several factors permits fibrinogen and other multivalent adhesive molecules to form cross-links between nearby platelets, resulting in platelet aggregation. Xenobiotics may interfere with the platelet response by causing thrombocytopenia or interfering with platelet function.

Thrombocytopenia Like anemia, thrombocytopenia may be due to decreased production or increased destruction. Thrombocytopenia is a common side effect of intensive chemotherapy because of the predictable effect of antiproliferative agents on hematopoietic precursors. Thrombocytopenia is a clinically significant component of idiosyncratic xenobiotic-induced aplastic anemia. Indeed, the initial manifestation of aplastic anemia may be mucocutaneous bleeding secondary to thrombocytopenia.

Exposure to xenobiotics may cause increased immune-mediated platelet destruction through any of several mechanisms. Some drugs, such as penicillin, function as haptens, binding to platelet membrane components and eliciting an immune response that is specific for the hapten. The responding antibody then binds to the hapten on the platelet surface, leading to removal of the antibody-coated platelet from the circulation.

A second mechanism of immune thrombocytopenia is initiated by a change in a platelet membrane glycoprotein caused by the xenobiotic. This altered protein then elicits an antibody response. The responding antibody binds to the altered platelet antigen in the presence of drug, resulting in removal of the platelet from the circulation by the mononuclear phagocytic system.

Thrombocytopenia is an uncommon but serious complication of inhibitors of factors involved in the clot-formation cascade. These inhibitors can change the comformation of those factors, causing exposure of certain peptides (called neoepitopes because they are newly exposed to the immune system) on the factors that react with endogenous antibodies. This leads to phagocytosis of the platelets associated with these factors. Thus, exposure of epitopes that react with naturally occurring antibodies represents a third mechanism of immune-mediated platelet destruction.

Heparin-induced thrombocytopenia represents a fourth mechanism of immune-mediated platelet destruction. When heparin (an anticoagulant) binds to certain clotting factors, a neoepitope is exposed, and an immune response then is mounted against the neoepitope. This results in platelet aggregation instead of heparin's normal function of preventing clot formation, which can lead to a risk of thrombosis (pieces of clots falling off and lodging in the microvasculature, impairing circulation).

Thrombotic thrombocytopenic purpura (TTP) is a syndrome characterized by the sudden onset of thrombocytopenia, a microangiopathic hemolytic anemia, and multisystem organ failure. The syndrome tends to occur after an infectious disease but also may occur after the administration of some pharmacologic agents. The pathogenesis of TTP appears to be related to the ability of a clotting factor called von Willebrand's factor (vWF) to activate platelets even in the absence of significant vascular damage. Acquired TTP is associated with the development of an antibody that inhibits the protease responsible for processing very large vWF multimers into smaller multimers; the large multimers inappropriately activate the platelets. The organ failure and hemolysis in TTP are due to the formation of platelet-rich microthrombi throughout the circulation. The development of TTP or TTP-like syndromes has been associated with drugs such as ticlopidine, clopidogrel, cocaine, mitomycin, and cyclosporine.

Toxic Effects on Platelet Function Platelet function is dependent on the coordinated interaction of a number of biochemical response pathways. Major drug groups that affect platelet function include nonsteroidal anti-

inflammatory agents; β-lactam-containing antibiotics; cardiovascular drugs, particularly beta blockers; psychotropic drugs; anesthetics; antihistamines; and some chemotherapeutic agents.

Xenobiotics may interfere with platelet function through a variety of mechanisms. Some drugs inhibit the phospholipase A_2/cyclooxygenase pathway and the synthesis of thromboxane A_2 (e.g., nonsteroidal anti-inflammatory agents). Other agents appear to interfere with the interaction between platelet agonists and their receptors (e.g., antibiotics, ticlopidine, clopidogrel). As the platelet response is dependent on a rapid increase in cytoplasmic calcium, any agent that interferes with the translocation of calcium may inhibit platelet function (e.g., calcium channel blockers). Occasionally, drug-induced antibodies bind to a critical platelet receptor and inhibit its function.

Toxic Effects on Fibrin Clot Formation

Coagulation Fibrin clot formation results from the sequential activation of a series of serine proteases that culminates in the formation of thrombin. Thrombin is a multifunctional enzyme that converts fibrinogen to fibrin; activates factors V, VIII, XI, and XIII, protein C, and platelets; and interacts with a variety of cells (e.g., leukocytes and endothelial cells), activating cellular signaling pathways.

Decreased Synthesis of Coagulation Proteins Most proteins involved in the coagulation cascade are synthesized in the liver. Therefore, any agent that impairs liver function may cause a decrease in the production of coagulation factors. The common tests of the coagulation cascade—prothrombin time (PT) and activated partial thromboplastin time (aPTT)—may be used to screen for liver dysfunction and a decrease in clotting factors.

Factors II, VII, IX, and X are dependent on vitamin K for their complete synthesis. Anything that interferes with the absorption of vitamin K from the intestine or with the reduction of vitamin K epoxide may lead to a deficiency of these factors and a bleeding tendency (Table 11-7).

Increased Clearance of Coagulation Factors Idiosyncratic reactions to xenobiotics include the formation of antibodies that react with coagulation proteins, forming an immune complex that is cleared rapidly from the circulation and resulting in deficiency of the factor. The

Table 11-7
Conditions Associated with Abnormal Synthesis of Vitamin K–Dependent Coagulation Factors

Warfarin and analogs	Intravenous α-tocopherol
Rodenticides (e.g., brodifacoum)	Dietary deficiency
	Cholestyramine resin
Broad-spectrum antibiotics	Malabsorption syndromes
N-Methyl-thiotetrazole cephalosporins	

factors that are affected by xenobiotics most often are listed in Table 11-8. In addition to causing increased clearance from the circulation, these antibodies often inhibit the function of the coagulation factor.

Table 11-8
Relationship between Xenobiotics and the Development of Specific Coagulation Factor Inhibitors

COAGULATION FACTOR	XENOBIOTIC
Thrombin	Topical bovine thrombin
	Fibrin glue
Factor V	Streptomycin
	Penicillin
	Gentamicin
	Cephalosporins
	Topical bovine thrombin
Factor VIII	Penicillin
	Ampicillin
	Chloramphenicol
	Phenytoin
	Methyldopa
	Nitrofurazone
	Phenylbutazone
Factor XIII	Isoniazid
	Procainamide
	Penicillin
	Phenytoin
	Practolol
Von Willebrand factor	Ciprofloxacin
	Hydroxyethyl starch
	Valproic acid
	Griseofulvin
	Tetracycline
	Pesticides

Lupus anticoagulants are antibodies that can potentiate procoagulant mechanisms and interfere with the protein C system, increasing the risk of thrombosis. The development of lupus anticoagulants has been seen in association with chlorpromazine, procainamide, hydralazine, quinidine, phenytoin, and viral infections.

Toxicology of Agents Used to Modulate Hemostasis

Oral Anticoagulants The therapeutic window for oral anticoagulants (warfarin) is relatively narrow, and there is considerable interindividual variation in the response to a given dose. The consequence of insufficient anticoagulant effect is an increased risk of thromboembolism, whereas the consequence of excessive anticoagulation is an increased risk of bleeding. Therapy with these agents must be monitored routinely with PT, with the results expressed in terms of the international normalized ratio (INR).

Oral anticoagulants are absorbed readily from the gastrointestinal tract and bind avidly to albumin in the circulation. Genetic polymorphisms influence the biotransformation and the response to oral anticoagulants.

A number of xenobiotics, including foods, have been found to affect the response to oral anticoagulants. Mechanisms for interference with oral anticoagulants include induction or inhibition of biotransformation; interference with the absorption of warfarin from the gastrointestinal tract; displacement of warfarin from albumin in plasma, which temporarily increases the bioavailability of warfarin until equilibrium is reestablished; diminished vitamin K availability; and inhibition of the reduction of vitamin K epoxide, which potentiates the effect of oral anticoagulants.

The administration of oral anticoagulants may affect the activity or the half-lives of other medications.

Oral anticoagulants have been associated with warfarin-induced skin necrosis. The development of microvascular thrombosis in skin occurs most commonly in patients who are deficient in protein C or protein S.

Vitamin K is also necessary for the synthesis of osteocalcin, a major component of bone. Long-term administration of warfarin has been associated with bone demineralization.

Administration of warfarin, particularly during the first 12 weeks of pregnancy, is associated with congenital anomalies in 25 to 30 percent of exposed infants. Many of the anomalies are related to abnormal bone formation. It is thought that warfarin may interfere with the synthesis of additional proteins that are critical for normal structural development.

Heparin Heparin is used widely for both prophylaxis and therapy for acute venous thromboembolism. The major complication associated with heparin therapy is bleeding. The aPTT commonly is used to monitor therapy with unfractionated heparin. Long-term administration of heparin is associated with an increased risk of clinically significant osteoporosis. Also, heparin administration may cause a transient rise in serum aminotransferases.

Fibrinolytic Agents Fibrinolytic agents dissolve the pathogenic thrombus by converting plasminogen, an inactive zymogen, to plasmin, an active proteolytic enzyme. Plasmin normally is tightly regulated and is not freely present in the circulation. However, the administration of fibrinolytic agents regularly results in the generation of free plasmin, leading to systemic fibrin(ogen)olysis, which is characterized by prolongation of PT, aPTT, and thrombin time. All these effects potentiate the risk of bleeding. Platelet inhibitors and heparin commonly are used in conjunction with fibrinolytic therapy to prevent recurrent thrombosis.

Streptokinase is a protein derived from group C β-hemolytic streptococci and is antigenic in humans. Antibody formation to streptokinase occurs commonly in association with streptococcal infections as well as exposure to streptokinase. Acute allergic reactions may occur in 1 to 5 percent of patients exposed to streptokinase. Allergic reactions also occur with other fibrinolytic agents that contain streptokinase (e.g., anisoylated plasminogen-streptokinase complex) and streptokinase-derived peptides.

Inhibitors of Fibrinolysis Inhibitors of fibrinolysis commonly are used to control bleeding in patients with congenital abnormalities of hemostasis, such as von Willebrand disease. Tranexamic acid and ε-aminocaproic acid are small molecules that block the binding of plasminogen and plasmin to fibrin. Aprotinin is a naturally occurring polypeptide inhibitor of serine proteases that is immunogenic when administered to humans.

RISK ASSESSMENT

Assessing the risk that exposure to new chemical products poses to humans in terms of significant toxic effects on hematopoiesis and the functional integrity of blood cells and hemostatic mechanisms is challenging. This is due in part to the complexity of hematopoiesis and the range of important tasks that these components perform.

Risk assessment includes preclinical testing of animals and clinical trials in humans. It is hoped that in preclinical trials, the test animals will react similarly to humans upon exposure to the xenobiotic, and the animals are examined in detail for signs of toxicity. Subsequent clinical trials are conducted in humans and measure myriad parameters of potential toxicity to determine the relative safety or toxicity of the test substance.

Tests used to assess blood and bone marrow in preclinical toxicology studies should provide information on the effects of single- and multiple-dose exposure on erythrocyte parameters (RBC, hemoglobin, packed cell volume, mean corpuscular volume, mean corpuscular hemoglobin concentration), leukocyte parameters (white blood cells and absolute differential counts), thrombocyte counts, coagulation tests (PT, aPTT), peripheral blood cell morphology, and bone marrow cytologic and histologic examinations. Additional tests should be employed in a problem-driven fashion as required to better characterize hematotoxicologic potential. Examples of these tests are listed in Table 11-9.

Patient or population-related risk factors include pharmacogenetic variations in drug metabolism and detoxification that lead to reduced clearance of the agent or the production of novel intermediate metabolites, histocompatibility antigens, interaction with drugs or other agents, increased sensitivity of hematopoietic precursors to damage, preexisting disease of the bone marrow, and

Table 11-9

Examples of Problem-Driven Tests Used to Characterize Hematologic Observations in Preclinical Toxicology

Reticulocyte count
Heinz body preparation
Cell-associated antibody assays (erythrocyte, platelet, neutrophil)
Erythrocyte osmotic fragility test
Erythrokinetic/ferrokinetic analyses
Cytochemical/histochemical staining
Electron microscopy
In vitro hematopoietic clonogenic assays
Platelet aggregation
Plasma fibrinogen concentration
Clotting factor assays
Thrombin time
Bleeding time

metabolic defects that predispose to oxidative or other stresses associated with the agent.

A central issue in drug and nontherapeutic chemical development is the *predictive value* of preclinical toxi-cology data and the expansive but inevitably limited clinical database for the occurrence of significant hema-totoxicity upon broad exposure of human populations.

BIBLIOGRAPHY

Beutler E, Lichtman MA, Coller BS, et al (eds): *Williams Hematology,* 6th ed. New York: McGraw-Hill, 2000.

Bloom JC (ed): *Toxicology of the Hematopoietic System,* vol 4, in Sipes IG, McQueen CA, Gandolfi AJ (eds): *Comprehensive Toxicology.* Oxford: Pergamon Press, 1997.

Handin RI, Lux SE, Stossel TP: *Blood. Principles and Practice of Hematology,* 2d ed. Philadelphia: Lippincott Williams & Wilkins, 2002.

Hillman R, Ault KA: *Hematology in Clinical Practice: A Guide to Diagnosis and Management.* New York: McGraw-Hill, 2001.

Young NS: Hematopoietic cell destruction by immune mechanisms in acquired aplastic anemia. *Semin Hematol* 37:3–14, 2000.

CHAPTER 12

TOXIC RESPONSES OF THE IMMUNE SYSTEM

Leigh Ann Burns-Naas, B. Jean Meade, and Albert E. Munson

KEY POINTS

- Immunity is a series of delicately balanced, complex, multicellular, and physiologic mechanisms that allow an individual to distinguish foreign material from "self" and neutralize and/or eliminate that foreign matter.

- Innate immunity, which eliminates most potential pathogens before significant infection occurs, includes physical and biochemical barriers both inside and outside the body as well as immune cells designed for specific responses.

- Acquired immunity involves producing a specific immune response to each infectious agent (*specificity*) and remembering that agent in order to mount a faster response to a future infection by the same agent (*memory*).

- Autoimmunity involves a breakdown in the mechanisms of self-recognition; immunoglobulins and T-cell receptors react with self-antigens, resulting in tissue damage and disease.

- Hypersensitivity reactions require prior exposure leading to sensitization to elicit a reaction upon a subsequent challenge.

- Xenobiotics that alter the immune system can upset the balance between immune recognition and destruction of foreign invaders and the proliferation of those microbes and/or cancer cells.

Immunity is a homeostatic process, a series of delicately balanced, complex, multicellular, and physiologic mechanisms that allow an individual to distinguish foreign material from "self" and neutralize and/or eliminate the foreign matter. Decreased immunocompetence (immunosuppression) may result in repeated, more severe, or prolonged infections as well as the development of cancer. Immunoenhancement may lead to immune-mediated diseases such as hypersensitivity responses or autoimmune disease.

THE IMMUNE SYSTEM

The immune system includes numerous lymphoid organs and many different cellular populations with a variety of functions. The bone marrow and the thymus support the production of mature T and B lymphocytes and myeloid cells such as macrophages and polymorphonuclear cells and are referred to as primary lymphoid organs.

Within the bone marrow, the cells of the immune system developmentally "commit" to either the lymphoid lineage or the myeloid lineage. Cells of the lymphoid lin-

eage make a further commitment to become either T cells or B cells. T-cell precursors are programmed to leave the bone marrow and migrate to the thymus, where they differentiate further.

Mature naive or virgin lymphocytes (T and B cells that have never undergone antigenic stimulation) are first brought into contact with exogenously derived antigens in the spleen and lymph nodes, otherwise known as the secondary lymphoid organs.

Lymphoid tissues associated with the skin and the mucosal lamina propria of the gut, respiratory tract, and genitourinary tract can be classified as tertiary lymphoid tissues. Tertiary lymphoid tissues are primarily effector sites where memory and effector cells exert immunologic and immunoregulatory functions.

Innate Immunity

General Considerations Innate immunity acts as a first line of defense against infectious agents, eliminating most potential pathogens before significant infection occurs. It includes physical and biochemical barriers both inside and outside the body as well as immune cells designed for specific responses. No immunologic memory is associated with innate immunity.

Most infectious agents enter the body through the respiratory system, gut, or genitourinary tract, whereas the skin provides an effective barrier. Innate defenses include mucus secreted along the nasopharynx, the presence of lysozyme in most secretions, and cilia lining the trachea and the main bronchi. In addition, reflexes such as coughing, sneezing, and elevation of body temperature are parts of innate immunity. Pathogens that enter the body through the digestive tract are met with severe changes in pH (acidic) in the stomach and a host of microorganisms living in the intestines.

Cellular Components: NK, PMN, Macrophage Two general types of cells are involved in nonspecific (innate) host resistance: natural killer (NK) cells and professional phagocytes. NK cells can recognize virally infected and malignant changes on the surface of cells as well as antibody-coated target cells. The latter form of recognition is utilized in cell-mediated immunity. Using surface receptors, the NK cell binds, expels cytolytic granules, and induces apoptosis of the target cell.

Phagocytic cells include polymorphonuclear cells (PMNs; neutrophils) and the monocyte/macrophage, which develop from pluripotent stem cells that have become committed to the myeloid lineage (Fig. 12-1). PMNs are excellent phagocytic cells and can eliminate most microorganisms and induce an inflammatory response.

Macrophages are terminally differentiated monocytes. Upon exiting the bone marrow, monocytes are distributed to the various tissues, where they can differentiate into macrophages. Within different tissues, macrophages have distinct properties and vary in the extent of their surface receptors, oxidative metabolism, and expression of major histocompatibility complex (MHC) class II.

If PMNs are unable to contain an infection, macrophages are recruited to the site of infection. Macrophages have both phagocytic and bactericidal functions and also can function as antigen-presenting cells. They are recruited to sites of inflammation by chemotactic factors, can be activated by cytokines to become more effective killers, and can produce cytokines. Macrophages also play a critical role as scavengers in the daily turnover of senescent tissues such as red cell nuclei from maturing red cells, PMNs, and plasma cells.

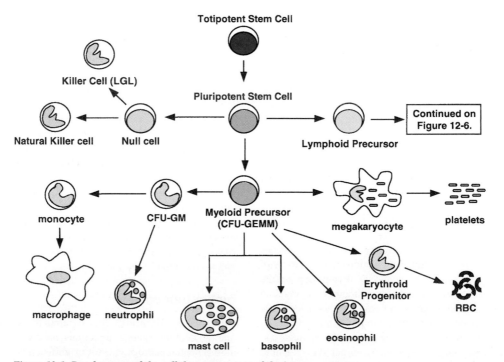

Figure 12-1. Development of the cellular components of the immune system.

Table 12-1
Innate versus Acquired Immunity

CHARACTERISTIC	INNATE IMMUNITY	ACQUIRED IMMUNITY
Cells involved	Polymorphonuclear cells (PMN)	T cells
		B cells
	Monocyte/macrophage	Macrophages
	NK cells	NK cells
Primary soluble mediators	Complement	Antibody
	Lysozyme	Cytokines
	Acute-phase proteins	
	Interferon-α/β	
	Other cytokines	
Specificity of response	None	Yes (very high specificity)
Response enhanced by repeated antigen challenge	No	Yes

Soluble Factors: Acute-Phase Proteins and Complement Soluble components of innate immunity (Table 12-1) are the acute-phase proteins and complement. Upon infection, macrophages become activated and secrete various cytokines, which are carried by the bloodstream to distant sites. This global response to foreign agents is termed the *acute-phase response* and consists of fever and large shifts in the types of serum proteins synthesized by hepatocytes. These proteins can bind to bacteria through a process called opsonization and facilitate the binding of complement and the subsequent uptake of the bacteria by phagocytic cells.

The complement system consists of about 30 serum proteins whose primary functions are the modification of membranes of infectious agents and the promotion of an inflammatory response. Complement activation occurs, with each component sequentially acting on others to coat the foreign cell and disrupt membrane integrity without harming the host cells. The complement-coated material is targeted for elimination by interaction with complement receptors on the surface of circulating immune cells.

Acquired (Adaptive) Immunity

General Considerations If the primary defenses against infection (innate immunity) are breached, the acquired arm of the immune system is activated and produces a specific immune response to each infectious agent. This branch of immunity can protect the host from future infection by the same agent. Therefore, two key features that distinguish acquired immunity are *specificity* and *memory*. This means that in a normal healthy adult, the speed and magnitude of the immune response to a foreign organism are greater for a secondary challenge than they are for the primary challenge (Table 12-1).

Essential to the development of specific immunity is the recognition of an antigen and the generation of an antibody that can bind to it. An antigen is defined functionally as a substance that can elicit the production of a specific antibody and can be specifically bound by that antibody. Small antigens are termed *haptens* and must be conjugated with carrier molecules (larger antigens) to elicit a specific response.

Antibodies, which are proteins classified as immunoglobulins, are produced by B cells and are defined functionally by the antigens with which they react (i.e., anti-sheep red blood cell IgM). There are five types of immunoglobulin that are related structurally (Table 12-2): IgM, IgG (and subsets), IgE, IgD, and IgA. All immunoglobulins are made up of heavy and light chains and have constant (Fc) and variable regions. It is the variable regions that determine antibody specificity. The variable region interacts with an antigen, whereas the Fc region mediates effector functions such as complement fixation and phagocyte binding (via Fc receptors). Antibodies also coat foreign cells to help with opsonization, initiate the complement cascade that leads to cell lysis, bind to viral particles, and bind to antigens on target cells to help NK cells and cytotoxic T lymphocytes destroy them.

During an immune response the cells of the immune system communicate by means of a vast network of soluble mediators: the cytokines. Nearly all immune cells

Table 12-2
Properties of Immunoglobulin Classes and Subclasses

CLASS	MEAN SERUM CONCENTRATION mg/mL	HUMAN HALF-LIFE days	BIOLOGICAL PROPERTIES
IgG			Complement fixation (selected subclasses) Crosses placenta Heterocytotropic antibody
Subclasses			
IgG$_1$	9	21	
IgG$_2$	3	20	
IgG$_3$	1	7	
IgG$_4$	1	21	
IgA	3	6	Secretory antibody
IgM	1.5	10	Complement fixation Efficient agglutination
IgD	0.03	3	Possible role in antigen-triggered lymphocyte differentiation
IgE	0.0001	2	Allergic responses (mast cell degranulation)

secrete cytokines, which may have local or systemic effects. Table 12-3 provides a brief summary of the sources and functions of cytokines.

Cellular Components: APCs, T Cells, B Cells To elicit a specific immune response to a particular antigen, that antigen must be taken up and processed by accessory cells called antigen-presenting cells (APCs) for presentation to lymphocytes. The macrophage plays a critical role as an APC in acquired immunity. Although thought about more for its ability to produce immunoglobulin, the B cell also can serve as an APC.

APCs and lymphocytes interact during the immune response. APCs absorb the antigen, cut it into pieces, and then display a piece of the antigen on its cell surface attached to a complex of proteins called MHC II.

Besides serving as APCs, B lymphocytes are the effector cells of humoral immunity, producing a number of isotypes of immunoglobulin (Ig) with varying specificities and affinities. Upon antigen binding to surface Ig, a mature B cell becomes activated and, after proliferation, undergoes differentiation into either a memory B cell or an antibody-forming cell (AFC; plasma cell), actively secreting antigen-specific antibody.

T cells undergo a complex process of maturation in which only cells that do not recognize self but do bind to MHC II proteins and recognize foreign antigens survive. These cells become either T-helper cells (which carry a certain protein on their surface called CD4$^+$ and work by facilitating the B-cell response) or T-cytotoxic cells (which carry CD8$^+$ and mediate cell killing).

Humoral and Cell-Mediated Immunity

The activation of antigen-specific T cells begins with the interaction of the T-cell receptor with MHC class II+ peptide. Upon activation and in the presence of interleukin-1 (IL-1) secreted by the APC, T cells begin to produce the T-cell growth factor IL-2 and express receptors for them. As T cells begin to proliferate, they secrete numerous lymphokines (Table 12-3), which can influence many aspects of the immune response. The next step in the generation of the humoral response is the interaction of activated T cells with B cells. This may be a direct interaction of a T cell with a B cell (antigen-specific) or may simply involve the production of lymphokines, which lead to B-cell growth and differentiation into antibody plaque-forming cells or memory B cells. A general diagram of the cellular interactions involved in the humoral immune response is presented in Fig. 12-2. The production of antigen-specific IgM requires 3 to 5 days

Table 12-3
Cytokines: Sources and Functions in Immune Regulation

CYTOKINE	SOURCE	PHYSIOLOGIC ACTIONS
IL-1	Macrophages	Activation and proliferation of T cells (Th2>Th1)
	B cells	Proinflammatory
	Several nonimmune cells	Induces fever and acute-phase proteins
		Induces synthesis of IL-8 and TNF-α
IL-2	T cells	Primary T-cell growth factor
		Growth factor for B cells and NK cells
		Enhances lymphokine production
IL-3	T cells	Stimulates the proliferation and differentiation of stromal cells, progenitors of the macrophage,
	Mast cells	granulocyte, and erythroid lineages
IL-4	T cells	Proliferation of activated T (Th2>Th1) and B cells
	Mast cells	B-cell differentiation and isotype switching may
	Stromal cells	inhibit some macrophage functions
	Basophils	Antagonizes IFN-γ
	CD4$^+$/NK1.1$^+$ cells	Inhibits IL-8 production
IL-5	T cells	Proliferation and differentiation of eosinophils
	Mast cells	Promotes B-cell isotype switching
		Synergizes with IL-4 to induce secretion of IgE
IL-6	Macrophages	Enhances B-cell differentiation and immunoglobulin
	Activated T cells	secretion
	B cells	Induction of acute phase proteins by liver
	Fibroblasts	Proinflammatory
	Keratinocytes	Proliferation of T cells and increased IL-2 receptor
	Endothelial cells	expression
	Hepatocytes	Synergizes with IL-4 to induce secretion of IgE
IL-7	Stromal cells	Proliferation of thymocytes (CD4$^-$/CD8$^-$)
	Epithelial cells	Proliferation of pro- and pre-B cells (mice)
		T-cell growth
IL-8	Macrophages	Activation and chemotaxis of monocytes, neutrophils,
	Platelets	basophils and T cells
	Fibroblasts	Proinflammatory
	NK cells	
	Keratinocytes	
	Hepatocytes	
	Endothelial cells	
IL-9	Th cells	T-cell growth factor (primarily CD4$^+$ cells)
		Enhances mast-cell activity
		Stimulates growth of early erythroid progenitors
IL-10	T cells	Inhibits macrophage cytolytic activity and macrophage
	Macrophages	activation of T cells
	B cells	General inhibitor of cytokine synthesis by Th1 cells
		(in presence of APCs)
		Enhances CD8$^+$ T cell cytolytic activity
		Enhances proliferation of activated B cells
		Mast-cell growth
		Anti-inflammatory
		Inhibits endotoxin shock

(continued)

Table 12-3
Cytokines: Sources and Functions in Immune Regulation *(continued)*

CYTOKINE	SOURCE	PHYSIOLOGIC ACTIONS
IL-11	Fibroblasts Stromal cells	Megakaryocyte growth factor Enhances T cell–dependent B-cell immunoglobulin synthesis Enhances IL-6–induced plasma cell differentiation Stimulates platelets, neutrophils, and erythrocytes Induces acute-phase proteins
IL-12	Macrophages B cells	Proliferation and cytolytic action of NK cells Activation, proliferation, and cytolytic action of CTL Stimulates production of IFN-γ Proliferation of activated T cells Decreases IgG$_1$ and IgE primary response
IL-13	T cells	Stimulates class II expression on APC Enhances antigen processing by APC Enhances B-cell differentiation and isotype switching Anti-inflammatory (inhibits synthesis of proinflammatory cytokines) Inhibits antibody-dependent cellular cytotoxicity (ADCC)
IL-14	T cells Some malignant B cells	Enhances B-cell proliferation Inhibition of immunoglobulin secretion Selective expansion of some B-cell subpopulations
IL-15	Activated monocytes Macrophages Several nonimmune cells	NK-cell activation T-cell proliferation Mast-cell growth
IL-16	T cells Mast cells Eosinophils	Chemoattractant for T cells, eosinophils, and monocytes Promotes CD4$^+$ T-cell adhesion Increases expression of IL-2 receptor Promotes synthesis of IL-3, GM-CSF, and IFN-γ Proinflammatory May exacerbate allergic reactions
IL-17	CD4$^+$ memory T cells	Induced production of IL-6, IL-8, G-CSF, and PGE$_2$ Enhances proliferation of activated T cells Inducer of stromal cell–derived proinflammatory cytokines Inducer of stromal cell–derived hematopoietic cytokines
IL-18	Hepatocytes	Synergizes with IL-12 to enhance the activity of Th1 cells Enhances production of IFN-γ
Interferon-α/β (IFN-α/β) (Type 1 IFN)	Leukocytes Epithelial cells Fibroblasts	Induction of class I expression Antiviral activity Stimulation of NK cells
Interferon-γ (IFN-γ)	T cells NK cells Epithelial cells Fibroblasts	Induction of class I and II Activates macrophages (as APC and cytolytic cells) Improves CTL recognition of virally infected cells
Tumor necrosis factor (TNF-α) and	Macrophages Lymphocytes Mast cells	Induces inflammatory cytokines Increases vascular permeability Activates macrophages and neutrophils

(continued)

Table 12-3
Cytokines: Sources and Functions in Immune Regulation *(continued)*

CYTOKINE	SOURCE	PHYSIOLOGIC ACTIONS
lymphotoxin (TNF-β)		Tumor necrosis (direct action)
		Primary mediator of septic shock
		Interferes with lipid metabolism (result is cachexia)
		Induction of acute-phase proteins
Transforming growth factor-β (TGF-β)	Macrophages Megakaryocytes Chondrocytes	Enhances monocyte/macrophage chemotaxis
		Enhances wound healing: angiogenesis, fibroblast proliferation, deposition of extracellular matrix
		Inhibits T- and B-cell proliferation
		Inhibits macrophage cytokine synthesis
		Inhibits antibody secretion
		Primary inducer of isotype switch to IgA
GM-CSF	T cells Macrophages Endothelial cells Fibroblasts	Stimulates growth and differentiation of monocytes and granulocytes
Migration inhibitory factor (MIF)	T cells Anterior pituitary cells Monocytes	Inhibits macrophage migration
		Proinflammatory (induces TNF-α production by macrophages)
		Appears to play a role in delayed hypersensitivity responses
		May be a counterregulator of glucocorticoid activity
Erythropoietin (EPO)	Endothelial cells Fibroblasts	Stimulates maturation of erythrocyte precursors

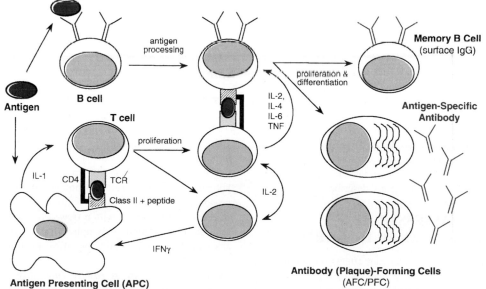

Figure 12-2. Cellular interactions in the antibody response.

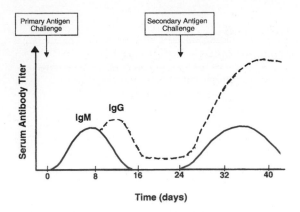

Figure 12-3. Kinetics of the antibody response.

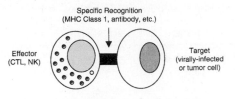

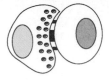

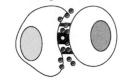

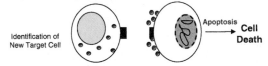

Figure 12-4. Cell-mediated cytotoxicity.

after the primary (initial) exposure to antigen (Fig. 12-3). Upon secondary antigen challenge, the B cells undergo isotype switching, producing primarily IgG antibody, which is of higher affinity. In addition, a higher serum antibody titer is associated with a secondary antibody response.

There are two general forms of cell-mediated immunity (CMI), referred to as delayed-type hypersensitivity and cell-mediated cytotoxicity. Delayed-type hypersensitivity is presented later in this chapter in the section "Immune-Mediated Disease." In cell-mediated cytotoxicity, the effector cell [cytotoxic T-lymphocytes (CTLs) or NK] binds in a specific manner to the target cell (Fig. 12-4), and the effector cell then releases the contents of its cytolytic granules onto the target cell, causing it to undergo programmed cell death.

Neuroendocrine Immunology

There is overwhelming evidence that cytokines, neuropeptides, neurotransmitters, and hormones are an integral and interregulated part of the central nervous system, the endocrine system, and the immune system. The triad of the influences these three systems exert on one another is bidirectional. Some selected outcomes of neuroendocrine actions on immunity are described in Table 12-4.

ASSESSMENT OF IMMUNOLOGIC INTEGRITY

Xenobiotics can have significant effects on the immune system. Among the unique features of immune cells is their ability to be removed from the body and function

in vitro. This unique quality offers the toxicologist an opportunity to evaluate the actions of xenobiotics on the immune system comprehensively.

Methods to Assess Immunocompetence

General Assessment All studies of immunocompetence should include toxicologic studies (such as organ weights, serum characteristics, hematologic parameters, and bone marrow function) to investigate the effects of immune modulation on other body organs. Histopathology of lymphoid organs also may provide insight into potential immunotoxicants. Moreover, the use of fluorescently labeled monoclonal antibodies to cell surface markers in conjunction with a flow cytometer allows an accurate enumeration of lymphocyte subsets and indicates whether a xenobiotic may affect maturation.

Functional Assessment *Innate Immunity* Innate immunity encompasses all the immunologic responses that

Table 12-4
Reported Influences of Neuroendocrine Factors on Immunity*

	CYTOKINE PRODUCTION	NK ACTIVITY	MACROPHAGE ACTIVITY	T CELL ACTIVITY	HUMORAL IMMUNITY
ACTH	↓	↓	↓	↓	↓
Prolactin	↑	?	↑	↑	↑
Growth Hormone	↑	↑	↑	↑	↑
α Endorphins	↑	↑	↑	↓	↓
β Endorphins	↑	↑	↑	↓	↑
Enkephalins	↑	↑	?	?	↓
Substance P	?	↑	↑	↑	↑
hCG	?	↓	?	↓	?
Chemical sympathectomy	↑	?	?	↑↓	↑
Norepinephrine	?	?	?	↓	↑↓
Epinephrine	?	?	?	↓	↑↓

KEY: ACTH, adrenocorticotropic hormone; hCG, human chorionic gonadotropin; ↑, generally enhanced responses; ↓, generally decreased responses; ↑↓, both enhanced and suppressed responses have been reported and may depend on receptor types or subclass of chemical or time of exposure relative to antigen challenge; ?, generally unknown.

do not require prior exposure to an antigen and that are nonspecific in nature. These responses include recognition of tumor cells by NK cells, phagocytosis of pathogens by macrophages, and the lytic activity of the complement system.

To evaluate phagocytic activity, macrophages are placed in culture plates and incubated with radiolabeled red blood cells. The cells that are not bound by the macrophages are removed, as are the cells that are bound but not phagocytized. The macrophages then are lysed to determine the number of cells that were phagocytized. This test provides information about both the binding and the phagocytizing activity of the macrophages and also can be performed in vivo by measuring the uptake of the radiolabeled red blood cells by certain tissue macrophages.

Another method for evaluating phagocytosis in vitro is to evaluate the uptake of latex spheres by macrophages. Evaluation of the ability of NK cells to lyse tumor cells is achieved by incubating radiolabeled target cells with NK cells and measuring the amount of radioactivity released into solution from the target cells.

Acquired Immunity—Humoral The plaque (antibody)-forming cell (PFC or AFC) assay tests the ability of the host to mount an antibody response to a specific antigen, which requires the coordinated interaction of several dif-

ferent immune cells: macrophages, T cells, and B cells. Therefore, an effect on any of these cells (e.g., antigen processing and presentation, cytokine production, proliferation, or differentiation) can have a profound impact on the ability of B cells to produce antigen-specific antibody.

A standard PFC assay involves immunizing mice with sheep red blood cells (sRBCs). The antigen is taken up in the spleen, and an antibody response occurs. Four days after immunization, spleens are removed and splenocytes are mixed with sRBCs, complement, and agar; the mixture is plated and incubated until the B cells secrete anti-sRBC IgM antibody. This antibody then coats the surrounding sRBCs, and areas of hemolysis (plaques) can be seen.

The PFC assay can be evaluated in vivo by using serum from the peripheral blood of immunized mice and an enzyme-linked immunosorbent assay (ELISA; Fig. 12-5).

Serum from mice immunized with sRBCs is incubated in microtiter plates that have been coated with sRBC membranes to serve as the antigen for sRBC-specific IgM or IgG to bind. After incubation, an enzyme-conjugated monoclonal antibody (the secondary antibody) against IgM (or IgG) is added. This antibody recognizes the IgM (or IgG) and binds specifically to that antibody. Then the enzyme substrate (chromogen) is added. When the substrate comes into contact with the

1. Bind antigen to plate. Wash.

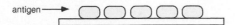

antigen ⟶

2. Add test sera and incubate. Wash.

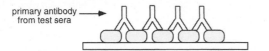

primary antibody
from test sera ⟶

3. Add enzyme-coupled secondary antibody. Wash.

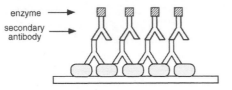

enzyme ⟶
secondary antibody ⟶

4. Add chromogen and develop color.

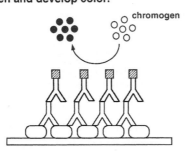

○ chromogen

Figure 12-5. Schematic diagram of a standard enzyme-linked immunosorbent assay (ELISA).

enzyme on the secondary antibody, a color change occurs that can be detected by measuring absorbance with a plate reader.

Humoral Immunity—Cell-Mediated   Among numerous assays of cell-mediated immunity, three routinely performed tests are the cytotoxic T-lymphocyte (CTL) assay, the delayed hypersensitivity response (DHR), and the T-cell proliferative response to antigens.

The CTL assay measures the in vitro ability of splenic T cells to recognize allogeneic or antigenically distinct target cells by evaluating the ability of the CTLs to proliferate and then lyse the target cells. CTLs are incubated with target cells that have been treated so that they cannot proliferate. The CTLs recognize the target cells and proliferate until they are harvested. Then they are incubated with radiolabeled target cells. CTLs that have acquired

memory recognize the foreign MHC class I on target cells and lyse them.

The DHR evaluates the ability of memory T cells to recognize a foreign antigen, proliferate and migrate to the site of the antigen, and secrete cytokines in vivo. Mice are sensitized by a subcutaneous injection of the chemical. Radiolabeled iodine is allowed to be incorporated into the mouse's mononuclear cells by injecting it into the mouse's bloodstream. Then some of the sensitizing chemical is injected into the ear, and after the mouse has been euthanized, the ear is evaluated for the presence of radiolabeled mononuclear cells.

There are several mechanisms for evaluating the proliferative capacity of T cells in cell-mediated immunity. The mixed lymphocyte response (MLR) measures the ability of T cells to recognize foreign MHC class I and undergo proliferation.

Host Resistance Assays   Host resistance assays represent a method of determining how xenobiotic exposure affects the ability of the host to handle infection by various pathogens.

Regulatory Approaches to the Assessment of Immunotoxicity

The NTP Tier Approach   The National Toxicology Program (NTP) screens for potential immunotoxic agents by using a tier approach. Tier I provides an assessment of general toxicity (immunopathology, hematology, body and organ weights) as well as endline functional assays (proliferative responses, PFC assay, and NK assay). Tier II was designed to further define an immunotoxic effect and includes tests for cell-mediated immunity (CTL and DHR), secondary antibody responses, enumeration of lymphocyte populations, and host resistance models.

Health Effects Test Guidelines   Guidelines for functional immunotoxicity assessments in regulatory studies recommend the conducting of three tests. Assessment of immunotoxicity begins by exposure for a minimum of 28 days to the chemical, followed by assessment of humoral immunity (PFC assay or anti-sRBC ELISA). If the chemical produces significant suppression of the humoral response, surface marker assessment by flow cytometry may be performed. If the chemical produces no suppression of the humoral response, an assessment of innate immunity (NK assay) may be performed.

Immunotoxicity Testing of Medical Devices Many medical devices may have intimate and prolonged contact with the body. Possible immunologic consequences of this contact could be envisioned to include immunosuppression, immune stimulation, inflammation, and sensitization.

Animal Models in Immunotoxicology

Rats and mice have been the animals of choice for studying the actions of xenobiotics on the immune system because (1) a vast database on the immune system is available, (2) rodents are less expensive to maintain than are larger animals, and (3) a wide variety of reagents (cytokines, antibodies, etc.) are available. Many reagents that are available for studying the human immune system also can be used in rhesus and cynomolgus monkeys. Chicken and fish are being used to evaluate the immunotoxicity of xenobiotics as alternative animal models because of heightened environmental consciousness.

Evaluation of Mechanisms of Action

Direct effects on the immune system may include chemical effects on immune function, structural alterations in lymphoid organs or on immune cell surfaces, and compositional changes in lymphoid organs or serum. Xenobiotics may exert an indirect action on the immune system as well. They may be metabolically activated to their toxic metabolites and also may have effects on other organ systems (e.g., liver damage) that then affect the immune system.

IMMUNOMODULATION BY XENOBIOTICS

Immunosuppression

Immunosuppression can be produced by numerous natural and synthetic chemicals (see Table 12-5).

Tobacco Smoke Pulmonary defenses against inhaled gases and particulates are dependent on both physical and immunologic mechanisms. Immune mechanisms primarily involve the complex interactions between PMNs and alveolar macrophages and their ability to phagocytize foreign material and produce cytokines.

In humans, the number of alveolar macrophages is increased three- to fivefold in smokers compared with nonsmokers, and the macrophages that are present appear to be in an activated state but have decreased phagocytic and bactericidal activity. Decreased serum immunoglobulin levels and decreased NK-cell activity have been reported. Concentration-dependent leukocytosis (increased numbers of T and B cells) is well defined in smokers compared with nonsmokers. Numerous immunologic studies conducted in animals exposed to cigarette smoke have demonstrated suppression of antibody responses.

Recombinant DNA–Derived Proteins Biologics (e.g., blood or vaccine products) and recombinant DNA–derived proteins result in some manner from living organisms. Any foreign protein may elicit the production of neutralizing antibodies. The effects of neutralizing antibodies also may lead to hypersensitivity reactions.

Ultraviolet Radiation Ultraviolet radiation (UVR) suppresses delayed hypersensitivity responses in both animals and humans and results in a decreased host resistance to infection. Induction of suppressor T cells and alterations in homing patterns have been suggested as possibilities. One plausible explanation is that UVR induces a switch from a predominantly Th1 response (favoring delayed hypersensitivity responses) to a Th2 response (favoring antibody responses).

Immune-Mediated Disease

The purpose of the immune system is to protect the individual from disease states—whether infectious, parasitic, or cancerous—through both cellular and humoral mechanisms. In doing this, the ability to distinguish "self" from "nonself" plays a predominant role. However, situations arise in which the individual's immune system responds in a manner that produces tissue damage, resulting in a self-induced disease: (1) hypersensitivity, or allergy, and (2) autoimmunity. Hypersensitivity reactions result because the immune system responds in an exaggerated or inappropriate manner. In the case of autoimmunity, mechanisms of self-recognition break down and immunoglobulins and T-cell receptors react with self-antigens, resulting in tissue damage and disease.

Hypersensitivity *Classification of Hypersensitivity Reactions* All four types of hypersensitivity reactions require prior exposure leading to sensitization to elicit a

Table 12-5
Xenobiotics Capable of Immunosuppression

Halogenated aromatic hydrocarbons	**Aromatic hydrocarbons**
Polychlorinated biphenyls	Carbon tetrachloride
Polybrominated biphenyls	Ethylene glycol monomethyl ether
Polychlorinated dibenzodioxins	2-Methoxyethanol
Polychlorinated dibenzofurans	**Mycotoxins**
Polycyclic aromatic hydrocarbons	Aflatoxin
Nitrosamines	Ochratoxin
Pesticides	Tricothecenes
Organophosphate pesticides	Vomitoxin
Organochlorine pesticides	**Estrogens**
Organotin pesticides	**Androgens**
Carbamate pestides	**Glucocorticoids**
Pyrethroids	**Immunosuppressive Drugs**
Metals	Cyclophosphamide
Lead	Azathioprine
Arsenic	Cyclosporin A
Mercury	Rapamycin
Cadmium	Leflunomide
Beryllium	Zidovudine (3′-azido-3′-deoxythymidine; AZT)
Platinum	Stavudine (2′,3′-didehydro-2′,3′-dideoxythymidine)
Gold	Zalcitabine (2′,3′-dideoxycytidine; ddC)
Nickel	Videx (2′,3′-dideoxyinosine; ddI)
Chromium	**Drugs of Abuse**
Cobalt	Cannabinoids
Inhaled substances	Cocaine
Urethane	Opioids: Heroin and Morphine
Tobacco Smoke	Ethanol
Asbestos	
Silica	
Formaldehyde	
Ethylenediamine	
Oxidant gases	
Ozone (O_3)	
Sulfur dioxide (SO_2)	
Nitrogen dioxide (NO_2)	
Phosgene	

reaction upon subsequent challenge. Figure 12-6 illustrates the mechanisms of hypersensitivity reactions as classified by Coombs and Gell.

Type I (Immediate Hypersensitivity) Sensitization occurs as a result of exposure to appropriate antigens through the respiratory tract, dermally, or by exposure through the gastrointestinal tract and is mediated by IgE production. IgE binds to appropriate cells and sensitizes an individual; reexposure to the antigen results in degranulation of

the mast cells, with the release of preformed mediators and cytokines that promote vasodilation, bronchial constriction, and inflammation.

Type II (Antibody-Dependent Cytotoxic Hypersensitivity) Type II hypersensitivity is IgG-mediated. Tissue damage may result from the direct action of cytotoxic cells or from antibody activation of the classic complement pathway. Complement activation may result in cell lysis.

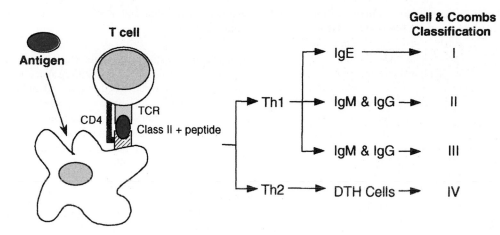

Figure 12-6. Schematic of classification of hypersensitivity reactions.

Type III (Immune Complex–Mediated Hypersensitivity) Type III hypersensitivity reactions also involve IgG immunoglobulins. Immunoglobulin may form complexes with soluble antigen, and the complex may deposit (lodge) in various tissues, causing tissue damage. The most common location is the vascular endothelium in the lung, joints, and kidneys. Macrophages, neutrophils, and platelets attracted to the deposition site contribute to the tissue damage.

Type IV (Cell-Mediated Hypersensitivity) Type IV is a delayed-type hypersensitivity (DTH) response. Contact hypersensitivity is initiated by topical exposure and consists of two phases: sensitization and elicitation. Sensitization results in the development of activated and memory T cells when the chemical is presented on an antigen-presenting cell to T-helper cells in local lymph nodes, leading to the generation of memory T cells.

Upon second contact, antigen-presenting Langerhans-dendritic cells present the processed hapten-carrier complex to memory T cells. The activated T cells then secrete cytokines that bring about further proliferation of T cells and facilitate the movement of inflammatory cells into the skin, resulting in erythema and the formation of papules and vesicles. Cells of the cell-mediated immune response may cause local tissue damage.

Whereas separation of hypersensitivity responses into types I to IV is helpful in understanding the involved mechanisms, it is important to realize that pathology often results from a combination of these mechanisms.

Assessment of Hypersensitivity Responses *Assessment of Respiratory Hypersensitivity in Experimental Ani-*

mals Methods for detecting pulmonary hypersensitivity can be divided into two types: (1) those for detecting immunologic sensitization and (2) those for detecting pulmonary sensitization. In the case of types I to III, immunologic sensitization occurs when antigen-specific immunoglobulin is produced in response to exposure to an antigen or, in the case of type IV, when a population of sensitized T lymphocytes is produced. Pulmonary sensitization is determined by a change in respiratory function after the challenge of a sensitized animal.

Guinea pig models have been the most frequently used because the lung is the major shock organ for anaphylactic response. Immunologic sensitization may be determined by obtaining sequential blood samples throughout the induction period and measuring antibody titer. Pulmonary sensitization is evaluated by detecting the presence of pulmonary reactivity (either visible respiratory distress or changes in respiratory function) after a challenge.

Assessment of IgE-Mediated Hypersensitivity Responses in Humans Two skin tests available for immediate hypersensitivity testing measure a "wheal and flare" reaction. The prick-puncture test introduces very small amounts of antigen under the skin. For test compounds that do not elicit a reaction in the less sensitive skin test, the intradermal test using dilute concentrations of antigen may be used, but there is a higher risk of systemic reactions.

In vitro serologic tests, ELISAs, and radioallergosorbent tests (RASTs) also may be used to detect the presence of antigen-specific antibody in a patient's serum.

Bronchial provocation tests may be performed by having the patient inhale an antigen into the bronchial tree and evaluating his or her pulmonary response.

Assessment of Contact Hypersensitivity in Experimental Animals The two most commonly utilized guinea pig models are the Büehler test and the guinea pig maximization test. In the Büehler test, the test article is applied to the shaven flank and covered with an occlusive bandage for 6 h once a week for 3 weeks. On day 28, a challenge dose of the test article is applied to a shaven area on the opposite flank; that area is evaluated for signs of edema and erythema for 2 days afterward. The guinea pig maximization test differs in that the test article is administered by intradermal injection, an adjuvant is employed, and irritating concentrations are used.

The assays described above evaluate the elicitation phase of the response in previously sensitized animals. The mouse local lymph node assay is a stand-alone alternative to the guinea pig assays for use in hazard identification of chemical sensitizers. Animals are dosed by topical application of the test article to the ears for 3 consecutive days. A few days later, the animals are injected with radiolabeled thymidine, which is incorporated into proliferating lymphocytes. Later, the animals are sacrificed and the local lymph nodes are assayed for radiolabeled lymphocytes to see whether the test article induced an immune response.

Assessment of Contact Hypersensitivity in Humans Human testing for contact hypersensitivity reactions is done by skin patch testing. Patches containing specified concentrations of the allergen in the appropriate vehicle are applied under an occlusive patch for 48 h. Once the patch is removed, the area is read for signs of erythema, papules, vesicles, and edema. Generally, the test is read again at 72 h, and in some cases, signs may not appear for up to 1 week or more.

Hypersensitivity Reactions to Xenobiotics Numerous xenobiotics illicit hypersensitivity reactions. Polyisocyanates, toluene diisocyanate in particular, which are used in the production of adhesives and coatings, are known to induce the full spectrum of hypersensitivity responses, types I to IV, as well as nonimmune inflammatory and neuroreflex reactions in the lung. Inhaled acid anhydrides, which are used in the manufacturing of paints, varnishes, coating materials, adhesives, and casting and sealing materials, may conjugate with serum albumin or erythrocytes, leading to type I, II, or III hypersensitivity reactions upon subsequent exposure.

Metals Metals and metallic substances, including metallic salts, are responsible for producing contact and pulmonary hypersensitivity reactions. Platinum, nickel, chromium, beryllium, and cobalt are the most commonly implicated salts.

Drugs Hypersensitivity responses to drugs are among the major types of unpredictable drug reactions. Drugs are designed to be reactive in the body, and multiple treatments are common. This type of exposure is conducive to producing an immunologic reaction. Immunologic mechanisms of hypersensitivity reactions to drugs include types I through IV. Penicillin is the agent most commonly involved in drug allergy.

Pesticides Pesticides have been implicated as causal agents in both contact and immediate hypersensitivity reactions.

Natural Rubber Latex Products Natural rubber latex is used in the manufacture of over 40,000 products, including examination and surgical gloves. Dermatologic reactions to latex include irritant dermatitis and contact dermatitis.

Cosmetics and Personal Hygiene Products Contact dermatitis and dermatoconjuctivitis may result from exposure to many cosmetic and personal hygiene products. These agents contain paraben esters, sorbic acid, phenolics, organomercurials, quaternary ammonium compounds, and formaldehyde.

Enzymes Subtilin and papain are enzymes that can elicit type I hypersensitivity responses. Subtilin is used in laundry detergents. Both individuals working where the product is made and those using the product may become sensitized. Subsequent exposure may produce signs of rhinitis, conjunctivitis, and asthma. Papain is another enzyme that is known to induce IgE-mediated disease. It is used most commonly as a meat tenderizer and a clearing agent in beer production.

Formaldehyde Formaldehyde exposure occurs in the cosmetics and textile industries and in the furniture, auto upholstery, and resins industries. Occupational exposure to formaldehyde has been associated with the occurrence of asthma.

Autoimmunity In cases of autoimmunity, self antigens are the target, and in the case of chemical-induced autoimmunity, the disease state is induced by a modification of host tissues or immune cells by the chemical, not by the chemical acting as an antigen/hapten.

Table 12-6
Chemical Agents Known to Be Associated with Autoimmunity

PROPOSED ANTIGENIC CHEMICAL	CLINICAL MANIFESTATIONS	DEPARTMENT
Drugs		
Methyldopa	Hemolytic anemia	Rhesus antigens
Hydralazine	SLE-like syndrome	Myeloperoxidase
Isoniazid	SLE-like syndrome	Myeloperoxidase
Procainamide	SLE-like syndrome	DNA
Halothane	Autoimmune hepatitis	Liver microsomal proteins
Nondrug chemicals		
Vinyl chloride	Scleroderma-like syndrome	Abnormal protein synthesized in liver
Mercury	Glomerular neuropathy	Glomerular basement membrane protein
Silica	Scleroderma	Most likely acts as an adjuvant

KEY: SLE, systemic lupus erythematosus.

Mechanisms of Autoimmunity   Three types of molecules are involved in the process of self-recognition: immunoglobulins (Igs), T-cell receptors (TCRs), and the products of the MHC. Igs and TCRs are expressed clonally on B and T cells, respectively, whereas MHC molecules are present on all nucleated cells.

The process of negative selection against autoreactive T cells in the thymus is important in the prevention of autoimmune disease. T cells that express receptors that bind to self antigens undergo apoptosis (negative selection), whereas those which do not recognize self proteins proliferate (positive selection) and migrate to the peripheral lymph organs. Some cells that recognize self molecules do not die but instead undergo anergy, in which they stay in the body but are inactive.

Several mechanisms may break down self-tolerance, leading to autoimmunity. First, if exposure to antigens is not available in the thymus during embryonic development, such as myelin, which is not produced until later in development, then antigen-specific T cell–reactive lymphocytes that are not subjected to negative selection can induce an autoimmune reaction. Breakdown of self-tolerance to these antigens may be induced by exposure to adjuvants, chemicals used to enhance immunogenicity, or another antigenically related protein. Second, T-cell anergy can be overcome with chronic lymphocyte stimulation. Third, interference with normal immunoregulation by $CD8^+$ T-cell suppressor cells may create an environment conducive to the development of autoimmune disease.

As is the case with hypersensitivity reactions, autoimmune disease often results from more than one mechanism working simultaneously. Therefore, pathology may be the result of antibody-dependent cytotoxicity, complement-dependent antibody-mediated lysis, or direct or indirect effects of cytotoxic T cells.

Autoimmune Reactions to Xenobiotics   Table 12-6 lists chemicals known to be associated with autoimmunity, showing the proposed self-antigenic determinant or stating adjuvancy as the mechanism of action. Table 12-7 shows chemicals that have been implicated in autoimmune

Table 12-7
Chemicals Implicated in Autoimmunity

MANIFESTATION	IMPLICATED CHEMICAL
Scleroderma	Solvents (toluene, xylene)
	Tryptophan
	Silicones
Systemic lupus erythematosus	Phenothiazines
	Penicillamine
	Propylthiouracil
	Quinidine
	L-Dopa
	Lithium carbonate
	Trichloroethylene
	Silicones

reactions, but in these cases the mechanism of auto-immunity has not been as clearly defined or confirmed.

Multiple Chemical Sensitivity Syndrome Multiple chemical sensitivity syndrome (MCS) has been associated with hypersensitivity responses to chemicals. The syndrome is characterized by multiple subjective symptoms that are related to more than one system. The more common symptoms are nasal congestion, headaches, lack of concentration, fatigue, and memory loss. Many mechanisms have been suggested to explain how chemicals cause these symptoms. A major hypothesis is that MCS occurs when chemical exposure sensitizes an individual, and, upon subsequent exposure to exceedingly small amounts of these or unrelated chemicals, the individual exhibits an adverse response.

NEW FRONTIERS AND CHALLENGES

New technology has brought more and more questions to be answered by immunotoxicology. A variety of new tools are available to assess these problems.

Molecular Biology Methods: Proteomics and Genomics

Proteomics (the study of all the expressed proteins in a particular cell and thus the functional expression of the genome) and genomics (the study of all the genes encoded by an organism's DNA), combined with bioinformatics, are making it possible to evaluate chemically induced alterations in entire pathways and signaling networks.

Animal Models: Transgenics and SCID

The manipulation of the embryonic genome, creating transgenic and knockout mice, may allow complex immune responses to be dissected into their components. In this way, the mechanisms by which immunotoxicants act can be better understood. Severe combined immunodeficient (SCID) mice have been used to study immune regulation, hematopoiesis, hypersensitivity, and autoimmunity.

Developmental Immunotoxicology

Developmental immunotoxicology involves an investigation of the effects xenobiotics have on the ontogeny of the immune system and includes prenatal (in utero), perinatal (<36 h of age), and neonatal periods of exposure.

Immune development in humans and other species may be altered after perinatal exposure to immunotoxic chemicals. It also has been suggested that these effects may be more dramatic or persistent than those which follow exposure during adult life.

Systemic Hypersensitivity

An adverse immune response, in the form of systemic hypersensitivity, is among the most common causes for the withdrawal of drugs that have made it to the market. These findings generally are unexpected in that they were not predicted in preclinical toxicology and immunotoxicology studies. Assays are needed that are more predictive of drug antigenicity, food allergy, and hypersensitivity in humans.

Computational Toxicology

Interest has grown in the use of computational toxicology methods to predict the potential biological/toxicologic activity of chemicals. The premise is that the structure of a chemical determines the physiochemical properties and reactivities that underlie its biological and toxicologic properties. The ability to predict potential adverse effects will aid in the designed development of new chemicals and could reduce the need for animal testing.

Biomarkers

True biomarkers indicate exposure to a specific chemical as well as susceptibility to an adverse effect and/or are predictive of disease associated with chemical exposure. The most desirable biomarkers would be those which indicate *exposure* in the absence of an immediate adverse effect. Biomarkers of *effect* would indicate subclinical effects of chemical exposure.

Risk Assessment

Assessments of the use of immunotoxicology data in animals as predictors of risk for human clinical effects have limitations, including the fact that no single immune test has been observed to be highly predictive of altered host resistance. Variability in the virulence of infectious agents in the human population, the complexity of the immune system, and the redundancy (multiple components capable of responding to a foreign challenge) in the immune system may all contribute to the difficulty in quantifying relationships between chemical-induced alterations in immune status and alterations in host resistance in humans.

CONCLUSIONS AND FUTURE DIRECTIONS

The balance between immune recognition and destruction of foreign invaders and the proliferation of those microbes and/or cancer cells can be a precarious one. Xenobiotics that alter the immune system can upset that balance, giving the advantage to the invader. Further-more, new xenobiotics continuously being introduced represent the potential for increased hypersensitivity and/or autoimmune responses. Validated methods are in place to detect xenobiotics that produce adverse effects related to the immune system. These methods must be improved continually by using the latest knowledge and technologies to provide a safe environment.

BIBLIOGRAPHY

Flaherty DK: *Immunotoxicology and Risk Assessment.* New York: Kluwer, 1999.

Lawrence DA (ed): *Toxicology of the Immune System,* vol 5, in Sipes IG, McQueen CA, Gandolfi AJ (eds-in-chief): *Comprehensive Toxicology.* New York: Elsevier, 1997.

Paul WE (ed): *Fundamental Immunology,* 4th ed. New York: Raven Press, 1999.

Smialowicz RJ, Holsapple MP: *Experimental Immunotoxicology.* Boca Raton, FL: CRC Press, 1996.

Voccia I, Blakley B, Brousseau P, Fournier M: Immunotoxicity of pesticides: A review. *Toxicol Ind Health* 15:119–132, 1999.

Zelikoff JT, Thomas P (eds): *Immunotoxicology of Environmental and Occupational Metals.* Bristol, PA: Taylor & Francis, 1998.

C H A P T E R   1 3

TOXIC RESPONSES OF THE LIVER

Mary Treinen-Moslen

KEY POINTS

- The liver's strategic location between the intestinal tract and the rest of the body facilitates its maintenance of metabolic homeostasis in the body.

- The liver extracts ingested nutrients, vitamins, metals, drugs, environmental toxicants, and waste products of bacteria from the blood for catabolism, storage, and/or excretion into bile.

- Formation of bile is essential for the uptake of lipid nutrients from the small intestine, protection of the small intestine from oxidative insults, and excretion of endogenous and xenobiotic compounds.

- Cholestasis is either a decrease in the volume of bile formed or an impaired secretion of specific solutes into bile that results in elevated serum levels of bile salts and bilirubin.

- Hepatocytes have a rich supply of phase I enzymes that often convert xenobiotics to reactive electrophilic metabolites and phase II enzymes that add a polar group to a molecule and thus enhance its removal from the body. The balance between phase I and phase II reactions determines whether a reactive metabolite will initiate liver cell injury or be detoxified safely.

INTRODUCTION

Numerous industrial compounds and therapeutic agents have been found to injure the liver. Factors are known that determine why the liver, as opposed to other organs, is the dominant target site of specific toxins. Scientists have identified mechanisms by which chemicals injure specific populations of liver cells. A basic understanding of hepatotoxicity requires appreciation of the (1) major functions of the liver, (2) structural organization of the liver, and (3) processes involved in the excretory function of the liver: bile formation.

PHYSIOLOGY AND PATHOPHYSIOLOGY

Hepatic Functions

The strategic location of the liver between the intestinal tract and the rest of the body facilitates the performance of its enormous task of maintaining metabolic homeostasis of the body. Venous blood from the stomach and intestines flows into the portal vein and then through the liver before entering the systemic circulation. The liver is the first organ to encounter ingested nutrients, vitamins, metals, drugs, and environmental toxicants as well as waste products of bacteria that enter portal blood. Efficient scavenging or uptake processes extract these absorbed materials from the blood for catabolism, storage, and/or excretion into bile.

All the major functions of the liver can be altered detrimentally by acute or chronic exposure to toxicants (Table 13-1). When toxicants inhibit or otherwise impede hepatic transport and synthetic processes, dysfunction can occur without appreciable cell damage (Fig. 13-1). Loss of function also occurs when toxicants kill an appreciable number of cells and when chronic insult leads to the replacement of cell mass by nonfunctional scar tissue.

Structural Organization

Classically, the liver was divided into hexagonal lobules oriented around terminal hepatic venules (also known as central veins). At the corners of the lobule are the portal triads (or portal tracts), which contain a branch of the

Table 13-1
Major Functions of Liver and Consequences of Impaired Hepatic Functions

TYPE OF FUNCTION	EXAMPLES	CONSEQUENCES OF IMPAIRED FUNCTIONS
Nutrient homeostasis	Glucose storage and synthesis	Hypoglycemia, confusion
	Cholesterol uptake	Hypercholesterolemia
Filtration of particulates	Products of intestinal bacteria (e.g., endotoxin)	Endotoxemia
Protein synthesis	Clotting factors	Excess bleeding
	Albumin	Hypoalbuminemia, ascites
	Transport proteins (e.g., very low density lipoproteins)	Fatty liver
Bioactivation and detoxification	Bilirubin and ammonia	Jaundice, hyperammonemia-related coma
	Steroid hormones	Loss of secondary male sex characteristics
	Xenobiotics	Diminished drug metabolism Inadequate detoxification
Formation of bile and biliary secretion	Bile acid–dependent uptake of dietary lipids and vitamins	Fatty diarrhea, malnutrition, Vitamin E deficiency
	Bilirubin and cholesterol	Jaundice, gallstones, hypercholesterolemia
	Metals (e.g., Cu and Mn)	Mn-induced neurotoxicity
	Xenobiotics	Delayed drug clearance

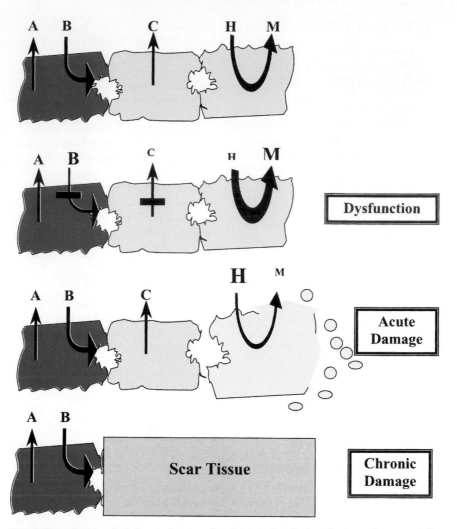

Figure 13-1. *Cartoon depicting toxicant-mediated events that lead to the loss of representative functions of hepatocytes, such as A, albumin secretion; B, bilirubin uptake and export into bile; C, clotting factor secretion; H and M, hormone uptake and bioactivation to metabolites.* Dysfunction without cell damage can occur when toxicants inhibit uptake and secretion or stimulate bioactivation excessively. The dysfunction can be selective when a toxicant impedes the secretion of only some compounds. Acute damage and chronic damage produce a loss of function in the cell population that dies or is replaced by scar tissue.

portal vein, a hepatic arteriole, and a bile duct (Fig. 13-2). The lobule is divided into three regions: the centrolobular, midzonal, and periportal regions. The preferred concept of a functional hepatic unit is the acinus. The base of the acinus is formed by the terminal branches of the portal vein and the hepatic artery, which extend out from the portal tracts. The acinus has three zones: Zone 1 is closest to the entry of blood, zone 3 abuts the terminal hepatic vein, and zone 2 is intermediate. The three zones

of the acinus roughly coincide with the three regions of the lobule (Fig. 13-2).

Acinar zonation is of considerable functional consequence in regard to gradients of components in both blood and hepatocytes. Blood entering the acinus consists of oxygen-depleted blood from the portal vein (60 to 70 percent of hepatic blood flow) and oxygenated blood from the hepatic artery (30 to 40 percent). En route to the terminal hepatic venule, oxygen rapidly leaves the

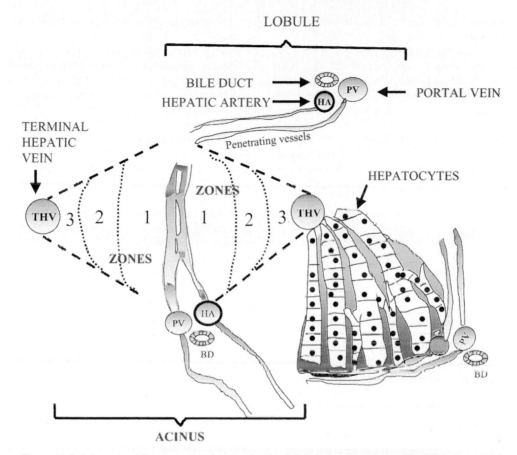

LOBULE

BILE DUCT

HEPATIC ARTERY

PORTAL VEIN

TERMINAL
HEPATIC
VEIN

Penetrating vessels

ZONES

HEPATOCYTES

THV 3 2 1 1 2 3 THV

ZONES

PV

HA

BD

PV

BD

ACINUS

Figure 13-2. Schematic of liver operational units: the classic lobule and the acinus.   The lobule is centered on the terminal hepatic vein (central vein), where the blood drains out of the lobule. The acinus has as its base the penetrating vessels, where blood supplied by the portal vein and hepatic artery flows down the acinus past the cords of hepatocytes. Zones 1, 2, and 3 of the acinus represent metabolic regions that are increasingly distant from the blood supply.

blood to meet the high metabolic demands of the parenchymal cells. Hepatocytes in zone 3 are exposed to substantially lower concentrations of oxygen than are hepatocytes in zone 1. In comparison to other tissues, zone 3 is hypoxic. Other well-documented acinar gradients exist for bile salts, bilirubin, and many organic anions.

Heterogeneities in protein levels of hepatocytes along the acinus generate gradients of metabolic functions. Hepatocytes in the mitochondria-rich zone 1 are predominant in fatty acid oxidation, gluconeogenesis, and ammonia detoxification to urea. Gradients of enzymes involved in the bioactivation and detoxification of xenobiotics have been observed along the acinus by immunohistochemistry. Notable gradients for hepatotoxins

are the higher levels of glutathione in zone 1 and the greater amounts of cytochrome P450 proteins in zone 3, particularly the CYP2E1 isozyme that is inducible by ethanol.

Hepatic sinusoids are the channels between cords of hepatocytes where blood percolates on its way to the terminal hepatic vein. The three major types of cells in the sinusoids are endothelial cells, Kupffer cells, and Ito cells. Sinusoids are lined by thin, discontinuous endothelial cells with numerous fenestrae (pores) that allow molecules smaller than 250 kDa to cross the interstitial space (the space of Disse) between the endothelium and the hepatocytes. The numerous fenestrae and the lack of basement membrane facilitate exchanges of fluids and molecules, such as albumin, between the sinusoid and the hepatocytes but hinder the movement of particles larger than chylomicron remnants.

Kupffer cells, the resident macrophages of the liver, constitute approximately 80 percent of the fixed macrophages in the body. Situated within the lumen of the sinusoid, Kupffer cells ingest and degrade particulate matter, are a source of cytokines, and can act as antigen-presenting cells.

Ito cells (also known by the more descriptive terms *fat-storing cells* and *stellate cells*) are located between endothelial cells and hepatocytes. Ito cells synthesize collagen and are the major storage site for vitamin A in the body.

Bile Formation

Bile is a yellow fluid containing bile salts, glutathione, phospholipids, cholesterol, bilirubin and other organic anions, proteins, metals, ions, and xenobiotics. The formation of this fluid is a specialized function of the liver. Adequate bile formation is essential for the uptake of lipid nutrients from the small intestine (Table 13-1), protection of the small intestine from oxidative insults, and excretion of endogenous and xenobiotic compounds. Hepatocytes begin the process by transporting bile salts, glutathione, and other solutes into the canalicular lumen. Tight junctions seal the canalicular lumen from materials in the sinusoid. Canaliculi form channels between hepatocytes that connect to a series of larger and larger channels or ducts within the liver. The large extrahepatic bile ducts merge into the common bile duct. Bile can be stored and concentrated in the gallbladder before its release into the duodenum.

The major driving force of bile formation is the active transport of bile salts and other osmolytes into the canalicular lumen. Transporters on the sinusoidal and canalicular membranes of hepatocytes are responsible for the uptake of bile salts, bilirubin, drugs, hormones, and xenobiotics from blood and then the transport of those solutes into the canalicular lumen (Fig. 13-3). Lipophilic cationic drugs, estrogens, and lipids are exported by the canalicular MDR (multiple-drug resistance) p-glycoproteins, one of which is exclusive for phospholipids. Conjugates of glutathione, glucuronide, and sulfate are exported by the canalicular multiple organic anion transporter (cMOAT).

Metals are excreted into bile by a series of partially understood processes that include (1) uptake across the sinusoidal membrane by facilitated diffusion or receptor-mediated endocytosis, (2) storage in binding proteins or lysosomes, and (3) canalicular secretion by lysosomes, a glutathione-coupled event, or a specific canalicular membrane transporter. Biliary excretion is important in the homeostasis of metals, notably copper, manganese, cadmium, selenium, gold, silver, and arsenic. Inability to export Cu into bile is a central problem in Wilson's disease, a rare genetic disorder characterized by the accumulation of Cu in the liver and then in other tissues.

Canalicular lumen bile is propelled forward into larger channels by dynamic, ATP-dependent contractions of the pericanalicular cytoskeleton. Bile ducts modify bile by absorbing and secreting solutes. Biliary epithelial cells also express phase I and phase II enzymes, which may contribute to the biotransformation of toxicants that are present in bile.

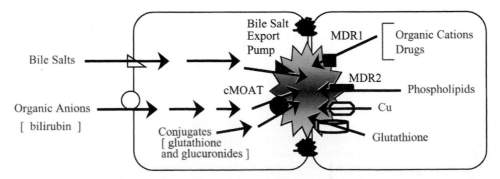

Figure 13-3. Processes involved in hepatocyte uptake and biliary secretion of endogenous solutes and toxicants.   Transporters localized to the sinusoidal membrane extract solutes from the blood. Exporters localized to the canalicular membrane move solutes into the lumen of the canaliculus. Exporters of particular relevance to canalicular secretion of toxic chemicals and their metabolites are the canalicular multiple organic anion transporter (MOAT) system and the family of multiple-drug-resistant (MDR) p-glycoproteins.

Secretion into biliary ducts is usually but not always a prelude to toxicant clearance by excretion in feces or urine. Exceptions occur when compounds are delivered repeatedly into the intestinal lumen in bile, absorbed efficiently from the intestinal lumen, and then redirected to the liver in portal blood, a process known as *enterohepatic cycling*.

Toxicant-related impairments of bile formation are more likely to have detrimental consequences in populations with other conditions in which biliary secretion is marginal. For example, neonates exhibit delayed development of bile salt synthesis and the expression of sinusoidal and canalicular transporters. Neonates are more prone to develop jaundice when treated with drugs that compete with bilirubin for biliary clearance.

Types of Injury and Toxic Chemicals

The hepatic response to insults by chemicals (Table 13-2) depends on the intensity of the insult, the population of cells affected, and whether the exposure is acute or chronic (Fig. 13-1).

Fatty Liver This change, which also is known as steatosis, consists of a buildup of lipids in the hepatocyte. Fatty liver can stem from disruptions in lipid metabolism. Steatosis is a common response to acute exposure to many hepatotoxins. Often toxin-induced steatosis is reversible and does not lead to the death of hepatocytes. The metabolic inhibitors ethionine, puromycin, and cycloheximide cause fat accumulation without causing the death of cells. Many other conditions besides toxin exposure, such as obesity, are associated with marked fat accumulation in the liver.

Cell Death Liver cells can die by two different modes: necrosis and apoptosis. Necrosis is characterized by cell swelling, leakage, nuclear disintegration, and an influx of inflammatory cells. Apoptosis is characterized by cell shrinkage, nuclear fragmentation, the formation of apoptotic bodies, and a lack of inflammation. When necrosis occurs in hepatocytes, the associated plasma membrane leakage can be detected biochemically by assaying plasma (or serum) for liver cytosol-derived enzymes such as alanine aminotransferase (ALT) and γ-glutamyltranspeptidase (GGT).

Hepatocyte death can occur in a focal, zonal, or panacinar (widespread) pattern. Focal cell death is characterized by the randomly distributed death of single hepatocytes or small clusters of hepatocytes. Zonal necrosis refers to death of hepatocytes in certain functional regions. Panacinar necrosis refers to massive death of hepatocytes with only a few or no remaining survivors.

Mechanisms of toxin-induced injury to liver cells include lipid peroxidation, binding to cell macromolecules, mitochondrial damage, disruption of the cytoskeleton, and massive calcium influx.

Canalicular Cholestasis Defined physiologically as a decrease in the volume of bile formed or an impaired secretion of specific solutes into bile, cholestasis is characterized biochemically by elevated serum levels of

Table 13-2
Types of Hepatobiliary Injury

TYPE OF INJURY OR DAMAGE	REPRESENTATIVE TOXINS
Fatty liver	CCl_4, ethanol, fialuridine, valproic acid
Hepatocyte death	Acetaminophen, Cu, dimethylformamide, ethanol, Ecstasy
Immune-mediated response	Diclofenac, ethanol, halothane, tienilic acid
Canalicular cholestasis	Chlorpromazine, cyclosporin A, 1,1-dichloroethylene, estrogens, Mn, phalloidin
Bile duct damage	Amoxicillin, α-naphthylisothiocyanate, methylene dianiline, sporidesmin
Sinusoidal disorders	Anabolic steroids, cyclophosphamide, microcystin, pyrrolidine alkaloids
Fibrosis and cirrhosis	Arsenic, ethanol, vitamin A, vinyl chloride
Tumors	Aflatoxin, androgens, thorium dioxide, vinyl chloride

compounds that normally are concentrated in bile, particularly bile salts and bilirubin. When biliary excretion of the yellowish bilirubin pigment is impaired, this pigment accumulates in the skin and eyes, producing jaundice, and spills into urine, which becomes bright yellow or dark brown. Toxin-induced cholestasis can be transient or chronic; when substantial, it is associated with cell swelling, cell death, and inflammation. Many different types of chemicals cause cholestasis (Table 13-2).

Bile Duct Damage Damage to the intrahepatic bile ducts (which carry bile from the liver to the gastrointestinal tract) is called *cholangiodestructive cholestasis*. A useful biochemical index of bile duct damage is a sharp elevation in serum alkaline phosphatase activity. In addition, serum levels of bile salts and bilirubin are elevated, as is observed with canalicular cholestasis. The initial lesions after a single dose of cholangiodestructive agents include swollen biliary epithelium, debris of damaged cells within lumens of the biliary tract, and inflammatory cell infiltration of portal tracts. Chronic administration of toxins that cause bile duct destruction can lead to biliary proliferation and fibrosis resembling biliary cirrhosis. Another response is the loss of bile ducts, a condition known as *vanishing bile duct syndrome*. This persisting problem has been reported in patients receiving antibiotics.

Sinusoidal Damage Functional integrity of the sinusoid (channels between hepatocytes that carry blood throughout the liver) can be compromised by dilation or blockade of its lumen or progressive destruction of its endothelial cell wall. Blockade occurs when red blood cells are caught in the sinusoids. These changes have been illustrated after large doses of the drug acetaminophen. A consequence of extensive sinusoidal blockade is that the liver becomes engorged with blood cells while the rest of the body goes into shock.

Progressive destruction of the endothelial wall of the sinusoid leads to gaps in and then ruptures of its barrier integrity, with entrapment of red blood cells. These disruptions of the sinusoid are considered the early structural features of the vascular disorder known as veno-occlusive disease, which occurs after exposure to pyrrolizidine alkaloids, which are found in some herbal teas and chemotherapeutic agents.

Cirrhosis Cirrhosis is characterized by the accumulation of extensive amounts of collagen fibers in response to direct injury or inflammation. With repeated chemical insults, destroyed hepatic cells are replaced by fibrotic scars. With continuing collagen deposition, the architecture of the liver is disrupted by interconnecting fibrous scars. When the fibrous scars subdivide the remaining liver mass into nodules of regenerating hepatocytes, fibrosis has progressed to cirrhosis and the liver has meager residual capacity to perform its essential functions. Cirrhosis is not reversible, has a poor prognosis for survival, and usually results from repeated exposure to chemical toxins.

Tumors Chemically induced neoplasia can involve tumors that are derived from hepatocytes or bile duct cells or the rare, highly malignant angiosarcomas derived from sinusoidal lining cells. Hepatocellular cancer has been linked to abuse of androgens and a high prevalence of aflatoxin-contaminated diets.

Thorotrast (radioactive thorium dioxide) accumulates in Kupffer cells, the resident macrophage of the sinusoid, and emits radioactivity throughout its very extended half-life. Multiple types of liver tumors are linked to thorium dioxide exposure.

FACTORS IN LIVER INJURY

Why is the liver the target site for so many chemicals of diverse structure? Why do many hepatotoxicants preferentially damage one type of liver cell? Our understanding of these fundamental questions is incomplete. The influences of several factors are of obvious importance (Table 13-3). Location and specialized processes for uptake and biliary secretion produce higher exposure levels in the liver than in other tissues of the body and strikingly high levels in certain types of liver cells. Then the abundant capacity for bioactivation reactions influences the rate of exposure to proximate toxicants. Subsequent events in the pathogenesis appear to be influenced critically by responses of sinusoidal cells and the immune system.

A number of experimental systems are useful for defining factors and mechanisms of liver injury. In vitro systems using the isolated perfused liver, isolated liver cells, and cell fractions allow observations at various levels of complexity without the confounding influences of other systems. Models that use cocultures or agents that inactivate a given cell type can document the contributions of and interactions between cell types. Whole-animal models are essential for assessment of the progression of injury and responses to chronic insult. The application of gene transfection or repression attenuates some of these interpretive problems. Knockout rodents provide extremely useful models for complex aspects of hepatotoxicity.

Table 13-3
Factors in the Site-Specific Injury of Representative Hepatotoxicants

SITE	REPRESENTATIVE TOXICANTS	POTENTIAL EXPLANATION FOR SITE-SPECIFICITY
Zone 1 hepatocytes (versus zone 3)	Fe (overload)	Preferential uptake and high oxygen levels
	Allyl alcohol	Higher oxygen levels for oxygen-dependent bioactivation
Zone 3 hepatocytes (versus zone 1)	CCl$_4$	More P450 isozyme for bioactivation
	Acetaminophen	More P450 isozyme for bioactivation and less GSH for detoxification
	Ethanol	More hypoxic and greater imbalance in bioactivation/detoxification reactions
Bile duct cells	Methylene dianiline, Sporidesmin	Exposure to the high concentration of reactive metabolites in bile
Sinusoidal endothelium (versus hepatocytes)	Cyclophosphamide, Monocrotaline	Greater vulnerability to toxic metabolites and less ability to maintain glutathione levels
Kupffer cells	Endotoxin, GdCl$_3$	Preferential uptake and then activation
Ito cells	Vitamin A	Preferential site for storage and then engorgement
	Ethanol (chronic)	Activation and transformation to collagen-synthesizing cell

Uptake and Concentration

Lipophilic drugs and environmental pollutants readily diffuse into hepatocytes because the fenestrated epithelium of the sinusoid enables close contact between circulating molecules and hepatocytes. The membrane-rich liver concentrates lipophilic compounds. Other toxins are extracted rapidly from blood because they are substrates for sinusoidal transporters. Phalloidin (from a mushroom) and microcystin (from a blue-green alga) are illustrative examples of hepatotoxins that target the liver as a consequence of extensive uptake into hepatocytes by sinusoidal transporters. Vitamin A hepatotoxicity initially affects the sinusoidal Ito cells, which actively extract and store this vitamin, and cadmium hepatotoxicity becomes manifest when cells exceed their capacity to complex cadmium with the metal-binding protein metallothionein.

Hepatocytes contribute to the homeostasis of Fe by extracting this essential metal from the sinusoid through a receptor-mediated process and maintaining a reserve of Fe within the storage protein ferritin. The cytotoxicity of free Fe is attributed to its function as an electron donor for the formation of reactive oxygen species, which initiate destructive oxidative stress reactions. Accumulation of excess Fe beyond the capacity for its safe storage in ferritin leads to liver damage. Chronic hepatic accumulation of excess iron in cases of hemochromatosis is associated with a spectrum of hepatic disease, including liver cancer.

Bioactivation and Detoxification

Hepatocytes have very high constitutive activities of the phase I enzymes that often convert xenobiotics to reactive electrophilic metabolites. Also, hepatocytes have a rich collection of phase II enzymes that add a polar group to a molecule and thus enhance its removal from the body. Phase II reactions usually yield stable, nonreactive metabolites. In general, the balance between phase I and phase II reactions determines whether a reactive metabolite will initiate liver cell injury or be detoxified safely.

Ethanol Genetic conditions of high clinical relevance to the bioactivation/detoxification balance are the polymorphisms in the enzymes that control the two-step metabolism of ethanol. Specifically, ethanol is bioactivated by alcohol dehydrogenase to acetaldehyde, a reactive aldehyde, which subsequently is detoxified to acetate by aldehyde dehydrogenase. Both enzymes exhibit genetic polymorphisms that result in higher concentrations of acetaldehyde—a "fast" activity isozyme of alcohol dehydrogenase [ALD2*2] and a physiologically very "slow" mitochondrial isozyme of aldehyde dehydrogenase [ALDH2*2]. Approximately 50 percent of Asian populations but virtually no white people have the slow aldehyde dehydrogenase; alcohol consumption by people with this slow polymorphism leads to uncomfortable symptoms of flushing and nausea caused by high systemic levels of acetaldehyde.

Cytochrome P450 Cytochrome P450–dependent bioactivation as a mechanism of hepatotoxicity is important even for assumedly *safe* compounds because some P450 isozymes generate reactive oxygen species during biotransformation reactions, and this can lead to liver damage. CYP2E1 generation of reactive oxygen species and other free radicals is a factor in the etiology of serious, end-stage liver damage.

Besides CYP2E1, the CYP3A isozyme has been linked to the hepatotoxicity caused by the folk medicine plant germander (*Teucrium chamaedrys L.*). Systematic experimental studies demonstrated a predominant role for the CYP3A bioactivation of germander constituents to reactive electrophiles.

Carbon Tetrachloride Cytochrome P450-dependent conversion of CCl_4 to $^{\bullet}CCl_3$ and then to $CCl_3OO^{\bullet}$ is the classic example of xenobiotic bioactivation to a free radical that initiates oxidative damage. Conditions in which cytochrome P450 is depleted lead to decreased liver damage when there is exposure to CCl_4.

Acetaminophen The hepatotoxicity of this extensively used analgesic is an exemplary instance of how acquired factors (e.g., diet, drugs, diabetes, obesity) can enhance hepatotoxicity. Typical therapeutic doses of acetaminophen are not hepatotoxic, because most of the acetaminophen gets glucuronidated or sulfated with little drug bioactivation. Injury after large doses of acetaminophen is enhanced by fasting and other conditions that deplete glutathione and is minimized by treatments with *N*-acetylcysteine that enhance hepatocyte synthesis of glutathione.

Alcoholics are vulnerable to the hepatotoxic effects of acetaminophen at doses within the high therapeutic range. This acquired enhancement often has been attributed to accelerated bioactivation of acetaminophen to the electrophilic *N*-acetyl-*p*-benzoquinone imine (NAPQI) intermediate by ethanol induction of CYP2E1 (Fig. 13-4). Inducers of CYP3A, including many drugs and dietary chemicals, potentially influence acetaminophen toxicity.

An attractive "two-hit" type of theory for the hepatotoxicity of acetaminophen suggests that adduction by a reactive drug metabolite "primes" the hepatocytes for destructive insults by reactive nitrogen species (e.g., peroxynitrite) (Fig. 13-4).

Activation of Sinusoidal Cells

Four kinds of observations collectively indicate roles for sinusoidal cell (immune cells present in the liver sinusoids) activation as primary or secondary factors in toxin-induced injury to the liver:

1. Kupffer cells and Ito cells exhibit an activated morphology after acute and chronic exposure to hepatotoxicants.
2. Pretreatments that activate or inactivate Kupffer cells appropriately modulate the extent of damage produced by classic toxicants. Kupffer cell activation by vitamin A profoundly enhances the acute toxicity of carbon tetrachloride; this enhancement did not occur when animals also were given an inactivator of Kupffer cells.
3. Activated Kupffer cells secrete appreciable amounts of soluble cytotoxins, including reactive oxygen and nitrogen species.
4. Acute and chronic exposure to alcohol directly or indirectly affects sinusoidal cells.

Figure 13-5 summarizes information presented in this section and earlier sections of this chapter about the multiplicity of toxin-induced interactions with and between various liver cells. The effect on a given cell type can be direct or may result from a cascade of signals and responses between cell types.

Inflammatory and Immune Responses

Migration of neutrophils, lymphocytes, and other inflammatory cells into regions of damaged liver is a well-recognized feature of the hepatotoxicity produced by many chemicals. In fact, the potentially confusing term *hepatitis* refers to hepatocyte damage by any insult in cases where hepatocyte death is associated with an influx of inflammatory cells.

The influx of inflammatory cells usually facilitates beneficial removal of debris from damaged liver cells.

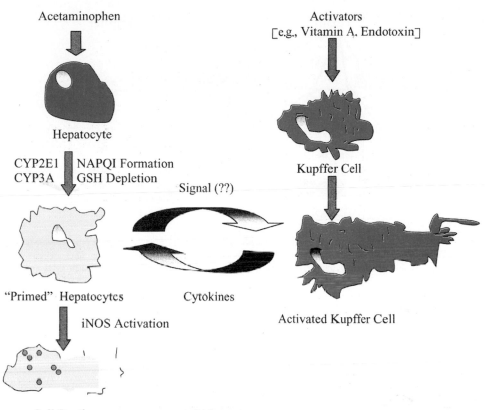

Figure 13-4. Schematic of key events in the bioactivation and hepatotoxicity of acetaminophen.   Bioactivation of acetaminophen by cytochrome P450 isozymes leads to the formation of the reactive intermediate *N* acetyl-*p*-benzoquinone imine (NAPQI), which can deplete glutathione or form covalent adducts with hepatic proteins. Experimental observations suggest that such effects "prime" hepatocytes for cytokines released by activated Kupffer cells. Progression to cell death is thought to involve activation of iNOS and other processes that produce reactive nitrogen species and oxidative stress. Agents that activate Kupffer cells exacerbate the toxicity. Exchange of signals between toxicant-primed and activated Kupffer cells probably is a factor in the acute hepatotoxicity produced by many compounds that damage hepatocytes.

However, detrimental effects are plausible, because activated neutrophils release cytotoxic proteases and reactive oxygen species.

Immune responses are considered factors in the hepatotoxicity occasionally observed after repeated exposure to chemicals, usually drugs. Individuals who develop infrequent, unpredictable responses are considered hypersensitive. An immune-mediated response is considered plausible when the problem subsides after therapy is halted and then recurs on drug challenge or the restoration of therapy. Although the concept is generally accepted, compelling evidence for immune-mediated responses is available only for ethanol, halothane, and a few other hepatotoxicants. Figure 13-6 depicts key features of the assumed scenario by which hepatic protein adducts could become antigenic and stimulate the production of antibodies. If, on reexposure, more drug-protein adducts are formed, cells with those adducts could be attacked by systemic antibodies.

Apparent immune-mediated injury has been observed in individuals taking the anti-arthritic non-steroidal anti-inflammatory drug (NSAID) diclofenac. Hepatic bioactivation of diclofenac leads to the formation of multiple adducts, which may localize to hepatocyte membrane proteins in which recognition by antibodies is feasible.

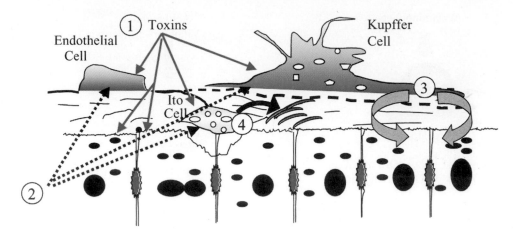

Figure 13-5. Schematic depicting the complex cascade of toxin-evoked interactions between hepatocytes and sinusoidal cells. Sinusoidal cell responses to toxins can lead to either injury or activation. One scenario could involve (1) toxin injury to hepatocytes, (2) signals from the injured hepatocyte to Kupffer and Ito cells, followed by (3) Kupffer cell release of cytotoxins and (4) Ito cell secretion of collagen. Activation of Kupffer cells is an important factor in the progression of injury evoked by many toxicants. Stimulation of collagen production by activated Ito cells is a proposed mechanism for toxicant-induced fibrosis.

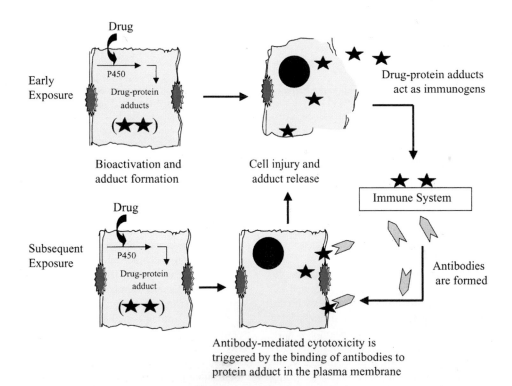

Figure 13-6. Proposed scenario of events leading to immune-mediated hepatotoxicity after repeated exposure to a toxicant that produces drug-protein adducts (★).

MECHANISMS OF LIVER INJURY

Liver cells are vulnerable to the same types of insults that injure other tissues. Preferential liver damage frequently ensues simply from the location of the liver and/or its high capacity for converting chemicals to reactive entities. Exceptions that merit explanation are toxins that target the cytoskeleton because of their uptake by hepatocytes and drugs that damage hepatic mitochondria. This section emphasizes mechanisms that produce cholestasis, because biliary secretion is a unique and vital function of the liver.

Disruption of the Cytoskeleton

Phalloidin and microcystin disrupt the integrity of hepatocyte cytoskeleton by affecting proteins that are vital to its dynamic nature by preventing disassembly of actin filaments. Phalloidin uptake into hepatocytes leads to an accentuated actin web of cytoskeleton, and the canalicular lumen dilates.

Microcystin uptake into hepatocytes leads to hyperphosphorylation of cytoskeletal proteins. Reversible phosphorylations of cytoskeletal structural and motor proteins are critical to the dynamic integrity of the cytoskeleton. As depicted in Fig. 13-7, extensive

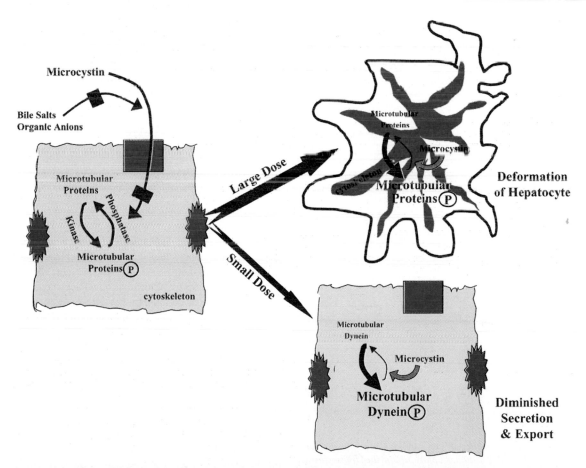

Figure 13-7. Schematic of events in the mechanism by which microcystin damages the structural and functional integrity of hepatocytes.   Microcystin is taken up exclusively into hepatocytes by a sinusoidal transporter in a manner inhibitable by bile salts and organic anions. Then microcystin inhibition of protein phosphatases leads to hyperphosphorylation of cytoskeletal proteins whose dynamic functions are dependent on reversible phosphorylations. Extensive hyperphosphorylation of microtubular proteins leads to a collapse of the microtubular actin filament scaffold into a spiky aggregate that produces a gross deformation of hepatocytes. More subtle changes in microtubule-mediated transport activities have been linked to the hyperphosphorylation of dynein, a cytoskeletal motor protein.

hyperphosphorylation produced by large amounts of microcystin leads to marked deformation of hepatocytes as a result of a unique collapse of the microtubular actin scaffold into a spiny central aggregate. Lower doses of microcystin interfere with vesicle transport by hyperphosphorylating the transport protein dynein.

Cholestasis

Bile formation is vulnerable to toxicant effects on the functional integrity of sinusoidal transporters, canalicular exporters, cytoskeleton-dependent processes for transcytosis, and the contractile closure of the canalicular lumen (Fig. 13-8). Changes that weaken the junctions that form the structural barrier between the blood and the canalicular lumen allow solutes to leak out of the canalicular lumen. These paracellular junctions provide a size and charge barrier to the diffusion of solutes between the blood and the canalicular lumen, whereas water and small ions diffuse across these junctions. One hepatotoxin that causes tight-junction leakage is α-napthylisothiocyanate.

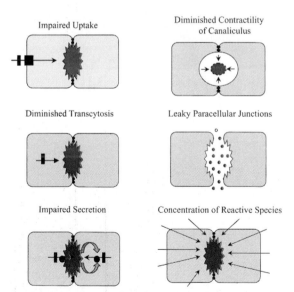

Figure 13-8. Schematic of six potential mechanisms for cholestasis involving inhibited uptake, diminished transcytosis, impaired secretion, diminished contractility of the canaliculus, leakiness of the junctions that seal the canalicular lumen from the blood, and detrimental consequences of high concentrations of toxic entities in the pericanalicular area. Note that impaired secretion across the canalicular membrane can result from inhibition of a transporter or retraction of a transporter away from the canalicular membrane.

Compounds that produce cholestasis do not necessarily act by a single mechanism or at just one site. Chlorpromazine impairs bile acid uptake and canalicular contractility. Multiple alterations have been well documented for estrogens, a well-known cause of reversible canalicular cholestasis. Estrogens decrease the uptake of bile salt by exerting effects at the sinusoidal membrane, including a decrease in the Na^+, K^+-ATPase necessary for Na-dependent transport of bile salts across the plasma membrane and changes in the lipid component of this membrane. At the canalicular membrane, estrogens diminish the transport of glutathione conjugates and reduce the number of bile salt transporters.

An additional mechanism for canalicular cholestasis is concentration of reactive forms of chemicals in the pericanalicular area (Fig. 13-8). Most chemicals that cause canalicular cholestasis are excreted in bile. Therefore, the proteins and lipids in the canalicular region encounter a high concentration of these chemicals. Observations consistent with this concentration mechanism have been reported for Mn, reactive thioether glutathione conjugates of 1,1-dichloroethylene, and sporidesmin.

Mitochondrial Damage

Mitochondrial DNA codes for several proteins in the mitochondrial electron transport chain. Nucleoside analog drugs for therapy for hepatitis B and AIDS infections cause mitochondrial DNA damage directly when incorporation of the analog base leads to miscoding or early termination of polypeptides. The severe hepatic mitochondrial injury produced by the nucleoside analog fialuridine is attributed to its higher affinity for the polymerase that is responsible for mitochondrial DNA synthesis than for the polymerases that are responsible for nuclear DNA synthesis. Mitochondrial DNA is also more vulnerable to miscoding (mutation) because of its limited capacity for repair.

Alcohol abuse causes mitochondrial injury by shifting the bioactivation/detoxification balance for ethanol, leading to an accumulation of its reactive acetaldehyde metabolite within mitochondria, because mitochondrial aldehyde dehydrogenase is the major enzymatic process for the detoxification of acetaldehyde. Bioactivation of large amounts of ethanol by alcohol dehydrogenase hampers the detoxification reaction, since the two enzymes require the common, depletable cofactor nicotinamide adenine dinucleotide (NAD). Any type of ethanol-induced change that enhances the leakiness of the mitochondrial transport chain will lead to an increased release of reactive oxygen species capable of attacking nearby mitochondrial constituents.

FUTURE DIRECTIONS

Our understanding of the mechanisms and critical factors in chemically mediated hepatotoxicity will continue to improve through the application of model systems that allow the observation of events at the level of the cell, organelle, and molecule. Advances in the area of cholestasis are possible through the use of highly puri- fied canalicular membranes, hepatocyte couplets that secrete bile, and cultures of primary bile duct cells. The consequences of damage to specific parts of the liver will be clarified through experiments with chemicals that have defined target sites. Important interrelationships between sinusoidal cells and other types of liver cells can be identified by using coculture systems or treatments that modify the functions of each type of sinusoidal cell. Knockout rodents and other applications of molecular biology will provide insight into the roles of bioactivation and excretion processes in hepatotoxicity.

BIBLIOGRAPHY

Arias IM (ed): *The Liver: Biology and Pathobiology,* 4th ed. Philadelphia: Lippincott Williams & Wilkins, 2001.

Crawford JM: The liver and the biliary tract, in Cotran RS, Kumar V, Collins T (eds): *Robbins: Pathologic Basis of Disease,* 6th ed. Philadelphia: Saunders, 1999, pp. 845–901.

Farrell GC (ed): *Drug-Induced Liver Disease.* Edinburgh: Churchill Livingstone, 1994.

McCuskey RS, Earnest DL: *Hepatic and Gastrointestinal Toxicology,* vol 9, in Sipes IG, McQueen CA, Gandolfi AJ (eds): *Comprehensive Toxicology.* New York: Pergamon Press, 1997

Selim K, Kaplowitz N: Hepatotoxicity of psychotrophic drugs. *Hepatology* 29:1347–1351, 1999.

Zimmerman HJ: *Hepatotoxicity: The Adverse Effects of Drugs and Other Chemicals on the Liver,* 2d ed. Philadelphia: Lippincott Williams & Wilkins, 1999.

TOXIC RESPONSES OF THE KIDNEY

Rick G. Schnellmann

KEY POINTS

- The kidney contributes to total body homeostasis through its role in the excretion of metabolic wastes, the synthesis and release of renin and erythropoietin, and the regulation of extracellular fluid volume, electrolyte composition, and acid–base balance.

- Xenobiotics in the systemic circulation are delivered to the kidney in relatively high amounts.

- The processes that concentrate urine also serve to concentrate potential toxicants in the tubular fluid.

- Renal transport, accumulation, and biotransformation of xenobiotics contribute to the susceptibility of the kidney to toxic injury.

- Numerous nephrotoxicants cause mitochondrial dysfunction through compromised respiration and ATP production or some other cellular process, leading to either apoptosis or necrosis.

The functional integrity of the mammalian kidney is vital to total body homeostasis because of the kidney's role in the excretion of metabolic wastes, synthesis and release of the hormones renin and erythropoietin, and regulation of extracellular fluid volume, electrolyte composition, and acid–base balance.

FUNCTIONAL ANATOMY

Gross examination of a sagittal section of the kidney reveals three clearly demarcated anatomic areas: the cortex, medulla, and papilla (Fig. 14-1). The cortex receives about 90 percent of blood flow, compared with the medulla (~6 to 10 percent) and the papilla (1 to 2 percent). The functional unit of the kidney, the nephron, may be divided into three portions: the vascular element, the glomerulus, and the tubular element.

Renal Vasculature and Glomerulus

The renal artery branches into afferent arterioles that supply the glomerulus (Fig. 14-1). Then blood leaves the glomerular capillaries through the efferent arteriole. Both the afferent and efferent arterioles control glomerular capillary pressure and the glomerular plasma flow rate. These arterioles are innervated by the sympathetic nerv-

ous system and respond to nerve stimulation, angiotensin II, vasopressin, endothelin, prostanoids, and cytokines. The efferent arterioles that drain the cortical glomeruli branch into a peritubular capillary network, whereas those which drain the juxtamedullary glomeruli form a capillary loop, the vasa recta, that supplies the medullary structures. These postglomerular capillary loops provide delivery of nutrients to the postglomerular tubular structures, delivery of wastes to the tubule for excretion, and return of reabsorbed electrolytes, nutrients, and water to the systemic circulation.

The glomerulus is a complex, specialized capillary bed that filters a portion of the blood into an ultrafiltrate that passes into the tubular portion of the nephron. The formation of such an ultrafiltrate is the net result of the balance between transcapillary hydrostatic pressure and colloid oncotic pressure. An additional determinant of ultrafiltration is the effective hydraulic permeability of the glomerular capillary wall, in other words, the ultrafiltration coefficient (K_f), which is determined by the total surface area available for filtration and the hydraulic permeability of the capillary wall.

Although the glomerular capillary wall permits a high rate of fluid filtration, it provides a significant barrier to the transglomerular passage of macromolecules; thus, small molecules such as inulin [molecular weight (MW) 5500] are freely filtered, whereas large molecules such

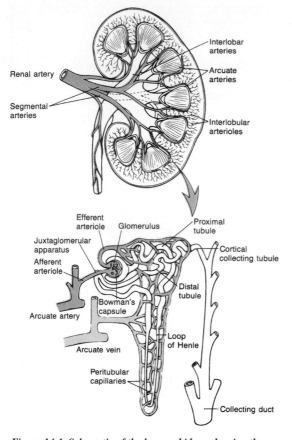

Figure 14-1. Schematic of the human kidney showing the major blood vessels and the microcirculation and tubular components of each nephron. [From Guyton AC, Hall JE (eds): *Textbook of Medical Physiology.* Philadelphia: Saunders, 1996, p. 318, with permission.]

as albumin (MW 56,000 to 70,000) are restricted. Filtration of anionic molecules tends to be restricted compared with that of neutral or cationic molecules of the same size.

Proximal Tubule

The proximal tubule consists of three discrete segments: the S_1 (pars convoluta), S_2 (transition between pars convoluta and pars recta), and S_3 (pars recta) segments. The volume and composition of the glomerular filtrate are altered progressively as fluid passes through each of the different tubular segments. The proximal tubule reabsorbs approximately 60 to 80 percent of solute and water filtered at the glomerulus, mostly by means of

numerous transport systems that are capable of driving the concentrative transport of many metabolic substrates. The proximal tubule also reabsorbs virtually all the filtered low-molecular-weight proteins by means of specific endocytotic protein reabsorption processes.

Loop of Henle

Approximately 25 percent of the filtered Na^+ and K^+ and 20 percent of the filtered water are reabsorbed by the segments of the loop of Henle. The tubular fluid entering the thin descending limb is isosmotic to the renal interstitium; water is freely permeable, and solutes such as electrolytes and urea may enter from the interstitium. In contrast, the thin ascending limb is relatively impermeable to water and urea, and Na^+ and Cl^- are reabsorbed by passive diffusion. The thick ascending limb is

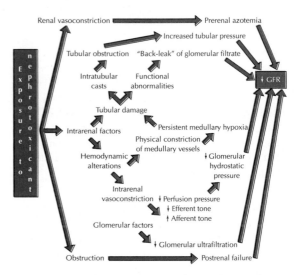

Figure 14-2. Mechanisms that contribute to decreased GFR in acute renal failure. After exposure to a nephrotoxicant, one or more mechanisms may contribute to a reduction in GFR. These mechanisms include renal vasoconstriction resulting in prerenal azotemia and obstruction caused by precipitation of a drug or endogenous compound within the kidney. Intrarenal factors include direct tubular obstruction and dysfunction resulting in tubular back leak and increased tubular pressure. Alterations in the levels of a variety of vasoactive mediators may result in decreased renal perfusion pressure or efferent arteriolar tone and increased afferent arteriolar tone, leading to decreased glomerular hydrostatic pressure. [From Schnellmann RG, Kelly KJ: Pathophysiology of nephrotoxic acute renal failure, in Berl T, Bonventre JV (eds): *Atlas of Diseases of the Kidney.* Philadelphia: Current Medicine, 1999, p. 15.4, with permission.]

impermeable to water, and electrolytes are reabsorbed by the active $Na^+/K^+/2Cl^-$ cotransport mechanism.

Distal Tubule and Collecting Duct

The macula densa contains specialized cells located between the end of the thick ascending limb and the early distal tubule, in close proximity to the afferent arteriole. Under normal physiologic conditions, increased solute delivery or concentration at the macula densa triggers a signal that results in afferent arteriolar constriction, leading to decreases in the glomerular filtration rate (GFR) (and hence decreased solute delivery). This regulatory mechanism is a volume-conserving mechanism that is designed to decrease GFR and prevent massive losses of fluid/electrolytes as a result of impaired tubular reabsorption. The renin-angiotensin system and other substances may be involved. The early distal tubule reabsorbs most of the remaining intraluminal Na^+, K^+, and Cl^- but is relatively impermeable to water.

The late distal tubule, cortical collecting tubule, and medullary collecting duct perform the final regulation and fine-tuning of urinary volume and composition. The remaining Na^+ is reabsorbed in conjunction with K^+ and H^+ secretion in the late distal tubule and the cortical collecting tubule. The combination of medullary and papillary hypertonicity generated by countercurrent multiplication and the action of antidiuretic hormone (vasopressin, ADH) enhances water permeability of the medullary collecting duct.

PATHOPHYSIOLOGIC RESPONSES OF THE KIDNEY

Acute Renal Failure

One of the most common manifestations of nephrotoxic damage is acute renal failure (ARF), which is characterized by an abrupt decline in GFR with resulting azotemia or a buildup of nitrogenous wastes in the blood. Figure 14-2 illustrates the pathways that lead to diminished GFR after chemical exposure. Table 14-1 provides a partial list of chemicals that produce ARF through different mechanisms.

The maintenance of tubular integrity is dependent on cell-to-cell and cell-to-matrix adhesion (Fig. 14-3). It has been hypothesized that after a chemical or hypoxic insult, adhesion of non–lethally damaged, apoptotic, and oncotic cells to the basement membrane is compromised, leading to gaps in the epithelial cell lining, potentially resulting in back leak of filtrate and diminished GFR. These detached cells may aggregate in the tubular lumen

Table 14-1
Mechanisms of Chemically Induced Acute Renal Failure

PRERENAL	VASOCONSTRICTION	CRYSTALLURIA	
Diuretics	Nonsteroidal anti-	Sulfonamides	
Interleukin-2	inflammatory drugs	Methotrexate	
Angiotensin-converting	Radiocontrast agents	Acyclovir	
enzyme inhibitors	Cyclosporine	Triamterene	
Antihypertensive	Tacrolimus	Ethylene glycol	
agents	Amphotericin B	Protease inhibitors	
TUBULAR TOXICITY	**ENDOTHELIAL INJURY**	**GLOMERULOPATHY**	**INTERSTITIAL NEPHRITIS**
Aminoglycosides	Cyclosporine	Gold	Multiple
Cisplatin	Mitomycin C	Penicillamine	
Vancomycin	Tacrolimus	Nonsteroidal anti-	
Pentamidine	Cocaine	inflammatory drugs	
Radiocontrast agents	Conjugated estrogens		
Heavy metals	Quinine		
Haloalkane- and			
haloalkene-cysteine			
conjugates			

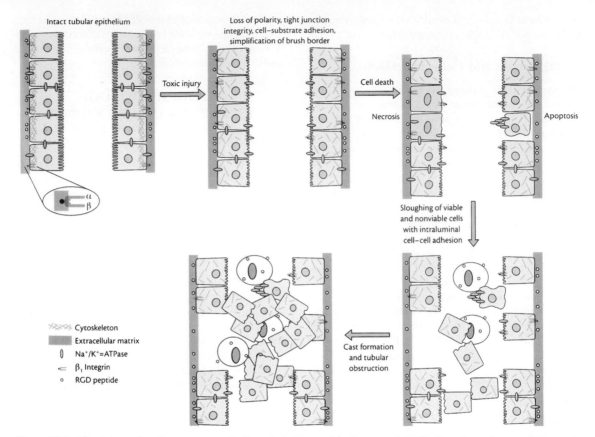

Figure 14-3. After injury, alterations can occur in the cytoskeleton and in the normal distribution of membrane proteins such as Na$^+$, K$^+$-ATPase and β$_1$ integrins in sublethally injured renal tubular cells. These changes result in loss of cell polarity, tight-junction integrity, and cell-substrate adhesion. Lethally injured cells undergo oncosis or apoptosis, and both dead and viable cells may be released into the tubular lumen. Adhesion of released cells to other released cells and to cells remaining adherent to the basement membrane may result in cast formation and tubular obstruction and further compromise the GFR. [From Schnellmann RG, Kelly KJ: Pathophysiology of nephrotoxic acute renal failure, in Berl T, Bonventre JV (eds): *Atlas of Diseases of the Kidney.* Philadelphia: Current Medicine, 1999, p. 15.5, with permission.]

(cell-to-cell adhesion) and/or adhere or reattach to adherent epithelial cells downstream, resulting in tubular obstruction.

Adaptation After a Toxic Insult

The kidney has a remarkable ability to compensate for a loss in renal functional mass. After unilateral nephrectomy, GFR of the remnant kidney increases by approximately 40 to 60 percent. Compensatory increases in single-nephron GFR are accompanied by proportionate increases in proximal tubular water and solute reabsorption; glomerulotubular balance therefore is maintained, and overall renal function appears normal on standard clinical tests. Consequently, chemically induced changes in renal function may not be detected until these compensatory mechanisms are overwhelmed by significant nephron loss and/or damage.

There are a number of cellular and molecular responses to a nephrotoxic insult. After a population of renal cells is exposed to a toxicant, a fraction of the cells will be severely injured and undergo cell death by apoptosis or oncosis (Fig. 14-4). Cells with nonlethal injuries may undergo cell repair and/or adaptation, which contribute to the structural and functional recovery of the nephron. In addition, there is a population of uninjured cells that may undergo compensatory hypertrophy, cellular adaptation, and cellular proliferation. The cellular

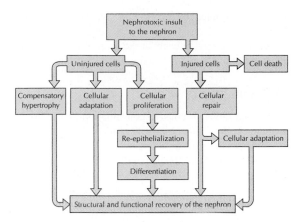

Figure 14-4. The response of the nephron to a nephrotoxic insult. After a population of cells is exposed to a nephrotoxicant, the cells respond; ultimately, the nephron recovers function, or, if cell death and loss are extensive, nephron function ceases. Terminally injured cells undergo cell death through oncosis or apoptosis. Cells injured sublethally undergo repair and adaptation in response to the nephrotoxicant. Cells not injured and adjacent to the injured area may undergo dedifferentiation, proliferation, migration or spreading, and differentiation. Cells that are not injured also may undergo compensatory hypertrophy in response to the cell loss and injury. Finally, the uninjured cells may also undergo adaptation in response to a nephrotoxicant exposure. [From Schnellmann RG, Kelly KJ: Pathophysiology of nephrotoxic acute renal failure, in Berl T, Bonventre JV (eds): *Atlas of Diseases of the Kidney.* Philadelphia: Current Medicine, 1999, p. 15.4, with permission.]

proliferation and compensatory hypertrophy contribute to the structural and functional recovery of the nephron.

Two of the most notable cellular adaptation responses are metallothionein induction and stress protein induction. The distribution of individual heat-shock proteins (Hsps) and glucose-regulated proteins (Grps) varies between different cell types in the kidney and within subcellular compartments. These proteins are involved in the maintenance of normal protein structure and the degradation of damaged proteins and provide a defense mechanism against toxicity by facilitating recovery and repair.

Chronic Renal Failure

Progressive deterioration of renal function may occur with long-term exposure to various chemicals. After nephron loss, adaptive increases in glomerular pressures and flows increase the single-nephron GFR of remnant viable nephrons, which serve to maintain whole-kidney GFR. With time, these alterations are maladaptive, and a focal glomerulosclerosis eventually develops that may lead to tubular atrophy and interstitial fibrosis. Compensatory increases in glomerular pressures and flows of the remnant glomeruli may result in mechanical damage to the capillaries, leading to altered permeabilities.

SUSCEPTIBILITY OF THE KIDNEY TO TOXIC INJURY

Incidence and Severity of Toxic Nephropathy

A wide variety of drugs, environmental chemicals, and metals can cause site-specific nephrotoxicity (Table 14-1). The consequences of ARF vary from recovery to permanent renal damage, which may require dialysis or renal transplantation.

Reasons for the Susceptibility of the Kidney to Toxicity

Although the kidneys constitute only 0.5 percent of total body mass, they receive about 20 to 25 percent of the resting cardiac output. Consequently, any drug or chemical in the systemic circulation is delivered to these organs in relatively high amounts. The processes involved in forming concentrated urine also serve to concentrate potential toxicants in the tubular fluid, thus driving passive diffusion of toxicants into tubular cells. Therefore, a nontoxic concentration of a chemical in the plasma may reach toxic concentrations in the kidney. Finally, renal transport, accumulation, and metabolism of xenobiotics contribute significantly to the susceptibility of the kidney to toxic injury.

In addition to intrarenal factors, the incidence and/or severity of chemically induced nephrotoxicity may be related to the sensitivity of the kidney to circulating vasoconstrictors (angiotensin II or vasopressin), whose actions normally are counterbalanced by the actions of increased vasodilatory prostaglandins. When prostaglandin synthesis is suppressed by nonsteroidal anti-inflammatory drugs (NSAIDs), renal blood flow (RBF) declines markedly and ARF ensues as a result of the unopposed actions of vasoconstrictors. Another example of predisposing risk factors relates to the clinical use of angiotensin-converting enzyme (ACE) inhibitors. Glomerular filtration pressure is dependent on angiotensin II–induced efferent arteriolar constriction. ACE inhibitors block this vasoconstriction, resulting in a precipitous decline in filtration pressure and ARF.

Glomerular Injury

The glomerulus is the initial site of chemical exposure in the nephron, and a number of nephrotoxicants alter glomerular permeability to proteins.

Cyclosporine, amphotericin B, and gentamicin impair glomerular ultrafiltration without a significant loss of structural integrity and decreased GFR. Amphotericin B decreases GFR by causing renal vasoconstriction and decreasing the glomerular capillary ultrafiltration coefficient (K_f). Gentamicin interacts with the anionic sites on the endothelial cells, decreasing K_f and GFR. Finally, cyclosporine not only causes renal vasoconstriction and vascular damage but is injurious to the glomerular endothelial cell.

Chemically induced glomerular injury also may be mediated by extrarenal factors. Circulating immune complexes may be trapped within the glomeruli. Neutrophils and macrophages commonly are observed within glomeruli in membranous glomerulonephritis, and the local release of cytokines and reactive oxygen species (ROS) may contribute to glomerular injury. Heavy metals, hydrocarbons, penicillamine, and captopril can produce this type of glomerular injury. A chemical may function as a hapten attached to a native protein or as a complete antigen and may elicit an antibody response. Antibody reactions with cell-surface antigens lead to immune deposit formation within the glomeruli, mediator activation, and subsequent injury to glomerular tissue.

Proximal Tubular Injury

The proximal tubule is the most common site of toxicant-induced renal injury. The proximal tubule has a leaky epithelium that favors the flux of compounds into proximal tubular cells. The nephrotoxic potential of xenobiotics depends on the intrinsic reactivity of the drug with subcellular or molecular targets. Both cytochrome P450 and cysteine conjugate β-lyase are localized almost exclusively in the proximal tubule, and bioactivation contributes at least in part to the proximal tubular lesions produced by chloroform (via cytochrome P450) and haloalkene S-conjugates (via cysteine β-lyase). Finally, proximal tubular cells appear to be more susceptible to ischemic injury than are distal tubular cells.

Loop of Henle/Distal Tubule/Collecting Duct Injury

Functional abnormalities at these sites manifest primarily as impaired concentrating ability and/or acidification defects. Amphotericin B, cisplatin, and methoxyflurane induce an ADH-resistant polyuria, suggesting that the concentrating defect occurs at the level of the medullary thick ascending limb and/or the collecting duct.

Papillary Injury

The initial target of abusive consumption of analgesics is the medullary interstitial cells, followed by degenerative changes in the medullary capillaries, loops of Henle, and collecting ducts. High papillary concentrations of potential toxicants and inhibition of vasodilatory prostaglandins compromise renal blood flow to the renal medulla/papilla and result in tissue ischemia.

ASSESSMENT OF RENAL FUNCTION

Both in vivo and in vitro methods are available for evaluation of the effects of a chemical on kidney function. Initially, nephrotoxicity can be assessed by evaluating serum and urine chemistries after treatment with the chemical in question. The standard battery of noninvasive tests includes the measurement of urine volume and osmolality, pH, and urinary composition (e.g., electrolytes, glucose, protein).

Chemically induced increases in urine volume accompanied by decreases in osmolality may suggest an impaired concentrating ability, possibly through a defect in ADH synthesis, release, and/or action. Glucosuria may reflect chemically induced defects in proximal tubular reabsorption of sugars or may be secondary to hyperglycemia. Urinary excretion of high-molecular-weight proteins such as albumin is suggestive of glomerular damage, whereas excretion of low-molecular-weight proteins such as β_2-microglobulin suggests proximal tubular injury. Urinary excretion of enzymes localized in the brush border (e.g., alkaline phosphatase, γ-glutamyl transferase) may reflect brush-border damage, whereas urinary excretion of other enzymes (e.g., lactate dehydrogenase) may reflect more generalized cell damage. Enzymuria is often a transient phenomenon, as chemically induced damage may result in an early loss of most of the enzyme available. Thus, the absence of enzymuria does not necessarily reflect an absence of damage.

GFR can be measured directly by determining creatinine or inulin clearance, both of which are essentially freely filtered and not reabsorbed or secreted. Therefore, the clearance of creatinine or inulin is about the same as the GFR. Creatinine is an endogenous compound that is released from skeletal muscle. Inulin is an exogenous compound. Creatinine or inulin clearance is determined by the following formula:

$$\text{Inulin clearance (mL/min)} =$$

$$\frac{\text{inulin concentration in urine}}{\text{Inulin concentration in serum (mg/L)}}$$

Indirect markers of GFR are serial blood urea nitrogen (BUN) and serum creatinine concentrations. However, a 50 to 70 percent decrease in GFR must occur before increases in serum creatinine and BUN develop. Chemically induced increases in BUN and/or serum creatinine may not necessarily reflect renal damage but instead may be secondary to dehydration, hypovolemia, and/or protein catabolism.

Histopathologic evaluation of the kidney after treatment is crucial in identifying the site, nature, and severity of a nephrotoxic lesion. Information on the biotransformation and toxicokinetics of the chemical should be used to direct further in vivo and in vitro studies.

Various in vitro techniques may be used to elucidate the underlying mechanisms. Freshly prepared isolated perfused kidneys, kidney slices, and renal tubular suspensions and cells exhibit the greatest degree of differentiated functions and similarity to the in vivo situation, but these models have limited life spans of 2 to 24 h. In contrast, primary cultures of renal cells and established renal cell lines have longer life spans. Once a mechanism has been identified in vitro, the postulated mechanism must be tested in vivo. Thus, appropriately designed in vivo and in vitro studies should provide a complete characterization of the biochemical, functional, and morphologic effects of a chemical on the kidney and an understanding of the underlying mechanisms in the target cell population(s).

BIOCHEMICAL MECHANISMS/MEDIATORS OF RENAL CELL INJURY

Cell Death

Cell death may occur through either oncosis or apoptosis. Apoptosis is a tightly controlled, organized process that usually affects scattered individual cells. Ultimately, the cell breaks into small fragments that are phagocytosed by adjacent cells or macrophages without producing an inflammatory response. In contrast, oncosis often affects many contiguous cells; the cells rupture, releasing

cellular contents, and inflammation follows. With many toxicants, lower but injurious concentrations produce cell death through apoptosis. As the concentration of the toxicant increases, oncosis plays a predominant role.

Mediators of Toxicity

A chemical can initiate cell injury by various mechanisms (Fig. 14-5). The chemical may initiate toxicity because of its intrinsic reactivity with cellular macromolecules, may require renal or extrarenal bioactivation to a reactive intermediate, or may initiate injury indirectly by inducing oxidative stress through increased production of ROS, such as superoxide anion, hydrogen peroxide, and hydroxyl radicals. ROS and reactive nitrogen species such as peroxynitrite ($ONOO^-$) can attack proteins, lipids, and DNA to induce toxicity.

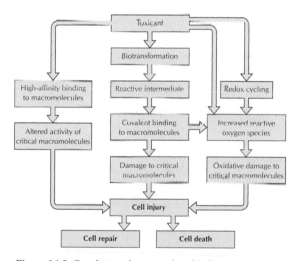

Figure 14-5. Covalent and noncovalent binding versus oxidative stress mechanisms of cell injury. Nephrotoxicants generally are thought to produce cell injury and death through one of two mechanisms, either alone or in combination. In some cases the toxicant may have a high affinity for a specific macromolecule or class of macromolecules that results in altered activity (increase or decrease) of these molecules and cell injury. Alternatively, the parent nephrotoxicant may not be toxic until it is biotransformed into a reactive intermediate that binds covalently to macromolecules and in turn alters their activity, resulting in cell injury. Finally, the toxicant may increase reactive oxygen species in the cells directly after being biotransformed into a reactive intermediate or through redox cycling. The resulting increase in reactive oxygen species causes oxidative damage and cell injury. [From Schnellmann RG, Kelly KJ: Pathophysiology of nephrotoxic acute renal failure, in Berl T, Bonventre JV (eds): *Atlas of Diseases of the Kidney.* Philadelphia: Current Medicine, 1999, p. 15.7, with permission.]

Cell Volume and Ion Homeostasis

Cell volume and ion homeostasis are tightly regulated and are critical for the reabsorptive properties of the tubular epithelial cells. Toxicants generally disrupt cell volume and ion homeostasis either by increasing ion permeability or by inhibiting energy production. The loss of ATP results in the inhibition of membrane transporters that maintain the internal ion balance.

Cytoskeleton and Cell Polarity

Toxicants may cause early changes in membrane integrity. These changes can result from toxicant-induced alterations in cytoskeleton components and cytoskeletal-membrane interactions or may be associated with perturbations in energy metabolism or calcium and phospholipid homeostasis. Under control conditions, the tubular epithelial cell is polarized with respect to certain transporters and enzymes. During in vivo ischemia and in vitro ATP depletion, there is a dissociation of Na^+, K^+-ATPase from the actin cytoskeleton and redistribution from the basolateral membrane to the apical domain in renal proximal tubule cells.

Mitochondria

Numerous nephrotoxicants cause mitochondrial dysfunction through compromised respiration and ATP production or another cellular process. It is clear that mitochondria play a critical role in determining whether cells die by apoptosis or oncosis, depending on cellular ATP levels. The mitochondrial permeability transition (MPT) occurs during cell injury and ultimately progresses to apoptosis if sufficient ATP is available or to oncosis if ATP is depleted. Furthermore, the release of cytochrome c after the MPT plays a key role in activating downstream caspases and executing apoptosis.

Lysosomes

Lysosomes, which are key subcellular targets of aminoglycosides, unleaded gasoline, and d-limonene, are believed to induce cellular injury through rupture and release of lysosomal enzymes and toxicants into the cytoplasm after excessive accumulation of reabsorbed toxicant(s) and lysosomal overload.

Ca^{2+} Homeostasis

The distribution of Ca^{2+} in renal cells is complex, involving binding to anionic sites on macromolecules and compartmentalization within subcellular organelles. The critical cellular Ca^{2+} pool for regulation is the free Ca^{2+} present in the cytosol at a concentration of approximately 100 nM. This level is maintained by a series of pumps and channels located on the plasma membrane and the endoplasmic reticulum (ER). Sustained elevations or abnormally large increases in cytosolic free Ca^{2+} can activate a number of degradative Ca^{2+}-dependent enzymes, such as phospholipases and proteinases, that can produce aberrations in the structure and function of cytoskeletal elements.

Phospholipases

The phospholipase A_2 (PLA$_2$) family of enzymes hydrolyzes phospholipids. A supraphysiologic increase in PLA$_2$ activity can result in the loss of membrane phospholipids and consequently impair membrane function.

Endonucleases

Endonuclease activation and the associated DNA cleavage have been suggested to play a role in renal cell oncosis and apoptosis after hypoxia/reoxygenation.

Proteinases

Supraphysiologic activation of proteinases can disrupt normal membrane and cytoskeleton function and lead to cell death. Under conditions of cell injury, the lysosomal membrane can rupture, releasing hydrolases into the cytosol to degrade susceptible proteins. The calpains are activated by calcium and have cytoskeletal proteins, membrane proteins, and enzymes as substrates. In addition, caspases are another class of cysteine proteinases that play a role in renal cell death. Caspases 1, 2, 3, and 6 have been identified in the rat kidney.

SPECIFIC NEPHROTOXICANTS

Heavy Metals

Many metals—including cadmium, chromium, lead, mercury, platinum, and uranium—are nephrotoxic. The nature and severity of metal nephrotoxicity vary with respect to its form. In addition, different metals have different primary targets in the kidney. Metals may cause renal cellular injury through their ability to bind to sulfhydryl groups of critical proteins in the cells and thus inhibit their normal function.

Mercury The kidneys are the primary target organs for the accumulation of Hg^{2+}. The acute nephrotoxicity induced by $HgCl_2$ is characterized by proximal tubular necrosis and ARF within 24 to 48 h after administration. Early markers of $HgCl_2$-induced renal dysfunction include an increase in the urinary excretion of brush-border enzymes such as alkaline phosphatase and γ-GT. Subsequently, when tubular injury becomes severe, intracellular enzymes such as lactate dehydrogenase and aspartate aminotransferase increase in the urine. As injury progresses, tubular reabsorption of solutes and water decreases.

Changes in mitochondrial morphology and function are very early events after $HgCl_2$ administration, supporting the hypothesis that mitochondrial dysfunction is an early and important contributor to inorganic mercury-induced cell death along the proximal tubule.

Cadmium Cadmium has a half-life of more than 10 years in humans and thus accumulates in the body over time. Approximately 50 percent of the body burden of cadmium can be found in the kidney. Cadmium produces proximal tubule dysfunction and injury that may progress to a chronic interstitial nephritis.

Chemically Induced α_{2u}-Globulin Nephropathy

A diverse group of chemicals—including unleaded gasoline, d-limonene, 1,4-dichlorobenzene, tetrachloroethylene, decalin, and lindane—cause α_{2u}-globulin nephropathy or hyaline droplet nephropathy in male rats. Binding to α_{2u}-globulin decreases lysosomal protease breakdown of α_{2u}-globulin. Chronic exposure to these compounds results in the progression of these lesions and ultimately in chronic nephropathy.

Humans are not at risk because (1) humans do not synthesize α_{2u}-globulin, (2) humans secrete less protein in general and in particular less low-molecular-weight protein in urine than does the rat, and (3) the low-molecular-weight proteins in human urine are not related structurally to α_{2u}-globulin.

Halogenated Hydrocarbons

Humans are exposed to halogenated hydrocarbons in the workplace and in the environment.

Chloroform The primary cellular target of chloroform is the proximal tubule, with no primary damage to the glomerulus or the distal tubule. Proteinuria, glucosuria, and increased blood urea nitrogen levels are all characteristic of chloroform-induced nephrotoxicity. The nephrotoxicity produced by chloroform is linked to its metabolism by renal cytochrome P450, which biotransforms chloroform to trichloromethanol, which is unstable and releases HCl to form phosgene, which reacts injuriously with cellular macromolecules.

Tetrafluoroethylene Tetrafluoroethylene is conjugated with glutathione in the liver, and the glutathione conjugate is secreted into the bile and small intestine, where it is degraded to the cysteine S-conjugate (TFEC), reabsorbed, and transported to the kidney. Although several metabolites are formed, the cysteine S-conjugate is the penultimate nephrotoxicant. After transport into the proximal tubule, the cysteine S-conjugate is a substrate for the cytosolic and mitochondrial forms of the enzyme cysteine conjugate β-lyase. The products of the reaction are ammonia, pyruvate, and a reactive thiol that is capable of binding covalently to cellular macromolecules, causing cellular damage. Functionally, increases in urinary glucose, protein, cellular enzymes, and BUN are noted.

Bromobenzene Biotransformation of bromobenzene and other halogenated benzenes is critical for their nephrotoxicity. Hepatic cytochrome P450 metabolizes bromobenzene, conjugates it to glutathione, and then releases it in a form that can cause nephrotoxicity. The diglutathione conjugate of the hydroquinone is approximately a thousandfold more potent than is bromobenzene in causing nephrotoxicity, producing the same pathologic changes in the S_3 segment and increasing the amount of protein, glucose, and cellular enzymes in the urine.

Mycotoxins

Fumonisins (mycotoxins produced by the fungus *Fusarium moniliforme* and other *Fusarium* species) commonly are found on corn and corn products and produce nephrotoxicity in rats and rabbits. Changes in renal function include increased urine volume, decreased osmolality, and increased excretion of low- and high-molecular-weight proteins. The fumonisins may produce toxicity through interference with sphingolipid metabolism.

Therapeutic Agents

Acetaminophen Acetaminophen (APAP) nephrotoxicity is characterized by proximal tubular necrosis with increases in BUN and plasma creatinine; decreases in GFR and clearance of para-aminohippurate; increases in the fractional excretion of water, sodium, and potassium; and increases in urinary glucose, protein, and brush-border enzymes. Renal cytochrome P450 plays a role in APAP activation and nephrotoxicity, and glutathione conjugates of APAP also may contribute to APAP nephrotoxicity.

Nonsteroidal Anti-Inflammatory Drugs At least three different types of nephrotoxicity have been associated with NSAID administration. ARF may occur within hours after a large dose of a NSAID, is usually reversible upon withdrawal of the drug, and is characterized by decreased RBF and GFR and by oliguria. When the normal production of vasodilatory prostaglandins is inhibited by NSAIDs, vasoconstriction induced by circulating catecholamines and angiotensin II is unopposed, resulting in decreased RBF and ischemia.

In contrast, chronic consumption of NSAIDs and/or APAP (>3 years) results in an often irreversible nephrotoxicity. The primary lesion in this nephropathy is papillary necrosis with chronic interstitial nephritis. The mechanism by which NSAIDs produce analgesic nephropathy is not known, but the process may result from chronic medullary/papillary ischemia secondary to renal vasoconstriction or from the genesis of a reactive intermediate that in turn initiates an oxidative stress or binds covalently to critical cellular macromolecules.

The third, albeit rare, type of nephrotoxicity associated with NSAIDs is an interstitial nephritis. These patients normally present with elevated serum creatinine and proteinuria. If NSAIDs are discontinued, renal function improves in 1 to 3 months.

Aminoglycosides Renal dysfunction caused by aminoglycosides is characterized by nonoliguric renal failure with reduced GFR, an increase in serum creatinine and BUN, and polyuria. The earliest lesion observed after clinically relevant doses of aminoglycosides is an increase in the size and number of lysosomes, which contain phospholipids. The renal phospholipidosis produced by the aminoglycosides is thought to occur through their inhibition of lysosomal hydrolases such as sphingomyelinase and phospholipases.

Amphotericin B Amphotericin B nephrotoxicity is characterized by antidiuretic hormone–resistant polyuria, renal tubular acidosis, hypokalemia, and acute or chronic renal failure. The functional integrity of the glomerulus and of the proximal and distal portions of the nephron is impaired, leading to decreases in RBF and GFR secondary to renal arteriolar vasoconstriction or activation of tubuloglomerular feedback.

Cyclosporine Cyclosporine-induced nephrotoxicity may manifest as (1) acute reversible renal dysfunction, (2) acute vasculopathy, and (3) chronic nephropathy with interstitial fibrosis. Acute renal dysfunction is characterized by dose-related decreases in RBF and GRF and increases in BUN and serum creatinine. The decrease in RBF and GFR is related to the marked vasoconstriction induced by cyclosporine.

Acute vasculopathy or thrombotic microangiopathy after cyclosporine treatment affects arterioles and glomerular capillaries without having an inflammatory component. Hyaline and/or fibroid changes, often with fibrinogen deposition, are observed in arterioles, whereas thrombosis with endothelial cell desquamation affects the glomerular capillaries. Long-term treatment with cyclosporine can result in chronic nephropathy with interstitial fibrosis.

Cisplatin Cisplatin nephrotoxicity includes acute and chronic renal failure, renal magnesium wasting, and polyuria. ARF is characterized by decreases in RBF and GFR, enzymuria, β_2-microglobulinuria, and inappropriate urinary losses of magnesium. The primary cellular target associated with ARF is the proximal tubule. The chronic renal failure observed with cisplatin is due to prolonged exposure and is characterized by focal necrosis in numerous segments of the nephron without a significant effect on the glomerulus. Cisplatin may produce nephrotoxicity through its ability to inhibit DNA synthesis as well as transport functions.

Radiocontrast Agents Iodinated contrast media used for the imaging of tissues have a very high osmolality (>1200 mOsm/L) and are potentially nephrotoxic, particularly in patients with existing renal impairment, diabetes, or heart failure and those who are receiving other nephrotoxic drugs. The newer nonionic contrast agents (e.g., iotrol, iopamidol) have lower nephrotoxicity. The nephrotoxicity of these agents is due to both hemodynamic alterations (vasoconstriction) and tubular injury (via ROS).

BIBLIOGRAPHY

Berl T, Bonventre JV (eds): *Atlas of Diseases of the Kidney.* Philadelphia: Current Medicine, 1999.

DeBroe ME, Porter GA, Bennett AM, Verpooten GA (eds): *Clinical Nephrotoxicants, Renal Injury from Drugs and Chemicals.* Amsterdam, Netherlands: Kluwer, 1998.

Goldstein RS (ed): *Renal Toxicology.* Vol. 7 in Sipes IG, McQueen CA, Gandolfi AJ (eds): *Comprehensive Toxicology.* New York: Elsevier, 1997.

Molitoris BA, Finn WF (eds): *Acute Renal Failure: A Companion to Brenner's and Rector's The Kidney.* Philadelphia: Saunders, 2001.

Zalups RK, Lash LH (eds): *Methods in Renal Toxicology.* Boca Raton, FL: CRC Press, 1996.

C H A P T E R   1 5

TOXIC RESPONSES OF THE RESPIRATORY SYSTEM

Hanspeter R. Witschi and Jerold A. Last

KEY POINTS

- Inhaled xenobiotics can affect lung tissues directly and can affect distant organs after absorption.
- Water solubility is a decisive factor in determining how deeply a given gas penetrates into the lung.
- Particle size is usually the critical factor that determines the region of the respiratory tract in which a particle or an aerosol will deposit.
- The lung contains most of the enzymes involved in xenobiotic biotransformation that have been identified in other tissues.
- Asthma is characterized by increased reactivity of the bronchial smooth muscle in response to exposure to irritants.
- In emphysema, destruction of the gas-exchanging surface area results in a distended, hyperinflated lung that no longer effectively exchanges oxygen and carbon dioxide.

Exposure to chemicals by inhalation can have two effects: on the lung tissues and on distant organs that are reached after chemicals enter the body by means of inhalation. Indeed, the term *inhalation toxicology* refers to the route of exposure, whereas *respiratory tract toxicology* refers to target-organ toxicity, that is, the abnormal changes in the respiratory tract produced by toxicants. Lung tissue can be injured directly or secondarily by metabolic products from organic compounds. However, the most important effect of many toxic inhalants is to place an undue oxidative burden on the lungs.

LUNG STRUCTURE AND FUNCTION

Nasal Passages

Air enters the respiratory tract through the nasal and oral regions (Figure 15-1). The nasal passages function as a filter for particles. Highly water-soluble gases are absorbed efficiently in the nasal passages, which reach from the nostril to the pharynx. Also, nasal epithelia can metabolize foreign compounds. Cytochrome P450 isozymes 1A1, 2B1, and 4B1 have been localized in the nose in several species.

Conducting Airways

The trachea and bronchi are covered with mucus that traps pollutants and debris. The action of the respiratory tract cilia continuously drives the mucous layer toward the pharynx, where it is removed from the respiratory system by swallowing or expectoration. The mucous layer also is thought to have antioxidant, acid-neutralizing, and free radical–scavenging functions that protect the epithelial cells.

Conducting airways have a characteristic branched bifurcating structure with a progressively decreasing internal diameter. Eventually a transition zone is reached where cartilaginous bronchi give way to noncartilaginous bronchioles, which in turn give way to gas-exchange regions, respiratory bronchioles, and alveoli.

Gas-Exchange Region

A ventilatory unit is the anatomic region that includes all alveolar ducts and alveoli distal to each bronchiolar-alveolar duct junction. Gas exchange occurs in the alveoli; adult human lungs contain an estimated 300 million alveoli. Within the alveolar septum, capillaries are organized in a single sheet. Capillaries are separated from the air space by a thin layer of tissue formed by epithelial, interstitial, and endothelial components.

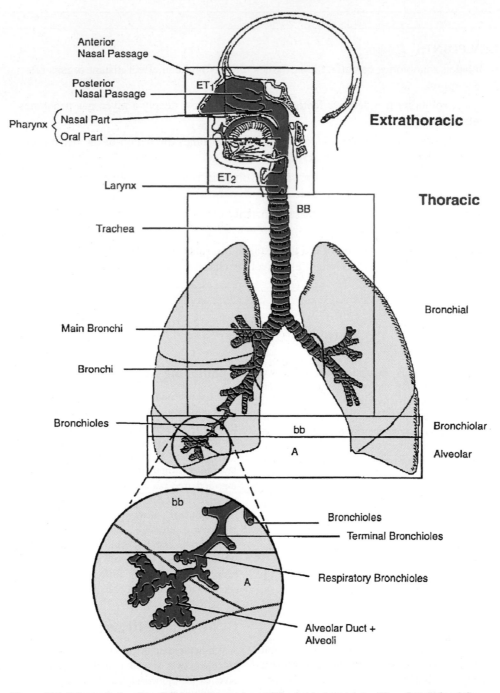

Figure 15-1. Schematic drawing of the anatomic regions of the respiratory tract. (From International Commission on Radiological Protection, Human Respiratory Tract Model for Radiological Protection. ICRP Publication 66; *Ann ICRP.* Oxford: Pergamon Press, 1994, p. 24.)

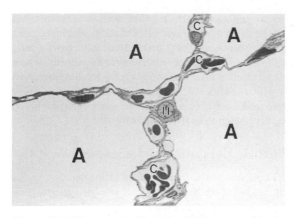

Figure 15-2. Micrograph of four alveoli (A) *separated by the alveolar septum.* The thin air-to-blood tissue barrier of the alveolar septal wall is composed of squamous alveolar type I cells and occasional alveolar type II cells (II), a small interstitial space, and the attenuated cytoplasm of the endothelial cells that form the wall of the capillaries (C). (Photograph courtesy of Dr. Kent E. Pinkerton, University of California, Davis.)

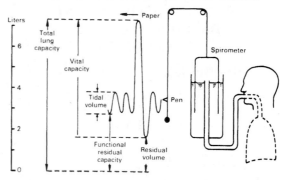

RESPONSES OF THE RESPIRATORY SYSTEM TO TOXIC AGENTS

Figure 15-3. Lung volumes. Note that the functional residual capacity and residual volume cannot be measured with a spirometer but require special procedures (e.g., nitrogen or helium outwash). (From West JB: *Respiratory Physiology—The Essentials.* Baltimore: Williams & Wilkins, 1994, with permission.)

Type I and type II alveolar cells represent approximately 25 percent of all the cells in the alveolar septum (Fig. 15-2). Type I cells cover a large surface area. Type II cells are cuboidal, have abundant perinuclear cytoplasm, produce surfactant, and in cases of damage to the type I epithelium may undergo mitotic division and replace damaged cells.

The mesenchymal interstitium consists of fibroblasts that produce collagen, elastin, other cell matrix components, and various effector molecules. Pericytes, monocytes, and lymphocytes also reside in the interstitium, as do macrophages before they enter the alveoli. Clara cells are located in the terminal bronchioles and have a high content of xenobiotic-metabolizing enzymes.

Gas Exchange

The principal function of the lung is gas exchange, which consists of ventilation, perfusion, and diffusion.

Ventilation During inhalation, fresh air moves into the lung through the upper respiratory tract and conducting airways and into the terminal respiratory units. After diffusion of oxygen into the blood and that of CO_2 from the blood into the alveolar spaces, the air (now enriched in CO_2) is expelled by exhalation.

The total volume of air in an inflated human lung represents the total lung capacity (TLC). After a maximum expiration, the lung retains the residual volume (RV). The air volume moved into and out of the lung with a maximum inspiratory and expiratory movement is called the vital capacity (VC). Under resting conditions, the fraction of the vital capacity moved into and out of the lung is called the tidal volume (TV) (Fig. 15-3). If an augmented metabolic demand of the body requires the delivery of increased amounts of oxygen, both the TV and the respiratory rate can be increased greatly.

Perfusion The lung receives the entire output from the right ventricle and thus may be exposed to substantial amounts of toxic agents carried in the blood. An agent entering the peripheral venous system ultimately comes into contact with the pulmonary capillary bed before distribution to other organs or tissues in the body.

Diffusion Gas exchange takes place across the entire alveolar surface. A variety of abnormal processes may thicken the alveolar septum and adversely affect the diffusion of oxygen to the erythrocytes. Those processes may include collection of liquid in the alveolar space, abnormal thickening of the pulmonary epithelium, accumulation of tissue constituents in the interstitial space, and increased formation and deposition of extracellular substances such as collagen.

GENERAL PRINCIPLES IN THE PATHOGENESIS OF LUNG DAMAGE CAUSED BY CHEMICALS

Oxidative Burden

An undue oxidative burden that often is mediated by free radicals, such as those generated by ozone, NO_2, tobacco smoke, and lung defense cells, contributes to lung damage. Because these oxidant species are potentially cytotoxic, they may mediate or promote the actions of pneumotoxicants such as paraquat and nitrofurantoin. When cellular injury of any type occurs, the release of otherwise contained cellular constituents such as microsomes and flavoproteins into the extracellular space may lead to extracellular generation of deleterious reactive O_2 species.

Neutrophils, monocytes, and macrophages seem to be particularly adept at converting molecular O_2 to reactive O_2 metabolites; this probably is related to their phagocytotic and antimicrobial activities. As a by-product of this capability, toxic O_2 species are released into surrounding tissues. As most forms of toxic pulmonary edema are accompanied by phagocyte accumulation in the lung microcirculation (pulmonary leukostasis) and parenchyma, oxidative damage may represent a significant component of pneumotoxic lung injury.

Phagocytic production of active oxygen species causes inactivation of proteinase inhibitors and degranulation of mast cells.

The lung can respond with specific defense mechanisms that may be stimulated by constant exposure to airborne microorganisms as well as to low- and high-molecular-weight antigenic materials. The immune system can mount either cellular or humorally mediated responses to these inhaled antigens. Direct immunologic effects occur when inhaled foreign material sensitizes the respiratory system to further exposure to the same material. Bronchoconstriction and chronic pulmonary disease can result from the inhalation of materials that appear to act wholly or partly through an allergic response.

Toxic Inhalants, Gases, and Dosimetry

The sites of deposition of toxicants in the respiratory tract define the pattern of their toxicity. Water solubility is the critical factor in determining how deeply a given gas penetrates into the lung. Highly soluble gases such as SO_2 do not penetrate farther than the nose and therefore are relatively nontoxic to animals. Relatively insoluble gases such as ozone and NO_2 penetrate deeply into the lung and reach the smallest airways and the alveoli, where they can elicit toxic responses. Very insoluble gases such as CO and H_2S efficiently pass through the respiratory tract and are taken up by the pulmonary blood supply to be distributed throughout the body.

Particle Deposition and Clearance

Particle size is usually the critical factor that determines the region of the respiratory tract in which a particle or an aerosol will be deposited.

Particle Size Larger particles usually are distributed to the upper air passages, and smaller particles are transported all the way to the alveoli (Fig. 15-4). Particle shape and density also may play a role in distribution. Inhaled aerosols are most frequently polydisperse in regard to size.

Deposition Mechanisms Deposition of particles occurs primarily by interception, impaction, sedimentation, and diffusion (Brownian movement). Interception occurs

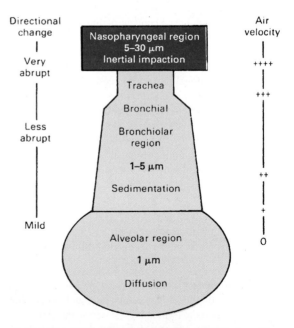

Figure 15-4. Parameters that influence particle deposition. [From Casarett LJ: The vital sacs: Alveolar clearance mechanisms in inhalation toxicology, in Blood FR (ed): *Essays in Toxicology,* vol. 3. New York: Academic Press, 1972, with permission.]

when the trajectory of a particle brings it close enough to a surface that the particle contacts the airway surface. As a result of inertia, particles suspended in air tend to continue to travel along their original path. In a bending airstream, such as at an airway bifurcation, a particle may be impacted on the surface.

Sedimentation brings about deposition in the smaller bronchi, the bronchioles, and the alveolar spaces. As a particle moves downward through air, buoyancy and the resistance of air act on the particle in an upward direction, while gravitational force acts on the particle in a downward direction. Eventually, the gravitational force equilibrates with the sum of the buoyancy and the air resistance, and the particle settles with a constant velocity known as the terminal settling velocity.

Diffusion is important in the deposition of submicrometer particles. A random motion is imparted to those particles by the impact of gas molecules.

An important factor in particle deposition is the pattern of breathing. During quiet breathing, a large proportion of the inhaled particles may be exhaled. During exercise, when larger volumes are inhaled at higher velocities, deposition in airways increases. Breath holding also increases deposition. Factors that modify the diameter of the conducting airways can alter particle deposition. In patients with chronic bronchitis, the mucous layer is greatly thickened and extended peripherally and may partially block the airways in some areas. Jets formed by air flowing through such partially occluded airways have the potential to increase the deposition of particles.

Particle Clearance   The clearance of deposited particles is an important aspect of lung defense. Rapid removal lessens the time available to cause damage to the pulmonary tissues or permit local absorption. Particles are cleared to (1) the stomach and gastrointestinal (GI) tract, (2) the lymphatics and lymph nodes, where they may be dissolved and enter the venous circulation, or (3) the pulmonary vasculature.

Nasal Clearance   Particles deposited in the nose are cleared by various mechanisms, depending on their site of deposition and solubility in mucus. Particles deposited in the anterior nose are removed by extrinsic actions such as wiping and blowing. The other regions of the nose are largely covered by a mucociliary epithelium that propels mucus toward the glottis, where it is swallowed.

Tracheobronchial Clearance   The mucous layer covering the tracheobronchial tree is moved upward by the

beating of the underlying cilia. This mucociliary escalator transports deposited particles and particle-laden macrophages to the oropharynx, where they are swallowed and pass through the GI tract.

Pulmonary Clearance   There are several primary ways in which particulate material is removed from the lower respiratory tract once it has been deposited:

1.   Particles may be trapped directly on the fluid layer of the conducting airways by impaction and cleared upward in the tracheobronchial tree by the mucociliary escalator.
2.   Particles may be phagocytized by macrophages and cleared by the mucociliary escalator.
3.   Particles may be phagocytized by alveolar macrophages and removed by lymphatic drainage.
4.   Material may dissolve from the surfaces of particles and be removed by the bloodstream or lymphatics.
5.   Small particles may directly penetrate epithelial membranes.

ACUTE RESPONSES OF THE LUNG TO INJURY

Airway Reactivity

Large airways are surrounded by bronchial smooth muscles, which help maintain airway tone and diameter during expansion and contraction of the lung. Bronchial smooth muscle tone normally is regulated by the autonomic nervous system. Bronchoconstriction can be provoked by irritants such as cigarette smoke and air pollutants and by cholinergic drugs such as acetylcholine, histamine, various prostaglandins and leukotrienes, substance P, and nitric oxide. Bronchoconstriction causes a decrease in airway diameter and a corresponding increase in resistance to airflow. Characteristic associated symptoms include wheezing, coughing, a sensation of chest tightness, and dyspnea. Exercise potentiates these problems.

Pulmonary Edema

Toxic pulmonary edema represents an acute, exudative phase of lung injury that alters ventilation-perfusion relationships and limits diffusive transfer of O_2 and CO_2 even in otherwise structurally normal alveoli.

Mechanisms of Respiratory Tract Injury

Airborne agents can contact cells lining the respiratory tract from the nostrils to the gas-exchanging region. Certain gases and vapors stimulate nerve endings in the nose, particularly those of the trigeminal nerve. The result is holding of the breath or changes in breathing patterns to avoid or reduce further exposure. If continued exposure cannot be avoided, many acidic or alkaline irritants produce cell necrosis and increased permeability of the alveolar walls. Other inhaled agents can be more insidious; inhalation of HCl, NO_2, NH_3, or phosgene may at first produce very little apparent damage in the respiratory tract. The epithelial barrier in the alveolar zone, after a latency period of several hours, begins to leak, flooding the alveoli and producing a delayed pulmonary edema that is often fatal.

A different pathogenetic mechanism is typical of highly reactive molecules such as ozone. It is unlikely that ozone as such can penetrate beyond the layer of fluid covering the cells of the lung. Instead, ozone lesions are propagated by a cascade of secondary reaction products and by reactive oxygen species that arise from free radical reactions.

Metabolism of foreign compounds can be involved in the pathogenesis of lung injury. The lung contains most of the enzymes involved in xenobiotic metabolism that have been identified in other tissues. Microsomal enzymes identified in lung include cytochrome P450 1A1, 2B1, 2F1, 4B1, and 3A4 as well as NADPH cytochrome P450 reductase, epoxide hydrolase, and flavin-containing monooxygenases. Two important cytosolic enzymes involved in lung xenobiotic metabolism are glutathione S-transferases and glutathione peroxidase.

Cell Proliferation

The effects of toxicants on the lung may be reversible or irreversible. The normal adult lung is an organ for which under normal circumstances very few cells appear to die and need to be replaced. When damaged by a toxic insult, the lung parenchyma is capable of repairing itself. Type I cell damage is followed by the proliferation of type II epithelial cells, which eventually transform into new type I cells; in the airways, the Clara cells proliferate and divide after injury. The migration of mobile blood cells such as leukocytes across the pulmonary capillaries into the alveolar lumen also may trigger a mitotic response. Other cells in the alveolar zone, such as capillary endothelial cells, interstitial cells, and alveolar

macrophages, also proliferate. The result is a normal-looking organ, although on occasion excessive proliferation of fibroblasts may result in lung disease. In general, the lung appears to have a high capacity to repair itself and thus to deal with the many toxic insults presented by the environment.

CHRONIC RESPONSES OF THE LUNG TO INJURY

Fibrosis

Fibrotic lungs from humans with acute or chronic pulmonary fibrosis contain increased amounts of collagen. In lungs damaged by toxicants, the response resembles adult or infant respiratory distress syndrome. Excess lung collagen usually is observed not only in the alveolar interstitium but also throughout the alveolar ducts and respiratory bronchioles.

Type I collagen and type III collagen are major interstitial components and are found in an approximate ratio of 2:1. There is an increase in type I collagen relative to type III collagen in patients with idiopathic pulmonary fibrosis and patients who are dying of acute respiratory distress syndrome. It is not known whether shifts in collagen types, compared with absolute increases in collagen content, account for the increased stiffness of fibrotic lungs. Because type III collagen is more compliant than is type I, increasing type I relative to type III collagen may result in a stiffer lung. Changes in collagen cross-linking in fibrotic lungs also may contribute to the increased stiffness.

Emphysema

In emphysema, the lungs become larger and overly compliant. Destruction of the gas-exchanging surface area results in a distended, hyperinflated lung that no longer effectively exchanges oxygen and carbon dioxide as a result of both loss of tissue and air trapping. The major cause of human emphysema is, by far, inhalation of cigarette smoke, although other toxicants also can elicit this response. A feature of toxicant-induced emphysema is severe or recurrent inflammation.

A unifying hypothesis that explains the pathogenesis of emphysema has emerged from studies conducted by several investigators. Alpha$_1$-antitrypsin (now called alpha$_1$-antiprotease) is one of the body's main defenses against uncontrolled proteolytic digestion by this class of enzymes, which includes elastase. Studies in smokers led to the hypothesis that neutrophil (and perhaps alveolar macrophage) elastases can break down lung elastin and thus cause emphysema; these elastases usually are kept in check by alpha$_1$-antiprotease that diffuses into the lung from the blood. As an individual ages, an accumulation of random elastolytic events can cause the emphysematous changes in the lungs that normally are associated with aging. Toxicants that cause inflammatory cell influx and thus increase the burden of neutrophil elastase can accelerate this process.

Asthma

Asthma is characterized clinically by attacks of shortness of breath, which is caused by narrowing of the large conducting airways (bronchi). The clinical hallmark of asthma is increased reactivity of the bronchial smooth muscle in response to exposure to irritants.

Lung Cancer

Lung cancer is the leading cause of death from cancer among men and women. Retrospective and prospective epidemiologic studies unequivocally show an association between tobacco smoking and lung cancer. Average smokers have a 10-fold and heavy smokers a 20-fold increased risk of developing lung cancer compared with nonsmokers. Many other agents also cause lung cancer (see Table 15-1).

Human lung cancers may have a latency period of 20 to 40 years, making the relationship to specific exposures difficult to establish. Many lung cancers in humans originate from the cells lining the airways, but during the last two decades, a significant increase in peripheral adenocarcinomas has occurred. Compared with cancer in the lung, cancer in the upper respiratory tract is less common.

The potential mechanisms of lung carcinogenesis center on damage to DNA. An activated carcinogen or its metabolic product may interact with DNA. DNA damage caused by active oxygen species is another potentially important mechanism. Ionizing radiation leads to the formation of superoxide. Cigarette smoke contains high quantities of active oxygen species and other free radicals.

AGENTS KNOWN TO PRODUCE LUNG INJURY IN HUMANS

During the last 20 years, a large body of knowledge about the cellular and molecular events that determine lung injury and repair has accumulated. Table 15-1 lists common toxicants that are known to produce acute and chronic lung injury in humans.

Airborne Agents That Produce Lung Injury in Humans

Lung Overload Caused by Particles Investigators have observed a slowing of the rate of alveolar clearance when deposited lung burdens are high. Clearance mechanisms in the deep lung that depend predominantly if not completely on phagocytosis and migration of pulmonary alveolar macrophages can be overwhelmed by quantities of respirable dusts that are far in excess of physiologic loads. As a consequence, lung burdens of these dusts persist for months or years, and completely unphysiologic mechanisms of disease pathogenesis may come into play.

Oxygen Oxygen toxicity is mediated through increased production of partially reduced oxygen products. In animals exposed to 95 to 100% oxygen, diffuse pulmonary damage develops and is usually fatal after 3 to 4 days. Type I epithelial cells and capillary endothelial cells develop necrotic changes. Capillary damage leads to leakage of proteinaceous fluid and formed blood elements into the alveolar space. Hyaline membranes formed by cellular debris and proteinaceous exudate are a characteristic sign of pulmonary oxygen toxicity. In animals that are returned to air after the development of acute oxygen toxicity, there is active cell proliferation.

Blood-Borne Agents That Cause Pulmonary Toxicity in Humans

Paraquat The bipyridylium herbicide paraquat produces extensive lung injury when ingested by humans. In patients who survive the first few days of acute paraquat poisoning, progressive and eventually fatal lung lesions characterized by diffuse interstitial and intraalveolar fibrosis can develop. After initial widespread necrosis, extensive proliferation of fibroblasts in the alveolar interstitium follows. Paraquat accumulates in the cells of the lung. Once it is inside the cells, paraquat continuously cycles from the oxidized form to the reduced form, with the concomitant formation of active oxygen species and eventual depletion of cellular NADPH.

Monocrotaline Monocrotaline is one of many structurally related naturally occurring products that have been identified in grains, honey, and herbal teas. These compounds produce hepatocellular necrosis and venoocclusive disease. Monocrotaline is metabolized in the liver by cytochrome P450 3A to a highly reactive pyrrole, a bifunctional alkylating agent, some of which is released from the liver and travels to other organs, such

Table 15-1
Industrial Toxicants That Produce Lung Disease

TOXICANT	COMMON NAME OF DISEASE	OCCUPATIONAL SOURCE	ACUTE EFFECT	CHRONIC EFFECT
Asbestos	Asbestosis	Mining, construction, shipbuilding, manufacture of asbestos-containing material		Fibrosis, pleural calcification, lung cancer, pleural mesothelioma
Aluminum dust	Aluminosis	Manufacture of aluminum products, fireworks, ceramics, paints, electrical goods, abrasives	Cough, shortness of breath	Interstitial fibrosis
Aluminum abrasives	Shaver's disease, corundum smelter's lung, bauxite lung	Manufacture of abrasives, smelting	Alveolar edema	Interstitial fibrosis, emphysema
Ammonia		Ammonia production, manufacture of fertilizers, chemical production, explosives	Upper and lower respiratory tract irritation, edema	Chronic bronchitis
Arsenic		Manufacture of pesticides, pigments, glass, alloys	Bronchitis	Lung cancer, bronchitis, laryngitis
Beryllium	Berylliosis	Ore extraction, manufacture of alloys, ceramics	Severe pulmonary edema, pneumonia	Fibrosis, progressive dyspnea, interstitial granulomatosis, lung cancer, cor pulmonale
Cadmium oxide		Welding, manufacture of electrical equipment, alloys, pigments, smelting	Cough, pneumonia	Emphysema, cor pulmonale
Carbides of tungsten, titanium, tantalum	Hard metal disease	Manufacture of cutting edges on tools	Hyperplasia and metaplasia of bronchial epithelium	Peribronchial and perivascular fibrosis
Chlorine		Manufacture of pulp and paper, plastics, chlorinated chemicals	Cough, hemoptysis, dyspnea, tracheobronchitis, bronchopneumonia	
Chromium (VI)		Production of Cr compounds, paint pigments; reduction of chromite ore	Nasal irritation, bronchitis	Lung cancer, fibrosis
Coal dust		Coal mining		Fibrosis
Cotton dust	Pneumoconiosis Byssinosis	Manufacture of textiles	Chest tightness, wheezing, dyspnea	Reduced pulmonary function, chronic bronchitis

(continued)

Table 15-1
Industrial Toxicants That Produce Lung Disease *(continued)*

TOXICANT	COMMON NAME OF DISEASE	OCCUPATIONAL SOURCE	ACUTE EFFECT	CHRONIC EFFECT
Hydrogen fluoride		Manufacture of chemicals, photographic film, solvents, plastics	Respiratory irritation, hemorrhagic pulmonary edema	
Iron oxides	Siderotic lung disease; silver finisher's lung, hematite miner's lung, arc welder's lung	Welding, foundry work, steel manufacture, hematite mining, jewelry making	Cough	Silver finisher's lung: subpleural and perivascular aggregations of macrophages; hematite miner's lung: diffuse fibrosis-like pneumoconiosis; arc welder's lung: bronchitis
Isocyanates		Manufacture of plastics, chemical industry	Airway irritation, cough, dyspnea	Asthma, reduced pulmonary function
Kaolin	Kaolinosis	Pottery making		Fibrosis
Manganese	Manganese pneumonia	Chemical and metal industries	Acute pneumonia, often fatal	Recurrent pneumonia
Nickel		Nickel ore extraction, smelting, electronic electroplating, fossil fuels	Pulmonary edema, delayed by 2 days (NiCO)	Squamous cell carcinoma of nasal cavity and lung
Oxides of nitrogen		Welding, silo filling, explosive manufacture	Pulmonary congestion and edema	Bronchiolitis obliterans
Ozone		Welding, bleaching flour, deodorizing	Pulmonary edema	Fibrosis
Phosgene		Production of plastics, pesticides, chemicals	Edema	Bronchitis, fibrosis
Perchloro-ethylene		Dry cleaning, metal degreasing, grain fumigating	Edema	Cancer, liver and lung
Silica	Silicosis, pneumoconiosis	Mining, stone cutting, construction, farming, quarrying, sand blasting	Acute silicosis	Fibrosis, silicotuberculosis
Sulfur dioxide		Manufacture of chemicals, refrigeration, bleaching, fumigation	Bronchoconstriction, cough, chest tightness	Chronic bronchitis
Talc	Talcosis	Rubber industry, cosmetics		Fibrosis
Tin	Stanosis	Mining, processing of tin		Widespread mottling of x-ray without clinical signs
Vanadium		Steel manufacture	Airway irritation and mucus production	Chronic bronchitis

as the lung by red blood cells (RBCs), where it initiates endothelial injury with resulting hypertension of the pulmonary arterial system and hypertrophy of the right side of the heart.

Bleomycin Bleomycin is a widely used cancer chemotherapeutic agent that also produces pulmonary fibrosis. The sequence of damage includes necrosis of capillary endothelial and type I alveolar cells, edema formation and hemorrhage, delayed (after 1 to 2 weeks) proliferation of type II epithelial cells, and eventually thickening of the alveolar walls by fibrotic changes.

Cyclophosphamide and 1,3-Bis-(2-Chloroethyl)-1-Nitrosourea (BCNU) Cyclophosphamide is widely used as an anticancer and immunosuppressive agent. The undesirable side effects include hemorrhagic cystitis and pulmonary fibrosis. Cyclophosphamide is metabolized by the cytochrome P450 system to two highly reactive metabolites—acrolein and phosphoramide mustard—which initiate lipid peroxidation. In humans, a dose-related pulmonary toxicity often is noticed first as a decrease in diffusion capacity, and subsequent pulmonary fibrosis can be fatal. Because BCNU inhibits pulmonary glutathione disulfide reductase, the GSH/GSSG ratio may be disturbed, leaving lung cells unable to cope with oxidant stress.

Cationic Amphophilic Drugs Several drugs with similar structural characteristics, such as the antiarrhythmic amiodarone and the anorexic chlorphentermine, elicit pulmonary lipidosis, presumably because these drugs inhibit phospholipases A and B. Degradation of pulmonary surfactant is impaired, and the material accumulates in phagocytic cells.

METHODS FOR STUDYING LUNG INJURY

Inhalation Exposure Systems

Monitoring and quantifying gaseous pollutants require either expensive detectors or very labor intensive wet chemical analysis procedures after sampled gases from the chambers are bubbled through traps. Particle generation is difficult. Exposure chambers must allow for rapid attainment of the desired concentrations of toxicants, maintenance of desired levels homogeneously throughout the chamber, adequate capacity for experimental animals, and minimal accumulation of undesired products associated with animal occupancy (usually ammonia, dander, heat, and carbon dioxide). As a general rule, the

total body volume of the animals should not exceed 5 percent of the chamber volume. Nose-only exposure chambers avoid some of these problems.

Pulmonary Function Studies

Commonly used tests include measurement of VC, TLC, functional residual volume, TV, airway resistance, and maximum flow (Fig. 15-5). Additional tests evaluate the distribution of ventilation, lung and chest wall compliance, diffusion capacity, and the oxygen and carbon dioxide content of the arterial and venous blood.

The FEV_1 (forced expiratory volume during the first second of an active exhalation) is an easy test to administer to humans, does not require sophisticated equipment or a hospital setting, and is completely noninvasive. A reduction in FEV_1 is usually indicative of impaired ventilation such as that found in restrictive (increased lung stiffness) or obstructive (obstructed airflow) lung disease.

Analysis of breathing patterns has been used widely to assess the effects of irritants. This technique allows one to differentiate between sensory or upper airway irritants and "pulmonary" irritants. Highly water soluble irritants such as ammonia, chlorine, and formaldehyde produce upper respiratory tract irritation, whereas less soluble gases such as nitrogen dioxide and ozone generate pulmonary irritation. The sensory irritant pattern has been described as slowing down respiratory frequency while increasing TV. Pulmonary irritants usually increase

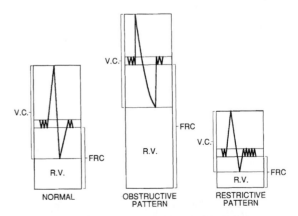

Figure 15-5. Typical lung volume measurements from individuals with normal lung function, obstructive airway disease, or restrictive lung disease. Note that there is (1) a slowing of forced expiration in addition to gas trapping (an increase in residual volume) in obstructive disease and (2) a general decrease in lung volumes in restrictive disease. Note that the measurements read from left to right.

respiratory frequency and decrease minute volume. The result is rapid, shallow breathing.

To accomplish proper oxygenation of venous blood and elimination of CO_2, the gases have to diffuse across the air-blood barrier. Gas exchange can be evaluated by measuring the arterial partial pressure of both oxygen and CO_2. In general, blood gas analysis is a comparatively insensitive assay for disturbed ventilation because of an organism's buffering and reserve capacities. Although it is a useful tool in clinical medicine, only the most severe obstructive or restrictive pulmonary alterations cause signs of impaired gas exchange in animals. Measurement of diffusion capacity with CO, a gas that binds with 250 times higher affinity to hemoglobin than does oxygen, is more sensitive and is used widely in toxicology studies.

Morphologic Techniques

The pathology of acute and chronic injury may be described after examination of the respiratory tract by gross inspection and under the microscope. Morphologic evaluation should include nasal passages and the larynx; major airways must be examined as well as the lung parenchyma. Careful consideration must be given to tissue fixation and preparation. The choice of a fixative depends on how the lung will be analyzed further.

Ordinary paraffin sections of respiratory tract tissue are suitable for routine histopathologic analysis; gross pathologic changes such as inflammation and the presence of cancerous tissue can be detected easily. Plastic or epon sections about 1 μm thick are required for proper identification of different cell types lining the airways or alveoli and for recognition of cytoplasmic changes in damaged Clara cells. Other structural alterations, such as degenerative changes and necrosis of type I epithelial cells or capillary endothelial cells, usually are detected on transmission electron microscopy. Scanning electron microscopy allows visualization of the surface of interior lung structures, reveals alterations in the tissue surface, and detects rearrangement of the overall cell population. Confocal microscopy allows examination of thick sections and discovery of specific cell types deep within the tissue; it is an ideal tool for three-dimensional reconstruction of normal and damaged lung.

Additional tools for the study of toxic lung injury include immunohistochemistry, in situ hybridization, and analysis of cell kinetics. Antibodies to a variety of enzymes, mediators, and other proteins are available. In situ hybridization allows one to visualize anatomic sites where a specific gene product is expressed, for example, collagen production in a fibrotic lung. Flow cytometry is valuable in the study of cell populations prepared from the lung. This technique requires dissociation of the lung parenchyma into its individual cell populations. Different lung cells then can be identified and isolated.

Pulmonary Lavage

Generally, the lungs of exposed and control animals are washed with multiple small volumes of isotonic saline. Current emphasis seems to be on the measurement of polymorphonuclear leukocytes, macrophages, and monocytes (and their phagocytotic capabilities) in the cellular fraction and the measurement of several types of enzymes and total protein levels. Measurement of apparent changes in the permeability of the air-blood barrier by quantification of intravenously injected tracer in lung lavage fluid represents another useful index of lung damage.

In Vitro Approaches

In vitro systems are particularly well suited for the study of mechanisms that cause lung injury. The following systems are used widely.

Isolated Perfused Lung The lung, in situ or excised, is perfused with blood or a blood substitute through the pulmonary arterial bed. At the same time, the lung is ventilated. Toxic agents can be introduced into the perfusate or the inspired air. Repeated sampling of the perfusate allows one to determine the rate of metabolism of drugs and the metabolic activity of the lung.

Lung Explants and Slices Slices and explants from the conducting airways or the lung parenchyma allow one to examine biochemical and morphologic changes in the lung parenchyma without intervening complications from cells migrating into the tissue (e.g., leukocytes). If the lung is first inflated with agar, the alveolar spaces remain open in the explant. Slices prepared in this way can be kept viable for several weeks, and the mechanisms of development of chronic lesions can be studied.

Microdissection Many inhalants act in circumscribed regions of the respiratory tract, such as the terminal bronchioles, a region especially rich in metabolically highly competent Clara cells. Microdissection of the airways consists of the stripping of small bronchi and terminal bronchioli from the surrounding parenchyma and maintenance of the isolated airways in culture. Specific biochemical reactions predominantly located in the cells of the small airways then can be studied with biochemical or morphologic techniques.

Organotypic Cell Culture Systems Tissue culture systems permit epithelial cells to maintain their polarity, differentiation, and normal function; this is similar to what is observed in vivo. Epithelial cell surfaces are exposed to air (or a gas phase containing an airborne toxic agent), and the basal portion is bathed by a tissue culture medium.

Isolated Lung Cell Populations Many specific lung cell types have been isolated and maintained as primary cultures in vitro. Alveolar macrophages can be obtained easily from human and animal lungs by lavage. Their function can be examined in vitro with or without exposure to appropriate toxic stimuli. Type II alveolar epithelial cells are isolated after digestion of the lung. Direct isolation of type I epithelial cells also has been successful. Systems for the isolation and culture of Clara cells and neuroepithelial cells are available. Lung fibroblasts can be grown easily and have been studied in coculture with epithelial cells. Multiple primary cell cultures and cell lines have been established from lung tumors found in experimental animals and humans.

BIBLIOGRAPHY

Barnes PJ, Chung KF, Page CP: Inflammatory mediators of asthma: An update. *Pharmacol Rev* 50:575–596, 1998.

Hecht SS: Tobacco smoke carcinogens and lung cancer. *J Natl Cancer Inst* 91:1194–1210, 1999.

Gardner DE, Crapo JD, McClellan RO (eds): *Toxicology of the Lung,* 3d ed. Philadelphia: Taylor & Francis, 1999.

National Cancer Institute: *Health Effects of Exposure to Environmental Tobacco Smoke: The Report of the California Environmental Protection Agency.* Smoking and Tobacco Control Monograph No. 10. NIH Pub. No. 99-4645. Bethesda, MD: U.S. Department of Health and Human Services, National Institutes of Health, National Cancer Institute, 1999.

Roth RA (ed): *Toxicology of the Respiratory System.* Vol 8, in Sipes IG, McQueen CA, Gandolfi AJ (eds): *Comprehensive Toxicology.* New York: Elsevier, 1997.

Swift DL, Foster WM (eds): *Air Pollutants and the Respiratory Tract.* New York: Marcel Dekker, 1999.

TOXIC RESPONSES OF THE NERVOUS SYSTEM

Douglas C. Anthony, Thomas J. Montine, William M. Valentine, and Doyle G. Graham

KEY POINTS

- The central nervous system is protected from the adverse effects of many potential toxicants by an anatomic blood-brain barrier.
- Neurons are highly dependent on aerobic metabolism because this energy is needed to maintain proper ion gradients.
- Individual neurotoxic compounds typically target the neuron, the axon, the myelinating cell, or the neurotransmitter system.
- Neuronopathy is the toxicant-induced irreversible loss of neurons, including the cytoplasmic extensions, dendrites, and axons, as well as the myelin ensheathing the axon.
- Neurotoxicants that result in *axonopathies* cause axonal degeneration and loss of the myelin surrounding the axon; however, the neuron cell body remains intact.
- Xenobiotic-induced myelinopathies include separation of the myelin lamellae, termed *intramyelinic edema,* or the selective loss of myelin, termed *demyelination.*
- Numerous naturally occurring toxins as well as synthetic chemicals may interrupt the transmission of impulses, block or accentuate transsynaptic communication, block reuptake of neurotransmitters, or interfere with second-messenger systems.

OVERVIEW OF THE NERVOUS SYSTEM

Several generalities that allow a basic understanding of the actions of neurotoxicants include (1) the privileged status of the nervous system (NS), with the maintenance of a biochemical barrier between the brain and the blood, (2) the importance of the high energy requirements of the brain, (3) the spatial extensions of the NS as long cellular processes and the requirements of cells with this complex geometry, (4) the maintenance of an environment rich in lipids, and (5) the transmission of information across extracellular space at the synapse.

Blood-Brain Barrier

The central nervous system (CNS) is protected from the adverse effects of many potential toxicants by an anatomic barrier between the blood and the brain, or a "blood-brain barrier." To gain entry to the NS, molecules must pass into the cell membranes of endothelial cells in the brain rather than between endothelial cells, as they do in other tissues (Fig. 16-1). The blood-brain barrier also contains xenobiotic transporters that transport some xenobiotics that have diffused through endothelial cells back into the blood. The penetration of toxicants or their metabolites into the NS is related largely to their lipid solubility. However, spinal and autonomic ganglia as well as a small number of other sites within the brain are not protected by blood-tissue barriers. The blood-brain barrier is incompletely developed at birth and even less developed in premature infants. This predisposes a premature infant to brain injury by toxicants that later in life are excluded from the NS.

Energy Requirements

Neurons are highly dependent on aerobic metabolism because they must use this energy to maintain proper ion gradients. The brain is extremely sensitive to even brief interruptions in the supply of oxygen or glucose.

Axonal Transport

Impulses are conducted over great distances at rapid speed, providing information about the environment to the organism in a coordinated manner that allows an organized response to be carried out at a specific site.

Systemic Capillaries   Brain Capillaries

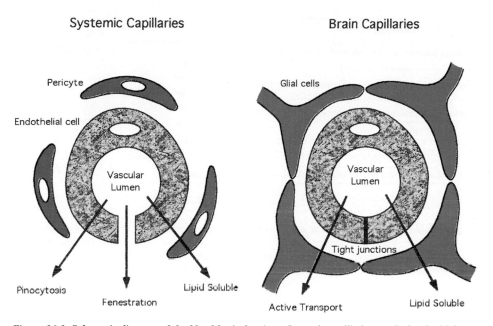

Figure 16-1. Schematic diagram of the blood-brain barrier.   Systemic capillaries are depicted with inter-cellular gaps, or fenestrations, which permit the passage of molecules incapable of crossing the endothelial cell. There is also more abundant pinocytosis in systemic capillaries, in addition to the transcellular passage of lipid-soluble compounds. In brain capillaries, tight junctions between endothelial cells and the lack of pinocytosis limit transport to compounds with active transport mechanisms and those which pass through cellular membranes by virtue of their lipid solubility.

However, the intricate organization of this complex network places an unparalleled demand on the cells of the NS. Single cells, rather than being spherical and a few micrometers in diameter, are elongated and may extend over a meter in length. Two immediate demands placed on the neuron are the maintenance of a much larger cellular volume requiring more protein synthesis and the transport of intracellular materials over great distances through the use of various mechanisms. These demands require ATP.

Axonal transport moves protein products from the cell body to the appropriate site in the axon. *Fast axonal transport* carries a large number of proteins from their site of synthesis in the cell body into the axon. Many proteins associated with vesicles migrate through the axon at a rate of 400 mm/day (Fig. 16-2). This process is dependent on microtubule-associated ATPase activity and the microtubule-associated motor proteins—kinesin and dynein—that provide both the mechanochemical force in the form of a microtubule-associated ATPase and the interface between microtubules as the track and vesicles as the cargo. Vesicles are transported rapidly in an anterograde direction by kinesin and are transported in a

retrograde direction by dynein. Although this mechanism of cytoplasmic transport toward the cell periphery and back toward the nucleus appears to be a general feature of cells, the process is amplified within the NS by the distances encompassed by the axonal extensions of neurons.

The transport of some organelles, including mitochondria, constitutes an intermediate component of axonal transport, moving at 50 mm/day. The slowest component of axonal transport is the movement of the cytoskeleton itself (Fig. 16-2). The cytoskeleton is composed of microtubules formed by the association of tubulin subunits and neurofilaments formed by the association of three neurofilament protein subunits. Each element of the cytoskeleton moves along the length of the axon at a specific rate. Overall, slow component A (SCa) represents retrograde axonal transport, whereas slow component B (SCb) consists of the movement of the axonal cytoskelton in an anterograde direction.

Neurofilaments and microtubules move at a rate of approximately 1 mm/day and make up the majority of SCa, the slowest-moving component of axonal transport. Moving at only a slightly more rapid rate of 2 to

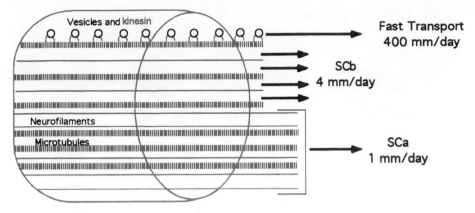

Figure 16-2. Schematic diagram of axonal transport. Fast axonal transport is depicted as spherical vesicles moving along microtubules with intervening microtubule-associated motors. The slow component A (SCa) represents the movement of the cytoskeleton, composed of neurofilaments and microtubules. Slow component B (SCb) moves at a faster rate than does SCa and includes soluble proteins, which apparently are moving between the more slowly moving cytoskeleton.

4 mm/day is SCb, which is composed of many proteins. Included in SCb are several structural proteins, such as the component of microfilaments (actin) and several microfilament-associated proteins (M2 protein and fodrin), as well as clathrin and many soluble proteins.

This continual transport of proteins from the cell body through the various components of forward-directed, or anterograde, axonal transport is the mechanism through which the neuron provides the distal axon with its complement of functional and structural proteins. Some vesicles also move in a retrograde direction and undoubtedly provide the cell body with information about the status of the distal axon.

Axonal Degeneration After axotomy (cutting of an axon), there is degeneration of the distal nerve stump, referred to as *Wallerian degeneration,* which is followed by the generation of a microenvironment that is supportive of regeneration. After the axon dies, active proteolysis digests the axolemma and axoplasm, leaving only a myelin sheath surrounding a swollen degenerate axon (Fig. 16-3), which then is digested by endogenous proteases. Schwann cells then provide physical guidance to direct the regrowth of a new axon and also release growth factors that stimulate growth. Schwann cells respond to the loss of axons by decreasing synthesis of myelin lipids, down-regulating genes that encode myelin proteins, and dedifferentiating to a premyelinating mitotic Schwann cell phenotype. In addition to providing physical guidance for regenerating axons, Schwann cells provide trophic support from nerve growth factor, brain-

derived nerve growth factor, insulin-like growth factor, and corresponding receptors produced by the associated Schwann cells. Resident and recruited macrophages and the denervated Schwann cells clear myelin debris so that a new axon can grow into the space.

Investigations have shown that degeneration of the distal axonal stump after transection is an active, synchronized process that can be delayed by decreasing temperature, preventing the entry of extracellular Ca^{2+} or inhibiting proteolysis by calpain II.

When a neuronal cell body has been lethally injured, it degenerates, along with all its cellular processes. This process is a *neuronopathy* and is characterized by loss of the cell body and all its processes, with no potential for regeneration. However, when the injury is at the level of the axon, the axon may degenerate while the neuronal cell body continues to survive, a condition known as an "axonopathy" (Fig. 16-4).

Myelin Formation and Maintenance

Myelin is formed in the CNS by oligodendrocytes and in the peripheral nervous system (PNS) by Schwann cells as concentric layers through the progressive wrapping of their cytoplasmic processes around the axon in successive loops (Fig. 16-5). These cells exclude cytoplasm from the inner surface of their membranes to form the major dense line of myelin. In a similar process, the extracellular space is reduced on the extracellular surface of the bilayers, and the lipid membranes are stacked together.

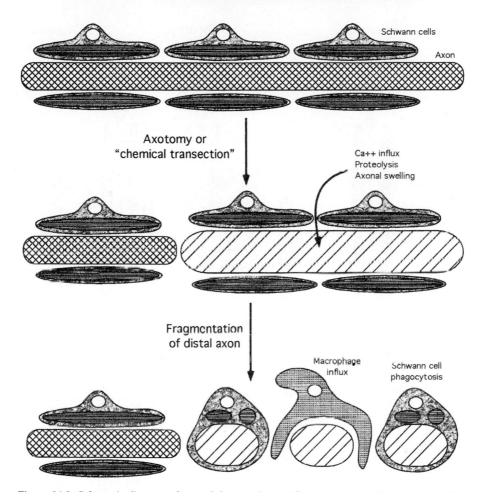

Figure 16-3. Schematic diagram of axonal degeneration.   After axotomy, or chemical injury of an axon, the distal portion of the axon undergoes a process of axonal degeneration. Initial stages of axonal swelling are followed by fragmentation of the distal axon and phagocytosis by resident Schwann cells and an influx of macrophages, which are derived largely from the circulation.

The maintenance of myelin is dependent on a number of membrane-associated proteins and on the metabolism of specific lipids present in myelin bilayers. Some toxic compounds interfere with this complex process of the maintenance of myelin and result in the toxic "myelinopathies" (Fig. 16-4). In general, the loss of myelin, with the preservation of axons, is referred to as *demyelination.*

Neurotransmission

Intercellular communication is achieved in the NS through the synapse. Neurotransmitters released from one axon act as the first messenger. Binding of the transmitter to the postsynaptic receptor is followed by modulation of an ion channel or activation of a second-messenger system, leading to changes in the responding cell. Various therapeutic drugs and toxic compounds affect the process of neurotransmission.

Development of the Nervous System

Replication, migration, differentiation, myelination, and synapse formation are the basic processes that underlie the development of the NS. Neuron and support cell

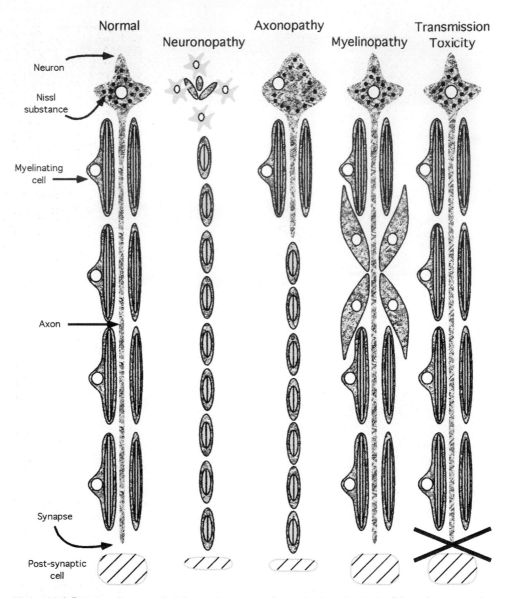

Figure 16-4. Patterns of neurotoxic injury. A neuronopathy results from the death of the entire neuron. Astrocytes often proliferate in response to the neuronal loss, creating both neuronal loss and gliosis. When the axon is the primary site of injury, the axon degenerates, whereas the surviving neuron shows only chromatolysis with margination of its Nissl substance and nucleus to the cell periphery. This condition is termed an axonopathy. Myelinopathies result from disruption of myelin or from selective injury to the myelinating cells. To prevent cross-talk between adjacent axons, myelinating cells divide and cover the denuded axon rapidly; however, the process of remyelination is much less effective in the CNS than in the PNS. Some compounds do not cause cell death but exert their toxic effects by interrupting the process of neurotransmission either by blocking excitation or by excessive stimulation.

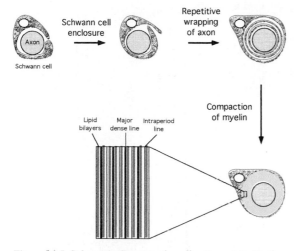

Figure 16-5. Schematic diagram of myelination. Myelination begins when a myelinating cell encircles an axon, either Schwann cells in the peripheral nervous system or oligodendrocytes in the central nervous system. Simple enclosure of the axon persists in unmyelinated axons. Myelin formation proceeds by a progressive wrapping of multiple layers of the myelinating cell around the axon, with extrusion of the cytoplasm and extracellular space to bring the lipid bilayers into close proximity. The intracellular space is compressed to form the major dense line of myelin, and the extracellular space is compressed to form the intraperiod line.

precursors replicate in an area called the neural tube and then migrate to different destinations throughout the body. Myelination begins in utero and continues through childhood. Synaptic connectivity, the basis of neurologic function, is a dynamic process throughout life.

The immature NS is especially vulnerable to certain agents. Ethanol exposure during pregnancy can result in abnormalities in the fetus, including abnormal neuronal migration and diffuse abnormalities in the development of neuronal processes. The clinical result of fetal alcohol exposure is often mental retardation, with malformations of the brain and delayed myelination of white matter.

FUNCTIONAL MANIFESTATIONS OF NEUROTOXICITY

Functional assessment uses functional test batteries to screen potentially neurotoxic compounds. A group of behavioral tests typically is performed to evaluate a variety of neurologic functions. There are two distinct tiers of functional testing of neurotoxicants: a first tier in which tests may be used to identify the presence of a neurotoxic substance and a second tier that involves characterization of the effects of the compound on sensory, motor, autonomic, and cognitive functions. The second tier is critical to the validation of the behavioral tests as behavioral changes are correlated with physiologic, biochemical, and pathologic identification of neurotoxic injury. Ultimately, neurotoxicants identified by behavioral methods are evaluated at a cellular and molecular level to provide an understanding of the events in the NS that cause the neurologic dysfunction detected by observational tests.

MECHANISMS OF NEUROTOXICITY

Individual neurotoxic compounds typically have one of four targets: the neuron, the axon, the myelinating cell, or the neurotransmitter system.

Neuronopathies

Certain toxicants are specific for neurons, resulting in their injury or death. Neuron loss is irreversible and includes degeneration of all of its cytoplasmic extensions, dendrites, and axons as well as the myelin ensheathing the axon (Fig. 16-4). Features of the neuron that place it at risk for the action of cellular toxicants include a high metabolic rate, a long cellular process that is supported by the cell body, and an excitable membrane that is depolarized and repolarized rapidly.

Although a large number of compounds are known to result in toxic neuronopathies (Table 16-1), all these toxicants share certain features. Each toxic condition results from a cellular toxicant that has a predilection for neurons. The initial injury to neurons is followed by apoptosis or necrosis, leading to permanent loss of the neuron. These agents tend to be diffuse in their action, although they may show some selectivity in the degree of injury of different neuronal subpopulations. The expression of these cellular events is often a diffuse encephalopathy with global dysfunctions.

Doxorubicin Doxorubicin (Adriamycin) injures neurons in the PNS, specifically those of the dorsal root ganglia and autonomic ganglia, by intercalating with DNA and interfering with transcription. The vulnerability of sensory and autonomic neurons appears to reflect the lack of protection of these neurons by a blood-tissue barrier within ganglia.

Table 16-1
Compounds Associated with Neuronal Injury (Neuronopathies)

NEUROTOXICANT	NEUROLOGIC FINDINGS	CELLULAR BASIS OF NEUROTOXICITY
Aluminum	Dementia, encephalopathy (humans), learning deficits	Spongiosis cortex, neurofibrillary aggregates, degenerative changes in cortex
6-Aminonicotinamide	Not reported in humans; hind limb paralysis (experimental animals)	Spongy (vacuolar) degeneration in spinal cord, brainstem, cerebellum, axonal degeneration of the peripheral nervous system (PNS)
Arsenic	Encephalopathy (acute), peripheral neuropathy (chronic)	Brain swelling and hemorrhage (acute), axonal degeneration in PNS (chronic)
Azide	Insufficient data (humans); convulsions, ataxia (primates)	Neuronal loss in cerebellum and cortex
Bismuth	Emotional disturbances, encephalopathy, myoclonus	Neuronal loss, basal ganglia and Purkinje cells of cerebellum
Carbon monoxide	Encephalopathy, delayed parkinsonism/dystonia	Neuronal loss in cortex, necrosis of globus pallidus, focal demyelination; blocks oxygen-binding site of hemoglobin and iron-binding sites of brain
Carbon tetrachloride	Encephalopathy (probably secondary to liver failure)	Enlarged astrocytes in striatum, globus pallidus
Chloramphenicol	Optic neuritis, peripheral neuropathy	Neuronal loss (retina), axonal degeneration (PNS)
Cyanide	Coma, convulsions, rapid death; delayed parkinsonism/dystonia	Neuronal degeneration, cerebellum and globus pallidus; focal demyelination; blocks cytochrome oxidase/ATP production
Doxorubicin	Insufficient data (humans); progressive ataxia (experimental animals)	Degeneration of dorsal root ganglion cells, axonal degeneration (PNS)
Ethanol	Mental retardation, hearing deficits (prenatal exposure)	Microcephaly, cerebral malformations
Lead	Encephalopathy (acute), learning deficits (children), neuropathy with demyelination (rats)	Brain swelling, hemorrhages (acute), axonal loss in PNS (humans)
Manganese	Emotional disturbances, parkinsonism/dystonia	Degeneration of striatum, globus pallidus
Mercury, inorganic	Emotional disturbances, tremor, fatigue	Insufficient data in humans (may affect spinal tracts; cerebellum)
Methanol	Headache, visual loss or blindness, coma (severe)	Necrosis of putamen, degeneration of retinal ganglion cells

(continued)

Table 16-1

Compounds Associated with Neuronal Injury (Neuronopathies) *(continued)*

NEUROTOXICANT	NEUROLOGIC FINDINGS	CELLULAR BASIS OF NEUROTOXICITY
Methylazoxymethanol acetate	Microcephaly (rats)	Developmental abnormalities of fetal brain (rats)
Methyl bromide	Visual and speech impairment; peripheral neuropathy	Insufficient data
Methyl mercury (organic mercury)	Ataxia, constriction of visual fields, paresthesias (adult)	Neuronal degeneration, visual cortex, cerebellum, ganglia
	Psychomotor retardation (fetal exposure)	Spongy disruption, cortex and cerebellum
1-Methyl-4-phenyl-1,2,3,6-tetrahydropyridine (MPTP)	Parkinsonism, dystonia (acute exposure) Early-onset parkinsonism (late effect of acute exposure)	Neuronal degeneration in substantia nigra Neuronal degeneration in substantia nigra
3-Nitropropionic acid	Seizures, delayed dystonia/grimacing	Necrosis in basal ganglia
Phenytoin (diphenyl-hydantoin; Dilantin)	Nystagmus, ataxia, dizziness	Degeneration of Purkinje cells (cerebellum)
Quinine	Constriction of visual fields	Vacuolization of retinal ganglion cells
Streptomycin (aminoglycosides)	Hearing loss	Degeneration of inner ear (organ of Corti)
Thallium	Emotional disturbances, ataxia, peripheral neuropathy	Brain swelling (acute), axonal degeneration in PNS
Trimethyltin	Tremors, hyperexcitability (experimental animals)	Loss of hippocampal neurons, amygdala pyriform cortex

Abou-Donia MB (ed): *Neurotoxicology.* Boca Raton, FL: CRC Press, 1993.

Chang LW, Dyer RS (eds): *Handbook of Neurotoxicology.* New York: Marcel Dekker, 1995.

Graham DI, Lantos PL (eds): *Greenfield's Neuropathology,* 5th ed. New York: Arnold, 1997.

Spencer PS, Schaumburg HH (eds): *Experimental and Clinical Neurotoxicology,* 2d ed. New York: Oxford University Press, 2000.

Methyl Mercury The neurons that are most sensitive to the toxic effects of methyl mercury are those which reside in the dorsal root ganglia, perhaps again reflecting the vulnerability of neurons not shielded by blood-tissue barriers. Methyl mercury exposure impairs glycolysis, nucleic acid biosynthesis, aerobic respiration, protein synthesis, and neurotransmitter release. In addition, there is evidence for enhanced oxidative injury and altered calcium homeostasis. Exposure to methyl mercury leads to widespread neuronal injury and subsequently to a diffuse encephalopathy.

Dopamine, 6-Hydroxydopamine, and Catecholamine Toxicity The oxidation of catecholamines by monoamine oxidase (MAO) yields H_2O_2, a known cytotoxic metabolite. The metal ion–catalyzed autoxidation of catecholamines, especially dopamine, results in the production of catecholamine-derived quinones as well as superoxide anion.

6-Hydroxydopamine produces chemical sympathectomy in peripheral nerves after systemic administration. 6-Hydroxydopamine is transported actively into nerve terminals, employing the uptake mechanism utilized by the structurally similar catecholamines in sympathetic terminals. Oxidation of this catecholamine analog leads to the production of reactive oxygen species with selective destruction of sympathetic innervation. The sympathetic fibers degenerate, resulting in an uncompensated parasympathetic tone, slowing of the heart rate, and hypermotility of the gastrointestinal system.

MPTP A contaminant formed during meperidine synthesis, 1-methyl-4-phenyl-1,2,3,6-tetrahydropyridine (MPTP), produces, over hours to days, the signs and symptoms of irreversible Parkinson's disease. Autopsy studies have demonstrated marked degeneration of dopaminergic neurons in the substantia nigra, with degeneration continuing for many years after exposure. It appears that MPTP is metabolized to a molecule that enters the dopaminergic neurons of the substantia nigra, resulting in their deaths.

Although not identical, MPTP neurotoxicity and Parkinson's disease are strikingly similar. The symptomatology of each condition reflects a disruption of the nigrostriatal pathway: Masked facies, difficulties in initiating and terminating movements, resting "pill-rolling" tremors, rigidity, and bradykinesias are all features of both conditions.

Environmental Factors Relevant to Neurodegenerative Diseases It has been observed that individuals who are exposed to insufficient MPTP to result in immediate parkinsonism develop early signs of the disease years later. Smaller exposures to MPTP may cause a decrement in the population of neurons in the substantia nigra. Such a loss most likely would be silent until approximately 80 percent of the substantia nigra neurons were lost. These individuals with a diminished number of neurons may be more vulnerable to further loss of dopaminergic neurons.

An epidemic of dialysis-related dementia with some pathologic resemblance to Alzheimer's disease appears to have been related to aluminum in the dialysate, and removal of aluminum has prevented further instances of dialysis dementia.

Axonopathies

The neurotoxic disorders termed *axonopathies* are those in which the primary site of toxicity is the axon itself. The axon degenerates, and with it the myelin surrounding that axon; however, the neuron cell body remains intact (Fig. 16-4). The toxicant results in a "chemical transection" of the axon at some point along its length, and the axon distal to the transection degenerates.

A critical difference exists in the significance of axonal degeneration in the CNS compared with that in the PNS: Peripheral axons can regenerate, whereas central axons cannot. In the PNS, glial cells and macrophages support axonal regeneration. In the CNS, the release of inhibitory factors from damaged myelin and astrocyte scarring actually interferes with regeneration. The clinical relevance of the disparity between the CNS and the PNS is that partial to complete recovery can occur after axonal degeneration in the PNS, whereas the same event is irreversible in the CNS.

Axonopathies can be considered to result from a chemical transection of the axon. The number of axonal toxicants is large and is increasing in number (Table 16-2). As the axons degenerate, sensations and motor strength are first impaired in the most distal extent of the axonal processes—the feet and hands—resulting in a "glove and stocking" neuropathy. With time and continued injury, the deficit progresses to involve more proximal areas of the body and the long axons of the spinal cord.

Gamma-Diketones Humans develop a progressive sensorimotor distal axonopathy when they are exposed to high concentrations of a simple alkane, *n*-hexane, day after day in work settings or after repeated intentional inhalation of hexane-containing glues.

Table 16-2
Compounds Associated with Axonal Injury (Axonopathies)

NEUROTOXICANT	NEUROLOGIC FINDINGS	CELLULAR BASIS OF NEUROTOXICITY
Acrylamide	Peripheral neuropathy (often sensory)	Axonal degeneration; axon terminal affected in earliest stages
p-Bromophenylacetyl urea	Peripheral neuropathy	Axonal degeneration in peripheral nervous system (PNS) and central nervous system (CNS)
Carbon disulfide	Psychosis (acute), peripheral neuropathy (chronic)	Axonal degeneration; early stages include neurofilamentous swelling
Chlordecone (Kepone)	Tremors, incoordination experimental animals)	Insufficient data (humans); axonal swelling and degeneration
Chloroquine	Peripheral neuropathy, weakness	Axonal degeneration, inclusions in dorsal root ganglion cells; also vacuolar myopathy
Clioquinol	Encephalopathy (acute), subacute myelooptic neuropathy (subacute)	Axonal degeneration, spinal cord, PNS, optic tracts
Colchicine	Peripheral neuropathy	Axonal degeneration, neuronal perikaryal filamentous aggregates; vacuolar myopathy
Dapsone	Peripheral neuropathy, predominantly motor	Axonal degeneration (both myelinated and unmyelinated axons)
Dichlorophenoxyacetate	Peripheral neuropathy (delayed)	Insufficient data
Dimethylaminopropionitrile	Peripheral neuropathy, urinary retention	Axonal degeneration (both myelinated and unmyelinated axons)
Ethylene oxide	Peripheral neuropathy	Axonal degeneration
Glutethimide	Peripheral neuropathy (predominantly sensory)	Insufficient data
Gold	Peripheral neuopathy (may have psychiatric problems)	Axonal degeneration, some segmental demyelination
Hexane	Peripheral neuropathy, severe cases have spasticity	Axonal degeneration, early neurofilamentous swelling, PNS and spinal cord
Hydralazine	Peripheral neuropathy	Insufficient data
3,3'-Iminodipropionitrile	No data in humans; excitatory movement disorder (rats)	Axonal swellings, degeneration of olfactory epithelial cells, vestibular hair cells
Isoniazid	Peripheral neuropathy (sensory), ataxia (high doses)	Axonal degeneration
Lithium	Lethargy, tremor, ataxia (reversible)	Insufficient data
Methyl n-butyl ketone	Peripheral neuropathy	Axonal degeneration, early neurofilamentous swelling, PNS and spinal cord

(continued)

Table 16-2
Compounds Associated with Axonal Injury (Axonopathies) *(continued)*

NEUROTOXICANT	NEUROLOGIC FINDINGS	CELLULAR BASIS OF NEUROTOXICITY
Metronidazole	Sensory peripheral neuropathy, ataxia, seizures	Axonal degeneration, mostly affecting myelinated fibers; lesions of cerebellar nuclei
Misonidazole	Peripheral neuropathy	Axonal degeneration
Nitrofurantoin	Peripheral neuropathy	Axonal degeneration
Organophosphorus compounds	Headache, abdominal pain (acute; anticholinesterase)	No anatomic changes (neurotransmitter effect)
	Delayed peripheral neuropathy (motor), spasticity	Axonal degeneration (delayed after single exposure), PNS and spinal cord
Paclitaxel (taxoids)	Peripheral neuropathy	Axonal degeneration; microtubule accumulation in early stages
Platinum (cisplatin)	Ototoxicity with tinnitus, sensory peripheral neuropathy	Axonal degeneration, axonal loss in posterior columns of spinal cord
Pyrethroids	Movement disorders (tremor, choreoathetosis)	Axonal degeneration (variable)
Pyridinethione (pyrithione)	No reported human toxicity; weakness (experimental animals)	Axonal degeneration, early stages with membranous arrays in axon terminals
Trichloroethylene	Cranial (most often trigeminal) neuropathy	Insufficient data
Vincristine (vinca alkaloids)	Peripheral neuropathy, variable autonomic symptoms	Axonal degeneration (PNS), neurofibrillary changes (spinal cord, intrathecal route)

Abou-Donia MB (ed): *Neurotoxicology.* Boca Raton, FL: CRC Press, 1993.

Chang LW, Dyer RS (eds): *Handbook of Neurotoxicology.* New York: Marcel Dekker, 1995.

Graham DI, Lantos PL (eds): *Greenfield's Neuropathology,* 6th ed. New York: Arnold, 1997.

Spencer PS, Schaumburg HH, (eds): *Experimental and Clinical Neurotoxicology,* 2d ed. New York: Oxford University Press, 2000.

The ω-1 oxidation of *n*-hexane results ultimately in the γ-diketone 2,5-hexanedione (HD), which reacts with amino groups in all tissues to form pyrroles that derivatize and cross-link neurofilaments, leading to the development of neurofilament aggregates of the distal, subterminal axon. The neurofilament-filled axonal swellings distort nodal anatomy and impair axonal transport. The pathologic processes of neurofilament accumulation and degeneration of the axon are followed by the emergence of a clinical peripheral neuropathy.

Carbon Disulfide Significant exposures of humans to CS_2 cause a distal axonopathy that is identical pathologically to that caused by hexane. Covalent cross-linking of neurofilaments occurs, and CS_2 is the ultimate toxicant.

The clinical effects of exposure to CS_2 in the chronic setting are very similar to those of hexane exposure, with the development of sensory and motor symptoms occurring initially in a stocking-and-glove distribution. In addition to this chronic axonopathy, CS_2 can lead to aberrations in mood and signs of diffuse encephalopathic disease.

IDPN β,β'-Iminodipropionitrile (IDPN) causes a bizarre "waltzing syndrome" that appears to result from degeneration of the vestibular sensory hair cells. In addition, administration of IDPN is followed by massive neurofilament-filled swellings of the proximal, instead of the distal, axon (Fig. 16-6).

DMHD (3,4-dimethyl-2,5-hexanedione) is an analog of 2,5-hexanedione that is 20 to 30 times more potent as a neurotoxicant, and the neurofilament-filled swellings occur in the proximal axon, as in IDPN intoxication. DMHD intoxication leads to limb paralysis, whereas IDPN intoxication results in muscle atrophy but not paralysis.

Acrylamide Acrylamide is a vinyl monomer that is used in the manufacture of paper products, as a flocculant in water treatment, as a soil-stabilizing and waterproofing agent, and for making polyacrylamide gels in research laboratories. The neuropathy induced by acrylamide is a toxic distal axonopathy that begins with degeneration of the nerve terminal. Continued intoxication results in degeneration of the more proximal axon and abnormal axonal transport.

Organophosphorus Esters These compounds, which are used as pesticides and as additives in plastics and petroleum products, inhibit acetylcholinesterase and create a cholinergic excess. However, tri-ortho-cresyl phosphate (TOCP) causes a severe axonopathy without inducing cholinergic poisoning.

Some hydrophobic organophosphorus compounds readily enter the NS, where they alkylate or phosphorylate macromolecules and lead to delayed-onset neurotoxicity. Whereas "nontoxic" organophosphorus esters inhibit most of the esterase activity in the NS, there is another esterase activity, or *neuropathy target esterase* (NTE), that is inhibited by the neurotoxic organophosphorus esters. Furthermore, there is a good correlation between the potency of a specific organophosphorus ester as an axonal toxicant and its potency as an inhibitor of NTE.

The degeneration of axons does not commence immediately after acute organophosphorus ester exposure but is delayed for 7 to 10 days between the acute high-dose exposure and the clinical signs of axonopathy. The axonal lesion in the PNS appears to be repaired readily, and the peripheral nerve becomes refractory to degeneration after repeated doses. By contrast, axonal degeneration in the long tracks of the spinal cord is progressive.

Pyridinethione Zinc pyridinethione has antibacterial and antifungal properties and is a component of shampoos that are effective in the treatment of seborrhea and dandruff. Only the pyridinethione moiety is absorbed after ingestion, with the majority of zinc eliminated in the feces. Pyridinethione appears to interfere with the fast axonal transport systems, impairs the turnaround of rapidly transported vesicles, and slows the retrograde transport of vesicles. Aberration of the fast axonal transport systems most likely contributes to the accumulation of tubular and vesicular structures in the distal axon (Fig. 16-6). As these materials accumulate in one region of the axon, the axon degenerates in its more distal regions beyond the accumulated structures. The earliest signs are diminished grip strength and changes in the axon terminal, leading to a peripheral neuropathy.

Microtubule-Associated Neurotoxicity The vinca alkaloids and colchicine, which bind to tubulin and inhibit the association of this protein subunit to form microtubules, produce peripheral neuropathies in patients. Paclitaxel, which stabilizes the assembled polymerized form of tubules, causes sensorimotor axonopathy and autonomic neuropathy in high doses.

The morphology of the axon is, of course, different in the two situations. In the case of colchicine, the axon appears to undergo atrophy and there are fewer microtubules within the axons. In contrast, after exposure to paclitaxel, microtubules are present in great numbers and are aggregated in arrays of microtubules. Both situations probably interfere with the process of fast axonal trans-

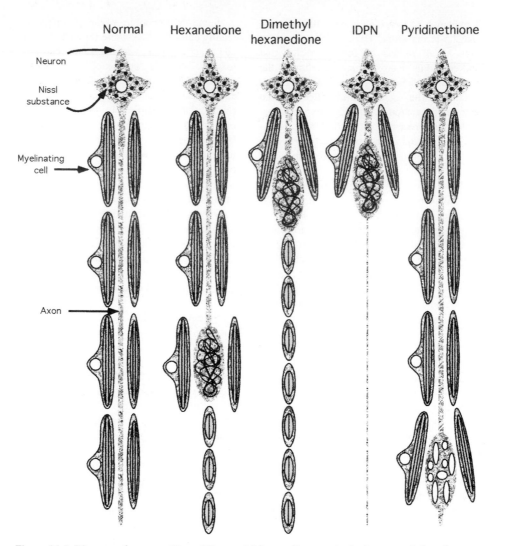

Figure 16-6. Diagram of axonopathies. Whereas 2,5-hexanedione results in the accumulation of neurofilaments in the distal regions of the axon, 3,4-dimethyl-2,5-hexanedione results in identical accumulation within the proximal segments. These proximal neurofilamentous swellings are quite similar to those which occur in the toxicity of β,β'-iminodipropionitrile (IDPN), although the distal axon does not degenerate in IDPN axonopathy but instead becomes atrophic. Pyridinethione results in axonal swellings that are distended with tubulovesicular material, followed by distal axonal degeneration.

port. In both situations, the resultant clinical condition is a peripheral neuropathy.

Myelinopathies

Myelin provides electrical insulation of neuronal processes, and its absence leads to a slowing of conduction and aberrant conduction of impulses between adjacent processes. Exposure to toxicants can result in either separation of the myelin lamellae, termed *intramyelinic edema,* or the selective loss of myelin, termed *demyelination* (Fig. 16-4). Remyelination in the CNS occurs to only a limited extent after demyelination. However, Schwann cells in the PNS are capable of remyelinating the axon.

The compounds listed in Table 16-3 all lead to a myelinopathy.

Table 16-3
Compounds Associated with Injury of Myelin (Myelinopathies)

NEUROTOXICANT	NEUROLOGIC FINDINGS	CELLULAR BASIS OF NEUROTOXICITY
Acetylethyltetramethyl tetralin (AETT)	Not reported in humans; hyperexcitability, tremors (rats)	Intramyelinic edema; pigment accumulation in neurons
Amiodarone	Peripheral neuropathy	Axonal degeneration and demyelination; lipid-laden lysosomes in Schwann cells
Cuprizone	Not reported in humans; encephalopathy (experimental animals)	Status spongiosis of white matter, intramyelinic edema (early stages); gliosis (late)
Disulfiram	Peripheral neuropathy, predominantly sensory	Axonal degeneration, swellings in distal axons
Ethidium bromide	Insufficient data (humans)	Intramyelinic edema, status spongiosis of white matter
Hexachlorophene	Irritability, confusion, seizures	Brain swelling, intramyelinic edema in CNS and PNS, late axonal degeneration
Lysolecithin	Effects only on direct injection into peripheral nervous system (PNS) or central nervous system (CNS) (experimental animals)	Selective demyelination
Perhexilene	Peripheral neuropathy	Demyelinating neuropathy, membrane-bound inclusions in Schwann cells
Tellurium	Hydrocephalus, hind-limb paralysis (experimental animals)	Demyelinating neuropathy, lipofuscinosis (experimental animals)
Triethyltin	Headache, photophobia, vomiting, paraplegia (irreversible)	Brain swelling (acute) with intramyelinic edema, spongiosis of white matter

Chang LW, Dyer RS (eds): *Handbook of Neurotoxicology*. New York: Marcel Dekker, 1995.
Graham DI, Lantos PL (eds): *Greenfield's Neuropathology*, 6th ed. New York: Arnold, 1997.
Spencer PS, Schaumburg HH (eds): *Experimental and Clinical Neurotoxicology*, 2d ed. New York: Oxford University Press, 2000.

Hexachlorophene Hexachlorophene, methylene 2,2′-methylenebis (3,4,6-trichlorophenol), caused neurotoxicity when newborn infants were bathed with the compound to avoid staphylococcal skin infections. After skin absorption of this hydrophobic compound, hexachlorophene enters the NS and results in intramyelinic edema, which leads to the formation of vacuoles, creating a "spongiosis" of the brain. Hexachlorophene causes intramyelinic edema that leads to segmental demyelination. Swelling of the brain causes increased intracranial pressure and axonal degeneration, along with degeneration of photoreceptors in the retina. Humans exposed acutely to hexachlorophene may have generalized weakness, confusion, and seizures. Progression may occur to include coma and death.

Tellurium The neurotoxicity of tellurium in young rats alters the synthesis of myelin lipids in Schwann cells because of various lipid abnormalities. As biochemical changes occur, lipids accumulate in Schwann cells, which eventually lose their ability to maintain myelin in the PNS.

Lead Lead exposure in animals results in a peripheral neuropathy with prominent segmental demyelination. In young children, acute massive exposures to lead result in severe cerebral edema, perhaps from damage to endothelial cells. Chronic lead intoxication in adults results in peripheral neuropathy, gastritis, colicky abdominal pain, anemia, and the prominent deposition of lead in particular anatomic sites, creating lead lines in the gums and in the epiphyses of long bones in children. Lead in the peripheral nerve of humans slows nerve conduction. The basis of lead encephalopathy is unclear, although an effect on the membrane structure of myelin and myelin membrane fluidity has been shown.

Neurotransmission-Associated Neurotoxicity

A wide variety of naturally occurring toxins as well as synthetic drugs interact with intercellular communication through the process of neurotransmission (Table 16-4). This group of compounds may interrupt the transmission of impulses, block or accentuate transsynaptic communication, block the reuptake of neurotransmitters, or interfere with second-messenger systems. As the targets of these drugs are located throughout the body, the responses are not localized; however, the responses are stereotyped in that each member of a class tends to have similar biological effects. In terms of toxicity, most of the side effects of these drugs may be viewed as short-term interactions that are easily reversible. However, long-term use is associated with irreversible tardive dyskinesias or facial grimaces.

Nicotine Nicotine exerts its effects by binding to a subset of nicotinic cholinergic receptors. Smoking and "pharmacologic" doses of nicotine accelerate heart rate, elevate blood pressure, and constrict blood vessels in the skin as a result of stimulation of the ganglionic sympathetic nervous system.

The rapid rise in circulating levels of nicotine after acute overdose leads to excessive stimulation of nicotinic receptors, a process that is followed rapidly by ganglionic paralysis. Initial nausea, rapid heart rate, and perspiration are followed shortly by marked slowing of heart rate with a fall in blood pressure. Somnolence and confusion may occur, followed by coma; if death results, it often results from paralysis of the muscles of respiration.

Exposure to lower levels for a longer duration, in contrast, is very common. The complications of smoking include cardiovascular disease, cancers, and chronic pulmonary disease. Chronic exposure to nicotine has effects on the developing fetus. Along with decreased birth weights, attention deficit disorders are more common in children whose mothers smoke cigarettes during pregnancy.

Cocaine and Amphetamines The euphoric and addictive properties of cocaine derive from enhanced dopaminergic neurotransmission by the blocking of the dopamine reuptake transporter. Acute toxicity resulting from excessive intake, or overdose, may result in unanticipated deaths.

Although cocaine increases maternal blood pressure during acute exposure in pregnant animals, the blood flow to the uterus actually diminishes. Depending on the level of the drug in the mother, the fetus may develop marked hypoxia. In one study, women who used cocaine during pregnancy had more miscarriages and placental hemorrhages (abruptions) than did drug-free women.

In addition to deleterious effects on fetal growth and development, cocaine abuse is associated with an increased risk of cerebrovascular disease, cerebral perfusion defects, and cerebral atrophy in adults, along with neurodegenerative changes.

Like cocaine, amphetamines exert their effects in the CNS, altering catecholamine neurotransmission by

Table 16-4
Compounds Associated with Neurotransmitter-Associated Toxicity

NEUROTOXICANT	NEUROLOGIC FINDINGS	CELLULAR BASIS OF NEUROTOXICITY
Amphetamine and methamphetamine	Tremor, restlessness (acute); cerebral infarction and hemorrhage; neuropsychiatric disturbances	Bilateral infarcts of globus pallidus, abnormalities in dopaminergic, serotonergic, cholinergic systems
Atropine	Restlessness, irritability, hallucinations	Acts at adrenergic receptors Block cholinergic receptors (anticholinergic)
Cocaine	Increased risk of stroke and cerebral atrophy (chronic users); increased risk of sudden cardiac death; movement and psychiatric abnormalities, especially during withdrawal	Infarcts and hemorrhages; alteration in striatal dopamine neurotransmission (binds to voltage-gated sodium channels)
Domoic acid	Decreased head circumference (fetal exposure) Headache, memory loss, hemiparesis, disorientation, seizures	Structural malformations in newborns Neuronal loss, hippocampus and amygdala, layers 5 and 6 of neocortex Kainate-like pattern of excitotoxicity
Kainate	Insufficient data in humans seizures in animals (selective lesioning compound in neuroscience)	Degeneration of neurons in hippocampus, olfactory cortex, amygdala, thalamus Binds AMPA/kainate receptors
β-N-Methylamino-L-alanine (BMAA)	Weakness, movement disorder (monkeys)	Degenerative changes in motor neurons (monkeys) Excitotoxic probably via NMDA receptors
Muscarine (mushrooms)	Nausea, vomiting, headache	Binds muscarinic receptors (cholinergic)
Nicotine	Nausea, vomiting, convulsions	Binds nicotinic receptors (cholinergic) low-dose stimulation; high-dose blocking
β-N-Oxalylamino-L-alanine (BOAA)	Seizures	Excitotoxic probably via AMPA class of glutamate receptors

Graham DI, Lantos PL (eds): *Greenfield's Neuropathology*, 6th ed: New York: Arnold 1997.
Hardman JG, Limbird LE, Molinoff PB, Ruddon RW (eds): *Goodman and Gilman's The Pharmacologic Basis of Therapeutics*, 9th ed. New York: McGraw-Hill, 1996.
Spencer PS, Schaumburg HH (eds): *Experimental and Clinical Neurotoxicology*, 2d ed. New York: Oxford University Press, 2000.

competing for uptake via plasma membrane transporters and by disrupting the vesicular storage of dopamine. Amphetamines have been associated with an increased risk of abnormal fetal growth and development, cerebrovascular disease, and psychiatric and neurologic problems in chronic abusers.

Excitatory Amino Acids Glutamate and certain other acidic amino acids are excitatory neurotransmitters in the CNS. The toxicity of glutamate can be blocked by certain glutamate antagonists, and the concept has emerged that the toxicity of excitatory amino acids may be related to conditions such as hypoxia, epilepsy, and neurodegenerative diseases.

Glutamate is the main excitatory neurotransmitter in the brain, and its effects are mediated by several subtypes of receptors (Fig. 16-7) called *excitatory amino acid receptors* (EAARs). The two major subtypes of glutamate receptors are those which are ligand-gated directly to ion channels (ionotropic) and those which are coupled with G proteins (metabotropic). Ionotropic receptors may be subdivided further by their specificity for binding kainate, quisqualate, α-amino-3-hydroxy-5-methylisoxazole-4-propionic acid (AMPA), and *N*-methyl-D-aspartate (NMDA). The entry of glutamate into the CNS is regulated at the blood-brain barrier, and glutamate exerts its effects in the circumventricular organ of the brain, in which the blood-brain barrier is least developed. In this site of limited access, glutamate injures neurons, apparently by opening glutamate-dependent ion channels, ultimately leading to neuronal swelling and neuronal cell death. The only known related human condition is the "Chinese restaurant syndrome," in which the consumption of large amounts of monosodium glutamate as a seasoning may lead to a burning sensation in the face, neck, and chest.

The cyclic glutamate analog kainate isolated from a seaweed in Japan is extremely potent as an excitotoxin, being a hundredfold more toxic than glutamate, and is selective at a molecular level for the kainate receptor. Like glutamate, kainate selectively injures dendrites and neurons and shows no substantial effect on the glia or axons. Injected into a region of the brain, kainate can destroy the neurons in that area without disrupting all the fibers that pass through that region.

Development of permanent neurologic deficits occurred in individuals accidentally exposed to high doses of the EAAR agonist domoic acid, an analog of glutamate. The acute illness most commonly presented as gastrointestinal disturbance, severe headache, and short-term memory loss. A subset of the more severely afflicted patients had chronic memory deficits and motor neuropathy. Neuropathologic investigation of patients who died within 4 months of intoxication showed neurodegeneration that was most prominent in the hippocampus and amygdala.

The expanding field of excitotoxic amino acids embodies many of the same attributes that characterize the entire discipline of neurotoxicology. Exposure to these excitotoxic amino acids leads to neuronal injury and sometimes neuronal death. However, the implications of these findings extend beyond the direct toxicity of the compounds in exposed populations. Kainate, an analog of glutamate, as is the case with many other neurotoxic compounds, has become a tool for neurobiologists who attempt to explore the anatomy and function of the NS. Kainate, through its selective action on neuronal cell bodies, has provided a greater understanding of the functions of cells in a specific region of the brain, whereas earlier lesioning techniques addressed only regional functions. This void in understanding and the epidemiologic evidence that some neurodegenerative diseases may have environmental contributors provide a heightened desire to appreciate more fully the effects of elements of our environment on the NS.

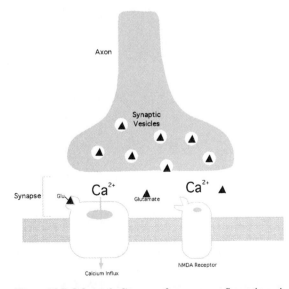

Figure 16-7. Schematic diagram of a synapse. Synaptic vesicles are transported to the axonal terminus and released across the synaptic cleft to bind to the postsynaptic receptors. Glutamate, as an excitatory neurotransmitter, binds to its receptor and opens a calcium channel, leading to the excitation of the postsynaptic cell.

BIBLIOGRAPHY

Albers JW, Berent S (eds): *Clinical Neurobehavioral Toxicology.* Philadelphia: Saunders, 2000.

Blain PG, Harris JB (eds): *Medical Neurotoxicology: Occupational and Environmental Causes of Neurological Dysfunction.* New York: Oxford University Press, 1999.

Lowndes HE, Reuhl K (eds): *Nervous System and Behavioral Toxicology.* Vol 11, in Sipes IG, McQueen CA, Gandolfi AJ (eds): *Comprehensive Toxicology.* New York: Elsevier, 1997.

Massaro EJ (ed): *Handbook of Neurotoxicology.* Totowa, NJ: Humana Press, 2002.

Pentreath VW (ed): *Neurotoxicology in Vitro.* London: Taylor & Francis, 1999.

C H A P T E R   1 7

TOXIC RESPONSES OF THE OCULAR AND VISUAL SYSTEM

Donald A. Fox and William K. Boyes

KEY POINTS

- Toxic chemicals and systemic drugs can affect all parts of the eye, including the cornea, iris, ciliary body, lens retina, and optic nerve.
- Ophthalmologic procedures for evaluating the health of the eye include routine clinical screening evaluations using a slit-lamp biomicroscope and ophthalmoscope and examination of the pupillary light reflex.
- Most electrophysiologic and neurophysiologic procedures for testing visual function after toxicant exposure involve stimulating the eyes with visual stimuli and electrically recording potentials generated by visually responsive neurons.

INTRODUCTION TO OCULAR AND VISUAL SYSTEM TOXICOLOGY

Environmental and occupational exposure to toxic chemicals, gases, and vapors, as well as the side effects of therapeutic drugs, frequently results in structural and functional alterations in the eye and the central visual system. The retina and the central visual system are especially vulnerable to toxic insult.

EXPOSURE TO THE EYE AND VISUAL SYSTEM

Ocular Pharmacodynamics and Pharmacokinetics

Toxic chemicals and systemic drugs can affect all parts of the eye (Fig. 17-1 and Table 17-1). The cornea, conjunctiva, and eyelids often are exposed directly to chemicals, gases, and particles. The first site of action is the tear film, a three-layered structure with both hydrophobic and hydrophilic properties. The outermost thin tear film layer is secreted by the meibomian (sebaceous) glands. This superficial lipid layer protects the underlying thicker aqueous layer that is produced by the lacrimal glands. The third layer is the very thin mucoid layer that is secreted by the goblet cells of the conjunctiva and acts as an interface between the hydrophilic layer of the tears and the hydrophobic layer of the corneal epithelial cells.

The avascular cornea is considered the external barrier to the internal ocular structures. Greater systemic absorption occurs through contact with the vascularized conjunctiva (Fig. 17-2). The human cornea has several distinct layers through which a chemical must pass to reach the anterior chamber. The first layer is the corneal epithelium of stratified squamous, nonkeratinized cells with tight junctions. The permeability of the corneal epithelium is low, and only lipid-soluble chemicals pass readily through this layer. The corneal stroma accounts for 90 percent of the corneal thickness and is composed of water, collagen, and glycosaminoglycans, permitting hydrophilic chemicals to dissolve easily in this thick layer. The inner edge of the corneal stroma is bounded by a thin basement membrane called Descemet's membrane that is secreted by the corneal endothelium. The innermost layer of the cornea, the corneal endothelium, is composed of a single layer of cells that are surrounded by lipid membranes. The permeability of the corneal endothelial cells to ionized chemicals is relatively low.

The two separate vascular systems in the eye are (1) the uveal blood vessels, which include the vascular beds of the iris, ciliary body, and choroid, and (2) the retinal vessels. In the anterior segment of the eye, there is a blood-aqueous barrier that has relatively tight junctions between the endothelial cells of the iris capillaries and nonpigmented cells of the ciliary epithelium. The major function of the ciliary epithelium is to produce aqueous humor from the plasma filtrate that is present in the ciliary processes.

In humans and several widely used experimental animals (e.g., monkeys, pigs, dogs, rats, mice), the retina has a dual circulatory supply: choroidal and retinal. The retina consists of the outer plexiform layer (OPL), inner

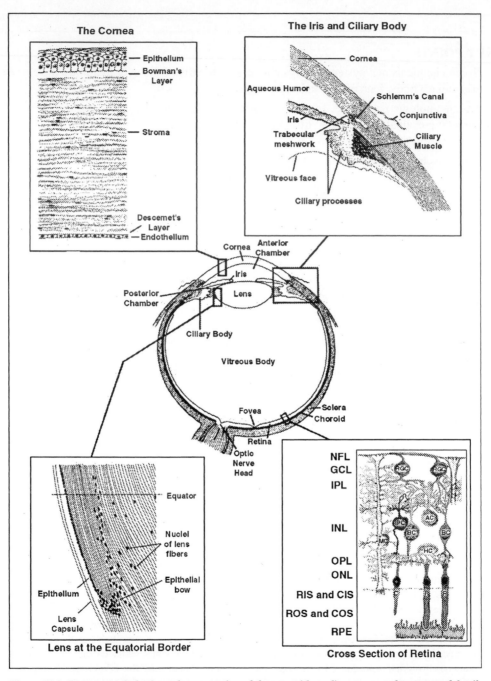

Figure 17-1. Diagrammatic horizontal cross section of the eye, with medium-power enlargement of details for the cornea, iris and ciliary body, lens, and retina.   The morphologic features; their role in ocular pharmacodynamics, pharmacokinetics, and drug metabolism; and the adverse effects of drugs and chemical agents on these sites are discussed in the text.

Table 17-1

Ocular and Central Visual System Sites of Action of Selected Xenobiotics After Systemic Exposure

XENOBIOTIC	CORNEA	LENS	OUTER RETINA: RPE	OUTER RETINA: RODS AND CONES	INNER RETINA: BCs, ACs, IPCs	RGCs AND OPTIC NERVE OR TRACT	LGN, VISUAL CORTEX
Acrylamide				−	−	++	++
Amiodarone	+	+				+	
Carbon disulfide				+	−	++	+
Chloroquine	+		+	+		+	
Chlorpromazine	+	+	+	+			
Corticosteroids		++				+	
Digoxin and digitoxin	+	+	+	++		+	+
Ethambutol				+		++	
Hexachlorophene				+		+	+
Indomethacin	+		+	+			
Isotretinoin	+						
Lead	+		+	++	+	+	+
Methanol			+	++	−	++	+
Methyl mercury, mercury				+	−	−	++
n-Hexane			+	+		+	
Naphthalene		+		+			
Organic solvents				+			+
Organophosphates		+		+		+	+
Styrene				+			
Tamoxifen	+			+		+	

KEY: RPE = retinal pigment epithelium; BC = bipolar cell; AC = amacrine cell; IPC = interplexiform cell; RGC = retinal ganglion cell; LGN = lateral geniculate nucleus.

nuclear layer (INL), inner plexiform layer (IPL), and ganglion cell layer (GCL). The endothelial cells of capillaries in the retinal vessels have tight junctions that form the blood-retinal barrier. However, at the level of the optic disk, the blood-retinal barrier is lacking, and thus hydrophilic molecules can enter the optic nerve (ON) head by diffusion from the extravascular space and cause selective damage at this site of action. The outer or distal retina, which consists of the retinal pigment epithelium (RPE), rod and cone photoreceptor outer segments (ROS, COS) and inner segments (RIS, CIS), and the photoreceptor outer nuclear layer (ONL), is avascular. These areas of the retina are supplied by the choriocapillaris, a dense, one-layered network of fenestrated vessels formed by the short posterior ciliary arteries that is located next to the RPE. Consistent with their known structure and function, these capillaries have loose endothelial junctions and abundant fenestrae; they are highly permeable to large proteins.

After systemic exposure to drugs and chemicals by the oral, inhalation, dermal, or parenteral route, these compounds are distributed to all parts of the eye by the blood in the uveal blood vessels and retinal vessels (Fig. 17-3). Most chemicals equilibrate rapidly with the extravascular space of the choroid, where they are separated from the retina and vitreous body by the RPE and endothelial cells of the retinal capillaries, respectively. Hydrophilic molecules with molecular weights less than 200 to 300 Da can cross the ciliary epithelium and iris capillaries and enter the aqueous humor. Thus, the corneal endothelium—the cells responsible for maintaining normal hydration and transparency of the corneal stroma—can be exposed to chemical compounds by the aqueous humor and limbal capillaries. Similarly, the anterior surface of the lens can be exposed as a result of its contact with the aqueous humor. The most likely retinal target sites after systemic drug and chemical exposure appear to be the RPE and photoreceptors, because

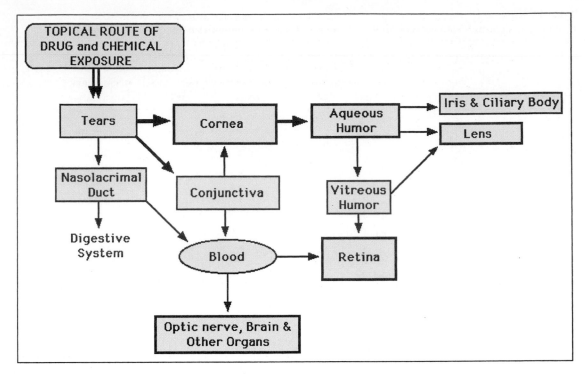

Figure 17-2. Ocular absorption and distribution of drugs and chemicals after the topical route of exposure. The details for movement of drugs and chemicals between compartments of the eye and subsequently to the optic nerve, brain, and other organs are discussed in the text.

the endothelial cells of the choriocapillaris are permeable to proteins smaller than 50 to 70 kDa. However, the cells of the RPE are joined on their basolateral surface by tight junctions that limit the passive penetration of large molecules into the neural retina.

Intraocular melanin plays a special role in ocular toxicology. First, it is found in several different locations in the eye: pigmented cells of the iris, ciliary body, RPE, and uveal tract. Second, it has a high binding affinity for polycyclic aromatic hydrocarbons, electrophiles, calcium, and toxic heavy metals such as aluminum, iron, lead, and mercury. Although this initially may play a protective role, the excessive accumulation, long-term storage, and slow release of numerous drugs and chemicals from melanin can influence toxicity.

Ocular Drug Metabolism

Metabolism of xenobiotics occurs in all compartments of the eye by well-known phase I and II xenobiotic-

biotransforming enzymes. Drug-metabolizing enzymes that are present in the tears, iris/ciliary body, choroid, and retina in many different species are listed in Table 17-2. The activity of these enzymes varies between species and ocular tissues; however, the whole lens has low biotransformational activity.

Central Visual System Pharmacokinetics

The penetration of potentially toxic compounds into visual areas of the central nervous system (CNS) is governed by the blood-brain barrier (Fig. 17-3). In some cases, toxic compounds may be transported actively into the brain by mimicking the natural substrates of active transport systems. One area of the brain that lacks a blood-brain barrier is the optic nerve near the lamina cribrosa, and that lack could cause this part of the central visual system to be vulnerable to exposures that do not affect much of the remainder of the brain.

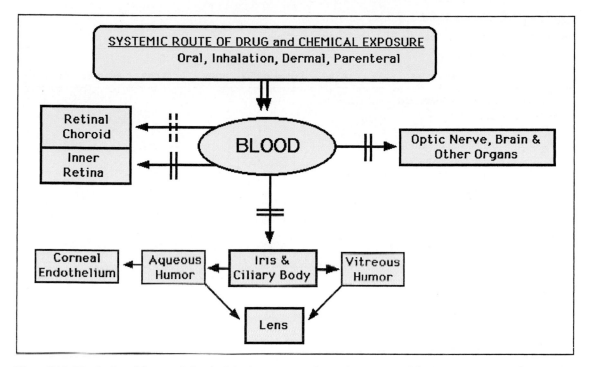

Figure 17-3. Distribution of drugs and chemicals in the anterior and posterior segments of the eye, optic nerve, brain, and other organs after the systemic route of exposure.   The details of the movement of drugs and chemicals between compartments of the eye are discussed in the text. The solid and dotted double lines represent the different blood-tissue barriers present in the anterior segment of the eye, retina, optic nerve, and brain. The solid double lines represent tight endothelial junctions, whereas the dotted double lines represent loose endothelial junctions.

TESTING VISUAL FUNCTION

Evaluation of Ocular Irritancy and Toxicity

Standard procedures for evaluating ocular irritation, the so-called Draize test, with some additions and revisions, has formed the basis of procedures employed for safety evaluations. Traditionally, albino rabbits are the subjects evaluated in the Draize test. The standard procedure involves instilling 0.1 mL of a liquid or 100 mg of a solid into the conjunctival sac of one eye and then gently holding the eye closed for 1 s. The untreated eye serves as a control. Both eyes are evaluated at 1, 24, 48, and 72 h after the treatment. If there is evidence of damage in the treated eye at 72 h, the examination time may be extended. The cornea, iris, and conjunctiva are evaluated and scored according to a weighted scale. The cornea is scored for both the degree of opacity and the area of in-

volvement, with each measure having a potential range from 0 (none) to 4 (most severe). The iris receives a single score (0 to 2) for irritation, including degree of swelling, congestion, and degree of reaction to light. The conjunctiva is scored for redness (0 to 3), chemosis (swelling) (0 to 4), and discharge (0 to 3). The individual scores then are multiplied by a weighting factor: 5 for the cornea, 2 for the iris, and 5 for the conjunctiva. The results are summed for a maximum total score of 110. In this scale, the cornea accounts for 73 percent of the total possible points in accordance with the severity associated with corneal injury.

The Draize test has been criticized on several grounds, including high interlaboratory variability, the subjective nature of the scoring, poor predictive value for human irritants, and undue pain and distress in the tested animals. These criticisms have spawned the development of alternative methods or strategies to evaluate compounds for their potential to cause ocular irritation.

Table 17-2
Distribution of Ocular Xenobiotic-Biotransforming Enzymes

	ENZYMES	TEARS	CORNEA	IRIS/CILIARY BODY	LENS	RETINA	CHOROID
Phase I reactions	Acetylcholinesterase (AChE)	+		+		+	+
	Alcohol dehydrogenase		+		−	+	+
	Aldehyde dehydrogenase		+		+	+	+
	Aldehyde reductase		+	+	+	+	+
	Aldose reductase		+		+	+	
	Carboxylesterase	+	+	+		+	+
	Catalase	−	+	+	+	+	+
	Cu/Zn superoxide dismutase	+	+		−/+	+	
	CYP1A1 or CYP1A2	+	+	+	−	+	+
	CYP4A1 or CYP4B2		+				
	MAO-A or B	+		+		+	+
Phase II reactions	Glutathione peroxidase	−	+	+	+	+	+
	Glutathione reductase		+		+	+	
	Glutathione S-transferase		+	+	+	+	
	N-Acetyltransferase		+	+	+	+	+

The Corrositex assay is an in vitro procedure in which compounds are tested for the ability to penetrate a biological barrier, a hydrated collagen matrix, and cause a color change in an underlying liquid chemical detection system. Chemicals that do not cause a color change in the chemical detection system when added directly in the absence of the biological barrier are not eligible for evaluation with this system. Application of the test is limited, however, by the fact that a number of potential test compounds do not cause a change in color when added directly to the fluid chemical detection system and therefore do not qualify for testing. The test also has a rate of false-positive results (30 percent) that may be too high for some applications.

Ophthalmologic Evaluations

There are many ophthalmologic procedures for evaluating the health of the eye. The procedures available range from fairly routine clinical screening evaluations to sophisticated techniques for very targeted purposes. Examination of the adnexa includes evaluating the eyelids, lacrimal apparatus, and palpebral (covering the eyelid) and bulbar (covering the eye) conjunctiva. The anterior structures or anterior segment include the cornea, iris, lens, and anterior chamber. The posterior structures, referred to as the *ocular fundus,* include the retina, retinal vasculature, choroid, ON, and sclera. The adnexa and the surface of the cornea can be examined initially with the naked eye and a hand-held light. Closer examination requires a slit-lamp biomicroscope, using a mydriatic drug (causes pupil dilation) if the lens is to be observed. The width of the reflection of a thin beam of light projected from the slit lamp is an indication of the thickness of the cornea and may be used to evaluate corneal edema. Lesions of the cornea can be visualized better with the use of fluorescein dye, which is retained in areas where there is an ulceration of the corneal epithelium. Examination of the fundus requires the use of a mydriatic drug and a direct or indirect ophthalmoscope.

An ophthalmologic examination of the eye also may involve an examination of the pupillary light reflex. The direct pupillary reflex involves shining a bright light into the eye and observing the reflexive pupil constriction in that eye. The consensual pupillary reflex is observed in the eye that is not stimulated. Both the direct and the consensual pupillary light reflexes are dependent on the function of a reflex arc involving cells in the retina, which travel through the ON, optic chiasm, and optic tract (OT) to project to neurons in the pretectal area. The absence of a pupillary reflex is indicative of damage somewhere in the reflex pathway, and differential impairment of the direct or consensual reflexes can indicate the location of the lesion. The presence of a pupillary light reflex, however, is not synonymous with normal visual function. Pupillary reflexes can be maintained even with substantial retinal damage. In addition, lesions in visual areas outside the reflex pathway, such as in the visual cortex, may leave the reflex function intact.

Electrophysiologic Techniques

Most electrophysiologic or neurophysiologic procedures for testing visual function in a toxicologic context involve stimulating the eyes with visual stimuli and electrically recording potentials generated by visually responsive neurons. The most commonly used procedures are the flash-evoked electroretinogram (ERG), visual-evoked potentials (VEPs), and, less often, the electrooculogram (EOG).

ERGs typically are elicited with a brief flash of light and recorded from an electrode placed in contact with the cornea. A typical ERG waveform includes an a-wave that reflects the activation of photoreceptors and a b-wave that reflects the activity of retinal bipolar cells and associated membrane potential changes in Müller cells. A standard set of ERG procedures includes the recording of (1) a response reflective of only rod photoreceptor function in the dark-adapted eye, (2) the maximal response in the dark-adapted eye, (3) a response developed by cone photoreceptors, (4) oscillatory potentials, and (5) the response to rapidly flickering light.

Flash-elicited VEPs are recorded from electrodes overlying visual (striate) cortex and reflect the activity of the retinogeniculostriate pathway and the activity of cells in the visual cortex. Pattern-elicited VEPs (PEPs), which are widely used in human clinical evaluations, have diagnostic value.

The EOG is generated by a potential difference between the front and the back of the eye that originates primarily in the RPE. The magnitude of the EOG is a function of the level of illumination and the health status of the RPE. Electrodes placed on the skin on a line lateral or vertical to the eye measure potential changes correlated with eye movements as the relative position of the ocular dipole changes. Thus, the EOG has applications in assessing RPE status and measuring eye

movements. The EOG also is used in monitoring eye movements during the recording of other brain potentials so that eye movement artifacts are not misinterpreted as brain-generated electrical activity.

Behavioral and Psychophysical Techniques

Behavioral testing procedures typically vary the parameters of the visual stimulus and then determine whether the subject can discriminate or perceive the stimulus. *Contrast sensitivity* refers to the ability to resolve small differences in luminance contrast, such as the difference between subtle shades of gray or a series of visual patterns that differ in pattern size or the luminance changes across the pattern in a sinusoidal profile. Contrast sensitivity functions are dependent primarily on the neural as opposed to the optical properties of the visual system. The assessment of visual acuity and contrast sensitivity has been recommended for field studies of humans potentially exposed to neurotoxic substances.

Color vision deficits are inherited or acquired. Most acquired deficits in color vision, such as those caused by drug and chemical exposure, begin with a reduced ability to perform blue-yellow discriminations. With increased or prolonged low-level exposure, the color confusion can progress to the red-green axis as well. Because of the rarity of inherited tritanopia, it generally is assumed that blue-yellow deficits, when observed, are acquired deficits. Generally, disorders of the outer retina produce blue-yellow deficits, whereas disorders of the inner retina and ON produce red-green perceptual deficits. Bilateral lesions in the visual cortex also can lead to color blindness (prosopagnosia).

Assessments of color vision in human toxicologic evaluations include the Farnsworth-Munson 100 Hue (FM-100) test and the simplified 15-chip tests using either the saturated hues of the Farnsworth D-15 or the desaturated hues of the Lanthony Desaturated Panel D-15. The Farnsworth-Munson procedure involves the arrangement of 85 chips in order of progressively changing color. The relative chromatic value of successive chips induces those with deficits in color perception to arrange the chips abnormally. The pattern is indicative of the nature of the color perception anomaly. The FM-100 is considered more diagnostically reliable but takes considerably longer to administer than the similar but more efficient Farnsworth and Lanthony tests. The desaturated hues of the Lanthony D-15 are designed to better identify subtle acquired deficits in color vision.

TARGET SITES AND MECHANISMS OF ACTION: CORNEA

The cornea has three essential functions. First, it must provide a clear refractive surface, and the curvature of the cornea must be correct for the visual image to be focused at the retina. Second, it provides tensile strength to maintain the appropriate shape of the globe. Third, it protects the eye from external factors, including potentially toxic chemicals.

The cornea is transparent to wavelengths of light ranging between 310 [ultraviolet (UV)] and 2500 nm [infrared (IR)]. Exposure to UV light below this range can damage the cornea. The cornea is most sensitive to wavelengths of approximately 270 nm. Excessive UV exposure leads to photokeratitis and corneal pathology, with the classic example being welder's-arc burns. Also, the cornea can be damaged by topical or systemic exposure to chemicals.

Direct chemical exposure to the eye requires emergency medical attention. Products at pH extremes ≤2.5 or ≥11.5 can cause severe ocular damage and permanent loss of vision. Damage that extends to the corneal endothelium is associated with poor repair and recovery. The most important therapy is immediate and adequate irrigation with large amounts of water or saline, whichever is most readily available. The extent of damage to the eye and the ability to achieve a full recovery are dependent on the nature of the chemical, the concentration and duration of exposure, and the speed and magnitude of the initial irrigation.

Acids

Among the most significant acidic chemicals in terms of the tendency to cause clinical ocular damage are hydrofluoric acid, sulfurous acid, sulfuric acid, and chromic acid, followed by hydrochloric acid and nitric acid and finally acetic acid. Injuries may be mild if contact is with weak acids or with dilute solutions of strong acids. Compounds with a pH between 2.5 and 7 produce pain or stinging, but with only brief contact, they cause no lasting damage. After mild burns, the corneal epithelium may become turbid as the corneal stroma swells (chemosis). Mild burns typically are followed by rapid regeneration of the corneal epithelium and full recovery. In more severe burns, the epithelium of the cornea and the conjunctiva become opaque and necrotic and may disintegrate over the course of a few days. In severe burns, there may be no sensation of pain because the corneal nerve endings are destroyed.

Bases or Alkalies

Compounds with a basic pH are potentially even more damaging to the eye than are strong acids. Among the compounds of clinical significance in terms of the frequency and severity of injuries are ammonia or ammonium hydroxide, sodium hydroxide (lye), potassium hydroxide (caustic potash), calcium hydroxide (lime), and magnesium hydroxide. One of the reasons caustic agents are so dangerous is their ability to penetrate the ocular tissues rapidly. The toxicity of these substances is a function of their pH; they are more toxic with increasing pH values. Rapid and extensive irrigation after exposure and removal of particles, if present, is the immediate therapy of choice.

Two phases of injury may be observed with caustic burns. There is an acute phase from exposure up to 1 week. Depending on the extent of injury, direct damage from exposure is observed in the cornea, adnexia, and possibly the iris, ciliary body, and lens. Strong alkali substances attack membrane lipids, causing necrosis, hydration of the collagen matrix, and corneal swelling. Intraocular pressure may increase. Conversely, if the alkali burn extends to involve the ciliary body, intraocular pressure may decrease as a result of reduced formation of aqueous humor. The acute phase of damage typically is followed by the initiation of corneal repair. The repair process may involve corneal neovascularization along with regeneration of the corneal epithelium. Approximately 2 to 3 weeks after alkali burns, however, damaging ulceration of the corneal stroma often occurs as a result of inflammatory infiltration of polymorphonuclear leukocytes and fibroblasts and the release of degratory proteolytic enzymes. Stromal ulceration usually stops when the corneal epithelium is restored.

Organic Solvents

When organic solvents are splashed into the eye, the result is typically a painful immediate reaction. Exposure of the eye to solvents should be treated rapidly with abundant water irrigation. Highly lipophilic solvents can damage the corneal epithelium and produce swelling of the corneal stroma. Most organic solvents cause minimal chemical burns to the cornea. In most cases, the corneal epithelium is repaired over the course of a few days and there is no residual damage. Exposure to solvent vapors may produce small transparent vacuoles in the corneal epithelium, which may be asymptomatic or associated with moderate irritation and tearing.

Surfactants

These compounds have water-soluble (hydrophilic) properties at one end of the molecule and lipophilic properties at the other end that help dissolve fatty substances in water and also serve to reduce water surface tension. The widespread use of these agents in soaps, shampoos, detergents, cosmetics, and similar consumer products leads to abundant opportunities for exposure to ocular tissues. Many of these agents may be irritating or injurious to the eye. In general, cationic surfactants tend to be stronger irritants and more injurious than are the other types, and anionic compounds are more injurious than neutral ones. Because these compounds are by design soluble in both aqueous and lipid media, they readily penetrate the sandwiched aqueous and lipid barriers of the cornea.

TARGET SITES AND MECHANISMS OF ACTION: LENS

The lens of the eye plays a critical role in focusing the visual image on the retina. The lens is a biconvex transparent body that is encased in an elastic capsule and is located between the pupil and the vitreous humor (Fig. 17-1). The mature lens has a dense inner nuclear region surrounded by the lens cortex. The high transparency of the lens to visible wavelengths of light is a function of its chemical composition—approximately two-thirds water and one-third protein—and the special organizational structure of the lenticular proteins. Nutrients are provided from the aqueous and vitreous fluids and are transported into the lens substance through a system of intercellular gap-type junctions. The lens is a metabolically active tissue that maintains careful electrolyte and ionic balance. The lens continues to grow throughout the life span, with new cells added to the epithelial margin of the lens as the older cells condense into a central nuclear region. The dramatic growth of the lens is illustrated by its increasing weight: from approximately 150 mg at 20 years of age to approximately 250 mg at 80 years of age.

Cataracts are decreases in the optical transparency of the lens that ultimately can lead to functional visual disturbances. Cataracts can occur at any age; they also can be congenital. Risk factors for the development of cataracts include aging, diabetes, low antioxidant levels, and exposure to a variety of environmental factors. Environmental factors include exposure to UV radiation and visible light, trauma, smoking, and exposure to a large variety of topical and systemic drugs and chemicals. Several different mechanisms of action have been hypothesized to account for the development of cataracts. The formation of high-molecular-weight aggregates involves the oxidation of protein thiol groups, which leads to a reduction in lens transparency and impairments in membrane transport and permeability.

Corticosteroids

Topical or systemic treatment with corticosteroids causes cataracts. There are two proposed mechanisms through which corticosteroids may cause cataracts. Corticosteroids alter lens epithelium electrolyte balance, which disrupts the normal lens epithelial cells' structure, causing gaps to appear between the lateral epithelial cell borders. Another theory is that corticosteroid molecules react with lens crystallin proteins, producing corticosteroid-crystallin adducts that are light-scattering complexes.

Light

The most important oxidizing agents are visible light and UV radiation, particularly UV-A (320 to 400 nm) and UV-B (290 to 320 nm), and other forms of electromagnetic radiation. Light- and UV-induced photooxidation leads to the generation of reactive oxygen species and oxidative damage that can accumulate over time. Higher-energy UV-C (100 to 290 nm) is even more damaging. At sea level, the atmosphere filters out virtually all UV-C and all but a small fraction of UV-B derived from solar radiance. The cornea absorbs about 45 percent of light with wavelengths below 280 nm but only about 12 percent of light with wavelengths between 320 and 400 nm. The lens absorbs much of the light between 300 and 400 nm and transmits light 400 nm and above to the retina. Absorption of light energy in the lens triggers a variety of photoreactions, including the generation of fluorophores and pigments that lead to the yellow-brown coloration of the lens. Sufficient exposure to infrared radiation, as occurs in glassblowers, or microwave radiation also produces cataracts through direct heating of the ocular tissues.

Naphthalene

Accidental exposure to naphthalene results in cortical cataracts and retinal degeneration. The metabolite 1,2-dihydro-1,2-dihydroxynaphthalene (naphthalene dihydrodiol) is the cataract-inducing agent. Studies have shown that aldose reductase in the rat lens is the enzyme responsible for the formation of naphthalene dihydrodiol and that treatment with aldose reductase inhibitors prevents naphthalene-induced cataracts.

Phenothiazines

Schizophrenics receiving phenothiazine drugs develop pigmented deposits in the eyes and skin. The phenothiazines combine with melanin to form a photosensitive product that reacts with sunlight, causing formation of the deposits in the lens and cornea. The amount of pigmentation is related to the dose of the drug, with the annual yearly dose being the most predictive dose metric. More recent epidemiologic evidence has demonstrated a dose-related increase in the risk of cataracts from the use of chlorpromazine and nonantipsychotic phenothiazines.

TARGET SITES AND MECHANISMS OF ACTION: RETINA

The adult mammalian retina contains 9 distinct layers plus the RPE, 10 major types of neurons, and 3 cells with glial functions (Fig. 17-1). The 9 layers of the neural retina are the internal limiting membrane, nerve fiber layer (NFL), ganglion cell layer (GCL), inner plexiform layer (IPL), inner nuclear layer (INL), outer plexiform layer (OPL), outer nuclear layer (ONL), rod and cone photoreceptor inner segment layer (RIS, CIS), and rod and cone photoreceptor outer segment layer (ROS, COS). The RPE is a single layer of cuboidal epithelial cells that lies on Bruch's membrane adjacent to the vascular choroid. Between the RPE and the photoreceptor outer segments lies the subretinal space, which is similar to the brain ventricles. The major types of neurons are the rod (R) and cone (C) photoreceptors, ON-rod and ON-cone bipolar cells (BCs), OFF-cone bipolar cells, horizontal cells (HCs), numerous subtypes of amacrine cells (ACs), an interplexiform cell (IPC), and retinal ganglion cells. The three cells with glial functions are the Müller cells (MCs), fibrous astrocytes, and microglia. The somas of the MCs are in the INL. The end feet of the MCs in the proximal or inner retina along with a basal lamina, form the internal limiting membrane of the retina, which is similar to the pial surface of the brain. In the distal retinal, the MC end feet join with the photoreceptors and the zonula adherens to form the external limiting membrane (ELM), which is located between the ONL and the RIS/CIS.

The mammalian retina is highly vulnerable to toxicant-induced structural and/or functional damage as a result of (1) the presence of a highly fenestrated choriocapillaris that supplies the distal or outer retina as well as a portion of the inner retina, (2) the very high rate of oxidative mitochondrial metabolism, especially in the photoreceptors, (3) high daily turnover of rod and cone outer segments, (4) high susceptibility of the rods and cones to degeneration caused by inherited retinal dystrophies as well as associated syndromes and metabolic disorders, (5) presence of specialized ribbon synapses and synaptic contact sites, (6) presence of numerous neurotransmitter and neuromodulatory systems, including extensive glutamatergic, GABAergic, and glycinergic systems, (7) presence of numerous and highly specialized gap junctions used in the information-signaling process, (8) presence of melanin in the choroid and RPE and also in the iris and pupil, (9) a very high choroidal blood flow rate, up to 10 times that of the gray matter of the brain, and (10) the additive or synergistic toxic actions of certain chemicals with ultraviolet and visible light.

Each of the retinal layers can have specific as well as general toxic effects. These alterations and deficits include but are not limited to visual field deficits, scotopic vision deficits such as night blindness and increases in the threshold for dark adaptation, cone-mediated (photopic) deficits such as decreased color perception, decreased visual acuity, macular and general retina edema, retinal hemorrhages and vasoconstriction, and pigmentary changes.

Retinotoxicity of Systemically Administered Therapeutic Drugs

Chloroquine and Hydroxychloroquine Chloroquine and hydroxychloroquine can cause irreversible loss of retinal function. Chloroquine, desethylchloroquine, and hydroxychloroquine have a high affinity for melanin; this results in the accumulation of these drugs in the choroid and RPE, ciliary body, and iris during and after drug administration. Prolonged exposure of the retina to these drugs, especially chloroquine, may lead to an irreversible retinopathy. Doses of hydroxychloroquine lower than 400 mg per day appear to produce little or no retinopathy even after prolonged therapy.

The clinical findings that accompany chloroquine retinopathy can be divided into early and late stages. The early changes include (1) the pathognomonic "bull's-eye retina" visualized as a dark, central pigmented area involving the macula, surrounded by a pale ring of depigmentation, which in turn is surrounded by another ring of pigmentation, (2) a diminished EOG, (3) possible granular pigmentation in the peripheral retina, and (4) visual complaints such as blurred vision and problems discerning letters or words. Late-stage findings, which can occur during or even after the cessation of drug exposure, include (1) a progressive scotoma, (2) constriction of the peripheral fields commencing in the upper temporal quadrant, (3) narrowing of the retinal artery, (4) color and night blindness, (5) absence of a typical retinal pigment pattern, and (6) very abnormal EOGs and ERGs. These late-stage symptoms are irreversible.

Digoxin and Digitoxin The cardiac glycosides digoxin and digitoxin induce visual system abnormalities such as decreased vision, flickering scotomas, and altered color vision. The photoreceptors are a primary target site of the cardiac glycosides digoxin and digitoxin. The retina has the highest number of Na^+, K^+ ATPase sites of any ocular tissue.

Indomethacin Chronic administration of 50 to 200 mg per day of indomethacin for 1 to 2 years has been reported to produce corneal opacities, discrete pigment scattering of the RPE perifoveally, paramacular depigmentation, decreases in visual acuity, altered visual fields, increases in the threshold for dark adaptation, blue-yellow color deficits, and decreases in ERG and EOG amplitudes. Decreases in the ERG a- and b-wave amplitudes, with larger changes observed under scotopic dark-adapted than under scotopic light-adapted conditions, have been reported. Upon cessation of drug treatment, the ERG waveforms and color vision changes return to near normal, although the pigmentary changes are irreversible. The mechanism of retinotoxicity is unknown.

Tamoxifen Chronic high-dose therapy (180 to 240 mg per day for ~2 years) produces widespread axonal degeneration in the macular and perimacular areas. Clinical symptoms include a permanent decrease in visual acuity and abnormal visual fields, as the axonal degeneration is irreversible. Chronic low-dose tamoxifen (20 mg per day) can result in a small increase in the incidence of keratopathy, with minimal alterations in visual function. After the cessation of low-dose tamoxifen therapy, most of the keratopathy and retinal alterations, except the corneal opacities and retinopathy, are reversible.

Retinotoxicity of Known Neurotoxicants

Inorganic Lead Lead poisoning [mean blood lead (BPb) $\geq$80 μg/dL] in humans produces amblyopia,

blindness, optic neuritis or atrophy, peripheral and central scotomas, paralysis of eye muscles, and decreased visual function. A low (BPb 10 to 20 μg/dL) to moderate (BPb 21 to 60 μg/dL) level of lead exposure produces scotopic and temporal visual system deficits in occupationally exposed factory workers and developmentally lead-exposed monkeys and rats. Occupational lead exposure produces concentration- and time-dependent alterations in the retina such that higher levels of lead directly and adversely affect both the retina and the ON, whereas lower levels appear to affect primarily the rod photoreceptors and the rod pathway. Furthermore, in a study, these retinal and oculomotor alterations in most cases were correlated with the blood lead levels and occurred in the absence of observable ophthalmologic changes, CNS symptoms, and abnormal performance test scores. Thus, these measures of temporal visual function may be among the most sensitive for the early detection of the neurotoxic effects of inorganic lead.

Methanol Formic acid is the toxic metabolite that mediates the metabolic acidosis as well as the retinal and ON toxicity observed in humans, monkeys, and rats with a decreased capacity for folate metabolism. Human and nonhuman primates are highly sensitive to methanol-induced neurotoxicity because of their limited capacity to oxidize formic acid. The toxicity occurs in several stages. It first occurs as a mild CNS depression, followed by an asymptomatic 12- to 24-h latent period, followed by a syndrome consisting of formic acidemia, uncompensated metabolic acidosis, ocular and visual toxicity, coma, and possibly death. Acute methanol poisoning results in profound and permanent structural alterations in the retina and ON and visual impairments ranging from blurred vision to decreased visual acuity and sensitivity to blindness. Formate is directly toxic to Müller glial cell function as well as rod and cone photoreceptors. The mechanism of formate toxicity appears to involve a disruption in oxidative phosphorylation in photoreceptors, Müller glial cells, and the ON.

Organic Solvents Organic solvents produce structural alterations in rods and cones as well as functional alterations such as color vision deficits, decreased contrast sensitivity, and altered visual-motor performance. Dose–response color vision loss and decreases in the contrast sensitivity function occur in workers exposed to organic solvents such as trichlorethylene, alcohols, xylene, toluene, *n*-hexane, mixtures of these, and others. Adverse effects usually occur only at concentrations above the occupational exposure limits.

Organophosphates Various organophosphates produce retinotoxicity and chronic ocular damage. The evidence for organophosphate-induced retinal toxicity is strongest for fenthion (dimethyl 3-methyl-4-methylthiophenyl phosphorothionate).

TARGET SITES AND MECHANISMS OF ACTION: OPTIC NERVE AND TRACT

The ON consists primarily of retinal ganglion cell (RGC) axons that carry visual information from the retina to several distinct anatomic destinations in the CNS. Disorders of the ON may be termed *optic neuritis, optic neuropathy,* or *ON atrophy,* referring to inflammation, damage, or degeneration, respectively, of the ON. *Retrobulbar neuritis* refers to inflammation or involvement of the orbital portion of the ON posterior to the globe. Among the symptoms of ON disease are reduced visual acuity, contrast sensitivity, and color vision. Toxic effects observed in the ON may originate from damage to the ON fibers themselves or to the RGC somas that provide axons to the ON. A number of toxic and nutritional disorders can affect the ON adversely. A deficiency of thiamine, vitamin B_{12}, or zinc results in degenerative changes in ON fibers. Occasional toxic and nutritional and toxic factors interact to produce ON damage. A condition referred to as *alcohol-tobacco amblyopia* or simply as *toxic amblyopia* is observed in habitually heavy users of these substances and is associated with nutritional deficiency.

Acrylamide

Exposure to acrylamide monomer produces a distal axonopathy in large-diameter axons of the peripheral nerves and spinal cord. The visual effects of acrylamide exposure occur at dose levels high enough to cause substantial peripheral neuropathy.

Carbon Disulfide

Carbon disulfide (CS_2) damages the peripheral and central nervous systems. In the visual system, workers exposed to CS_2 experience loss of visual function accompanied by observable lesions in the retinal vasculature. Central scotoma, depressed visual sensitivity in the peripheral visual field, optic atrophy, pupillary disturbances, blurred vision, and disorders of color perception all have been reported. The retinal and ON pathologies produced by CS_2 probably are direct neuropathologic actions, not indirect results of vasculopathy.

Ethambutol

The dextro isomer of ethambutol produces dose-related alterations in the visual system such as blue-yellow and red-green dyschromatopsias, decreased contrast sensitivity, reduced visual acuity, and visual field loss. The earliest visual symptoms appear to be a decrease in contrast sensitivity and color vision, although impaired red-green color vision is the most commonly observed and reported complaint. The symptoms are associated primarily with one of two forms of retrobulbar neuritis (i.e., optic neuropathy). The most common form, which is seen in almost all cases, involves the central ON fibers, typically results in a central or paracentral scotoma in the visual field, and is associated with impaired red-green color vision and decreased visual acuity, whereas the second form involves the peripheral ON fibers and typically results in a peripheral scotoma and visual field loss.

TARGET SITES AND MECHANISMS OF ACTION: THE CENTRAL VISUAL SYSTEM

Many areas of the cerebral cortex are involved in the perception of visual information. The primary visual cortex—called V1, Brodmann's area 17, or the striate cortex—receives the primary projections of visual information from the thalamus and also from the superior colliculus. Neurons from the thalamus project to the visual cortex, maintaining a topographic representation of the receptive field origin in the retina.

Lead

In addition to the well-documented retinal effects of lead (see above), lead exposure during adulthood or perinatal development produces structural, biochemical, and functional deficits in the visual cortex of humans, nonhuman primates, and rats. Quantitative morphometric studies in monkeys exposed to high levels of lead from birth or from infancy to 6 years of age revealed a decrease in visual cortex (areas V1 and V2), cell volume density, and the number of initial arborizations among pyramidal neurons. These alterations could contribute partially to the alterations in the amplitude and latency measures of the flash and pattern-reversal evoked potentials in lead-exposed children, workers, monkeys, and rats and the alterations in tasks assessing visual function in lead-exposed children.

Methyl Mercury

Visual deficits are a prominent feature of methyl mercury intoxication in adult humans. Methyl mercury–poisoned individuals experience a striking and progressive con-striction of the visual field (peripheral scotoma). The narrowing of the visual world gives the impression that one is looking through a long tunnel, hence the term *tunnel vision.* The damage is most severe in the regions of primary visual cortex that subserved the peripheral visual field, with relative sparing of the cortical areas representing the central vision. Methyl mercury–poisoned individuals also experience poor night vision that is also attributable to peripheral visual field losses.

BIBLIOGRAPHY

Ballantyne B: Toxicology related to the eye, in Ballantyne B, Marrs TC, Syversen T (eds): *General and Applied Toxicology.* New York: McGraw-Hill, 1999, pp 737–774.

Bartlett JD, Jaanus SD: *Clinical Ocular Pharmacology.* Boston: Butterworth-Heinemann, 3d ed. 1995.

Hart WM: *Adler's Physiology of the Eye,* 10th ed. St. Louis: Mosby–Year Book, 2002.

Lupulus P, Garaffo RG. Ocular pharmacokinetics, in Hockwin O, Green K, Rubin LF (eds): *Manual of Oculotoxicity Testing of Drugs.* Stuttgart, Germany: Gustav Fischer Verlag, 1992, pp 119–136.

Leibowitz HM, Waring GO (eds): *Corneal Disorders, Clinical Diagnosis and Management,* 2d ed. Philadelphia: Saunders, 1998.

Spector A: Oxidative stress and disease. *J Ocul Pharmacol Ther* 16:193–201, 2000.

C H A P T E R   1 8

TOXIC RESPONSES OF THE HEART AND VASCULAR SYSTEMS

Kenneth S. Ramos, Russell B. Melchert, Enrique Chacon, and Daniel Acosta, Jr.

KEY POINTS

- Typical chemical-induced disturbances in cardiac function consist of effects on heart rate (chronotropic), contractility (inotropic), conductivity (dromotropic), and excitability (bathmotropic).

- Any xenobiotic that disrupts ion movement or homeostasis may induce a cardiotoxic reaction that consists principally of disturbances in heart rhythm.

- All toxicants absorbed into the circulatory system contact vascular cells before reaching other sites in the body.

- Common mechanisms of vascular toxicity include (1) alterations in membrane structure and function, (2) redox stress, (3) vessel-specific bioactivation of protoxicants, and (4) preferential accumulation of the active toxin in vascular cells.

INTRODUCTION

The cardiovascular system has two major components: the myocardium and a diverse network of vascular vessels consisting of arteries, capillaries, and veins. Both components supply the tissues and cells of the body with appropriate nutrients, respiratory gases, hormones, and metabolites and remove the waste products of tissue and cellular metabolism as well as foreign matter such as invading microorganisms. In addition, the cardiovascular system is responsible for maintaining the optimal internal homeostasis of the body as well as for critical regulation of body temperature and maintenance of tissue and cellular pH.

OVERVIEW OF CARDIAC PHYSIOLOGY

Figure 18-1 illustrates the basic anatomy of the heart. The main purpose of the heart is to pump blood to the

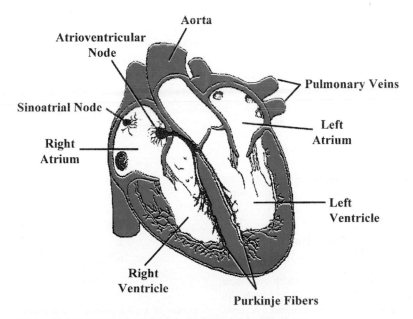

Figure 18-1. Diagram illustrating the basic anatomy of the heart.

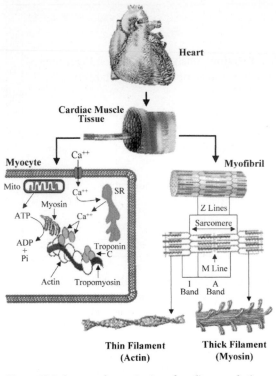

Figure 18-2. Structural organization of cardiac muscle tissue.

lungs and the systemic arteries to provide oxygen and nutrients to all body tissues.

Review of Cardiac Structure

The structural organization of myocardial tissue is shown in Fig. 18-2. The primary contractile unit is the cardiac muscle cell, or cardiac myocyte. Cardiac myocytes are composed of contractile elements known as myofibrils, which consist of a number of thick and thin myofilaments. The thick filaments are special assemblies of the protein myosin, whereas the thin filaments primarily consist of the protein actin. Cardiac myocytes are joined end to end by intercalated disks. Within those disks, there are tight gap junctions that facilitate action potential propagation and intercellular communication.

Cellular Phenotypes within the Heart

The heart contains cardiac myocytes, which contribute to the majority of cardiac mass, cardiac fibroblasts, vascular cells, Purkinje cells, and other connective tissue cells. From a toxicologic perspective, the heart is vul-

nerable to injury because of the limited proliferative capacity of cardiac myocytes and the promotion of cardiac fibroblast proliferation and cardiac remodeling after injury.

Cardiac Electrophysiology

Review of the Action Potential The characteristic appearance of the cardiac action potential demonstrates how ion currents result in changes in membrane potential (Fig. 18-3). In a resting cell, the density of the electrical charge on both sides of the sarcolemma is referred to as phase 4, or diastolic membrane potential (inside negative with respect to the outside of the cell). When an action potential is initiated, sodium (Na^+) channels open, and the rapid influx of Na^+ gives rise to upstroke of the action potential (phase 0). Closure of Na^+ channels and activation of outward potassium (K^+) channels initiate phase 1. As the Na^+ current dissipates, Ca^{2+} continues to enter the cell, giving rise to the characteristic plateau appearance of phase 2. Final repolarization (phase 3) of the cell results from closure of Ca^{2+} channels and K^+ efflux.

Electrical Conduction in the Heart The cardiac cycle begins in pacemaker cells that spontaneously depolarize and pass a depolarizing electrical current to neighboring cells. Pacemaker cells do not contract. Spontaneous depolarization can be found in the sinoatrial (SA) node, the atrioventricular (AV) node, the bundle of His (atrioventricular bundle), and Purkinje fibers. Under physiologic conditions, SA nodal cells set the pace of the heart. If the SA node is damaged or inhibited, the next fastest

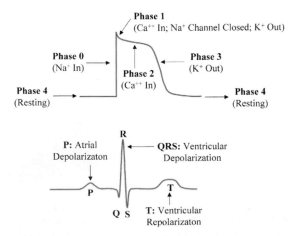

Figure 18-3. Characteristic cardiac action potential and electrocardiogram (ECG).

depolarizing cells (AV node) assume the pacemaking activity. However, normal cardiac function is compromised as a result of slower spontaneous depolarization rates.

Normally, the cardiac cycle begins with the spontaneous depolarization of cells in the SA node. The electrical impulse propagates through the atrial muscle and converges on the AV node. The dense fibrous tissue of the AV node causes the electrical impulse to slow down. This delayed transfer of current between the atria and the ventricles allows the atria to complete contraction before depolarization of the ventricles. The AV node impulse then is sent down the bundle of His, the bundle branches, and the Purkinje network, causing depolarization and contraction of the ventricles.

Electrical cardiac activity is regulated by the autonomic nervous system (ANS). Norepinephrine and similar sympathomimetics stimulate an increase in cardiac rate and the contractility of the myocardium. The major effect of parasympathomimetics is to decrease the rate of depolarization with only a slight decrease in ventricular contractility.

Excitation-Contraction Coupling For contraction to occur, both ATP and Ca^{2+} must be readily available. Mechanical contraction of cardiac myocytes occurs when Ca^{2+} binds to the protein troponin C with tropomyosin. After a Ca^{2+}-induced conformational change in troponin C and tropomyosin, ATP is hydrolyzed, inducing a conformational change in myosin and subsequently allowing myosin to bind actin, thus producing "cross-bridge cycling" and contraction. Relaxation of cardiac myocytes requires reductions in the free Ca^{2+} pool available for interaction with troponin C. As the active ion pump sarcoplasmic reticulum (SR) Ca^{2+} ATPase (SERCA) reduces the cytoplasmic free Ca^{2+} available for interaction with troponin C, the actin-myosin interaction ceases and the cell relaxes.

Cardiac Function

Electrocardiogram The electrocardiogram (ECG) records electrical currents generated during depolarization and repolarization. On the ECG shown in Fig. 18-3, deflections (or waves) are recorded that correspond to atrial depolarization (P wave), ventricular depolarization (QRS complex), and ventricular repolarization (T wave); however, atrial repolarization normally is not observed on the ECG because it is obscured by the large QRS complex. Useful intervals noted on the ECG include the PR interval, corresponding primarily to conduction

through the AV node; QRS duration, corresponding to ventricular depolarization; the ST interval, corresponding to ventricular repolarization; and the QT interval, corresponding to ventricular depolarization and repolarization.

Cardiac Output The primary indicator of cardiac function is *cardiac output,* which is the volume of blood pumped by the ventricles per minute. Cardiac output is dependent on heart rate and stroke volume (the amount of blood ejected by the ventricles during systole). Normal cardiac output at rest is approximately 5 L/min in an average adult human, and that value may increase three- to fourfold during strenuous exercise. Toxicants may alter cardiac output through numerous mechanisms and effects on the heart, vasculature, and/or nervous system.

DISTURBANCES IN CARDIAC FUNCTION

Abnormal Heart Rhythm

Typical chemically induced disturbances in cardiac function consist of effects on heart rate (chronotropic), contractility (inotropic), conductivity (dromotropic), and/or excitability (bathmotropic). The normal human heart rate at rest is approximately 70 beats per minute. A rapid resting heart rate (i.e., above 100 beats per minute) is known as tachycardia, whereas a slow heart rate (i.e., below 60 beats per minute) is known as bradycardia. Any variation from normal rhythm is termed an arrhythmia, and arrhythmias are often complications secondary to other ongoing disturbances in cardiac function.

Supraventricular arrhythmias may be based on defects in AV nodal reentry circuits or anatomic bypass tracts and atrial muscle injury. Ventricular arrhythmias are almost always symptomatic and lead to loss of consciousness within a few seconds and even to death if they are unresolved or untreated. Ventricular arrhythmias may arise from muscle injury secondary to ischemia, infarction, and subsequent scarring and fibrosis or from ventricular hypertrophy. Heart block is due to impairments in the cardiac conducting system. Typically, the atria maintain regular beating rates, but the ventricles occasionally fail to depolarize.

Ischemic Heart Disease

Ischemic heart disease (IHD) may be produced by various pathologic conditions and/or xenobiotics that disturb the balance of myocardial perfusion and myocardial oxygen and nutrient demand. A major cause of

IHD is coronary artery atherosclerosis and the resulting arterial obstruction. Prolonged ischemia may lead to myocardial infarction, or death of myocardial cells because of lack of blood flow. Areas of the heart that are permanently damaged by myocardial infarction are replaced with scar tissue. The *cardiac remodeling* process thus includes initial myocyte loss and subsequent connective tissue cell activation and scar production, hypertrophy of remaining myocytes, altered cardiac geometry, and microcirculatory changes within the heart.

Cardiac Hypertrophy and Heart Failure

Cardiac hypertrophy is an important component of cardiac remodeling after IHD. However, cardiac hypertrophy is often a compensatory response of the heart to an increased workload. For example, prolonged hypertension contributes to load-induced left ventricular hypertrophy. Cardiac hypertrophy in and of itself does not necessarily result in a disturbance in cardiac function. With regard to cardiac remodeling after injury, hypertrophy of the surviving myocytes may be necessary to sustain cardiac output for life support. At some point in the progression of IHD, however, the hypertrophic myocardium may "decompensate" by unknown mechanisms, resulting in failure. During failure, ventricular contractility and/or compliance are reduced such that cardiac output is diminished. Failure may present as left- or right-sided failure or both. When left-sided failure is the primary pathology, blood pools in the lungs and pulmonary edema develops. When right-sided failure is the primary pathology, blood pools in the extremities and pitting edema is found in the lower legs.

Cardiomyopathies

The term *cardiomyopathy* essentially refers to any disease state that alters myocardial function. Therefore, causes of cardiomyopathy include IHD (ischemic cardiomyopathy), cardiac hypertrophy, infectious diseases (e.g., viral cardiomyopathy), drug- or chemical-induced cardiomyopathy, and unknown causes (idiopathic cardiomyopathy). *Dilated cardiomyopathy* is produced by progressive cardiac hypertrophy, decompensation, ventricular dilation, and eventual systolic dysfunction or impaired contractility. *Hypertrophic cardiomyopathy* is produced by progressive cardiac hypertrophy, with impaired compliance of the ventricular walls and reduced diastolic ventricular filling.

GENERAL MECHANISMS OF CARDIOTOXICITY

Interference with Ion Homeostasis

Cardiac function is dependent on tight regulation of ion channel activity and ion homeostasis. Therefore, any xenobiotic that disrupts ion movement or homeostasis may induce a cardiotoxic reaction that consists principally of disturbances in heart rhythm.

Inhibition of Na^+,K^+-ATPase

Na^+,K^+-ATPase reduces intracellular Na^+ in exchange for extracellular K^+. Inhibition of cardiac Na^+,K^+-ATPase increases resting intracellular Na^+ concentrations. This in turn increases intracellular Ca^{2+} concentrations through Na^+/Ca^{2+} exchange, and the elevated intracellular Ca^{2+} and Ca^{2+} stores thus contribute to the inotropic actions of these inhibitors.

Na^+ Channel Blockade Agents that inhibit Na^+ channels in cardiac cells alter cardiac excitability by requiring greater membrane depolarization for the opening of Na^+ channels. The effects of Na^+ channel blockade include reduction of conduction velocity, prolonged QRS duration, decreased automaticity, and inhibition of triggered activity from delayed or early afterdepolarizations.

K^+ Channel Blockade Many different K^+ channels are expressed in the human heart. Blockade of K^+ channels increases the duration of the action potential and increases refractoriness (the cell undergoing repolarization is refractory to depolarization).

Ca^{2+} Channel Blockade The L-type Ca^{2+} channel contributes to excitation-contraction coupling, whereas the T-type Ca^{2+} channels contribute to pacemaker potential in the SA node. Blockade of Ca^{2+} channels in the heart produces a negative inotropic effect as a result of reductions in Ca^{2+}-induced Ca^{2+} release.

Altered Coronary Blood Flow

Coronary Vasoconstriction Xenobiotic-induced constriction of the coronary vasculature induces symptoms consistent with IHD. Catecholamines such as epinephrine normally enhance coronary blood flow indirectly through increased release of metabolic vasodilators and through a relative increase in diastolic duration at higher heart rates. Epinephrine stimulation of β-adrenergic receptors increases heart rate, contractility, and myocardial oxygen consumption. In contrast, the direct effect of sympathomimetics on the coronary vasculature includes coronary vasospasm through activation of α-adrenergic receptors. When β-adrenergic receptors are blocked or during underlying pathophysiologic conditions of the heart, the direct actions of sympathomimetics may predominate, leading to coronary vasoconstriction.

Ischemia-Reperfusion Injury Relief of the offending cause of ischemia (e.g., thrombolytic therapy after acute myocardial infarction) provides reperfusion of the myocardium. However, depending on the duration of ischemia, a reversible contractile dysfunction remains for a day to several days after reperfusion. Reperfusion of the myocardium leads to subsequent tissue damage that may be reversible or permanent, a phenomenon is known as ischemia-reperfusion (I/R) injury.

Intracellular acidosis, inhibition of oxidative phosphorylation, and ATP depletion are consequences of myocardial ischemia. Mechanisms proposed to account for the reperfusion injury include the generation of toxic oxygen radicals, Ca^{2+} overload, changes in cellular pH, uncoupling of mitochondrial oxidative phosphorylation, and physical damage to the sarcolemma.

Oxidative Stress

Reactive oxygen species are generated during myocardial ischemia and at the time of reperfusion. In patients with atherosclerosis, oxidative alteration of low-density lipoprotein is thought to be involved in the formation of atherosclerotic plaques. Figure 18-4 summarizes the adverse effects of reactive oxygen radicals generated during myocardial ischemia and reperfusion. Xenobiotics such as doxorubicin and ethanol may induce cardiotoxicity through the generation of reactive oxygen species.

Organellar Dysfunction

Sarcolemmal Injury, SR Dysfunction, and Ca^{2+} Overload All cells contain elaborate systems for the regulation of intracellular Ca^{2+} because calcium is an important second messenger. Because extracellular Ca^{2+} concentrations are typically several orders of magnitude higher than resting intracellular free Ca^{2+}, the sarcolemmal membrane must prevent a rapid influx of Ca^{2+} and subsequent Ca^{2+} overload (sustained elevated intracellular free Ca^{2+} concentration). The principal Ca^{2+} regulatory organelle in cardiac myocytes is the sarcoplasmic reticulum (SR). Alterations of cardiac Ca^{2+} homeostasis by toxicants may perturb the regulation of cellular functions.

Mitochondrial Injury ATP is the immediate energy source required for work in most biological systems and is obtained mainly through the oxidative phosphorylation of adenine diphosphate (ADP) in the mitochondria. Oxidative phosphorylation can be affected at various sites along the respiratory chain through the use of different chemical inhibitors, such as rotenone, cyanide, and antimycin A. Conversely, uncouplers such as 2,4-dinitrophenol stimulate electron flow and respiration but prevent the formation of ATP by short-circuiting the normal flow of protons through the ATP synthetase.

Apoptosis and Oncosis

In the early periods after myocardial infarction, ishemic injury, I/R injury, or toxicant-induced injury, cardiac myocyte death probably occurs through apoptotic pathways, whereas necrosis occurs at later time points after the insult. Several peptides and cytokines directly activate apoptotic signaling pathways and the death of cardiac myocytes in vitro. Atrial natriuretic peptide (ANP), angiotensin II (also a hypertrophic growth stimulus), tumor necrosis factor-α (TNF-α), and Fas ligand are elevated in the blood and myocardium during the progression of various cardiac diseases. Xenobiotics that are associated with the induction of cardiac myocyte apoptosis in vitro include cocaine, daunorubicin, doxorubicin, isoproterenol, norepinephrine, and staurosporine.

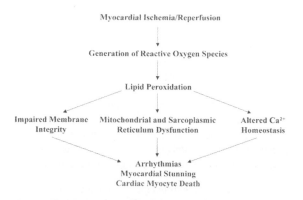

Figure 18-4. Deleterious effects of reactive oxygen species in myocardial ischemia and reperfusion.

CARDIOTOXICANTS

Pharmaceutical Agents

The cardiotoxicity of a cardiovascular drug often represents an overexpression of its principal pharmacologic effect on the heart. For example, digitalis, quinidine, and procainamide may induce cardiac arrhythmias as an exaggerated pharmacologic action of those drugs. In contrast, drugs may produce cardiotoxicity by actions that are not necessarily related to their intended therapeutic use and principal pharmacologic effects. Table 18-1 summarizes key pharmaceutical agents and their prominent cardiotoxic effects and proposed mechanisms of toxicity.

Alcohol The acute toxicity of ethanol includes reduced conductivity and a decreased threshold for ventricular fibrillation (rapid, repetitive excitation of the ventricles). Chronic consumption of ethanol by humans has been associated with myocardial abnormalities, arrhythmias, and a condition known as alcoholic cardiomyopathy that may present symptoms similar to those of congestive heart failure. Metabolites from the metabolism of ethanol may lead to lipid peroxidation of cardiac myocytes or oxidation of cytosolic and membraneous protein thiols. For example, the direct effects of acetaldehyde on the myocardium include inhibition of protein synthesis, inhibition of Ca^{2+} sequestration by the SR, alterations in mitochondrial respiration, and disturbances in the association of actin and myosin.

Antiarrhythmic and Inotropic Agents

Cardiac Glycosides Cardiac glycosides (digoxin and digitoxin) used for the treatment of congestive heart failure inhibit Na^+,K^+-ATPase, elevate intracellular Na^+, activate Na^+/Ca^{2+} exchange, and increase the availability of intracellular Ca^{2+} for contraction. Cardiotoxicity may result from Ca^{2+} overload, and arrhythmias may occur. Cardiac glycosides also may reduce resting membrane potential (less negative) and induce delayed afterdepolarizations and premature ventricular contractions. Cardiac glycosides also exhibit parasympathomimetic activity through vagal stimulation; however, at higher doses, sympathomimetic effects may occur as sympathetic outflow is enhanced. The principal adverse cardiac effects of cardiac glycosides include slowed AV conduction with potential block, ectopic beats, and bradycardia. During an overdose, ventricular tachycardia may develop and progress to ventricular fibrillation.

Catecholamines and Sympathomimetics Catecholamine-induced cardiotoxicity includes increased heart rate, enhanced myocardial oxygen demand, and an overall increase in systolic arterial blood pressure. These actions may cause myocardial hypoxia and, if severe enough, lead to the production of necrotic lesions in the heart. High concentrations of catecholamines also produce coronary insufficiency resulting from coronary vasospasm, decreased levels of high-energy phosphate stores caused by mitochondrial dysfunction, increased sarcolemmal permeability that leads to electrolyte alterations, altered lipid metabolism that results in the accumulation of fatty acids, intracellular Ca^{2+} overload, and apoptosis of cardiac myocytes.

Anthracyclines and Other Antineoplastic Agents

Doxorubicin and daunorubicin are antineoplastic agents whose clinical usefulness is limited because of cardiotoxicity. The acute effects mimic anaphylactic-type responses such as tachycardia and various arrhythmias. These effects are usually manageable and most likely are due to the potent release of histamine from mast cells that sometimes is observed in acute dosing. Long-term exposure to anthracyclines often results in the development of cardiomyopathies and, in severe stages, congestive heart failure. Major hypotheses that have been suggested to account for the onset of anthracycline-induced cardiomyopathy are listed in Table 18-1.

Centrally Acting Drugs

Tricyclic Antidepressants Standard tricyclic antidepressants have significant cardiotoxic actions, particularly in cases of overdose, that include ECG abnormalities and sudden cardiac death. As a result of peripheral α-adrenergic blockade, postural hypotension is a prevalent cardiovascular effect. Although many adverse effects are related to the anticholinergic effects and adrenergic actions of these agents, the tricyclics also may have direct cardiotoxic actions on cardiac myocytes and Purkinje fibers, depressing inward Na^+ and Ca^{2+} and outward K^+ currents.

Antipsychotic Agents Many antipsychotic agents exert profound cardiovascular effects, particularly orthostatic hypotension. Antipsychotic drugs may alter cardiovascular function through indirect actions on the autonomic and central nervous systems and through direct actions on the myocardium. The most prominent adverse cardiovascular effect of antipsychotic agents is orthostatic hypotension. Direct effects on the myocardium include negative inotropic actions and quinidine-like effects.

General Anesthetics Inhalational general anesthetics may reduce cardiac output by 20 to 50 percent, depress contractility, and produce arrhythmias. These anesthetics

Table 18-1
Cardiotoxicity of Key Pharmaceutical Agents

AGENTS	CARDIOTOXIC MANIFESTATIONS	PROPOSED MECHANISMS OF CARDIOTOXICITY
Ethanol	↓ Conductivity (acute) Cardiomyopathy (chronic)	Acetaldehyde (metabolite) Altered $[Ca^{2+}]_i$ homeostasis Oxidative stress Mitochondrial injury
Antiarrhythmic drugs		
Class I (disopyramide, encainide, flecainide, lidocaine, mexiletine, moricizine, phenytoin, procainamide, propafenone, quinidine, tocainide)	↓ Conduction velocity Proarrhythmic	Na^+ channel blockade
Class II (acebutolol, esmolol, propranolol, sotalol)	Bradycardia, heart block	β-adrenergic receptor blockade
Class III (amiodarone, bretylium, dofetilide, ibutilide, quinidine, sotalol)	↑ Action potential duration QT interval prolongation Proarrhythmic	K^+ channel blockade
Class IV (diltiazem, verapamil)	↓ AV conduction Negative inotropic effect Negative chronotropic effect Bradycardia	Ca^{2+} channel blockade
Inotropic drugs and related agents		
Cardiac glycosides (digoxin, digitoxin)	Action potential duration AV conduction Parasympathomimetic (low doses) Sympathomimetic (high doses)	Inhibition of Na^+,K^+-ATPase, ↑ $[Ca^{2+}]_i$
Ca^{2+} sensitizing agents (adibendan, levosimendan, pimobendan)	↓ Diastolic function? Proarrhythmic?	↑ Ca^{2+} sensitivity, Inhibition of phosphodiesterase
Other Ca^{2+} sensitizing agents (allopurinol, oxypurinol)	?	Inhibition of xanthine oxidase
Catecholamines (dobutamine, epinephrine, isoproterenol, norepinephrine)	Tachycardia Cardiac myocyte death	β_1-adrenergic receptor activation Coronary vasoconstriction Mitochondrial dysfunction ↑ $[Ca^{2+}]_i$ Oxidative stress Apoptosis

(continued)

Table 18-1
Cardiotoxicity of Key Pharmaceutical Agents (continued)

AGENTS	CARDIOTOXIC MANIFESTATIONS	PROPOSED MECHANISMS OF CARDIOTOXICITY
Bronchodilators (albuterol, bitolterol, fenoterol, formeterol, metaproterenol, pirbuterol, procaterol, salmeterol, terbutaline)	Tachycardia	Nonselective activation of β_1-adrenergic receptors
Nasal decongestants (ephedrine, ephedrine alkaloids, ma huang, phenylephrine, phenylpropanolamine, pseudoephedrine)	Tachycardia	Nonselective activation of β_1-adrenergic receptors
Appetite suppressants (amphetamines, fenfluramine, phentermine)	Tachycardia, Pulmonary hypertension Valvular disease	↑ Serotonin? Na^+ channel blockade?
Antineoplastic drugs		
Anthracyclines (daunorubicin, doxorubicin, epirubicin)	Cardiomyopathy Heart failure	Altered $[Ca^{2+}]_i$ homeostasis Oxidative stress Mitochondrial injury Apoptosis
5-Fluorouracil	Proarrhythmic	Coronary vasospasm?
Cyclophosphamide	Cardiac myocyte death	4-Hydroxycyclophosphamide (metabolite) Altered ion homeostasis
Antibacterial drugs		
Aminoglycosides (amikacin, gentamicin, kanamycin, netilmicin, streptomycin, tobramycin)	Negative inotropic effect	↓ $[Ca^{2+}]_i$
Macrolides (azithromycin, clarithromycin, dirithromycin, erythromycin)	↑ Action potential duration QT interval prolongation Proarrhythmic	K^+ channel blockade
Fluoroquinolones (grepafloxacin, moxifloxacin, sparfloxacin)	↑ Action potential duration QT interval prolongation Proarrhythmic	K^+ channel blockade
Tetracycline	Negative inotropic effect	↓ $[Ca^{2+}]_i$
Chloramphenicol	Negative inotropic effect	↓ $[Ca^{2+}]_i$
Antifungal drugs		
Amphotericin B	Negative inotropic effect	Ca^{2+} channel blockade? Na^+ channel blockade? ↑ Membrane permeability?

(continued)

Table 18-1
Cardiotoxicity of Key Pharmaceutical Agents *(continued)*

AGENTS	CARDIOTOXIC MANIFESTATIONS	PROPOSED MECHANISMS OF CARDIOTOXICITY
Flucytosine	Proarrhythmic Cardiac arrest	5-Fluorouracil metabolite Coronary vasospasm?
Antiviral drugs		
Nucleoside analog reverse transcriptase inhibitors (stavudine, zalcitabine, zidovudine)	Cardiomyopathy	Mitochondrial injury Inhibition of mitochondrial DNA polymerase Inhibition of mitochondrial DNA synthesis Inhibition of mitochondrial ATP synthesis
Centrally acting drugs		
Tricyclic antidepressants (amitriptyline, desipramine, doxepin, imipramine, protriptyline)	ST segment elevation QT interval prolongation Proarrhythmic Cardiac arrest	Altered ion homeostasis Ca^{2+} channel blockade Na^+ channel blockade K^+ channel blockade
Selective serotonin reuptake inhibitors (fluoxetine)	Bradycardia, Atrial fibrillation	Ca^{2+} channel blockade Na^+ channel blockade
Phenothiazine antipsychotic drugs (chlorpromazine, thioridazine)	Anticholinergic effects Negative inotropic effect QT interval prolongation PR interval prolongation	Ca^{2+} channel blockade?
Other antipsychotic drugs (clozapine)	Blunting of T waves ST segment depression	
General inhalational anesthetics (enflurane, desflurane, halothane, isoflurane, methoxyflurane, sevoflurane)	Negative inotropic effect Decreased cardiac output Proarrhythmic	Ca^{2+} channel blockade Altered Ca^{2+} homeostasis β-adrenergic receptor sensitization
Other general anesthetics (propofol)	Negative inotropic effect	Ca^{2+} channel blockade Altered Ca^{2+} homeostasis, β-adrenergic receptor sensitization
Local anesthetics		
Cocaine	Sympathomimetic effects Ischemia/myocardial infarction Proarrhythmic Cardiac arrest Cardiac myocyte death	Na^+ channel blockade Coronary vasospasm, Altered Ca^{2+} homeostasis Mitochondrial injury Oxidative stress Apoptosis

(continued)

Table 18-1
Cardiotoxicity of Key Pharmaceutical Agents *(continued)*

AGENTS	CARDIOTOXIC MANIFESTATIONS	PROPOSED MECHANISMS OF CARDIOTOXICITY
Other local anesthetics (bupivacaine, etidocaine, lidocaine, procainamide)	Decreased excitability ↓ Conduction velocity Proarrhythmic	Na^+ channel blockade
Antihistamines (astemizole, terfenadine)	↑ Action potential duration QT interval prolongation Proarrhythmic	K^+ channel blockade
Immunosuppressants (rapamycin, tacrolimus)	Cardiomyopathy Heart failure	Altered Ca^{2+} homeostasis
Miscellaneous drugs Cisapride	↑ Action potential duration QT interval prolongation Proarrhythmic	K^+ channel blockade
Methylxanthines (theophylline)	↑ Cardiac output Tachycardia Proarrhythmic	Altered Ca^{2+} homeostasis, Inhibition of phosphodiesterase
Sildenafil	?	Inhibition of phosphodiesterase
Radiocontrast agents (diatrizoate-meglumine, iohexol)	Proarrhythmic Cardiac arrest	Apoptosis?

may sensitize the heart to the arrhythmogenic effects of endogenous epinephrine or to β-receptor agonists. Halothane, as a prototype, may block Ca^{2+} channels, disrupt Ca^{2+} homeostasis associated with the SR, and modify the responsiveness of contractile proteins to activation by Ca^{2+}.

Local Anesthetics Local anesthetics interfere with the transmission of nerve impulses in other excitable organs, including the heart and the circulatory system.

Cocaine The cardiotoxicity of cocaine includes its ability to act as a local anesthetic and block nerve conduction by reversibly inhibiting Na^+ channels. In the heart, cocaine decreases the rate of depolarization and the amplitude of the action potential, slows conduction speed, and increases the effective refractory period. Cocaine also inhibits norepinephrine and dopamine reuptake into sympathetic nerve terminals. The net effect of these two pharmacologic

actions is to elicit and maintain ventricular fibrillation. In addition, a combination of actions involving inhibition of Na^+ channels, altered Ca^{2+} homeostasis, promotion of oxidative stress, inhibition of mitochondrial function, and induction of hypertrophy and apoptosis may contribute to direct injury of the myocardium by cocaine.

Antihistamines The second-generation antihistamines terfenadine and astemizole have been associated with life-threatening torsades de pointes arrhythmias. Electrophysiologic effects include altered repolarization, notched inverted T waves, a prolonged QT interval, AV block, ventricular tachycardia, and fibrillation.

Naturally Occurring Substances

Table 18-2 summarizes the cardiotoxicity of various naturally occurring substances, including cardiotoxic manifestations and proposed mechanisms of toxicity.

Table 18-2
Cardiotoxicity of Naturally Occurring Substances

AGENTS	CARDIOTOXIC MANIFESTATIONS	PROPOSED MECHANISMS OF CARDIOTOXICITY
Estrogens		
Natural estrogens (17β-estradiol, estrone, estriol)	QT interval prolongation?	Gender differences in K^+ channel expression?
Synthetic estrogens (diethylstilbestrol, equilin, ethinyl estradiol, mestranol, quinestrol)	Cardioprotection?	Antiapoptotic effects? Antioxidant activity? ↑ Na^+,K^+-ATPase activity? Ca^{2+} channel blockade? Other mechanisms?
Nonsteroidal estrogens (bisphenol A, diethylstilbestrol, DDT, genistein)		
Progestins (desogestrel, hydroxyprogesterone, medroxyprogesterone, norethindrone, norethynodrel, norgestimate, norgestrel, progesterone)	Enhanced toxicity of cocaine?	Mechanisms?
Androgens		
Natural androgens (androstenedione, dehydroepi-androsterone, dihydrotestosterone, testosterone)	Myocardial infarction Cardiac hypertrophy	Mitochondrial injury? Altered Ca^{2+} homeostasis? Other mechanisms?
Synthetic androgens (boldenone, danazol, fluoxymesterone, methandrostenolone, methenolone, methyltestosterone, nandrolone, oxandrolone, oxymetholone, stanozolol)		
Glucocorticoids		
Natural glucocorticoids (corticosterone, cortisone, hydrocortisone)	Cardiac hypertrophy Cardiac fibrosis	Increased collagen expression Other mechanisms?

(continued)

Table 18-2
Cardiotoxicity of Naturally Occurring Substances *(continued)*

AGENTS	CARDIOTOXIC MANIFESTATIONS	PROPOSED MECHANISMS OF CARDIOTOXICITY
Synthetic glucocorticoids (e.g., dexamethasone, methylprednisolone, prednisolone, prednisone)		
Mineralocorticoids (aldosterone)	Cardiac fibrosis, Heart failure	Increased collagen expression, Other mechanisms?
Thyroid hormones (thyroxine, triiodothyronine)	Tachycardia, Positive inotropic effect, Increased cardiac output, Cardiac hypertrophy, Proarrhythmic	Altered Ca^{2+} homeostasis
Cytokines Interleukin-1β	Negative inotropic effect Cardiac myocyte death	$\uparrow$ Nitric oxide synthase expression Apoptosis
Interleukin-2	Negative inotropic effect	$\uparrow$ Nitric oxide synthase expression
Interleukin-6	Negative inotropic effect	$\uparrow$ Nitric oxide synthase expression
Interferon-γ	Cardiomyopathy Proarrhythmic	$\uparrow$ Nitric oxide synthase expression Altered ion homeostasis
Tumor necrosis factor-α	Negative inotropic effect Cardiac myocyte death	$\uparrow$ Nitric oxide synthase expression $\uparrow$ Sphingosine production $\downarrow$ Ca^{2+} transients Apoptosis

Steroids and Related Hormones The myocardium expresses steroid receptors, and the heart serves as a target organ for steroid effects. Also, cardiac tissue can synthesize steroid hormones, although the capacity for synthesis may be much lower than it is in more classic steroid-synthesizing tissue.

Estrogens Estrogens alter cardiac fibroblast proliferation; they have been shown to both increase and decrease proliferation of these cells. Furthermore, antiapoptotic effects of estrogen in cardiac myocytes have been reported.

Progestins Naturally occurring and synthetic progestins play a role opposite to that of estrogens. The effects of progestins on lipid metabolism are similar to those of androgens. Very little is known about the direct effects of progestins on the heart.

Androgens Anabolic steroids increase low-density lipoprotein (LDL) and decrease high-density lipoprotein (HDL) cholesterol. Increasing evidence suggests that the anabolic-androgenic steroids may exert direct cardiotoxic actions, including mitochondrial swelling, dissolution of sarcomeric contractile units, and rapid Ca^{2+}

fluxes (both directions) in cardiac myocytes. In humans, high-dose use of anabolic-androgenic steroids has been associated with cardiac hypertrophy and myocardial infarction.

Glucocorticoids Chronic glucocorticoid therapy often results in elevated total, LDL, and HDL cholesterols. Furthermore, glucocorticoids are known to cause Na^+ and water retention through mineralocorticoid receptor activation, which could produce hypertension during chronic therapy. Glucocorticoids appear to stimulate cardiac fibrosis directly by regulating cardiac collagen expression independently of hemodynamic alterations. Moreover, glucocorticoids may induce hypertrophic growth and alter the expression of several ion transporters.

Thyroid Hormones Triiodothyronine and thyroxine exert profound effects on the cardiovascular system. Hypothyroid states are associated with decreased heart rate, contractility, and cardiac output, whereas hyperthyroid states are associated with increased heart rate, contractility, cardiac output, ejection fraction, and heart mass. Peripheral vascular resistance is unchanged or decreased regardless of thyroid status. Thyroid hormones promote hypertrophic growth of cardiac myocytes, alter the expression of cardiac sarcoplasmic reticulum Ca^{2+} handling proteins, and may promote arrhythmias.

Cytokines The cardiovascular effects of cytokines can be classified as proinflammatory, anti-inflammatory, or cardioprotective. Many of these cytokines are elevated during cardiovascular diseases such as I/R injury, myocardial infarction, and congestive heart failure. In addition, cardiac myocytes may serve as the synthetic source of many of these cytokines.

Interleukin-1β IL-1β is known to exert negative inotropic actions and induce apoptosis of cardiac myocytes. The effects of IL-1β on cardiac myocytes probably are mediated through induction of nitric oxide synthase and/or increased production of nitric oxide.

Tumor Necrosis Factor-α TNF-α induces apoptotic death of target cells, including cardiac myocytes. TNF-α also exerts negative inotropic effects on cardiac myocytes.

Industrial Agents

Table 18-3 provides a summary of selected industrial agents with their prominent cardiotoxic effects and proposed mechanisms of cardiotoxicity.

Solvents Industrial solvents act on the nervous system, which is responsible for regulating cardiac electrical activity. Because of their high lipid solubility, solvents may disperse into cell membranes and affect membrane fluidity, signal transduction, and oxidative phosphorylation. Their influence on cardiac function also may involve the release of circulating hormones such as catecholamines, vasopressin, and serotonin. From a more general perspective, industrial solvents typically produce a depressant effect on the central nervous system (CNS) and an attenuation of myocardial contractility.

Halogenated Alkanes Halogenated alkanes encompass a wide range of industrial and pharmaceutical agents. Their highly lipophilic nature allows them to cross the blood-brain barrier readily, where they produce CNS depression. Halogenated hydrocarbons depress heart rate, contractility, and conduction.

Heavy Metals Cadmium, lead, and cobalt exhibit negative inotropic and dromotropic effects and also can produce cardiac hypertrophy. The cardiotoxic effects of heavy metals are attributed to their ability to form complexes with intracellular macromolecules and to antagonize intracellular Ca^{2+}.

OVERVIEW OF VASCULAR PHYSIOLOGY

As a complex network of vessels of varying size and complexity, the vascular system delivers oxygen and nutrients to tissues throughout the body and removes the waste products of cellular metabolism. Oxygenated blood returning from the lungs to the heart is emptied into the aorta, which gradually branches off, giving rise to smaller vessels that reach individual organs (Fig. 18-5). Blood returns to the heart for reoxygenation through the venous system before the reinitiation of subsequent cycles.

Vascular endothelial cells play an integral role in the regulation of hemostasis, vascular tone, and angiogenesis. Angiogenesis involves the formation of blood vessels secondary to the migration, proliferation, and differentiation of vascular cells.

DISTURBANCES OF VASCULAR STRUCTURE AND FUNCTION

Human epidemiologic studies have established a positive correlation between injury to a blood vessel wall and the occurrence of vascular diseases such as atherosclerosis and hypertension. Atherosclerosis is a major structural

Table 18-3
Cardiotoxicity of Selected Industrial Agents

AGENTS	CARDIOTOXIC MANIFESTATIONS	PROPOSED MECHANISMS OF CARDIOTOXICITY
Solvents		
Toluene (paint products)	Proarrhythmic	↓ Parasympathetic activity ↑ Adrenergic sensitivity Altered ion homeostasis
Halogenated hydrocarbons		
(carbon tetrachloride,	Proarrhythmic	↓ Parasympathetic activity
chloroform,	Negative inotropic effect	↑ Adrenergic sensitivity
chloropentafluoroethane,	Decreased cardiac output	Altered ion homeostasis
1,2-dibromotetra-		Altered coronary blood flow
fluoromethane,		
dichlorodifluoromethane,		
cis-dichloroethylene		
trans-dichloroethylene		
dichlorotetrafluoroethane,		
difluoroethane,		
ethyl bromide,		
ethyl chloride,		
fluorocarbon 502,		
heptafluoro-1-iodopropane		
1,2-hexafluoroethane,		
isopropyl chloride,		
methyl bromide,		
methyl chloride,		
methylene chloride,		
monochlorodifluoroethane,		
monochlorodifluoromethane,		
octafluorocyclobutane,		
propyl chloride,		
1,1,1-trichloroethane,		
trichloroethane,		
trichloroethylene,		
trichlorofluoromethane,		
trichloromonofluoroethylene,		
trichlorotrifluoroethane,		
trifluoroiodomethane,		
trifluorobromomethane)		
Ketones		
(e.g., acetone, methyl ethyl ketone)	Proarrhythmic	↓ Parasympathetic activity ↑ Adrenergic sensitivity Altered ion homeostasis
Heavy metals		
(cadmium, cobalt, lead)	Negative inotropic effect Cardiac hypertrophy Proarrhythmic	Complex formation, Altered Ca^{2+} homeostasis
(barium, lanthanum, manganese, nickel)	Proarrhythmic	Ca^{2+} channel blockade

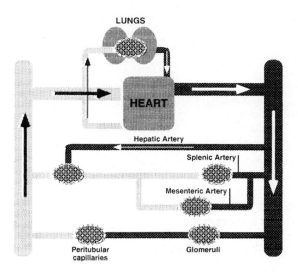

Figure 18-5. Schematic diagram of vascular supply to selected organs. The capillary beds are represented by a meshwork connecting the arteries (*right*) with the veins (*left*); the distribution of the vasculature in several organs (liver, kidney, lung) indicates the importance of the vascular system in toxicology.

change in the vessel wall that involves focal intimal thickenings formed after the migration of smooth muscle cells to the intima and uncontrolled proliferation. Extracellular matrix components such as collagen and elastin, intra- and extracellular lipids, complex carbohydrates, blood products, and calcium accumulate to varying degrees as the lesion advances. The plaque also contains inflammatory cells, such as infiltrated monocytes and leukocytes, which participate in the progression of the pathologic response. The principal consequence of atheroma formation is a progressive narrowing of the arterial lumen that leads to a restricted blood supply to distal sites. Such changes can result in renal hypertension, stroke, and myocardial ischemia and infarction.

Changes in blood pressure often are seen during acute poisonings. Hypotension, a sustained reduction in systemic arterial pressure, is common in poisonings with CNS depressants or antihypertensive agents as well as during anaphylactic reactions. Postural hypotension, particularly in elderly people, can be induced by therapeutic agents such as drugs that lower cardiac output or decrease blood volume.

Hypertension may result from an increased concentration of circulating vasoconstrictors such as angiotensin II and catecholamines or from disturbances of local regulation mediated by metabolic, myogenic, or angiogenic mechanisms. Increased vascular resistance has

been associated with an overall increase in wall thickness that is caused in part by hypertrophy and the proliferation of smooth muscle cells. A sustained elevation in blood pressure also has been associated with destruction of capillaries at the tissue level and compensatory angiogenesis. Sustained hypertension is the most important risk factor that predisposes a person to coronary and cerebral atherosclerosis. The mechanisms by which hypertension produces vascular degenerative lesions involve increased vascular permeability that leads to the entry of blood constituents into the vessel wall.

Thrombosis, which is the formation of a semisolid mass from blood constituents in the circulation, can occur in both arteries and veins as a result of exposure to toxicants. Predisposition to thrombosis occurs by means of induction of platelet aggregation, an increase in their adhesiveness, or the creation of a state of hypercoagulability through an increase in or activation of clotting factors. Sudden changes in blood flow can trigger arterial thrombosis, whereas venous stasis contributes to the development of venous thrombosis. Table 18-4 provides a partial list of thrombogenic agents and their putative mechanisms of action. Portions of a thrombus may be released and travel in the vascular system until they are arrested as an embolus in a vessel with a caliber even smaller than that of its origin. The consequence depends on the site of arrest, but a thrombus can result in death. The most important drugs known to produce thromboembolisms are the contraceptive steroids.

GENERAL BIOCHEMICAL MECHANISMS OF VASCULAR TOXICITY

Chemicals absorbed through the gastrointestinal, respiratory, cutaneous, and intravenous routes contact vascular cells before reaching other sites in the body. This property alone puts the vascular system at increased risk of toxic insult. Many target organ toxicities have a significant microvascular component. Chemicals can produce degenerative or inflammatory changes in blood vessels as a direct consequence of an excessive pharmacologic effect or secondary to the interaction of chemicals or their metabolites with components of the vessel wall.

Endothelial cells represent the first cellular barrier to the movement of blood-borne toxins from the lumen of the vessel to deeper layers of the wall. These cells are particularly susceptible to toxic insult. Toxic chemicals that reach the subendothelial space may cause injury to medial smooth muscle cells and/or adventitial fibroblasts.

Table 18-4
Compounds Producing Thrombosis

AGENT	MECHANISM OF ACTION SPECIFIC EFFECTS
Endothelial damage	
Homocysteine	Deendothelialization
Endotoxin	Deendothelialization
Sodium acetriozate	Disseminated thrombosis in capillaries and veins
Pathophysiologic circulatory dynamics	
Ergotamine	Profound vasoconstriction in peripheral arteries
Pitressin	Profound vasoconstriction in coronary and mesenteric arteries
Oral contraceptives	Venous stasis in lower extremities
ACh and autonomic blockers	Hypovolemic hypotension and stasis
Sympathomimetic agents	Elevated blood pressure; distentions of vessels to produce endothelial damage
Effects on platelets	
Serotonin	Increase in platelet count (above $10^6/mm^3$)
Progesterone	
Testosterone	
Somatotropic hormone	
Vinblastine	
Vincristine	
Congo Red	
Ristocetin	
Thrombin	
Epinephrine	
Adenosine diphosphate	Increase in platelet adhesiveness
Thrombin	
Evans blue	
Effects on clotting factors	
Epinephrine	Increase in factors VIII and IX
Guanethidine	Secondary effects due to release of epinephrine
Debrisoquine	
Tyramine	
Lactic acid (IV infusion)	Activation of Hageman factor
Long-chain fatty acids (IV infusion)	Activation of contact factors
Catecholamines	Elevation in circulating levels of fatty acids
ACTH	
Thymoleptics	
Nicotine	
Oral contraceptives	Decrease in antithrombin III levels
Mercuric chloride	Inhibition of fibrinolysis
Corticosteroids	
ε-Aminocaproic acid	Plasminogen antiactivator
Aprotinine	Proteinase inhibitors

The vasculotoxic response is also dependent on the influence of (1) extracellular matrix proteins that influence cell behavior, (2) coagulation factors that dictate the extent of hemostatic involvement, (3) hormones and growth factors that regulate vascular function, and (4) plasma lipoproteins, some of which modulate cellular metabolism and facilitate the transport and delivery of hydrophobic substances.

Common mechanisms of vascular toxicity include (1) alterations in membrane structure and function, (2) redox stress leading to disruption of gene regulatory mechanisms, compromised antioxidant defenses, and generalized loss of homeostasis, (3) vessel-specific bioactivation of protoxicants, and (4) preferential accumulation of the active toxin in vascular cells. Multiple mechanisms often operate simultaneously in the course of the toxic response. Interestingly, the modulation of growth and differentiation in vascular cells is a common endpoint of vasculotoxic injury.

Vascular reactivity is regulated by the transfer of signals from the surface to the interior of the cell and/or direct modulation of the structure and function of contractile proteins. Usually, disorders of vascular reactivity involve disturbances of ionic regulation. Vascular toxicity also may be due to deficiencies in the capacity of target cells to detoxify the active toxin or handle prooxidant states.

Oxidative metabolism of plasma lipoproteins is critical in the initiation and progression of atherosclerosis. LDLs are oxidized by oxygen free radicals that are released by arterial cells. Modified LDLs attract macrophages and prevent their migration from the tissues. Oxidation of LDLs generates activated oxygen species, which can directly injure endothelial cells and increase adherence and the migration of monocytes and T lymphocytes into the subendothelial space. Subsequent release of growth modulators from endothelial cells and/or macrophages can promote smooth muscle cell proliferation and the secretion of extracellular matrix proteins.

Vascular toxicity may be due to the accumulation of chemicals in the vascular wall. Aromatic hydrocarbons and other ubiquitous environmental contaminants partition into the lipid phase of the atherosclerotic plaques. The consequences of vasculotoxic insult are dictated by the interplay between vascular and nonvascular cells and by noncellular factors such as extracellular matrix proteins, coagulation factors, hormones, immune complexes, and plasma lipoproteins. Furthermore, toxic responses can be modulated by mechanical and hemodynamic factors such as arterial pressure, shear stress, and blood viscosity.

CLASSIFICATION OF VASCULOTOXIC AGENTS

A summary of selected agents and their vascular effects is presented in Tables 18-5 through 18-7. A few specific examples are discussed below.

Pharmaceutical Agents

Autonomic Agents *Nicotine* The plant alkaloid nicotine at pharmacologic doses increases heart rate and blood pressure as a result of stimulation of sympathetic ganglia and the adrenal medulla.

Cocaine Cardiovascular disorders commonly are associated with cocaine abuse. The central actions of cocaine trigger an increase in circulating levels of catecholamines and a generalized state of vasoconstriction. Hypertension and cerebral strokes are notable vascular complications. In pregnant women, cocaine-induced vascular changes have been associated with spontaneous abortions.

Oral Contraceptives Oral contraceptive steroids can produce thromboembolic disorders such as deep vein phlebitis and pulmonary embolism. Intracranial venous thrombosis and secondary increases in the risk of stroke also have been noted.

Natural Products

Bacterial Endotoxins Bacterial endotoxins produce various toxic effects in many vascular beds. In the liver, they cause swelling of endothelial cells and adhesion of platelets to sinusoid walls. In the lung, endotoxins produce increased vascular permeability and pulmonary hypertension. Changes in coronary vessels include disappearance (exfoliation) of endothelial cells followed by necrosis of medial smooth muscle cells. The terminal phase of the effects of an endotoxin on the systemic vasculature results in marked hypotension.

Vitamin D Vitamin D hypervitaminosis causes medial degeneration, calcification of the coronary arteries, and proliferation of smooth muscle cells in laboratory animals.

Industrial Agents

Heavy Metals Food- and water-borne elements (lead, selenium, chromium, copper, mercury, cadmium, and zinc) as well as airborne elements (vanadium and lead)

Table 18-5
Vasculotoxic Agents: Industrial and Environmental Agents

AGENT	SOURCES	PROMINENT VASCULAR EFFECTS	ASSOCIATED DISEASES
Allylamine	Synthetic precursor	Bioactivation of parent compound by amine oxidase to acrolein and hydrogen peroxide results in smooth muscle cell injury; intimal smooth muscle cell proliferation in large arteries	Atherosclerosis
β-Aminopropionitrile		Damage to vascular connective tissue; aortic lesions; atheroma formation, aneurysm	
Boron		Hemorrhage; edema; increase in microvascular permeability of the lung	Pulmonary edema
Butadiene	Synthetic precursor	Hemangiosarcomas in several organs	
Carbamylhydrazine		Tumors of pulmonary blood vessels	Cancer
Carbon disulfide	Fumigant/solvent	Microvascular effect on ocular fundus and retina; direct injury to endothelial cells; atheroma formation	Coronary vascular disease Atherosclerosis
Chlorophenoxy herbicides			Hypertension
Dimethylnitrosamine		Decreased hepatic flow; hemorrhage; necrosis	Occlusion of veins
Dinitrotoluenes	Synthetic precursor		
4-Fluoro-10-methyl-12-benzyanthracene		Pulmonary artery lesions; coronary vessel lesion	
Glycerol		Strong renal vasoconstriction	Acute renal failure
Hydrogen fluoride		Hemorrhage; edema in the lungs	Pulmonary edema
Hydrazinobenzoic acid	Constituent of *A. bisporus*		
Paraquat		Vascular damage in lungs and brain	Cerebral purpura
Polycyclic aromatic hydrocarbons	Environmental tobacco smoke		
Pyrrolidine alkaloids		Pulmonary vasculitis; damage to vascular smooth muscle cells; proliferation of endothelium and vascular connective tissue in the liver	Pulmonary hypertension; hepatic venoocclusive disease
Organophosphate pesticides			Cerebral arteriosclerosis
T-2 toxin	*Fusarium* mycotoxin		
Vinyl chloride		Portal hypertension; tumors of hepatic blood vessels	Cancer

Table 18-6
Vasculotoxic Agents: Gases

AGENT	SOURCES	PROMINENT VASCULAR EFFECTS	ASSOCIATED DISEASE
Auto exhaust		Hemorrhage and infarct in cerebral hemispheres; atheroma formation in aorta	Atherosclerosis
Carbon monoxide	Environmental	Damage to intimal layer; edema; atheroma formation	Atherosclerosis
Nitric oxide		Vacuolation of arteriolar endothelial cells; edema, thickening of alveolar-capillary membranes	Pulmonary edema
Oxygen		Vasoconstriction—retinal damage; increased retinal vascular permeability—edema; increased pulmonary vascular permeability—edema	Blindness in neonate; shrinking of visual field in adults; edema
Ozone		Arterial lesion in the lung	Pulmonary edema

Table 18-7
Vasculotoxic Agents: Therapeutic Agents and Related Compounds

CLASS (AGENT)	SOURCES	PROMINENT VASCULAR EFFECTS	ASSOCIATED DISEASES
Antibiotics/antimitotics			
Cyclophosphamide		Lesions of pulmonary endothelial cells	
5-Fluorodeoxyuridine		GI tract hemorrhage; portal vein thrombosis	
Gentamicin		Long-lasting renal vasoconstriction	Renal failure
Vasoactive agents			
Amphetamine		Cerebrovascular lesions secondary to drug abuse	Disseminated arterial lesions similar to periarteritis nodosa
Dihydroergotamine		Spasm of retinal vessels	
Ergonovine		Coronary artery spasm	Angina
Ergotamine		Vasospastic phenomena with and without medial atrophy	Gangrene of the thrombosis; peripheral tissues
Epinephrine		Peripheral arterial thrombi in hyperlipemic rats	Participates in thrombogenesis
Histamine		Coronary spasm; damage to endothelial cells in hepatic portal vein	
Methysergide		Intimal proliferation; vascular occlusion of coronary arteries	Coronary artery disease
Nicotine	Tobacco	Alteration of cytoarchitecture of aortic endothelium; increase in microvilli	
Nitrites and nitrates		"Aging" of coronary arteries	Repeated vasodilation
Norepinephrine		Spasm of coronary artery; endothelial damage	

(continued)

Table 18-7
Vasculotoxic Agents: Therapeutic Agents and Related Compounds *(continued)*

CLASS (AGENT)	SOURCES	PROMINENT VASCULAR EFFECTS	ASSOCIATED DISEASES
Metabolic affectors			
Alloxan		Microvascular retinopathy	Diabetes; blindness
Chloroquine		Retinopathy	
Fructose		Microvascular lesions in retina	Diabetes-like condition
Iodoacetates		Vascular changes in retina	
Anticoagulants			
Sodium warfarin: warfarin		Spinal hematoma; subdural hematoma; vasculitis	Uncontrolled bleeding; hemorrhage
Radiocontrast dyes			
Metrizamide; metrizoate		Coagulation; necrosis in celiac and renal vasculature	
Cyanoacrylate adhesives			
2-Cyano-acrylate-*n*-butyl		Granulation of arteries with fibrous masses	
Ethyl-2-cyanoacrylate		Degeneration of vascular wall with thrombosis	
Methyl-2-cyanoacrylate		Vascular necrosis	
Miscellaneous			
Aminorex fumarate		Intimal and medial thickening of pulmonary arteries	Pulmonary hypertension
Aspirin		Endothelial damage, gastric erosion obliteration of small vessels, ischemic infarcts	
Cholesterol, oxygenated		Atheroma formation; arterial damage	Atherosclerosis derivatives of cholesterol: noncholesterol steroids
Homocysteine		Increase of vascular fragility, loss of endothelium, proliferation of smooth muscle cells, promotion of atheroma formation	Atherosclerosis; synthesis
Oral contraceptives		Thrombosis in cerebral and peripheral vasculature	Thromboembolic disorders
Penicillamine		Vascular lesion in connective tissue matrix of arterial wall, glomerular immune complex deposits; inhibits synthesis of vascular connective tissue	Glomerulonephritis
Talc and other silicates		Pulmonary arteriolar thrombosis, emboli	
Tetradecylsulfate Na		Sclerosis of veins	
Thromboxane A_2		Extreme cerebral vasoconstriction	Cerebrovascular ischemia
Vitamin D	Dietary		

react with sulfhydryl, carboxyl, or phosphate groups. Metals such as cobalt, magnesium, manganese, nickel, cadmium, and lead also block calcium channels. Intracellular calcium-binding proteins such as calmodulin are biologically relevant targets of mercury and lead. Epidemiologic studies have shown that a large percentage of patients with essential hypertension have increased body stores of lead, and the direct vasoconstrictor effect of lead may be related to this. Inorganic mercury produces vasoconstriction of preglomerular vessels and disrupts the integrity of the blood-brain barrier. The opening of the blood-brain barrier results in extravasation of plasma protein across vascular walls and into adjoining brain tissues. Acute arsenic poisoning causes capillary dilation, which contributes to transudation of plasma and decreased intravascular volume. Chromium appears to play an important role in the maintenance of vascular integrity.

Aromatic Hydrocarbons Aromatic hydrocarbons, including polycyclic aromatic hydrocarbons, readily associate with plasma lipoproteins, and this may play a critical role in vascular toxicity. Benzo [*a*] pyrene and its metabolites elicit alterations in smooth muscle cell proliferation through several mechanisms, including enhanced transcription of growth-related genes through aryl hydrocarbon receptor–mediated pathways, interaction and inactivation of protein kinase C, and conversion of the parent molecule to metabolites that can form covalent DNA adducts.

Gases *Carbon Monoxide* Carbon monoxide induces focal intimal damage and edema in laboratory animals at concentrations arising from environmental sources such as automobile exhaust, tobacco smoke, and fossil fuels. However, it is not clear which of the many chemicals present in these mixtures mediate the atherogenic effect (endothelial injury, changes in lipid profiles, and proliferation of smooth muscle cells). The toxic effects of carbon monoxide have been attributed to the formation of carboxyhemoglobin because carboxyhemoglobin decreases the oxygen-carrying capacity of blood, causing functional anemia.

Oxygen The administration of oxygen to a premature newborn can cause irreversible vasoconstriction and obliteration of retinal vasculature, resulting in permanent blindness.

1,3-Butadiene A chemical used in the production of styrene, 1,3-butadiene increases the incidence of cardiac hemangiosarcomas, which are tumors of endothelial origin. The toxic effects of 1,3-butadiene are dependent on its metabolic activation by cytochrome P450 to toxic epoxide metabolites.

BIBLIOGRAPHY

Acosta D (ed): *Cardiovascular Toxicology,* 3d ed. New York: Taylor & Francis, 2001.

Bishop SP, Kerns WD: *Cardiovascular Toxicology.* Vol 6, in Sipes IG, McQueen CA, Gandolfi AJ (eds): *Comprehensive Toxicology.* New York: Elsevier, 1997.

C H A P T E R   1 9

TOXIC RESPONSES OF THE SKIN

David E. Cohen and Robert H. Rice

SKIN AS A BARRIER

　Skin Histology

　Percutaneous Absorption

　　Transdermal Drug Delivery

　　Measurements of Penetration

　Biotransformation

CONTACT DERMATITIS

　Irritant Dermatitis

　Chemical Burns

　Allergic Contact Dermatitis

　Testing Methods

　　Predictive

　　Diagnostic

PHOTOTOXICOLOGY

　**Adverse Responses to Electromagnetic
　Radiation**

Photosensitivity

　Phototoxicity

　Photoallergy

ACNE

　Chloracne

PIGMENTARY DISTURBANCES

GRANULOMATOUS DISEASE

URTICARIA

TOXIC EPIDERMAL NECROLYSIS

CARCINOGENESIS

　Radiation

　Polycyclic Aromatic Hydrocarbons

　Arsenic

　Mouse Skin Tumor Promotion

KEY POINTS

- The skin participates directly in thermal, electrolyte, hormonal, metabolic, and immune regulation.

- Percutaneous absorption depends on a xenobiotic's hydrophobicity, which affects its ability to partition into epidermal lipid, and rate of diffusion through this barrier.

- The cells of the epidermis and pilosebaceous units express biotransformation enzymes.

- Irritant dermatitis is a non-immune-related response caused by the direct action of an agent on the skin.

- Allergic contact dermatitis represents a delayed (type IV) hypersensitivity reaction by which minute quantities of material elicit overt reactions.

SKIN AS A BARRIER

The skin protects the body against external insults to maintain internal homeostasis. It participates directly in thermal, electrolyte, hormonal, metabolic, and immune regulation. Rather than merely repelling noxious physi-

cal agents, the skin may react to them with various defensive mechanisms that prevent internal or widespread cutaneous damage. If an insult is severe or intense enough to overwhelm the protective function of the skin, acute or chronic injury becomes readily manifest. The specific presentation depends on a variety of intrinsic and ex-

Table 19-1
Factors Influencing Cutaneous Responses

VARIABLE	COMMENT
Body site	
Palms/soles	Thick stratum corneum—good physical barrier
	Common site of contact with chemicals
	Occlusion with protective clothing
Intertriginous areas (axillae, groin, neck, finger webs, umbilicus, genitalia)	Moist, occluded areas
	Chemical trapping
	Enhanced percutaneous absorption
Face	Exposed frequently
	Surface lipid interacts with hydrophobic substances
	Chemicals frequently transferred from hands
Eyelids	Poor barrier function—thin epidermis
	Sensitive to irritants
Postauricular region	Chemical trapping
	Occlusion
Scalp	Chemical trapping
	Hair follicles susceptible to metabolic damage
Predisposing cutaneous illnesses	
Atopic dermatitis	Increased sensitivity to irritants
	Impaired barrier function
Psoriasis	Impaired barrier function
Genetic factors	Predisposition to skin disorders
	Variation in sensitivity to irritants
	Susceptibility to contact sensitization
Temperature	Vasodilation—improved percutaneous absorption
	Increased sweating—trapping
Humidity	Increased sweating—trapping
Season	Variation in relative humidity
	Chapping and wind-related skin changes

trinsic factors, including body site, duration of exposure, and other environmental conditions (Table 19-1).

Skin Histology

The skin consists of two major components—the outer epidermis and the underlying dermis—which are separated by a basement membrane (Fig. 19-1). The junction ordinarily is not flat but has an undulating appearance (rete ridges). In addition, epidermal appendages (hair follicles, sebaceous glands, and eccrine glands) span the epidermis and are embedded in the dermis. In regard to thickness, the dermis makes up approximately 90 percent of the skin and has largely a supportive function. Separating the dermis from underlying tissues is a layer of adipocytes whose accumulation of fat has a cushion-

ing action. The blood supply to the epidermis originates in the capillaries located in the rete ridges at the dermal-epidermal junction. Capillaries also supply the bulbs of the hair follicles and the secretory cells of the eccrine (sweat) glands. The ducts from these glands carry a dilute salt solution to the surface of the skin, where its evaporation provides cooling.

The interfollicular epidermis is a stratified squamous epithelium consisting primarily of keratinocytes, which are tightly attached to each other and to the basement membrane. Melanocytes are distributed sparsely in the dermis, with occasional concentrations beneath the basal lamina and in the papillae of hair follicles. In the epidermis, these cells are stimulated by ultraviolet light to produce melanin granules. The granules are extruded and taken up by the surrounding epidermal cells, which thus

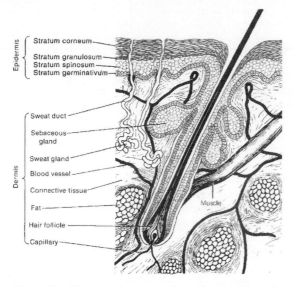

Figure 19-1. Diagram of a cross section of human skin.   The epidermis and pilosebaceous unit are shown in blue.

become pigmented. Migrating through the epidermis are numerous Langerhans cells, which are important participants in the immune response of skin to foreign agents.

Keratinocytes of the basal layer make up the germinative compartment. When a basal cell divides, one of the progeny detaches from the basal lamina and migrates outward. As cells move toward the skin surface, they undergo a remarkable program of terminal differentiation. They gradually express new protein markers and accumulate keratin proteins. At the granular layer, the cells become flattened and increase nearly 40-fold in volume. Lipid granules fuse with the plasma membrane, replacing the aqueous environment in the intercellular space with their contents. Meanwhile, the plasma membranes of these cells become permeable, cell organelles are degraded, and a protein envelope is synthesized immediately beneath the plasma membrane. The membrane is altered characteristically by the loss of phospholipid and the addition of sphingolipid.

This program of terminal differentiation, beginning as keratinocytes leave the basal layer, produces the outermost layer of the skin: the stratum corneum. No longer viable, the mature cells (called *corneocytes*) are approximately 80 percent keratin in content. They are shed gradually from the surface and replaced from beneath. The process typically takes 2 weeks for basal cells to reach the stratum corneum and another 2 weeks for them to be shed from the surface. In instances in which the outer layer is deficient because of disease or physical or chem-

ical trauma, the barrier to the environment the skin provides is inferior to that provided by normal, healthy skin.

Percutaneous Absorption

The stratum corneum is the primary barrier to percutaneous absorption. Diseases (e.g., psoriasis) and other conditions (e.g., abrasion, wounding) that compromise this barrier can permit greatly increased uptake of poorly permeable substances. The viable layer of epidermis provides a much less effective barrier, because hydrophilic agents diffuse readily into the intercellular water, whereas hydrophobic agents can partition into cell membranes, and each can diffuse readily to the blood supply in the rete ridges of the dermis.

The stratum corneum prevents water loss from underlying tissues by evaporation. Its hydrophobic character reflects the lipid content of the intercellular space. The lipids, a major component of which are sphingolipids, have a high content of long-chain ceramides, the removal of which seriously compromises barrier function as measured by transepidermal water loss. The stratum corneum ordinarily is hydrated (typically 20 percent water), with the moisture residing in corneocyte protein, but it can take up a great deal more water upon prolonged immersion, thus reducing the effectiveness of the barrier to agents with a hydrophilic character. Indeed, occlusion of the skin with plastic wrap, permitting the retention of perspiration underneath the plastic, is a commonly employed technique to enhance the uptake of agents applied to the skin surface. Penetration from the air is generally too low to be of concern.

Uptake through the skin is incorporated in pharmacokinetic modeling to estimate potential risks from exposures. The degree of uptake depends on the details of exposure conditions, being proportional to solute concentration (assuming it is dilute), time, and the amount of skin surface exposed. In addition, two intrinsic factors contribute to the absorption rate of a given compound: its hydrophobicity, which affects its ability to partition into epidermal lipid, and its rate of diffusion through this barrier. A measure of the first property is the commonly used octanol/water partitioning ratio (K_{ow}). This is particularly relevant for exposure to contaminated water such as that which occurs during bathing or swimming. However, partitioning of an agent into the skin is affected greatly by its solubility in or adhesion to the medium in which it is applied (including soil). The second property is an inverse function of molecular weight (MW) or molecular volume. Thus, hydrophobic agents of low MW permeate the skin better than do those of high MW or those which are hydrophilic. For small molecules, hydrophobicity is a dominant factor in penetration.

Diffusion through the epidermis is considerably faster at some anatomic sites than it is at others. A list in order of decreasing permeability under steady-state conditions gives the following hierarchy: foot sole > palm > scrotum > forehead > abdomen. Absorption through the epidermal appendages generally is neglected despite the ability of agents to bypass the stratum corneum by this route because the combined appendageal surface area constitutes such a small fraction of the total available for uptake. However, penetration through the appendages can be appreciable.

Transdermal Drug Delivery Specially designed patches are currently in use to deliver clonidine, estradiol, testosterone, nitroglycerin, scopolamine, fentanyl, and nicotine for therapeutic purposes, and others are under development. The advantages of this approach over oral dosing include providing a steady infusion for extended periods (typically 1 to 7 days), thus avoiding large variations in plasma concentration; preventing exposure to the acidic pH of the stomach; and avoiding first-pass removal by the gastrointestinal tract or liver.

Measurements of Penetration Volunteers are dosed, plasma and/or urine concentrations are measured at suitable intervals, and the amounts excreted from the body are estimated. For in vitro work, excised split-thickness skin can be employed in special diffusion chambers, though care is needed to preserve the viability of the living layer of epidermis. The agent is removed for measurement from the underside by a fluid into which it partitions, thus permitting continued penetration. A simpler setup that is commonly employed uses cadaver skin with the lower dermis removed. This material lacks biotransformation capability but retains the barrier function of the stratum corneum. To simplify determination of penetration kinetics, skin flaps may be employed and the capillary blood flow may be monitored to measure penetration. Pig skin has particular utility for this purpose. A promising variation that minimizes species differences is to use skin grafts on experimental animals for these measurements. Human skin persists well on athymic mice and retains its normal barrier properties.

Biotransformation

The ability of the skin to metabolize agents that diffuse through it contributes to its barrier function. This influences the potential biological activity of xenobiotics and topically applied drugs, leading to their degradation or their activation as skin sensitizers or carcinogens. The epidermis and pilosebaceous units are the major sites of such activity in the skin. Enzymes participating in biotransformation that are expressed in skin include multiple forms of cytochrome P450, epoxide hydrolase, UDP-glucuronosyltransferase, quinone reductase, and glutathione transferases. Other metabolic enzyme activites that are detected in human epidermal cells include sulfatases, β-glucuronidase, N-acetyltransferases, esterases, and reductases. The intercellular region of the stratum corneum has catabolic activities (e.g., proteases, lipases, glycosidases, phosphatase).

CONTACT DERMATITIS

Among all occupational skin diseases, contact dermatitis accounts for over 90 percent of reported causes. It includes two distinct inflammatory processes caused by adverse exposure of the skin: irritant and allergic contact dermatitis. These syndromes have indistinguishable clinical characteristics. Classically, erythema (redness), induration (thickening and firmness), scaling (flaking), and vesiculation (blistering) are present on areas in direct contact with the chemical agent.

Irritant Dermatitis

Irritant dermatitis is a non-immune-related response caused by the direct action of an agent on the skin. Extrinsic variables such as concentration, pH, temperature, duration, repetitiveness of contact, and occlusion have a significant impact on the appearance of the eruption. Strong acids, bases, solvents, and unstable or reactive chemicals rank high among the many possible human irritants.

Strongly noxious substances such as those with extreme pH can produce an immediate irreversible and potentially scarring dermatitis after a single exposure. This acute irritant phenomenon is akin to a chemical burn and has been described as an "etching" reaction. More commonly, single exposures to potentially irritating chemicals do not produce significant reactions; repeated exposures eventually result in either an eczematous dermatitis with clinical changes characteristic of allergic contact dermatitis or a fissured, thickened eruption without a substantial inflammatory component. Chemicals that induce these two reactions are termed *marginal irritants*.

Divergent etiologies make it difficult to assign a specific mechanism for the pathophysiology of irritant dermatitis. Direct corrosives, solvents, oxidizing and reducing agents, and dehydrating agents act as irritants by disrupting the keratin ultrastructure or directly injuring critical cellular macromolecules or organelles. Marginal irritants require multifactorial variables to create disease and may not be capable of producing reactions under all circumstances. The varying time courses necessary to produce dermatitis by different known irritants result from differing rates of percutaneous absorption and also depend on the specific agent selected.

No single testing method has been successful in determining the irritancy potential of specific chemicals. Several tests exploit various contributory factors necessary to elicit irritant contact dermatitis. These tests involve either a single application or repeated applications of the same material to the skin. The use of animals in the testing of potentially irritant chemicals is based on a variety of epicutaneous (epidermal surface) methods and has been done for decades. Generally, both intact skin and abraded skin of albino rabbits is tested with various materials under occluded patches. The patches are removed in 24 h, and the tested areas of the skin are evaluated at that time and again in 1 to 3 days.

The in vitro Corrositex assay tests the ability of a chemical to penetrate a hydrated collagen matrix barrier and produce a color change in the underlying aqueous chemical detection system. The relative corrosiveness of a chemical is determined by the time required to penetrate the collagen and enter the liquid buffer with pH indicator dyes.

In the Repeat Insult Patch Test, which is used in humans primarily for the evaluation of potential allergic sensitization, chemicals are placed on the skin under occlusion for 3 to 4 weeks. The test materials are replaced every 2 to 3 days to maintain an adequate reservoir in the patch site. The test is functionally similar to the Cumulative Irritancy Test, in which daily patches are applied under occlusion for 2 weeks in parallel with control substances. The Chamber Scarification Test modifies the tests mentioned above by abrading the skin to expose the upper dermis. All these provocative tests rely on overt clinical changes such as erythema and induration (hardening) at the site of challenge with a potential irritant.

Chemical Burns

Extremely corrosive and reactive chemicals may produce immediate coagulative necrosis that results in substantial tissue damage, with ulceration and sloughing. This is distinct from irritant dermatitis, since the lesion is a direct result of the chemical insult and does not rely heavily on secondary inflammation to manifest the cutaneous signs of injury. In addition to the direct effects of the chemical, necrotic tissue can act as a chemical reservoir, resulting in either continued cutaneous damage or percutaneous absorption and systemic injury after exposure. Table 19-2 lists selected corrosive chemicals that are important clinically.

Allergic Contact Dermatitis

Allergic contact dermatitis represents a delayed (type IV) hypersensitivity reaction. Only minute quantities of material are necessary to elicit overt reactions. This is distinct from irritant contact dermatitis, in which the intensity of the reaction is proportional to the dose applied. An estimated 20 percent of all cases of contact dermatitis are allergic in nature. Currently, 3700 chemicals have been described as potential allergens.

For allergic contact dermatitis to occur, one first must be sensitized to the potential allergen. Subsequent contact elicits the classic clinical and pathologic findings. To mount an immune reaction to a sensitizer, one must be genetically prepared to become sensitized, have sufficient contact with a sensitizing chemical, and then have repeated contact later.

Contact dermatitis may occur upon exposure to one or any number of the thousands of allergens to which people are potentially exposed daily. Table 19-3 lists common allergens based on common exposure patterns. Contact with esoteric allergens frequently occurs in the workplace.

Inspection of the chemicals listed in Table 19-3 indicates that common causes of allergic contact dermatitis are ubiquitous in the materials that touch human skin regularly. There are, however, several allergens—such as nickel, chromium, cobalt, and some food flavorings—that also are ingested with great frequency. In cases in which an individual has a contact sensitivity to an agent that is administered systemically (orally), a generalized skin eruption with associated symptoms such as headache, malaise, and arthralgia may occur. Less dramatic eruptions may include flaring of a previous contact dermatitis to the same substance, vesicular hand eruptions, and an eczematous eruption in flexural areas. Systemic contact dermatitis may produce a delayed-type hypersensitivity reaction and/or the deposition of immunoglobulins and complement components in the skin. These deposits are potent inducers of a secondary inflammatory response and are responsible for the initial pathophysiology of many blistering and connective tissue diseases of the skin.

Table 19-2
Selected Chemicals Causing Skin Burns

CHEMICAL	COMMENT
Ammonia	Potent skin corrosive
	Contact with compressed gas can cause frostbite
Calcium oxide (CaO)	Severe chemical burns
	Extremely exothermic reaction—dissolving in water can cause heat burns
Chlorine	Liquid and concentrated vapors cause cell death and ulceration
Ethylene oxide	Solutions and vapors may burn
	Compressed gas can cause frostbite
Hydrogen chloride (HCl)	Severe burning with scar formation
Hydrogen fluoride (HF)	Severe, painful, slowly healing burns in high concentration
	Lower concentration causes delayed cutaneous injury
	Systemic absorption can lead to electrolyte abnormalities and death
	Calcium-containing topical medications and quaternary ammonium compounds are used to limit damage
Hydrogen peroxide	High concentration causes severe burns and blistering
Methyl bromide	Liquid exposure produces blistering, deep burns
Nitrogen oxides	Moist skin facilitates the formation of nitric acid, causing severe yellow-colored burns
Phosphorus	White phosphorus continues to burn on skin in the presence of air
Phenol	Extremely corrosive even in low concentrations
	Systemic absorption through burn sites may result in cardiac arrhythmias, renal disease, and death
Sodium hydroxide	High concentration causes deep burns, readily denatures keratin
Toluene diisocyanate	Severe burns with contact
	Skin contact rarely may result in respiratory sensitization

Cross-reactions between chemicals may occur if they share similar functional groups that are critical to the formation of complete allergens (hapten plus carrier protein). These reactions may cause difficulties in controlling contact dermatitis, since avoidance of known allergens and potentially cross-reacting substances is necessary for improvement. Table 19-4 lists common cross-reacting substances. Proper diagnosis can be hampered by concomitant sensitization to two different chemicals in the same product or simultaneous sensitization to two chemicals in different products.

Testing Methods

Predictive As with irritant dermatitis, animals have been used to determine the allergenicity of chemicals in the hope of correlating the data to humans. The Draize test is an intradermal test in which the induction of sensitization is accomplished by means of 10 intracutaneous injections of a specific test material. Subsequent challenges are performed by using the same method, and local reactions are graded by their clinical appearance. The Guinea Pig Maximization Test attempts to induce allergy through serial intradermal injections of an agent with the addition of Freund's complete adjuvant, an immune enhancer that consists of mycobacterial proteins. Subsequent challenge with the agent alone under an occluded chamber is graded clinically. For chemicals with higher allergenicity, epicutaneous skin testing can be performed, obviating the need for percutaneous (through the epidermis) sensitization. The Buehler test, Guinea Pig Maximization Test, and Epicutaneous Maximization Test use

Table 19-3
Common Contact Allergens

SOURCE	COMMON ALLERGENS	
Topical medications/hygiene products	**Antibiotics**	**Therapeutics**
	Bacitracin	Benzocaine
	Neomycin	Fluorouracil
	Polymyxin	Idoxuridine
	Aminoglycosides	α-Tocopherol (vitamin E)
	Sulfonamides	Corticosteroids
	Preservatives	**Others**
	Benzalkonium chloride	Cinnamic aldehyde
	Formaldehyde	Ethylenediamine
	Formaldehyde releasers	Lanolin
	Quaternium-15	p-Phenylenediamine
	Imidazolidinyl urea	Propylene glycol
	Diazolidinyl urea	Benzophenones
	DMDM hydantoin	Fragrances
	Methylchloroisothiazolone	Thioglycolates
Plants and trees	Abietic acid	Pentadecylcatechols
	Balsam of Peru	Sesquiterpene lactone
	Rosin (colophony)	Tuliposide A
Antiseptics	Chloramine	Glutaraldehyde
	Chlorhexidine	Hexachlorophene
	Chloroxylenol	Thimerosal (Merthiolate)
	Dichlorophene	Mercurials
	Dodecylaminoethyl glycine HCl	Triphenylmethane dyes
Rubber products	Diphenylguanidine	Resorcinol monobenzoate
	Hydroquinone	Benzothiazolesulfenamides
	Mercaptobenzothiazole	Dithiocarbamates
	p-Phenylenediamine	Thiurams
Leather	Formaldehyde	Potassium dichromate
	Glutaraldehyde	
Paper products	Abietic acid	Rosin (colophony)
	Formaldehyde	Triphenyl phosphate
	Nigrosine	Dyes
Glues and bonding agents	Bisphenol A	Epoxy resins
	Epichlorohydrin	p-(t-Butyl)formaldehyde resin
	Formaldehyde	Toluene sulfonamide resins
	Acrylic monomers	Urea formaldehyde resins
	Cyanoacrylates	
Metals	Chromium	Mercury
	Cobalt	Nickel

animals with intact and abraded skin to induce sensitization and subsequent elicitation upon rechallenge to predict the allergenicity of strongly sensitizing substances
in human beings. However, weaker allergens often are
not discovered until they reach a large human population.

Diagnostic Determining the cause of a contact dermatitis requires a careful evaluation of possible chemical exposures, the history of the illness, and the distribution of
lesions. This evaluation is imperative, because without
strict avoidance, the dermatitis will continue. Diagnostic

Table 19-4
Common Cross-Reacting Chemicals

CHEMICAL	CROSS REACTOR
Abietic acid	Pine resin (colophony)
Balsam of Peru	Pine resin, cinnamates, benzoates
Bisphenol A	Diethylstilbestrol, hydroquinone monobenzyl ether
Canaga oil	Benzyl salicylate
Chlorocresol	Chloroxylenol
Diazolidinyl urea	Imidazolidinyl urea, formaldehyde
Ethylenediamine di-HCl	Aminophylline, piperazine
Formaldehyde	Arylsulfonamide resin, chloroallyl-hexaminium chloride
Hydroquinone	Resorcinol
Methyl hydroxybenzoate	Parabens, hydroquinone monobenzyl ether
p-Aminobenzoic acid	p-Aminosalicylic acid, sulfonamide
Phenylenediamine	Parabens, p-aminobenzoic acid
Propyl hydroxybenzoate	Hydroquinone monobenzyl ether
Phenol	Resorcinol, cresols, hydroquinone
Tetraethylthiuram disulfide	Tetraethylthiuram mono- and disulfide

patch testing utilizes standardized concentrations of material dissolved or suspended in petrolatum or water that are placed on stainless steel chambers adhering to acrylic tape. The chambers are left in place for 48 h, and an initial reading is performed when the patches are removed. A subsequent reading 24 to 96 h later also is made, since delayed reactions commonly occur. Reactions are graded as positive if erythema (redness) and induration (skin thickening) occur at the test site. Strict adherence to established protocols is necessary to draw conclusions about the clinical relevance of the reactions. Avoidance and substitution of the offending agent will lead to improvement in the majority of cases in a few weeks.

PHOTOTOXICOLOGY

In the course of a lifetime, the skin is exposed to radiation that spans the electromagnetic spectrum, including ultraviolet (UV), visible, and infrared radiation from the sun, artificial light sources, and heat sources. In general, the solar radiation reaching the earth that is most capable of inducing skin changes extends from 290 to 700 nm, the ultraviolet and visible spectra. For any form of electromagnetic radiation to produce a biological change, it first must be absorbed. The absorption of light in deeper, more vital structures of the skin is dependent on chromophores, epidermal thickness, and water content that differ from region to region on the body. The chromophores melanin and amino acids are capable of absorbing UV-B (290 to 320 nm) radiation. Biologically,

the most significant chromophore is DNA, because the resultant damage from radiation can have lasting effects on the structure and function of the tissue.

Adverse Responses to Electromagnetic Radiation

After exposure, the most evident acute feature of UV radiation exposure is erythema (redness or sunburn). The minimal erythema dose (MED), the smallest dose of UV light needed to induce an erythematous response, varies greatly from person to person. The vasodilation responsible for the color change is accompanied by significant alterations in inflammatory mediators such as prostaglandins D2, E2, and F2α; leukotriene B$_4$; and prostacyclin I$_2$. Also, interleukin-1 (IL-1), released from local inflammatory cells as well as from injured keratinocytes, may be responsible for several of the systemic symptoms associated with sunburn, such as fever, chills, and malaise. UV-B (290 to 320 nm) is the most effective solar band in causing erythema in human skin. Environmental conditions that affect UV-induced injury include duration of exposure, season, altitude, body site, skin pigmentation, and previous exposure. A substantially greater dosage of UV-A (320 to 400 nm) reaches the earth compared with UV-B (up to 100-fold); however, its efficiency in generating erythema in humans is about 1000-fold less than that of UV-B. Overt pigment darkening is another typical response to UV exposure. This may be accomplished by enhanced melanin production by melanocytes or by the photooxidation of melanin. Tanning or increased pigmentation usually occurs within 3 days of exposure to UV light, whereas photooxidation is evident immediately. The tanning response is produced most readily by exposure in the UV-B band. The tanning response serves to augment the protective effects of melanin in the skin. However, the immediate pigment-darkening characteristic of UV-A and visible light exposure does not confer improved photoprotection.

Commensurate with melanogenesis, UV radiation provokes skin thickening primarily in the stratum corneum, and this response confers a significant defense against subsequent UV insult. Chronic exposure to radiation may induce a variety of characteristic skin changes that depend greatly on the baseline skin pigmentation of the individual as well as the duration and location of the exposure. Lighter-skinned people tend to suffer from chronic skin changes with greater frequency than do darker individuals, and locations such as the head, neck, hands, and upper chest are involved more readily because of their routine exposures. Pigmentary changes such as freckling and hypomelanotic areas, wrinkling, telangiectasias (fine superficial blood vessels), actinic keratoses (precancerous lesions), and malignant skin lesions such as basal and squamous cell carcinomas and malignant melanomas are all consequences of chronic exposure to UV light. A significant pathophysiologic response of chronic exposure to UV light is the pronounced decrease in epidermal Langerhans cells, which may result in lessened immune surveillance of neoantigens on malignant cells, allowing such transformation to proceed unabated. Exposures to ionizing radiation may produce a different spectrum of disease, depending on the dose delivered. Large acute exposures result in local redness, blistering, swelling, ulceration, and pain. After a latent period or after subacute chronic exposures, characteristic changes such as epidermal thinning, freckling, telangiectasias (dilated capillaries), and nonhealing ulcerations may occur. Also, a variety of skin malignancies have been described years after exposure of the skin to radiation.

Aside from the toxic nature of electromagnetic radiation, natural and environmental exposures to certain bands of light are vital for survival. Ultraviolet radiation is critical for the conversion of 7-dehydrocholesterol to previtamin D_3, a required precursor for normal endogenous production of vitamin D. Blue light in the 420- to 490-nm range can photoisomerize bilirubin (a red blood cell breakdown product) in the skin, causing urinary excretion of this neurotoxic metabolite by infants with elevated serum bilirubin. In addition, the toxic effects of UV light have been exploited for decades through artificial light sources for the treatment of hyperproliferative skin disorders such as psoriasis.

Photosensitivity

An abnormal sensitivity to UV and visible light, photosensitivity may result from endogenous or exogenous factors. Various genetic diseases and the autoimmune disease lupus erythematosus impair a cell's ability to repair UV light–induced damage. In hereditary or chemically induced porphyrias, enzyme abnormalities disrupt the biosynthetic pathways that produce heme, leading to the accumulation of porphyrin precursors or derivatives throughout the body. These compounds in general fluoresce when exposed to light of 400 to 410 nm (Soret band) and in this excited state interact with cellular macromolecules or with molecular oxygen to generate toxic free radicals. Chlorinated aromatic hydrocarbons induce this syndrome.

Phototoxicity Phototoxic reactions from exogenous chemicals may be produced by systemic or topical administration or exposure. In acute reactions, the skin may appear red and blister within minutes to hours after ultraviolet light exposure and resemble a bad sunburn. Chronic phototoxic responses may result in hyperpigmention and thickening of the affected areas. UV-A (320 to 400 nm) is most commonly responsible; UV-B (290 to 320 nm) occasionally may be involved.

The agents most often associated with phototoxic reactions are listed in Table 19-5. These chemicals readily absorb UV light and assume a higher-energy excited state. The oxygen-dependent photodynamic reaction is the most common as these excited molecules return to the ground state. Here excited triplet-state molecules transfer their energy to oxygen, forming singlet oxygen, or are reduced and form other highly reactive free radicals. These reactive products are capable of damaging cellular components and macromolecules and causing cell death. The resulting damage elaborates a variety of immune mediators from keratinocytes and local white blood cells that recruit more inflammatory cells to the skin and thus produce the clinical signs of phototoxicity.

Nonphotodynamic mechanisms have been described in the pathogenesis of phototoxicity, with psoralens being prime examples. Upon entering the cell, psoralens intercalate with DNA. Subsequent excitation with UV-A provokes a photochemical reaction that ultimately results in a covalently linked cycloadduct between the psoralen

Table 19-5
Selected Phototoxic Chemicals

Furocoumarins
   8-Methoxypsoralen
   5-Methoxypsoralen
   Trimethoxypsoralen
Polycyclic aromatic hydrocarbons
   Anthracene
   Fluoranthene
   Acridine
   Phenanthrene
Tetracyclines
   Demethylchlortetracycline
Sulfonamides
Chlorpromazine
Nalidixic acid
Nonsteroidal anti-inflammatory drugs
   Benoxaprofen
Amyl O-dimethylaminobenzoic acid
Dyes
   Eosin
   Acridine orange
Porphyrin derivatives
   Hematoporphyrin

and pyrimidine bases. This substantially inhibits DNA synthesis and repair, resulting in clinical phototoxic reactions. Psoralens may be found in sufficiently high concentrations in limes and celery and can cause a significant blistering eruption called phytophotodermatitis. Psoralen-induced phototoxicity may be harnessed and controlled pharmacologically. Topically and orally administered psoralens are used therapeutically to enhance the effects of controlled delivery of UV-A. PUVA (psoralens plus UV-A) is administered to control keratinocyte and lymphocyte hyperproliferative diseases such as psoriasis, eczema, and cutaneous T-cell lymphomas.

Photoallergy In contrast to phototoxicity, photoallergy represents a true type IV delayed hypersensitivity reaction. Hence, while phototoxic reactions can occur with the first exposure to the offending chemical, photoallergy requires prior sensitization. Induction and subsequent elicitation of reactions may result from topical or systemic exposure to the agent. If the exposures are topical, the reactions are termed *photocontact dermatitis,* whereas systemic exposures are termed *systemic photoallergy.* Generally, the mechanisms of photocontact

dermatitis and even that of systemic photoallergy are the same as those described above for allergic contact dermatitis. However, UV light is necessary to convert a potentially photosensitizing chemical into a hapten that elicits an allergic response.

Testing for photoallergy is similar to patch testing for allergic contact dermatitis. Duplicate allergens are placed on the back under occlusion with stainless steel chambers. Approximately 24 h later, one set of patches is removed and irradiated with UV-A. All the patches are removed and clinical assessments of patch-test sites are made 48 h and 4 to 7 days after placement. A reaction to an allergen solely on the irradiated side is termed photocontact dermatitis. Reactions occurring simultaneously on the irradiated and nonirradiated sides are consistent with an allergic contact dermatitis. There is disagreement about the presence of coexisting allergic contact and photocontact dermatitis to the same agent, because a photo patch test occasionally may exhibit greater reactivity on the irradiated side compared with the nonirradiated side. Table 19-6 lists potential photoallergens.

ACNE

Acne is a pleomorphic disease with a multifactorial etiology. The influence of sebum, hormones, bacteria, genetics, and environmental factors is well known. In many situations, one of these factors has an overwhelmingly greater influence in the genesis of lesions than do the others. Among the literally dozens of different kinds of acne that have been described over the decades, this section concentrates on acne venenata.

Chemicals that are termed *comedogenic* induce comedone lesions, which may be open or closed (blackhead or whitehead, respectively, in the vernacular). Additionally, papules, pustules, cysts, and scars may complicate the process. Hair follicles and associated sebaceous glands become clogged with compacted keratinocytes that are bathed in sebum. The pigmentary change most evident in open comedones comes from melanin.

Chloracne

Chloracne, one of the most disfiguring forms of acne in humans, is caused by exposure to halogenated aromatic hydrocarbons. Table 19-7 lists several chloracnegens. Chloracne is a relatively rare disease; however, its recalcitrant nature and preventability make it an important occupational and environmental illness. Typically, comedones and straw-colored cysts are present behind the ears,

Table 19-6
Photoallergen Series for Photo Patch Testing

p-Aminobenzoic acid
Bithionol (thiobis-dichlorophenol)
Butyl methoxydibenzoylmethane
Chlorhexidine diacetate
Chlorpromazine hydrochloride
Cinoxate
Dichlorophen
4,5-Dibromosalicylanide
Diphenhydramine hydrochloride
Eusolex 8020 (1-(4-Isopropylphenyl)-3-phenyl-
　1,3-propandione)
Eusolex 6300 (3-(4-Methylbenzyliden)-camphor)
Fenticlor (thiobis-chlorophenol)
Hexachlorophene
Homosalate
Menthyl anthranilate
6-Methylcoumarin
Musk ambrette
Octyl dimethyl p-aminobenzoic acid
Octyl methoxycinnamate
Octyl salicylate
Oxybenzone
Petrolatum control
Promethazine
Sandalwood oil
Sulfanilamide
Sulisobenzone
Tetrachlorocarbanilide
Thiourea
Tribromosalicylanilide
Trichlorocarbanilide
Triclosan

SOURCE: New York University Medical Center (January 2000).

Table 19-7
Causes of Chloracne

Polyhalogenated dibenzofurans
　Polychlorodibenzofurans (PCDFs), especially
　　tri-, tetra- (TCDFs), penta- (PCDFs), and
　　hexachlorodibenzofuran
　Polybromodibenzofurans (PBDFs), especially
　　tetrabromodibenzofuran (TBDF)
Polychlorinated dibenzodioxins (PCDDs)
　2,3,7,8-Tetrachlorodibenzo-p-dioxin (TCDD)
　Hexachlorodibenzo-p-dioxin
Polychloronaphthalenes (PCNs)
Polyhalogenated biphenyls
　Polychlorobiphenyls (PCBs)
　Polybromobiphenyls (PBBs)
3,3′,4,4′-Tetrachloroazoxybenzene (TCAOB)
3,3′,4,4′-Tetrachloroazobenzene (TCAB)

around the eyes, and on the shoulders, back, and genitalia. In addition to acne, hypertrichosis (increased hair in atypical locations), hyperpigmentation, brown discoloration of the nail, conjunctivitis, and eye discharge may be present.

PIGMENTARY DISTURBANCES

Several factors influence the appearance of pigmentation on the skin. Melanin is produced through a series of enzymatic pathways that begin with tyrosine. Errors in this pathway or exposure to tyrosine analogs may result in abnormal pigmentation. Hyperpigmentation results from increased melanin production or deposition of endogenous or exogenous pigment in the upper dermis. Exogenous hyperpigmentation can arise from deposition of metals and drugs in dermal tissue. Conversely, hypopigmentation is a loss of pigmentation resulting from melanin loss, melanocyte damage, or vascular abnormalities. Leukoderma and depigmentation denote complete loss of melanin from the skin, imparting a porcelain-white appearance. Table 19-8 lists chemicals that can cause alterations in pigmentation.

GRANULOMATOUS DISEASE

A number of dermatologic illnesses produce the histopathologic findings of granulomatous inflammation. In general, a granuloma is an immune mechanism that "walls off" an adverse injury. It is seen in the skin in infectious diseases (i.e., leprosy, tuberculosis), foreign-body reactions, and idiopathic illnesses. Foreign-body reactions may be secondary to a primary irritant phenomenon such as the traumatic introduction of talc, silica, or wood into the dermis. More rarely, sensitization may drive a granulomatous reaction, as is the case for beryllium, zirconium, cobalt, mercury, and chromium, sometimes occurring in response to tattoo dyes.

URTICARIA

Urticaria (hives) is an immediate type I hypersensitivity reaction driven primarily by histamine and vasoactive peptide release from mast cells. Potential nonimmune

Table 19-8
Selected Causes of Cutaneous Pigmentary Disturbances

I. Hyperpigmentation
    Ultraviolet light exposure
    Postinflammatory changes (melanin and/or
      hemosiderin deposition)
    Hypoadrenalism
    Internal malignancy
    Chemical exposures
      Coal tar volatiles
      Anthracene
      Picric acid
      Mercury
      Lead
      Bismuth
      Furocoumarins (psoralens)
      Hydroquinone (paradoxical)
    Drugs
      Chloroquine
      Amiodarone
      Bleomycin
      Zidovudine (AZT)
      Minocycline
II. Hypopigmentation/depigmentation/leukoderma
    Postinflammatory pigmentary loss
      Vitiligo
    Chemical leukoderma/hypopigmentation
      Hydroquinone
      Monobenzyl, monoethyl, and monomethyl
        ethers of hydroquinone
      p-(t-Butyl)phenol
      Mercaptoamines
      Phenolic germicides
      p-(t-Butyl)catechols
      Butylated hydroxytoluene

Table 19-9
Selected Substances Reported to Elicit Contact Urticaria

CHEMICALS	FOODS
Anhydrides	Animal viscera
Methylhexahydrophthalic anhydride	Apple
Hexahydrophthalic anhydride	Artichoke
Antibiotics	Asparagus
Bacitracin	Beef
Streptomycin	Beer
Cephalosporins	Carrot
Penicillin	Chicken
Rifamycin	Deer
Benzoic acid	Egg
Cobalt chloride	Fish
Butylhydroxyanisol (BHA)	Lamb
Butylhydroxytoluene (BHT)	Mustard
Carboxymethylcellulose	Paprika
Cyclopentolate hydrochloride	Potato
Diphenyl guanidine	Pork
Epoxy resin	Rice
Formaldehyde	Strawberry
Fragrances	Turkey
Balsam of Peru	
Cinnamic aldehyde	
Isocyanates	
Diphenylmethane-4,4-diisocyanate	
Maleic anhydride	
Menthol	
Plants, woods, trees, and weeds	
Latex	
Phenylmercuric acetate	
Xylene	

releasers of histamine from mast cells include curare, aspirin, azo dyes, benzoates, and toxins from plants and animals. The majority of urticarial responses result either from systemically ingested substances to which a person has a specific allergy or from completely idiopathic mechanisms. Localized urticaria may be elicited by certain substances in the area of epicutaneous contact and is referred to as *contact urticaria*. Some reported causes are described in Table 19-9.

A syndrome of contact urticaria, rhinitis, conjunctivitis, asthma, and rarely anaphylaxis and death has been associated with latex proteins found in rubber. The

allergens in natural latex rubber are incompletely characterized water-soluble proteins that are capable of inducing type I allergic responses in sensitized individuals. Contact with rubber products such as gloves can cause hives solely in the area of contact with the skin; however, more allergic individuals may experience generalized hiving, asthma, anaphylaxis, and death. This syndrome is distinct from allergic contact dermatitis to rubber components such as accelerators and antioxidants, which cause delayed-type hypersensitivity/contact dermatitis. Risk factors that have been elucidated in epidemiologic studies include a history of eczema, hay fever or asthma, spina bifida, a history of hand dermititis, and female gender.

TOXIC EPIDERMAL NECROLYSIS

Toxic epidermal necrolysis (TEN) represents one of the most immediately life-threatening dermatologic diseases and often is caused by drugs and chemicals. It is characterized by full-thickness necrosis of the epidermis accompanied by widespread detachment of this necrotic material. After the epidermis has sloughed, only dermis remains, severely compromising heat, fluid, and electrolyte homeostasis. A study evaluating TEN induced by the anticonvulsant carbamazepine revealed reduced lymphocyte capacity to metabolize cytotoxic carbamazepine intermediates. Abnormalities in epoxide hydrolase and glutathione transferase may be responsible for the metabolism of the purported toxin, which may be an arene oxide. The inflammatory reaction of CD8 lymphocytes and a role of nitric oxide metabolites as mediators of epidermal necrosis in TEN suggest a metabolic pathogenesis rather than a strictly immunologic one.

CARCINOGENESIS

Radiation

Skin cancer is the most common neoplasm in humans. At present, the major cause of skin cancer is sunlight, which damages epidermal cell DNA. UV-B (290 to 320 nm) induces pyrimidine dimers, thus eliciting mutations in critical genes. The *p53* tumor suppressor gene has been targeted in nearly all squamous cell carcinomas. Because the p53 protein arrests cell cycling until DNA damage is repaired and may induce apoptosis, its loss destabilizes the genome of initiated cells and gives them a growth advantage. UV light also has immunosuppressive effects that may help skin tumors survive. The incidence of skin cancer is highest in the tropics and in pale-complexioned whites. Even when it does not cause cancer in normal individuals, sun exposure leads to premature aging of the skin. For this reason, sunbathing is discouraged and the use of sun-block lotions is encouraged.

Polycyclic Aromatic Hydrocarbons

Substances rich in polycyclic aromatic hydrocarbons (coal tar, creosote, pitch, and soot) are skin carcinogens in humans and animals. Oxidative biotransformation of polycyclic aromatic compounds produces electrophilic epoxides that can form DNA adducts. Phenols, produced by rearrangement of the epoxides, can be oxidized further to quinones, yielding active oxygen species, and are also toxic electrophiles. Occupations at risk of skin cancer from exposure to these compounds (e.g., roofing) often involve considerable sun exposure, an additional risk factor.

Arsenic

High exposures from smelting operations and from well water derived from rock strata with a high arsenic content are associated with arsenical keratoses (premalignant lesions), blackfoot disease (a circulatory disorder that reflects endothelial cell damage), and squamous cell carcinoma of the skin and several other organs (bladder, lung, liver). Arsenite (+3 oxidation state) avidly binds vicinal thiols and is thought to inhibit DNA repair, whereas arsenate (+5 oxidation state) can replace phosphate in macromolecules such as DNA, but the resulting esters are unstable. Arsenic also alters DNA methylation, suppresses keratinocyte differentiation markers, and enhances growth factor secretion in the epidermis. Methylation has been considered the most likely detoxification method, since the observed mono- and dimethyl arsenates isolated in urine from exposed humans and animals are indeed much less toxic.

Mouse Skin Tumor Promotion

Mouse skin has been developed as an important target for carcinogenicity testing. The observed incidence of squamous cell carcinomas in mouse skin is taken as evidence of a more general carcinogenic risk for humans. Much has been learned about the pathogenesis of squamous cell carcinomas in mouse skin that has general applicability to human squamous cell carcinomas. An advantage of the mouse skin carcinogenesis model is the ability to separate the neoplastic process into stages of initiation, promotion, and progression, depending on experimental design.

BIBLIOGRAPHY

Maibach HI: *Toxicology of the Skin.* New York: Taylor & Francis, 2000.

Marzulli FN, Maibach HI: *Dermatotoxicology Methods: The Laboratory Worker's Ready Reference.* New York: Hemisphere, 1997.

Roberts MS, Walters KA (eds): *Dermal Absorption and Toxicity Assessment.* New York: Marcel Dekker, 1998.

TOXIC RESPONSES OF THE REPRODUCTIVE SYSTEM

Michael J. Thomas and John A. Thomas

KEY POINTS

* The gonads have a dual function: an endocrine function involving the secretion of sex hormones and a nonendocrine function consisting of the production of germ cells (gametogenesis).

* Gametogenic and secretory functions of both the ovary or the testes are dependent on the secretion of follicle-stimulating hormone and luteinizing hormone from the pituitary.

* The blood-testis barrier between the lumen of an interstitial capillary and the lumen of a seminiferous tubule impedes or prevents the free exchange of chemicals and drugs between the blood and the fluid inside the seminiferous tubules.

* Xenobiotics can act directly on the hypothalamus and the adenohypophysis, leading to alterations in the secretion of hypothalamic-releasing hormones and/or gonadotropins.

* Steroid hormone biosynthesis can occur in several endocrine organs, including the adrenal cortex, ovary, and testes.

* Female reproductive processes of oogenesis, ovulation, the development of sexual receptivity, coitus, gamete and zygote transport, fertilization, and implantation of the conceptus may be sites of xenobiotic interference.

* Xenobiotics may influence the structure of male reproductive organs, spermatogenesis, androgen hormone secretion, and accessory organ function.

INTRODUCTION

The endocrine function of the gonads is primarily involved in the perpetuation of the species. Genes in the chromosomes of the germ cells transmit genetic information and modulate cell differentiation and organogenesis. Germ cells ensure the maintenance of structure and function in the organism in its own lifetime and from generation to generation.

Exposure to endocrine-disrupting chemicals has been linked with diminished fertility in birds, fish, shellfish, and mammals and with demasculatinization and feminization in fish, gastropods, and birds. In general, the mechanism(s) of endocrine disruption caused by non-heavy-metal agents is due to competition for receptors or inhibition of steroidogenesis.

In the human, it is estimated that one in five couples are involuntarily sterile; over one-third of early embryos die, and about 15 percent of recognized pregnancies abort spontaneously. Among the surviving fetuses at birth, approximately 3 percent have developmental defects (not always anatomic); with increasing age, over twice that many become detectable. Even under normal physiologic conditions, the reproductive system does not function in an optimal state. Not surprisingly, the imposition of xenobiotics on this system can interfere with a number of reproductive processes or events.

GENERAL REPRODUCTIVE BIOLOGY

The developing gonad is very sensitive to chemical insult and to changes in its environment whether those changes are caused by exposure to foreign chemicals or exposure to certain viruses. The development of normal reproductive capacity may offer particularly susceptible targets for toxins. Environmental factors may alter the genetic determinants of gonadal sex, the hormonal determinants of phenotypic sex, fetal gametogenesis, and reproductive tract differentiation as well as postnatal integration of endocrine functions and other processes essential for the propagation of the species.

Sexual Differentiation

An understanding of reproductive physiology requires consideration of the process of sexual differentiation, or the pattern of development of the gonads, genital ducts, and external genitalia. Male sexual differentiation is critically dependent on the physiologic action of androgens. Thus, an imbalance in the androgen/estrogen ratio can affect sexual differentiation. Environmental xenoestrogens that mimic estrogens (certain herbicides, pesticides, plasticizers, nonylphenols, etc.) and environmental antiandrogens (p,p'-DDE, vinclozolin, linuron, etc.) that perturb endocrine balance may cause demasculinizing and feminizing effects in a male fetus.

Gonadal Sex A testes-determining gene [the sex-determining region of the Y chromosome (SRY)] on the Y chromosome is responsible for determining gonadal sex. It converts undifferentiated gonads into testes. The testes produces two separate hormones: the müllerian inhibiting factor and testosterone. Testosterone-induced masculine differentiation is modulated by androgen receptors that are regulated by genes on the X chromosome. Failure of the sex chromosomes of either parent to separate during gametogenesis is called nondisjunction and can result in gonadal agenesis. Klinefelter's syndrome is characterized by testicular dysgenesis with male morphology and an XXY karyotype; Turner's syndrome includes ovarian agenesis with female morphology (XO karyotype).

Hermaphroditism (true and pseudo) may occur secondary to nondisjunction of sex chromosomes during the initial cleavage mitosis of the egg. This condition usually is due to an XY karyotype and sometimes to sex mosaics of XY/XX or XY/XO. Pseudohermaphrodites are characterized by secondary sex characteristics that differ from those predicted by genotype.

Genotypic Sex The normal female chromosome complement is 44 autosomes and 2 sex chromosomes, XX. The two X chromosomes contained in the germ cells are necessary for the development of a normal ovary. The Y chromosome is consistent with the male determinant. The normal male has a chromosome complement of 44 autosomes and 2 sex chromosomes, X and Y. Genetic coding on the X chromosome may be involved in transforming the gonad into a testis.

Phenotypic (Genital) Sex During the early stages of fetal development, sexual differentiation does not require any known hormonal products. The differentiation of the genital ducts and the external genitalia, however, requires hormones. The onset of testosterone synthesis by the male gonad is necessary for the initiation of male differentiation. Female characteristics develop in the absence of androgen secretion.

Two principal types of hormones are secreted by the fetal testes: an androgenic steroid responsible for development of the male reproductive tract and a nonsteroid factor that causes regression of the müllerian ducts. The embryonic testis suppresses the development of the müllerian ducts, allows the development of the wolffian duct and its derivatives, and thus imposes the male phenotype on the embryo.

Factors that reduce the ability of testosterone to be synthesized and activated, enter the cell, and/or affect the ability of the cell nucleus to regulate the synthesis of androgen-dependent proteins can alter sexual differentiation. Chemicals capable of exerting a testosterone-depriving effect on the developing systems influence the feedback regulation of gonadotropin secretion, gonadotropin effectiveness, testosterone and dihydrotestosterone synthesis, and plasma binding as well as cytoplasmic receptor and nuclear chromatin binding.

Insufficient amounts of androgens can feminize a male fetus with otherwise normal testes and an XY karyotype. Slight deficiencies affect only the later stages of differentiation of the external genital organs, whereas a severe androgen deficiency (or resistance) allows external female genital organs to coexist with ectopic testes and normal male efferent ducts. Sexual behavior also appears to be "imprinted" in the central nervous system by androgens from the testis and can be affected by endogenous and exogenous chemicals.

GONADAL FUNCTION

Central Modulation

The gonads have a dual function: an endocrine function involving the secretion of sex hormones and a nonendocrine function, the production of germ cells (gametogenesis). The testes secrete male sex steroids, including testosterone, dihydrotestosterone, and small amounts of estrogens. The ovaries, depending on the phase of the menstrual cycle, secrete various amounts of estrogens and progesterone. The corpus luteum and the placenta are also primary sites of the secretion of progesterone.

Gametogenic and secretory functions of the ovary and the testes are dependent on the secretion of follicle-stimulating hormone (FSH) and luteinizing hormone (LH) from the pituitary. FSH in a female stimulates follicular development and maturation in the ovary. FSH in a male stimulates the process of spermatogenesis. LH provokes the process of steroidogenesis in the testes.

The onset of puberty results in the cyclic secretion of pituitary gonadotropins in females. This establishes the normal menstrual cycle. In males, puberty is advanced by the continuous and noncyclic secretion of gonadotropins.

Testicular Function

During the fertile phase of the life span of mammals, the function of the gonads is hormonally controlled. Tissue selectivity of toxicants can stem from the apoptotic or necrotic thresholds at which different cells die. Physiologically, apoptosis serves to limit the number of germ cells in the seminiferous epithelium. During the process of spermatogenesis, clonal proliferation of germ cells occurs during the many mitotic divisions, leading to a significantly expanding population of germ cells. Left unchecked, the number of germ cells would quickly outgrow the supportive capacity of the Sertoli cells. Hence, a delicate balance exists in the testes between proliferation and apoptosis. About three-fourths of the potential population of mature germ cells in the testes may be lost by active elimination. Sertoli cells appear to regulate germ cell apoptosis directly through a paracrine mechanism.

Spermatogenesis The germinal epithelium plays a dual role in spermatogenesis: It must produce millions of spermatozoa each day and also continuously replace the population of cells that give rise to the process: the spermatogonia. Spermatogenesis starts at puberty and continues almost throughout the life span. Male germ cells are transformed into haploid spermatozoa within the seminiferous tubules (Fig. 20-1). As sperm traverse the tubules of the testes and the epididymides, sperm acquire the capacity for fertilization and become more motile (Fig. 20-2).

Sertoli Cells The Sertoli cell plays an important role in spermatogenesis. In early fetal life, the Sertoli cells secrete antimüllerian hormone (AMH). After puberty, these cells secrete the hormone inhibin, which may aid in modulating pituitary FSH. Also, Sertoli cells provide germ cells with nutrients, structural support, and regulatory/paracrine factors. Sertoli cells secrete tissue plasminogen activator, androgen-binding protein (ABP), inhibin, AMH, transferrin, and other proteases. ABP acts as a carrier for testosterone and dihydrotestosterone. The Sertoli cell junctions form the blood-testis barrier. Normal spermatogenesis requires Sertoli cells. Many chemicals that affect spermatogenesis act on the Sertoli cell.

Interstitium (Leydig Cells) The Leydig, or interstitial, cells are the primary sites of testosterone synthesis. LH stimulates testicular steroidogenesis. Androgens are

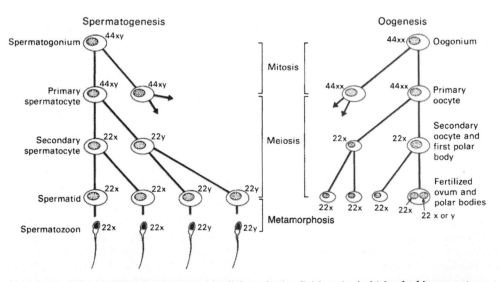

Figure 20-1. Cellular replication (mitosis) and cellular reductive divisions (meiosis) involved in spermatogenesis, oogenesis, and fertilization.

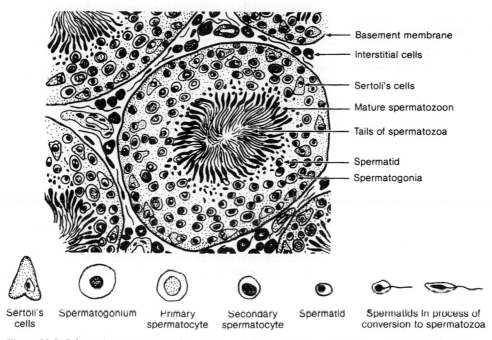

Basement membrane
Interstitial cells
Sertoli's cells
Mature spermatozoon
Tails of spermatozoa
Spermatid
Spermatogonia

| Sertoli's cells | Spermatogonium | Primary spermatocyte | Secondary spermatocyte | Spermatid | Spermatids in process of conversion to spermatozoa |

Figure 20-2. Schematic cross section of seminiferous tubules of testes.   Morphology of the Sertoli cell along with the cellular events involved in spermatogenesis (spermatogonium through spermatid).

essential to spermatogenesis, epididymal sperm maturation, the growth and secretory activity of accessory sex organs, somatic masculinization, male behavior, and various metabolic processes. Table 20-1 lists a number of diverse chemicals and drugs that can cause Leydig cell hyperplasia and neoplasia.

Posttesticular Processes

The end product of testicular gametogenesis is immature sperm. Posttesticular processes involve ducts (the rete testes and the epididymis) that move maturing sperm from the testis to storage sites where the sperm await ejaculation. A number of secretory processes control fluid production and ion composition; secretory organs (the seminal vesicles and the prostate gland) contribute to the chemical composition (including specific proteins) of the semen.

Erection and Ejaculation These physiologic processes are controlled by the central nervous system (CNS) and modulated by the autonomic nervous system. Parasympathetic nerve stimulation results in dilatation of the arterioles of the penis, which initiates an erection.

Ejaculation is a two-stage spinal reflex that involves emission and ejaculation. Emission is the movement of the semen into the urethra; ejaculation is the propulsion of the semen out of the urethra at the time of orgasm. Emission is a sympathetic response that is effected by contraction of the smooth muscle of the vas deferens and seminal vesicles. Semen is ejaculated out of the urethra by contraction of the bulbocavernosus muscle.

Little is known about the effects of chemicals on erection or ejaculation. Pesticides, particularly the organophosphates, are known to affect the neuroendocrine processes involved in erection and ejaculation. Many drugs act on the autonomic nervous system and affect potency (Table 20-2).

Ovarian Function

Oogenesis About 400,000 follicles are present at birth in each human ovary. After birth, many undergo atresia, and those which survive are continuously reduced in number (Fig. 20-3). Follicles remain in a primary follicle stage after birth and until puberty, when a number of follicles start to grow during each ovarian cycle. Each month, one not yet fully developed oocyte (called a

Table 20-1
Chemicals/Drugs Causing Leydig Cell Hyperplasia/Neoplasia in Rodents

AGENT/CHEMICAL/DRUG	AGENT CLASS OR BIOLOGIC ACTIVITY
Cadmium	Heavy metal
Estrogen	Hormone
Linuron	Herbicide
SOZ-200-110, isradine	Calcium channel blocker
Flutamide	Antiandrogen
Gemfibrozil	Hypolipidemic agent
Finasteride	5α-Reductase inhibitor
Cimetidine	Histamine (H_2) receptor blocker
Hydralazine	Antihypertensive agent
Carbamazepine	Anticonvulsant/analgesic
Vidarabine	Antiviral agent
Mesulergine	Dopamine (D_2) agonist-antagonist
Clomiphene	Treatment of infertility
Perfluoroctanoate	Industrial ingredient (plasticizers, lubricant/wetting agents)
Dimethylformide	Industrial use (tannery and leather goods, metal dyes)
Diethylstilbestrol	Synthetic hormone
Nitrosamine	Industrial uses
Methoxychlor	Pesticide with estrogenic properties
Oxolinic acid	Antimicrobial agent
Reserpine	Antihypertensive
Metronidazole	Antiprotozoal
Cyclophosphamide	Antineoplastic
Methylcholanthrene	Experimental carcinogen

Table 20-2
Drug-Induced Impotence

	AGENT	CNS	ANS	ENDO
Narcotics	Morphine	+	+	?
	Ethanol	+		
Psychotropics	Chlorpromazine		+	
	Diazepam	+		
	Tricyclic antidepressants		+	?
	MAO inhibitors		+	
Hypotensives	Methyldopa	+	+	+
	Clonidine	+	+	
	Reserpine	+	+	
	Guanethidine		++	
Hormones/antagonists	Estrogens			+
	Cyproterone			+

KEY: CNS, central nervous system; ANS, autonomic nervous system; ENDO, endocrine.

SCHEMATIC REPRESENTATION OF OVARIAN MORPHOLOGY

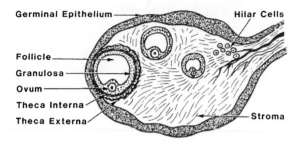

Figure 20-3. Schematic representation of ovarian morphology.

secondary oocyte) is released from the ovary. This oocyte completes its last cell division when it is fertilized by a sperm.

Ovarian Cycle The cyclic release of pituitary gonadotropins involving the secretion of ovarian progesterone and estrogen is depicted in Fig. 20-4. These female sex steroids determine ovulation and prepare the female accessory sex organs to receive the male sperm. Sperm

HORMONAL REGULATION OF MENSTRUAL FUNCTION

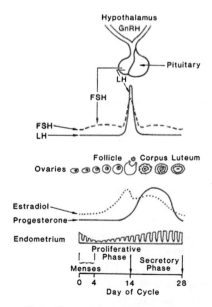

Figure 20-4. Hormonal regulation of menstrual function. FSH, follicle-stimulating hormone; GnRH, gonadotropin-releasing hormone; LH, luteinizing hormone.

that are ejaculated into the vagina must make their way through the cervix into the uterus, where they are capacitated. Sperm then migrate into the oviducts, where fertilization takes place. The conceptus then returns from the oviducts to the uterus and is implanted into the endometrium.

Uterus Uterine endometrium reflects the cyclicity of the ovary as it is prepared to receive and support the conceptus for the entire gestational period.

Fertilization During fertilization, the ovum contributes the maternal complement of genes to the nucleus of the fertilized egg and provides food reserves for the early embryo. From a single fertilized cell (the zygote), cells proliferate and differentiate until more than a trillion cells of about a hundred different types are present in the adult organism.

Implantation The developing embryo migrates through the oviduct and into the uterus. Upon contact with the endometrium, the blastocyst implants. Placental circulation then is established.

Generally, the placenta is quite impermeable to chemicals and drugs with molecular weights of 1000 Da or more. Because most medications have molecular weights of 500 Da or less, molecular size rarely affects a drug's crossing the placenta and entering the embryo/fetus. Placental permeability to a chemical is affected by placental characteristics, including thickness, surface area, carrier systems, and lipid-protein concentration of the membranes. The inherent characteristics of the chemical itself, such as its degree of ionization, lipid solubility, protein binding, and molecular size, also affect its transport across the placenta.

INTEGRATIVE PROCESSES

Hypothalamo-Pituitary-Gonadal Axis

FSH and LH are glycoproteins that are synthesized and released from the pituitary gland. Hypothalamic neuroendocrine neurons secrete specific releasing or release-inhibiting factors into the hypophyseal portal system, which carries them to the adenohypophysis (the anterior pituitary), where they act to stimulate or inhibit the release of anterior pituitary hormones. Gonadotropin-releasing hormone (GnRH) acts on gonadotropic cells, thus stimulating the release of FSH and LH.

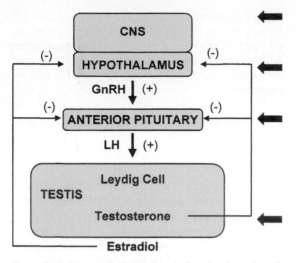

Figure 20-5. Hormonal relationships in the adenohypophyseal-hypothalamic-gonadal axis. Inhibitory actions (−) and stimulatory actions (+) are depicted along with sites of chemical/drug perturbation (*large black arrows*).

The neuroendocrine neurons have nerve terminals that contain monoamines (norepinephrine, dopamine, serotonin) that impinge on them. Reserpine, chlorpromazine, and monoamine oxidase (MAO) inhibitors modify the content or actions of brain monoamines that affect gonadotropins.

FSH probably acts primarily on the Sertoli cells but also appears to stimulate the mitotic activity of spermatogonia. LH stimulates steroidogenesis. A defect in the production of spermatozoa or testosterone tends to be reflected in increased levels of FSH and LH in serum because of the lack of the "negative feedback" effect of testicular hormones (Fig. 20-5).

The hypothalamo-pituitary-gonadal feedback system is a very delicately modulated hormonal process (Fig. 20-5). Gonadotoxic agents may act on neuroendocrine processes in the brain or act directly on the target organ (e.g., gonad). Toxicants that adversely or otherwise alter the hepatic and/or renal biotransformation of endogenous sex steroid may be expected to interfere with the pituitary feedback system.

Puberty

From the early newborn period to the onset of puberty, the testes remain hormonally dormant. The onset of puberty begins with the secretion of increasing levels of gonadotropins. The physiologic trigger for puberty is poorly understood, but somehow a hypothalamic gona-

dostat changes the rate of secretion of GnRH, resulting in increases in LH. As puberty approaches, a pulsatile pattern of LH and FSH secretion is observed.

SEXUAL BEHAVIOR AND LIBIDO

Physiologic processes that account for sexual behavior are poorly understood. The external environment greatly affects sexual behavior, and libido components of reproductive activity depend on a close interplay between neural and endocrine events.

GENERAL TOXICOLOGIC/ PHARMACOLOGIC PRINCIPLES

Many of the principles that govern the absorption, distribution, metabolism, and excretion of a chemical or drug also apply to the reproductive system. There are, however, unique barriers that affect a chemical's action on the mammalian reproductive system. The maternal-fetal interface occurring at the placenta represents a barrier to chemicals coming in contact with the developing embryo. Unfortunately, the placenta is not so restrictive that it prevents most chemicals from crossing the placenta. Unlike the female gonad, the male gonad has a somewhat specialized barrier. This specialized biological barrier is referred to as the blood-testis barrier.

Blood-Testis Barrier

The blood-testis barrier is situated somewhere between the lumen of an interstitial capillary and the lumen of a seminiferous tubule. Several anatomically related features intervene between the two luminal spaces, including the capillary endothelium, capillary basal lamina, lymphatic endothelium, basal lamina of the seminiferous tubule, and Sertoli cells. The barrier that impedes or denies the free exchange of chemicals/drugs between the blood and the fluid inside the seminiferous tubules is located in one or more of these structures. The degrees of lipid solubility and ionization are important determinants of whether a substance can permeate the blood-testis barrier.

Biotransformation of Exogenous Chemicals

Testes The mammalian gonad is capable of metabolizing a host of foreign chemicals that have traversed the

Table 20-3
Biotransformation of Drugs, Chemicals, and Their Metabolites—
Ability to Exert Toxic Actions on the Male Gonad

PARENT COMPOUND	METABOLITE
Amiodarone (antiarrhythmic drug)	Desethylamiodarone
Cephalosporin analogs (antimicrobial drug)	N-Methyletetrazolethiol*
Valproic acid (antiepileptic drug)	Isomers of 2-ethyl hexanol (?)†
Diethylhexyl phthalate (DEHP; plasticizer)	Mono-ethylhexyl phthalate and 2-ethyl hexanol (?)†
Dibromochloropropane‡ (DBCP; fungicide)	Dichloropropene(s) derivatives (?)†
Ethylene glycol monoethyl ether (industrial solvent)	2-Methoxyacetaldehyde
n-Hexane (environmental toxicant)	2,5-Hexanedione
Acrylamide (industrial use)	N-Methylacrylamide, N-isopropylacrylamide
Vinclozolin (fungicide)	Butanoic acid derivative and an enanilide metabolite

*Only substituent is a testicular toxin, not cephalosporin.
†Questionable testicular toxin but probably teratogenic.
‡Radiometabolites of (^{3}H)-DBCP are not preferentially labeled in the testes.

blood-testis barrier. Whether biotransformation occurs gonadally or extragonadally, the end result can be interference with spermatogenesis and/or steroidogenesis. Table 20-3 lists xenobiotics and their metabolites that exert male gonadal toxicity.

Ovary Like the testes, the ovary has the metabolic capability to biotransform certain exogenous substrates. Furthermore, the process of ovarian steroidogenesis, like those of the testes and the adrenal cortex, is susceptible to different agents that interfere with the biosynthesis of estrogens. Less is known about how chemicals or drugs interfere with ovarian metabolism. The ovary has not been studied as extensively because of its more difficult and complex hormonal relationships. Nevertheless, several chemotherapeutic agents can inhibit ovarian function (Table 20-4).

DNA Repair

Depending on the species, there are varying degrees of capacity of spermatogenic cells to repair DNA damage

resulting from environmental toxicants. Unscheduled DNA repair in spermatogenic cells is dose- and time-dependent. Spermiogenic cells are less able to repair DNA damage resulting from alkylating agents.

Drug-induced unscheduled DNA synthesis in mammalian oocytes reveals that female gametes have an excision repair capacity. Unlike mature sperm, the mature oocyte maintains a DNA repair ability. However, this ability decreases at the time of meiotic maturation.

Table 20-4
Chemotherapeutic Agents and Ovarian Dysfunction

Prednisone	Busulfan
Vincristine	Methotrexate
Vinblastine	Cytosine arabinoside
6-Mercaptopurine	L-Asparaginase
Nitrogen mustard	5-Fluorouracil
Cyclophosphamide	Adriamycin
Chlorambucil	

TARGETS FOR CHEMICAL TOXICITY

CNS

There are several sites of interference by chemicals in the mammalian reproductive system (Fig. 20-5). Drugs and chemicals can act directly on the hypothalamus and the adenohypophysis, leading to alterations in the secretion of hypothalamic-releasing hormones and/or gonadotropins. Synthetic steroids are very effective in suppressing gonadotropin secretion and thus block ovulation.

Gonads

The gonads are also targets for a host of drugs and chemicals (Table 20-5). The majority of these agents are cancer chemotherapeutic agents. Alkylating agents are effective against rapidly dividing cells. Not surprisingly, the division of germ cells also is affected, leading to the arrest of spermatogenesis.

Different cell populations of the mammalian testis exhibit somewhat different thresholds of sensitivity to different toxicants. The germ cells are most sensitive to chemical insult (i.e., spermatogenesis). The Sertoli cells have a somewhat intermediate sensitivity to chemical inhibition; Leydig cells are quite resistant to environmental toxicants.

Steroidogenesis Steroid biosynthesis can occur in several endocrine organs, including the adrenal cortex, ovary, and testes. In the ovary, the granulosa cells secrete estrogens in response to FSH. The thecal cells of the ovary secrete progesterone (as does the corpus luteum)

Table 20-5
Drugs That Are Gonadotoxic in Humans

MALES	FEMALES
Busulfan	Busulfan
Chlorambucil	Chlorambucil
Cyclophosphamide	Cyclophosphamide
Nitrogen mustard	Nitrogen mustard
Doxorubicin	
Corticosteroids	
Cytosine-arabinoside	
Methotrexate	
Procarbazine	
Vincristine	
Vinblastine	Vinblastine

(see Fig. 20-3). In the testes, the Leydig cell (or the interstitial cell) in response to LH [or interstitial cell-stimulating hormone (ICSH)] secretes androgens (e.g., testosterone and dihydrotestosterone).

Several drugs, hormones, and chemicals can affect steroidogenesis by interfering with or inhibiting specific enzymes. Also, anti-LH peptides can affect Leydig cell steroidogenesis. GnRH analogs (e.g., buserelin) can interfere with both ovarian and testicular function.

EVALUATING REPRODUCTIVE CAPACITY

A number of hormone assays are available to assess endocrine function. The endocrine system of the female is more complex and dynamic than that of the male. Hence, evaluating reproductive function in females is more difficult.

The fact that such a wide variety of chemicals and drugs can perturb the reproductive system adds another dimension of difficulty in attempting to evaluate reproductive toxicity. Not only is there considerable diversity in the chemical configuration of toxicants, the sites and mechanisms of action can be very different.

TESTING MALE REPRODUCTIVE CAPACITY

A host of tests have been used or proposed for evaluating the male reproductive system (Table 20-6). Multiple exposures extended over some length of time most likely are required to detect male reproductive toxicity. In humans, the noninvasive approaches involve sperm counts, blood gonadotrophin levels, and a nonbarren marriage. Testicular biopsy can be used in selected circumstances to evaluate spermatogenesis. Azoospermia can be caused by certain chemical agents, genetic disorders (e.g., Klinefelter's syndrome), infections (e.g., mumps), irradiation, and hormonal defects. Dietary deficiencies of manganese; vitamins A, B_6, and E; and zinc are well known to cause spermatogenic arrest. Similarly, lead can produce infertility, sterility, and varying abnormalities in sperm function and morphology. Other heavy metals, such as cobalt, iron, cadmium, mercury, molybdenum, and silver, can affect spermatogenesis and accessory sex organ function adversely. Dietary zinc deficiency can produce sterility. Mechanisms of heavy metal toxicity vary and include not only different cell sensitivities but also direct versus indirect actions. Furthermore, it appears that primary damage to one cell type may affect other cell types in the testes secondarily.

Table 20-6
Potentially Useful Tests of Male Reproductive Toxicity for Laboratory Animals and/or Humans

Testis
    Size in situ
    Weight
    Spermatid reserves
    Gross and histologic evaluation
    Nonfunctional tubules (%)
    Tubules with lumen sperm (%)
    Tubule diameter
    Counts of leptotene spermatocytes

Epididymis
    Weight and histology
    Number of sperm in distal half
    Motility of sperm, distal end (%)
    Gross sperm morphology, distal end (%)
    Detailed sperm morphology, distal end (%)
    Biochemical assays

Accessory sex glands
    Histology
    Gravimetric

Semen
    Total volume
    Gel-free volume
    Sperm concentration
    Total sperm/ejaculate
    Total sperm/day of abstinence
    Sperm motility, visual (%)
    Sperm motility, videotape (% and velocity)
    Gross sperm morphology
    Detailed sperm morphology

Endocrine
    Luteinizing hormone
    Follicle stimulating hormone
    Testosterone
    Gonadotropin-releasing hormone

Fertility
    Ratio exposed: pregnant females
    Number of embryos or young per pregnant female
    Ratio viable embryos: corpora lutea
    Number 2–8 cell eggs
    Sperm per ovum

In vitro
    Incubation of sperm in agent
    Hamster egg penetration test

Other tests considered
    Tonometric measurement of testicular consistency
    Qualitative testicular histology
    Stage of cycle at which spermiation occurs
    Quantitative testicular histology

Sperm motility
    Time-exposure photography
    Multiple-exposure photography
    Cinemicrography
    Videomicrography
    Sperm membrane characteristics
    Evaluation of sperm metabolism
    Fluorescent Y bodies in spermatozoa
    Flow cytometry of spermatozoa
    Karyotyping human sperm pronuclei
    Cervical mucus penetration test

The sensitivity of the various parameters used to evaluate the male reproductive system varies considerably. Testicular weight is a rapid quantitative index of testicular toxicity, but this measurement is less sensitive than are sperm counts. In normal males, the number of sperm produced per day per testis is determined largely by testicular size. Fertility as an index is quite insensitive, although it does incorporate all reproductive functions. Fertility profiles using serial mating studies to assess the biological status of sperm cells have been a useful test for both dominant lethal mutations and male reproductive capacity. Testicular histology provides information on target cell morphology. Leydig cell function is determined by evaluating androgen levels (or gonadotropins) or, in the case of Sertoli cells, by measuring ABP.

Thus, there are essentially two approaches to establishing whether a chemical can exert an adverse effect on spermatogenesis: (1) evaluation of testicular morphology and (2) functional evaluation of spermatogenesis. Included in the assessment are the detection of abnormalities in spermatogenesis/testicular morphology, stage-dependent germ cell degeneration, and impairment of normal sperm release.

Flow Cytometry

Flow cytometric analyses of the testes can be used to evaluate specific cell populations. In particular, the effects of toxicants on cell size, cell shape, cytoplasmic granularity and pigmentation, measurements of surface antigens, DNA/RNA, and chromatin structure can be ascertained. The dual parameters of DNA stainablility versus RNA content provide resolution of testicular cell types.

Sex Accessory Organs

The epididymis and the sex accessory organs also can be used to evaluate the status of male reproductive processes. Although the epididymis plays an important physiologic role in the male reproductive tract, it is less useful as a parameter for assessing gonadotoxins. Its histologic integrity may be examined, but the most meaningful determinations are the number of sperm stored within the cauda epididymis and a measure of sperm motility and morphology. Sex accessory organs, usually the prostate and the seminal vesicles, provide a rapid and quantitative measure of male reproductive processes that are androgen-dependent.

Semen Analyses

Semen analysis can be used as an index of testicular and posttesticular organ function. Both quantitative and qualitative characteristics of more than one ejaculate must be evaluated to ensure that conclusions about testicular function are valid. Because semen receives contributions from accessory sex glands as well as the testes and epididymides, only the total number of sperm in an ejaculate provides a reliable estimate of sperm production.

There have been recent advances in the automation of semen analysis. Semiautomated indirect methods of sperm analysis estimate the mean swimming speed of cells by measuring properties of the whole sperm suspension. Spectrometry and turbidimetric methods record changes in optical density. Direct methods involve visual assessment of individual sperm cells and stem from early efforts to quantitate the swimming speed of sperm. These direct measurements may include photographic methods such as timed-exposure photography, multiple-exposure photography, and cinematography.

Sperm Counts and Motility

Several factors affect the number of sperm in an ejaculate, including age, testicular size, frequency of ejaculation, degree of sexual arousal, and season (particularly in domestic animals). Although ejaculatory frequency, or the interval since the last ejaculation, alters the total number of sperm per ejaculate, it does not influence daily sperm production.

Androgens and Their Receptors

The androgen receptor (AR) is a member of the steroid/nuclear receptor superfamily, all the members of which share a basic and functional homology. AR action is highly specific in spite of the homology between AR and other steroid receptors. The two predominant naturally occurring ligands of the AR are testosterone and dihydrotestosterone.

Androgen receptors for testosterone and dihydrotestosterone (DHT) also have been used to evaluate the effects of various gonadotoxins. A number of divalent metal ions (Zn, Hg, Cu, Cd, etc.) can inhibit androgen-receptor binding in rodent prostate glands. In addition to heavy metals interfering with androgen binding, DDT and *p,p′*-DDE are potent androgen receptor antagonists and can affect male reproduction.

Hormonally active androgens promote reproductive and anabolic (myotropic) functions, which are mediated by their interaction with AR. Androgen target cells (e.g., prostate gland, seminal vesicles) contain steroid-modifying enzymes that can activate, inactivate, and alter the receptor specificity of androgens.

Other Secretory Biomarkers

Efforts have been made to identify so-called testicular marker enzymes as indicators of normal or abnormal cellular differentiation in the gonad, such as hyaluronidase and sorbitol dehydrogenase. A number of secretory products of the Sertoli cell (e.g., transferrin, ceruloplasmin, tissue plasminogen activator, sulfated glycoproteins) have some potential for evaluating male reproductive function. Among the secretory products of the Sertoli cell, ABP perhaps has received the most attention as a potential indicator for detecting gonadal injury.

TESTING FEMALE REPRODUCTIVE CAPACITY

The evaluation of mammalian reproductive processes is far more complex in the female than it is in the male. Female reproductive processes involve oogenesis, ovulation, the development of sexual receptivity, coitus, gamete and zygote transport, fertilization, and implantation of the conceptus. All these processes or events offer potential opportunities for chemical or drug interference.

Reproductive endpoints that indicate dysfunction in the female include perinatal parameters (Table 20-7) as well as developmental toxicity endpoints (Table 20-8). Neonates are particularly sensitive to a variety of drugs and chemicals. Gross pathology and histopathology should be evaluated on a wide variety of endpoints and at different anatomic sites and can include biochemical, hormonal, and morphologic parameters.

Oogenesis/Folliculogenesis

Methods to assess directly the effects of test compounds on oogenesis and/or folliculogenesis include histologic determination of oocytes and/or follicle number. Chemical effects on oogenesis can be measured indirectly by determining the fertility of the offspring.

Morphologic tests can quantify and assess primordial germ cell number, stem cell migration, oogonial

Table 20-7
Potentially Useful Tests of Female Reproductive Toxicity

Body Weight	*Uterus*
	Cytology and histology
Ovary	Luminal fluid analysis (xenobiotics,
Organ weight	proteins)
Histology	Decidual response
Number of oocytes	Dysfunctional bleeding
Rate of follicular atresia	
Follicular steroidogenesis	*Cervix/vulva/vagina*
Follicular maturation	Cytology
Oocyte maturation	Histology
Ovulation	Mucus production
Luteal function	Mucus quality (sperm
	penetration test)
Hypothalamus	
Histology	*Fertility*
Altered synthesis and release of	Ratio exposed: pregnant females
neurotransmitters, neuromodulators,	Number of embryos or young per
and neurohormones	pregnant female
	Ratio viable embryos: corpora lutea
Pituitary	Ratio implantation: corpora lutea
Histology	Number 2–8 cell eggs
Altered synthesis and release of trophic	
hormones	*In vitro*
	In vitro fertilization of superovulated
Endocrine	eggs, either exposed to chemical in
Gonadotropin	culture or from treated females
Chorionic gonadotropin levels	
Estrogen and progesterone	
Oviduct	
Histology	
Gamete transport	
Fertilization	
Transport of early embryo	

Table 20-8
Developmental Toxicity Endpoints

Type I changes
> (Outcomes permanent, life-threatening, and frequently associated with gross malformations)
> Reduction of number of live births (litter size)
> Increased number of stillbirths
> Reduced number of live fetuses (litter size)
> Increased number of resorptions
> Increased number of fetuses with malformations

Type II changes
> (Outcomes nonpermanent, non-life-threatening, and not associated with malformations)
> Reduced birth weights
> Reduced postnatal survival
> Decreased postnatal growth, reproductive capacity
> Increased number of fetuses with retarded development

proliferation, and urogenital ridge development. In vitro techniques can be used to evaluate primordial germ cell proliferation, migration, ovarian differentiation, and folliculogenesis.

Serial oocyte counts can monitor oocyte and/or follicle destruction in experimental animals. This approach is a reliable means of quantifying the effects of chemicals on oocytes and follicles.

Follicular growth may be assayed in experimental animals by using (^{3}H)-thymidine uptake, ovarian response to gonadotropins, and follicular kinetics. These approaches identify both direct and indirect effects on follicular growth and identify drugs and other environmental chemicals that are ovotoxic.

Estrogens and Their Receptors

Estrogen influences the growth, differentiation, and functioning of several target organs. Those organs include the mammary gland, the uterus, the vagina, the ovary, and several male reproductive system organs (testes, prostate gland, etc.). Estrogens affect osteogenesis and the CNS and seem to play a role in the homeostasis of the cardiovascular system. Estrogens migrate in and out of cells but are retained with high affinity and specificity in certain target tissues by an intranuclear binding protein called the estrogen receptor (ER). The receptors for

estrogen (and progesterone) are members of a large superfamily of nuclear proteins.

The activation of steroid hormone receptors (e.g., estrogen) regulates the transcriptional activity of specific genes, thus mediating the classic or genomic actions of steroid hormones. However, not all steroid effects can be explained by such a classic model of steroid–target cell interaction. Instead, signal-generating steroid receptors on the cell surface have been referred to as nonclassic, nongenomic steroid effects. Most nongenomic actions of steroids seem to involve Ca^{2+} as a second messenger. It is possible that nongenomic and genomic actions synergize, resulting in both a rapid onset and long-lasting or persistent actions.

Serum levels of estrogen and estrogenic effects on target tissues are indicators of normal follicular function. Tissue and organ responses include time of vaginal opening in immature rats, uterine weight, endometrial morphology, and/or serum levels of FSH and LH. Granulosa cell culture techniques provide direct screens of the ability of chemicals to inhibit cell proliferation and/or estrogen production. The biosynthesis of estradiol and its metabolism to estrone and estriol by the ovary constitute another indicator of the reproductive process.

Nuclear and cytoplasmic estrogen/progesterone may provide important toxicologic applications. Estradiol and progesterone receptors are especially important because chemicals (e.g., DDT and other organochlorine pesticides) compete for these receptors and may alter their molecular conformation.

Ovulation/Fertilization/ Implantation

Several steroidal and nonsteroidal agents can interfere with ovulation, fertilization, and implantation. The formation, maturation, and union of germ cells compose a complex physiologic event that is sensitive to foreign substances. Reproductive performance is best assessed by pregnancy, and this represents a successful index for evaluating endocrine toxicity (or the lack thereof).

REPRODUCTIVE TESTS AND REGULATORY REQUIREMENTS

Testing procedures to simulate human exposure have taken two different paths. One is based on the premise that specific injury from a chemical/drug can be more readily established by administering that agent only during certain periods of gestation. The second path was devised for compounds that are likely to involve chronic exposure and for which there may be a concentration factor when they are administered during several generations. Over the years, many efforts have been undertaken to harmonize testing guidelines (see also Chap. 10).

Endpoints—Females

Endpoints in studies of female reproductive toxicity include the following:

- Female fertility index
  [(number of pregnancies/number of matings) $\times$ 100]
- Gestation index
  [(number of litters—live pups/number of pregnancies) $\times$ 100]
- Live-born index
  [(number of pups born alive/total number of pups born) $\times$ 100]
- Weaning index
  [(number of pups alive at day 21/number of pups alive and kept on day 4) $\times$ 100]
- Sex ratio and percentage by sex
- Viability index
  [(number of pups alive on day 7/number of pups alive and kept on day 4) $\times$ 100]

Endpoints—Males

The endpoints of male reproductive toxicity include the following:

- Evaluation of testicular spermatid numbers
- Sperm evaluation for motility, morphology, and numbers

Both the U.S. Food and Drug Administration (FDA) and the U.S. Environmental Protection Agency (EPA) have established study protocols to assess the reproductive risks of chemicals and drugs. The FDA imposes guidelines for drugs that includes three different protocols: Segment I evaluates fertility and reproduction function in males and females, Segment II examines developmental toxicology and teratology, and Segment III determines perinatal and postnatal effects.

HUMAN RISK FACTORS AFFECTING FERTILITY

Most humans are exposed to a vast number of chemicals that may be hazardous to their reproductive capacity. Many chemicals have been identified as reproductive hazards in laboratory studies. Although the extrapolation of data from laboratory animals to humans is inexact, a number of these chemicals also have been shown to exert detrimental effects on human reproductive performance.

Male

It also has been suggested that the human male is more vulnerable to environmental and occupational toxins than other mammals are. Reproductive hazards and reproductive risks have led to the formulation of protection policies in certain occupations.

It is noteworthy that chronic illness may have a profound affect on gonadal function. Systemic illnesses that reduce spermatogenesis include thyrotoxicosis hypothyroidism, renal failure, mumps, and Crohn's disease. A large number of nonhormonal diseases likewise can decrease serum testosterone as well as gonadotrophins. Aging, nutritional deficiencies, and obesity also can affect fertility.

Female

Many physiologic, sociological, and psychological factors can affect the normality of the female reproductive system, as evidenced by variations in the menstrual process. The factors known to affect menstruation that are for the most part unrelated to occupational settings include age, body weight extremes, liver disease, thyroid dysfunction, intrauterine contraceptive devices, stress, exercise, and marital status. Menstruation can be influenced by therapeutic drugs, so-called recreational drugs, and potentially toxic substances that are present in occupational environments. Even the choice of control populations in studies involving adverse effects on the reproductive system can affect the risk estimates.

BIBLIOGRAPHY

Korach KS (ed): *Reproductive and Developmental Toxicology.* New York: Marcel Dekker, 1998.

Schettler T: *Generations at Risk: Reproductive Health and the Environment.* Cambridge, MA: MIT Press, 1999.

C H A P T E R   2 1

TOXIC RESPONSES OF THE ENDOCRINE SYSTEM

Charles C. Capen

KEY POINTS

- Endocrine glands are collections of specialized cells that synthesize, store, and release their secretions directly in the bloodstream.
- Each type of endocrine cell in the adenohypophysis is under the control of a specific releasing hormone from the hypothalamus.
- Toxicants can influence the synthesis, storage, and release of hypothalamic releasing hormones, adenohypophyseal releasing hormones, and the endocrine gland–specific hormones.

INTRODUCTION

Endocrine glands synthesize, store, and release their secretions directly into the bloodstream. They are sens ing and signaling devices located in the extracellular fluid compartment that are capable of responding to changes in the internal and external environments and coordinating multiple activities that maintain homeostasis.

PITUITARY GLAND

Normal Structure and Function

The pituitary gland (hypophysis) is divided into two major compartments: (1) the adenohypophysis (anterior lobe), which is composed of the pars distalis, pars tuberalis, and pars intermedia, and (2) the neurohypophyseal system, which includes the pars nervosa (posterior lobe), infundibular stalk, and hypothalamic nuclei (supraoptic and paraventricular) containing the neurosecretory neurons, which synthesize and package the neurohypophyseal hormones into secretory granules. The pars intermedia forms the thin cellular zone between the adenohypophysis and the neurohypophysis. The arterial blood supply to the pituitary gland forms a capillary plexus that drains into the hypophyseal portal veins, which supply the adenohypophysis. The hypothalamic-hypophyseal portal system transports the hypothalamic releasing and release-inhibiting hormones directly to the adenohypophysis, where they interact with their specific populations of trophic hormone-producing cells.

The pars distalis of the adenohypophysis is composed of multiple populations of endocrine cells that secrete the pituitary trophic hormones. The secretory cells are surrounded by abundant capillaries that are derived from the hypothalamic-hypophyseal portal system. The pars tu-

beralis functions primarily as a scaffold for the capillary network of the hypophyseal portal system during its course from the median eminence to the pars distalis.

Secretory cells in the adenohypophysis can be classified functionally into somatotrophs that secrete growth hormone (GH; somatotrophin), luteotrophs that secrete luteotropic hormone (LTH; prolactin), gonadotrophs that secrete luteinizing hormone (LH) and follicle-stimulating hormone (FSH), thyrotrophs that secrete thyroid-stimulating hormone (TSH), and chromophobes that are involved in the synthesis of adrenocorticotrophic hormone (ACTH) and melanocyte-stimulating hormone (MSH) in some species.

Each type of endocrine cell in the adenohypophysis is under the control of a specific releasing hormone from the hypothalamus (Fig. 21-1). These releasing hormones are small peptides that are synthesized and secreted by neurons of the hypothalamus and are conveyed by the hypophyseal portal system to specific trophic hormone-secreting cells in the adenohypophysis. Each hormone stimulates the rapid release of preformed secretory granules that contain a specific trophic hormone. Specific releasing hormones have been identified for TSH, FSH and LH, ACTH, and GH. Prolactin (PRL) secretion is stimulated by a number of factors, the most important of which appears to be thyrotropin-releasing hormone (TRH). Dopamine acts as the major prolactin-inhibitory factor and suppresses prolactin secretion and ACTH production. Somatostatin (somatotropin-release inhibiting hormone; SRIH) inhibits the secretion of both growth hormone and TSH. Control of pituitary trophic hormone secretion also is affected by negative feedback by the circulating concentration of target organ hormones.

The neurohypophyseal hormones (i.e., oxytocin and antidiuretic hormone) are synthesized in the cell body of

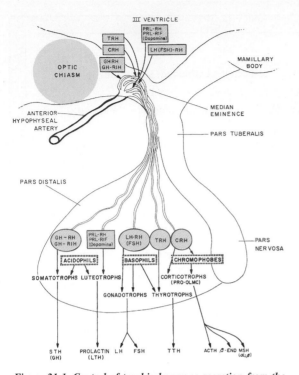

Figure 21-1. Control of trophic hormone secretion from the adenohypophysis by hypothalamic releasing hormones (RH) and release-inhibiting hormones (RIH). The releasing and release-inhibiting hormones are synthesized by neurons in the hypothalamus, transported by axonal processes, and released into the capillary plexus in the median eminence. They are transported to the adenohypophysis by the hypothalamic-hypophyseal portal system, where they interact with specific populations of trophic hormone-secreting cells to govern the rate of release of preformed hormones such as growth hormone (GH), somatotropic hormone (STH), luteotropic hormone (LTH), luteinizing hormone (LH), follicle-stimulating hormone (FSH), thyrotropic hormone (TTH), adrenocorticotropic hormone (ACTH), and melanocyte-stimulating hormone (MSH). There are RIHs for trophic hormones (e.g., prolactin and growth hormone) that do not directly influence the activity of target cells and result in the production of a final endocrine product (hormone) that could exert negative feedback control.

hypothalamic neurons, packaged into secretory granules, transported by long axonal processes to the pars nervosa, and released into the bloodstream. As the biosynthetic precursor molecules travel along the axons in secretion granules from the neurosecretory neurons, the precursors are cleaved into the active hormones and their respective neurophysins.

In addition to the specific trophic hormone-secreting cells, a population of supporting cells is present in the adenohypophysis. These cells, which are referred to as stellate (follicular) cells, appear to provide a phagocytic or supportive function in addition to producing a colloid-like material that accumulates in follicles.

Mechanisms of Toxicity

Pituitary tumors can be induced readily by sustained uncompensated hormonal derangements that lead to increased synthesis and secretion of pituitary hormones. The absence of negative feedback inhibition from pituitary cells leads to unrestrained proliferation (hyperplasia initially and neoplasia later). For example, surgical removal or radiation-induced ablation of the thyroid or interference with the production of thyroid hormones by the use of specific chemical inhibitors of thyroid hormone synthesis leads to stimulation of TSH synthesis and secretion with elevated blood levels. The thyrotrophic cells in the adenohypophysis undergo prominent hypertrophy. Similarly, estrogens, caffeine, *N*-methylnitrosourea, and the neuroleptic agent sulpiride have been reported to cause the development of pituitary tumors.

Morphologic Alterations and Proliferative Lesions of Pituitary Cells

Calcitonin is produced in the posterior hypothalamus and median eminence, where it normally exerts an effect on the hypothalamus-pituitary axis. Calcitonin receptors have been identified in the hypothalamus, and lower numbers of receptors are found in the pituitary gland. Several strains of rats are highly predisposed to develop pituitary tumors compared with humans.

There is a high frequency of spontaneous pituitary adenomas in laboratory rats in most long-term toxicologic studies. The incidence of pituitary tumors is determined by many factors, including strain, age, sex, reproductive status, and diet. Moreover, the separation between focal hyperplasia, adenoma, and carcinoma through the use of histopathologic techniques is difficult in the pituitary gland. There appears to be a continuous spectrum of proliferative lesions between diffuse or focal hyperplasia and adenomas derived from a specific population of secretory cells. Prolonged stimulation of a population of secretory cells commonly predisposes to the subsequent development of a higher than expected incidence of focal hyperplasia and tumors.

Focal ("nodular") hyperplasia in the adenohypophysis appears as multiple small areas that are well demarcated but not encapsulated from adjacent normal cells. Adenomas usually are solitary nodules that are larger than the often multiple areas of focal hyperplasia. Carcinomas usually are larger than adenomas in the pituitary and usually result in a macroscopically detectable enlargement.

ADRENAL CORTEX

Normal Structure and Function

The adrenal (suprarenal) glands in mammals are flattened bilobed organs that are in close proximity to the kidneys. The cortex is histologically characterized by the zona glomerulosa, zona fasciculata, and zona reticularis. The mineralocorticoid-producing zona glomerulosa contains cells that produce mineralocorticoids (aldosterone). Degeneration of this zone or an interference of the secretion of aldosterone results in a life-threatening retention of potassium and hypovolemic shock associated with the excessive urinary loss of sodium, chloride, and water. The large zona fasciculata is responsible for the secretion of glucocorticoid hormones (e.g., corticosterone and cortisol). The innermost zona reticularis secretes minute quantities of adrenal sex hormones.

The adrenal cortical cells contain large cytoplasmic lipid droplets that consist of cholesterol and other steroid hormone precursors. The lipid droplets are in close proximity to the smooth endoplasmic reticulum and large mitochondria, which contain the specific hydroxylase and dehydrogenase enzyme systems required to synthesize the different steroid hormones. There are no secretory granules in the cytoplasm, because there is direct secretion without significant storage of preformed steroid hormones.

The common biosynthetic pathway from cholesterol involves the formation of pregnenolone, the basic precursor for the three major classes of adrenal steroids. Pregnenolone is formed after two hydroxylation reactions at the carbon 20 and 22 positions of cholesterol and a subsequent cleavage between those two carbon atoms. In the zona fasciculata, pregnenolone first is converted to progesterone by two microsomal enzymes. Three subsequent hydroxylation reactions occur involving, in order, carbon atoms at the 17, 21, and 11 positions. The resulting steroid is cortisol.

The mineralocorticoids (e.g., aldosterone) are secreted from the zona glomerulosa under the control of the renin–angiotensin system. The mineralocorticoids have effects on ion transport by epithelial cells, particularly renal cells, resulting in conservation of sodium (chloride and water) and loss of potassium. In the distal convoluted tubule of the mammalian nephron, a cation exchange exists that promotes the resorption of sodium from the glomerular filtrate and the secretion of potassium into the lumen.

The principal control for the production of glucocorticoids is exerted by ACTH, a polypeptide hormone produced in the adenohypophysis of the pituitary gland. ACTH release is controlled largely by the hypothalamus through the secretion of corticotropin-releasing hormone (CRH). An increase in ACTH production results in an increase in circulating levels of glucocorticoids and under certain conditions also can result in weak stimulation of aldosterone secretion. Negative feedback control normally occurs when the elevated blood levels of cortisol act on the hypothalamus, the anterior pituitary, or both to cause a suppression of ACTH secretion.

Mechanisms of Toxicity

The adrenal cortex is predisposed to the toxic effects of xenobiotics for at least two reasons. First, adrenal cortical cells of most animal species contain large stores of lipids used primarily as a substrate for steroidogenesis. Many adrenal cortical toxic compounds are lipophilic and therefore can accumulate in these lipid-rich cells. Second, adrenal cortical cells have enzymes capable of metabolizing xenobiotic chemicals.

Classes of chemicals toxic for the adrenal cortex include short-chain (three- or four-carbon) aliphatic compounds, lipidosis inducers, and amphiphilic compounds. The most potent aliphatic compounds include acrylonitrile, 3-aminopropionitrile, 3-bromopropionitrile, 1-butanethiol, and 1,4-butanedithiol. By comparison, lipidosis inducers can cause accumulations of neutral fats, which may cause a reduction in or loss of organellar function and eventual cell destruction. Compounds causing lipidosis include aminoglutethimide, amphenone, and anilines. Biologically active cationic amphiphilic compounds, including chloroquine, triparanol, and chlorphentermine, produce a generalized phospholipidosis and microscopic phospholipid-rich inclusions that affect the functional integrity of lysosomes.

Many chemicals that cause morphologic changes in the adrenal glands also affect cortical function. Chemically induced changes in adrenal function result from blockage of the action of adrenocorticoids at peripheral sites or inhibition of the synthesis and/or secretion of hormone. In the first mechanism, many antisteroidal compounds (antagonists) act by competing with or binding to steroid hormone–receptor sites, thus reducing the number of available receptor sites or altering their binding affinity. Cortexolone (11α-deoxycortisol), an antiglucocorticoid, and spironolactone, an antimineralocorticoid, are two examples of peripherally acting adrenal cortical hormone antagonists.

Xenobiotic chemicals may affect adrenal steroidogenesis. For example, chemicals that cause increased lipid droplets often inhibit the utilization of steroid precursors, including the conversion of cholesterol to pregnenolone. Chemicals that affect the fine structure of mitochondria and smooth endoplasmic reticulum often impair the activity of 11α-, 17α-, and 21-hydroxylases, respectively, and are associated with lesions primarily in the zonae reticularis and fasciculata. Atrophy of the zona glomerulosa may reflect specific inhibition of aldosterone synthesis or secretion either directly (e.g., inhibition of 18α-hydroxylation) or indirectly (e.g., suppression of the renin–angiotensin system) by chemicals such as spironolactone and captopril.

Pathologic Alterations and Proliferative Lesions in Cortical Cells

Cortical hypertrophy resulting from impaired steroidogenesis or hyperplasia caused by long-term stimulation often is present when the adrenal cortex is increased in size. Small adrenal glands often are indicative of degenerative changes or trophic atrophy of the adrenal cortex. Nodular lesions that distort and enlarge one adrenal gland or both adrenal glands suggest that a neoplasm is present.

Lesions of adrenal cortical cells associated with chemical injury may be classified as follows: endothelial damage with acrylonitrile; mitochondrial damage with DMNM, o,p'-DDD, amphenone; endoplasmic reticulum disruption with triparanol; lipid aggregation with aniline; lysosomal phospholipid aggregation with chlorophentermine; and secondary effects caused by embolization by medullary cells with acrylonitrile. Damage to mitochondria and smooth endoplasmic reticulum occurs after exposure to chemical agents that inhibit steroidogenesis.

ADRENAL MEDULLA

Normal Structure and Function

The bulk of the medulla is composed of chromaffin cells, which synthesize and store catecholamines. Human adrenal medullary cells may contain both norepinephrine and epinephrine within a single chromaffin cell. The adrenal medulla also contains variable numbers of ganglion cells and the small granule–containing cells or small intensely fluorescent (SIF) cells. SIF cells lie intermediate between chromaffin cells and ganglion cells and may function as interneurons. The adrenal medullary cells also contain serotonin and histamine as well as several neuropeptides, including enkephalins, neurotensin, and neuropeptide Y.

Mechanisms of Toxicity

Proliferative lesions of the medulla develop as a result of various mechanisms. For example, the long-term administration of GH is associated with an increased incidence of pheochromocytomas as well as tumors at other sites. In addition, several neuroleptic compounds that increase prolactin secretion by inhibiting dopamine production have been associated with an increased incidence of proliferative lesions of medullary cells in rats. Drugs that increase the incidence of adrenal medullary proliferative lesions include nicotine, reserpine, zomepirac, isotretinoin, and nafarelin [a luteinizing hormone–releasing hormone (LHRH) analog], atenolol, terazosin, ribavirin, and pamidronate (bisphosphonate).

Environmental and dietary factors may be more important than genetic factors as determinants of the incidence of adrenal medullary proliferative lesions in rats. The incidence can be reduced by lowering the carbohydrate content of the diet. Several agents, including sugar alcohols, that increase the incidence of adrenal medullary lesions increase the absorption of calcium from the gut. The fact that vitamin D is the most potent in vivo stimulus identified for medullary chromaffin cell proliferation supports the hypothesis that altered calcium homeostasis is involved in pheochromocytoma pathogenesis.

THYROID GLAND (FOLLICULAR CELLS)

Species Differences in Thyroid Hormone Economy

Long-term perturbations of the pituitary-thyroid axis by xenobiotics, iodine deficiency, partial thyroidectomy, and natural goitrogens in food are likely to predispose rats to a higher incidence of proliferative lesions in response to chronic TSH stimulation than is the case in human thyroids. This greater sensitivity of the rodent thyroid is related to the shorter plasma half-life of thyroxine T_4 in rats compared with humans.

Mechanisms of Thyroid Tumorigenesis

Chronic treatment of rodents with goitrogenic compounds results in the development of follicular cell adenomas. Thiouracil and its derivatives, brassica seeds, erythrosine (FD&C Red No. 3), sulfonamides, and other compounds directly interfere with thyroid hormone synthesis or secretion in the thyroid gland, increase thyroid hormone catabolism and subsequent excretion into the bile, or disrupt the peripheral conversion of thyroxine (T_4) to triiodothyronine (T_3). The ensuing decrease in circulating thyroid hormone levels results in a compensatory increased secretion of pituitary TSH. TSH stimulation of the thyroid gland leads to proliferative changes in follicular cells that include hypertrophy, hyperplasia, and ultimately neoplasia in rodents.

Chemicals That Directly Inhibit Thyroid Hormone Synthesis

Blockage of Iodine Uptake Thyroid hormone biosynthesis occurs extracellularly in the follicular lumen. Essential raw materials such as iodide are transported rapidly against a concentration gradient into the lumen and are oxidized by a thyroid peroxidase to reactive iodine (I_2) (Fig. 21-2). This transport of iodide ion is linked to the transport of Na^+. The iodine transport system in

the thyroid gland can be inhibited selectively by competitive anion inhibitors, blocking the ability of the gland to iodinate tyrosine residues in thyroglobulin and synthesize thyroid hormones.

Inhibition of Thyroid Peroxidase Resulting in an Organification Defect The stepwise binding of iodide to the tyrosyl residues in thyroglobulin requires oxidation of inorganic iodide to molecular iodine (I_2) by thyroid peroxidase (Fig. 21-2). Classes of chemicals that inhibit the organification of thyroglobulin include (1) the thionamides (such as thiourea, thiouracil, propylthiouracil, methimazole, carbimazole, and goitrin), (2) aniline derivatives (e.g., sulfonamides, paraaminobenzoic acid, paraaminosalicylic acid, and amphenone), (3) substituted phenols (such as resorcinol, phloroglucinol, and 2,4-dihydroxybenzoic acid), and (4) miscellaneous inhibitors (e.g., aminotriazole, antipyrine, and iodopyrine). Many of these chemicals inhibit thyroid peroxidase, which disrupts both the iodination of tyrosyl residues in thyroglobulin and the coupling reaction of monoiodothyronine (MIT) and di-iodothyronine (DIT) to form T_3 and T_4 (Fig. 21-3). In addition, inhibition of gap-junction intercellular communication by propylthiouracil (PTU) or a low-iodine diet may increase thyroid follicular cell proliferation by disrupting the passage of regulatory substance(s) through these channels.

Blockage of Thyroid Hormone Release by Excess Iodide and Lithium

Relatively few chemicals selectively inhibit the secretion of thyroid hormone from the thyroid gland (Fig. 21-2).

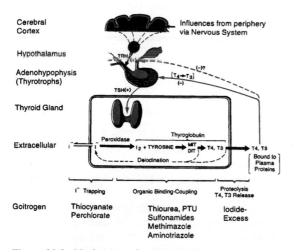

Figure 21-2. Mechanism of action of goitrogenic chemicals on thyroid hormone synthesis and secretion.

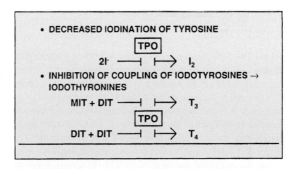

Figure 21-3. Mechanisms by which xenobiotic chemicals decrease thyroid hormone synthesis by inhibiting thyroperoxidase (TPO) in follicular cells.

An excess of iodine inhibits secretion of thyroid hormone and occasionally can result in goiter and subnormal function (hypothyroidism) in animals and human patients. Lithium carbonate inhibits the release of thyroid hormones and occasionally results in the development of goiter.

Hepatic Microsomal Enzyme Induction

Glucuronidation is the rate-limiting step in the biliary excretion of T_4 and sulfation for the excretion of T_3. Chemicals that induce these enzyme pathways may result in chronic stimulation of the thyroid by disrupting the hypothalamic-pituitary-thyroid axis (Fig. 21-4). Microsomal enzyme inducers are more effective in reducing serum T_4 than in reducing serum T_3. Xenobiotics that induce liver microsomal enzymes and disrupt thyroid function in rats include drugs that act on the central nervous system (CNS) (e.g., phenobarbital, benzodiazepines), calcium channel blockers (e.g., nicardipine, bepridil), spironolactone, retinoids, chlorinated hydrocarbons (e.g., chlordane, DDT, TCDD), and polyhalogenated biphenyls (PCB, PBB), among others. Most hepatic microsomal enzyme inducers have no apparent intrinsic carcinogenicity or mutagenicity. Their promoting effect on thyroid tumors usually is greater in rats than in mice, with males developing a higher incidence of tumors more often than females do.

There is no convincing evidence that humans treated with drugs or exposed to chemicals that induce hepatic microsomal enzymes are at increased risk for the development of thyroid or liver cancer. In fact, relatively high microsomal enzyme–inducing doses of phenobarbital have been used chronically as an anticonvulsant, sometimes for lifetime exposures, to control seizure activity in human beings without the onset of thyroid cancer.

Secondary Mechanisms of Thyroid Tumorigenesis and Risk Assessment

Many chemicals disrupt one or more steps in the synthesis and secretion of thyroid hormones, resulting in subnormal levels of T_4 and T_3 and an associated increased secretion of pituitary TSH (Fig. 21-4). In the secondary mechanism of thyroid oncogenesis in rodents, the specific xenobiotic or physiologic perturbation evokes the chronic hypersecretion of TSH that promotes the development of proliferative lesions derived from follicular cells.

In contrast to rats and mice, humans are relatively resistant to the development of thyroid cancer. A few human patients with congenital defects in thyroid hormone synthesis and elevated circulating TSH levels as well as thyrotoxic patients with Graves' disease appear to be at greater risk of developing thyroid tumors. The literature suggests that prolonged stimulation of the human thyroid by TSH induces neoplasia only in exceptional circumstances, possibly by acting together with some other metabolic or immunologic abnormality.

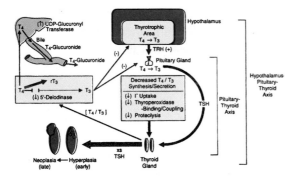

Figure 21-4. Multiple sites of disruption of the hypothalamic-pituitary-thyroid axis by xenobiotic chemicals. Chemicals can exert direct effects by disrupting thyroid hormone synthesis or secretion and indirectly influence the thyroid through an inhibition of 5'-deiodinase or by inducing hepatic microsomal enzymes (e.g., T_4-UDP glucuronyltransferase). All these mechanisms can lower circulating levels of thyroid hormones (T_4 and/or T_3), resulting in a release from negative-feedback inhibition and increased secretion of thyroid-stimulating hormone (TSH) by the pituitary gland. The chronic hypersecretion of TSH predisposes the sensitive rodent thyroid gland to develop an increased incidence of focal hyperplastic and neoplastic lesions (adenomas) by a secondary (epigenetic) mechanism.

THYROID C CELLS

Normal Structure and Function

Calcitonin (CT) is secreted by C cells (parafollicular or light cells) in the mammalian thyroid gland. C cells contain numerous small membrane-limited secretory granules in the cytoplasm in which the calcitonin activity is localized.

Calcitonin is a polypeptide hormone that is secreted continuously under conditions of normocalcemia. The rate of secretion of CT is increased greatly in response to elevations in blood calcium. C cells store substantial amounts of CT in their secretory granules. In response to hypercalcemia, there is a rapid discharge of stored hormone from C cells into interfollicular capillaries. The hypercalcemic stimulus, if sustained, is followed by hypertrophy of C cells. Hyperplasia of C cells occurs in response to long-term hypercalcemia.

Calcitonin exerts its function by interacting with target cells, primarily in bone and kidney. CT antagonizes the action of parathyroid hormone in mobilizing calcium from bone but synergistically decreases the renal tubular reabsorption of phosphorus. Calcitonin and parathyroid hormone, acting in concert, provide a dual negative feedback control mechanism to maintain the life-sustaining concentration of calcium ion in extracellular fluids within narrow limits.

Morphologic Alterations and Proliferative Lesions of Thyroid C Cells

There are two types of C-cell hyperplasia: diffuse and focal (nodular) (Fig. 21-5). In diffuse hyperplasia, the numbers of C cells are increased throughout the thyroid lobe to a point where they may be more numerous than follicular cells. In focal C-cell hyperplasia, the accumulations of proliferating C cells are of a lesser diameter than five average colloid-containing thyroid follicles, with minimal evidence of compression of adjacent follicles. C-cell adenomas are discrete, expansive masses of

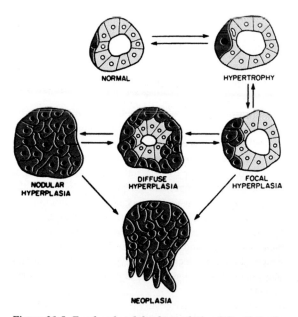

Figure 21-5. Focal and nodular hyperplasia of C cells in the thyroid often precedes the development of C-cell neoplasms.

C cells larger than five average colloid-containing thyroid follicles. The C cells composing an adenoma may be subdivided by fine connective tissue septae and capillaries into small neuroendocrine packets. Occasional amyloid deposits may be found both in nodular hyperplasia and in adenomas.

C-cell carcinomas often result in enlargement of one or both thyroid lobes as a result of the extensive proliferation of C cells. Immunoperoxidase reactions for calcitonin generally are more intense in diffuse or nodular hyperplasia, whereas in adenomas and carcinomas, calcitonin immunoreactivity varies between tumors and in different regions of a tumor. Hyperplastic C cells adjacent to adenomas and carcinomas usually are intensely positive for calcitonin.

PARATHYROID GLAND

To maintain a constant concentration of calcium despite marked variations in intake and excretion, endocrine control consists of the interactions of three major hormones: parathyroid hormone (PTH), calcitonin (CT), and cholecalciferol (vitamin D) (Fig. 21-6).

Normal Structure and Function of Chief Cells

Biosynthesis of Parathyroid Hormone Parathyroid chief cells in humans and many animal species store relatively small amounts of preformed hormone, but they respond quickly to variations in the need for hormone by changing the rate of hormone synthesis (Fig. 21-7). Under certain conditions of increased demand (e.g., a low calcium ion concentration in the extracellular fluid compartment), PTH may be released directly from chief cells without being packaged into secretion granules.

Control of Parathyroid Hormone Secretion The parathyroids have a unique feedback that is controlled by the concentration of calcium (and to a lesser extent magnesium) ion in serum. Serum Ca^{2+} binds to a Ca receptor on the chief cell, permitting the serum Ca^{2+} to regulate chief cell function. The concentration of blood phosphorus has no direct regulatory influence on the synthesis and secretion of PTH; however, an elevated blood phosphorus level may lead indirectly to parathyroid stimulation by virtue of its ability to lower blood calcium primarily by decreasing the production of the active form of vitamin D [1, 25-$(OH)_2$-cholecalciferol], thus diminishing the rate of intestinal calcium absorption.

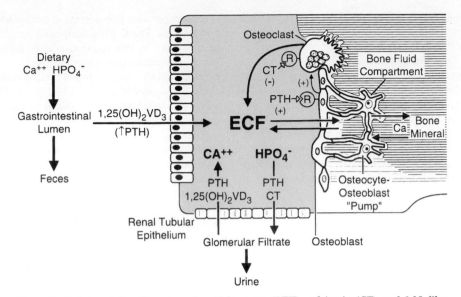

Figure 21-6. Interrelationship of parathyroid hormone (PTH), calcitonin (CT), and 1,25-dihy-droxycholecalciferol [1,25(OH)₂VD₃] in the regulation of calcium (Ca) and phosphorus in extra-cellular fluids. Receptors for PTH are on osteoblasts and those for CT on osteoclasts in bone. PTH and CT are antagonistic in their action on bone but synergistic in stimulating the renal excretion of phosphorous. Vitamin D exerts its action primarily on the intestine to enhance the absorption of both calcium and phosphorus.

Xenobiotic Chemical-Induced Toxic Injury of Parathyroids

Ozone One to five days after ozone exposure, many chief cells undergo compensatory hypertrophy and hy-

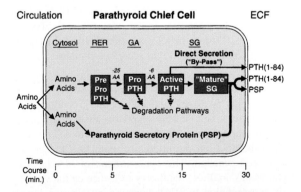

Figure 21-7. Biosynthesis of parathyroid hormone (PTH) and parathyroid secretory protein (PSP) by parathyroid chief cells. Active PTH is synthesized as a larger biosynthetic precursor molecule (preproPTH) that undergoes rapid posttranslational processing to proPTH before secretion from chief cells as active PTH (amino acids 1 to 84).

perplasia, with areas of capillary endothelial cell proliferation, interstitial edema, degeneration of vascular endothelium, formation of platelet thrombi, leukocyte infiltration of the walls of larger vessels in the gland, and disruption of basement membranes. Inactive chief cells with few secretory granules predominate in the parathyroids in the later stages of exposure to ozone.

Aluminum Patients with chronic renal failure who are treated by hemodialysis with aluminum-containing fluids or orally administered drugs containing aluminum often have normal or minimal elevations of immunoreactive parathyroid hormone (iPTH), little histologic evidence of osteitis fibrosa in bone, and a depressed response by the parathyroid gland to acute hypocalcemia. Aluminum appears to decrease diglyceride synthesis, as is reflected in a corresponding decrease in the synthesis of phosphatidylcholine and triglyceride. The mechanism by which aluminum decreases diglycerides and maintains phosphatidylinositol synthesis in parathyroid cells is not known.

L-Asparaginase Parathyroid chief cells appear to be destroyed selectively by L-asparaginase. In several studies, chief cells were predominantly inactive and degranulated, with large autophagic vacuoles present in the cytoplasm of degenerating cells. Cytoplasmic organelles involved with the synthesis and packaging of secretory products were poorly developed in chief cells. Rabbits developed hyperphosphatemia, hypomagnesemia, hyperkalemia, and azotemia in addition to acute hypocalcemia. The development of hypocalcemia and a tetany response may not be limited to the rabbit, because some human patients receiving the drug also have developed hypocalcemia.

Proliferative Lesions of Parathyroid Chief Cells

Parathyroid adenomas are solitary nodules that are sharply demarcated from adjacent parathyroid parenchyma. Adenomas are usually endocrinologically inactive in adult-age rats in chronic toxicity studies. The parathyroid glands that do not contain a functional adenoma also undergo trophic atrophy in response to the hypercalcemia.

Few chemicals or experimental manipulations increase the incidence of parathyroid tumors. Parathyroid adenomas have been encountered infrequently after the administration of the pesticide rotenone in 2-year bioassay studies in Fischer rats. Irradiation significantly increases the incidence of parathyroid adenomas in inbred Wistar albino rats.

TESTIS

Leydig (interstitial) cell tumors are among the most frequently occurring endocrine tumors in rodents in chronic carcinogenicity studies. In contrast, the incidence of Leydig cell tumors in human patients is extremely low, on the order of 1 in 5 million, with age peaks at approximately 30 and 60 years.

Structure and Endocrinologic Regulation of Leydig (Interstitial) Cells

The endocrinologic regulation of Leydig cells involves the coordinated activity of the hypothalamus and anterior pituitary with negative feedback control exerted by the blood concentration of gonadal steroids (Fig. 21-8). Hypothalamic gonadotrophin-releasing hormone (GnRH) stimulates the pulsatile release of both LH and FSH from the adenohypophysis. Luteinizing hormone is the major trophic factor controlling the activity of Leydig cells and the synthesis of testosterone. The blood levels of testosterone exert negative feedback on the hypothalamus and, to a lesser extent, the adenohypophysis. Follicle stimulating hormone binds to receptors on Sertoli cells in the seminiferous tubules and, along with the local concentration of testosterone, is critical in spermatogenesis. Testosterone, by controlling GnRH release, is an important regulator of FSH secretion by the pituitary

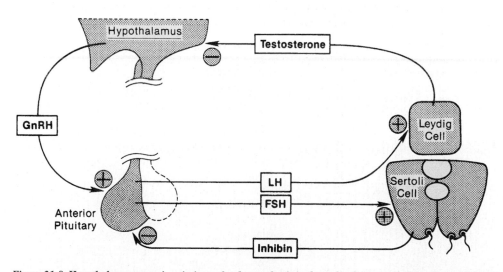

Figure 21-8. Hypothalamus–anterior pituitary gland–gonad axis in the endocrine control of Leydig and Sertoli cells by luteinizing hormone (LH) and follicle stimulating hormone (FSH).

gland. The seminiferous tubules also produce a gly-copeptide, designated inhibin, which exerts negative feedback on the release of FSH.

Pathology of Leydig (Interstitial) Cell Tumors

To standardize the classification of focal proliferative lesions of Leydig cells between studies with different xenobiotic chemicals and different testing laboratories, the following diagnostic criteria were established:

1. Hyperplasia was defined as a focal collection of Leydig cells with little atypia and a diameter of less than one seminiferous tubule.

2. An adenoma was defined as a mass of Leydig cells larger in diameter than one seminiferous tubule with some cellular atypia and compression of adjacent tubules.

Mechanisms of Leydig (Interstitial) Cell Tumor Development

Pathogenic mechanisms important in the development of proliferative lesions of Leydig cells include irradiation, the species and strain differences mentioned previously, cryptorchidism, a compromised blood supply to the testis, and heterotransplantation into the spleen. Hor-

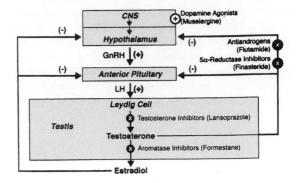

Figure 21-9. Regulation of the hypothalamic-pituitary-testis (HPT) axis and control points for potential disruption by xenobiotic chemicals. Symbols: (+) feedback stimulation; (−) feedback inhibition; ⊕ receptor stimulation; ⊗ enzyme or receptor inhibition.

monal imbalances include increased estrogenic steroids in mice and hamsters and elevated pituitary gonadotrophins resulting from the chronic administration of androgen receptor antagonists, 5α-reductase inhibitors, GnRH agonists, and aromatase inhibitors. Loss of negative feedback control and the resulting overproduction of LH cause the proliferative changes in Leydig cells (Fig. 21-9). Xenobiotics that increase the incidence of proliferative lesions of Leydig cells in chronic carcinogenicity studies in rats are listed in Table 21-1.

Table 21-1
Selected Examples of Drugs that Increase the Incidence of Proliferative Lesions of Leydig Cells in Chronic Exposure Studies in Rats or Mice

NAME	SPECIES	CLINICAL INDICATION
Indomethacin	R	Anti-inflammatory
Lactitol	R	Laxative
Metronidazole	R	Antibacterial
Mesulergine	R	Parkinson's disease
Buserelin	R	Prostatic and breast carcinoma, endometriosis
Cimetidine	R	Reduction of gastric acid secretion
Flutamide	R	Prostatic carcinoma
Gemfibrozil	R	Hypolipidemia
Spironolactone	R	Diuretic
Nararelin	R	LH-RH analog
Tamoxifen	M	Antiestrogen
Vidarabine	R	Antiviral
Clofibrate	R	Hypolipidemia
Finasteride	M	Prostatic hyperplasia

Although several hormonal imbalances result in an increased incidence of Leydig cell tumors in rodents, several disease conditions associated with chronic elevations in serum LH (including Klinefelter's syndrome and gonadotroph adenomas of the pituitary gland) in human patients have not been associated with an increased development of this type of rare testicular tumor. Likewise, compounds similar to those listed in Table 21-1 have not resulted in an increased incidence of Leydig cell neoplasia in humans. In summary, Leydig cell tumors are a frequently occurring tumor in rats that often are associated mechanistically with hormonal imbalances; however, they are not an appropriate model for assessing the risk to human males of developing this testicular tumor.

OVARY

Ovarian tumors in rodents can be subdivided into epithelial tumors, sex cord–stromal tumors, germ cell tumors, tumors derived from nonspecialized soft tissues of the ovary, and tumors metastatic to the ovary from distant sites. Epithelial tumors of the ovary include cystadenomas and cystadenocarcinomas, tubulostromal adenomas, and mesotheliomas. The tubular (or tubulostromal) adenomas are the most important ovarian tumors in mice; they are uncommon in rats, rare in other animal species, and not recognized in the ovaries of women.

Ovarian tumors derived from the sex cords and/or ovarian stroma include the granulosal cell tumors, luteomas, thecomas, Sertoli cell tumors, tubular adenoma (with contributions from ovarian stroma), and undifferentiated sex cord–stromal tumors. The granulosal cell tumor is the most common in this group, which accounts for 27 percent of naturally occurring ovarian tumors in mice. Granulosal cell tumors may develop within certain tubular or tubulostromal adenomas after a long-term perturbation of endocrine function associated with genic deletion, irradiation, oocytotoxic chemicals, and neonatal thymectomy.

Case Study: Ovarian Tumors Associated with Xenobiotic Chemicals

Nitrofurantoin When fed at high doses to mice for 2 years, nitrofurantoin increased the incidence of ovarian tumors of the tubular or tubulostromal type. Nitrofurantoin caused sterility as a result of destruction of ovarian follicles and subsequent hormonal imbalances. Mice ad-

ministered nitrofurantoin had a consistent change in the ovarian cortex, termed *ovarian atrophy,* that was characterized by an absence of graafian follicles, developing ova, and corpora lutea; focal or diffuse hyperplasia; and varying numbers of polygonal, often vacuolated sex cord–derived stromal cells between the tubular profiles. The ovaries were small with irregular surfaces and had scattered eosinophilic stromal cells between tubular profiles.

Selective Estrogen Receptor Modulators Selective estrogen receptor modulators (SERMs) are compounds that have estrogen agonist effects on some tissues and estrogen antagonist actions on other tissues. The SERM tamoxifen has estrogen antagonist effects in the breast and an estrogen agonist effect on bone and also may stimulate the uterine endometrium. The SERM raloxifene has estrogen agonist effects on bone and serum lipids but estrogen antagonist actions on the uterus and breast. Tamoxifen, toremifene, and raloxifene have been reported to increase the incidence of ovarian tumors when administered chronically to mice. However, there is no evidence of an increased risk of ovarian cancer in women administered SERMs, since tamoxifen has been used clinically since 1978.

Summary: Ovarian Tumorigenesis in Rodents

Examination of the literature supports the hypothesis that the unique intense hyperplasia of ovarian surface epithelium and stromal cells, leading eventually to tubular adenomas and occasionally granulosa cell tumors, develops secondarily to chronic pituitary gonadotrophic hormone stimulation (Fig. 21-10). Factors that destroy or greatly diminish the numbers of ovarian follicles—such as senescence, genetic deletion of follicles, x-irradiation, drugs, nitrofurantoin, and early thymectomy with the development of autoantibodies to oocytes—are known to diminish the secretion of sex steroid hormones by the ovary. This results in elevated circulating levels of gonadotrophins, especially LH, as a result of decreased negative feedback on the hypothalamic-pituitary axis by estrogens and possibly other humoral factors produced by the graafian follicles. The long-term stimulation of stromal (interstitial) cells, which have receptors for LH, and, indirectly, the ovarian surface epithelium appears to place the mouse ovary at increased risk of developing the unique tubular or tubulostromal adenomas.

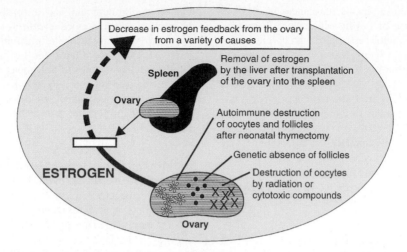

Figure 21-10. Multiple pathogenic mechanisms in ovarian tumorigenesis of mice, resulting in decreased negative feedback by diminished levels of gonadal steroids, particularly estrogen.

Studies using sterile mutant mice support the concept of a secondary (hormonally mediated) mechanism of ovarian carcinogenesis. Multiple pathogenetic factors that either destroy or diminish the numbers of graafian follicles in the ovary result in decreased secretion of sex hormones (especially estradiol-17β), leading to a compensatory overproduction of pituitary gonadotrophins (particularly LH) (Fig. 21-10), and this places the mouse ovary at an increased risk for developing tumors (Fig. 21-11). The intense proliferation of ovarian surface epithelium and stromal (interstitial) cells with the development of unique tubular adenomas in response to sterility does not appear to have a counterpart in the ovaries of human adult females.

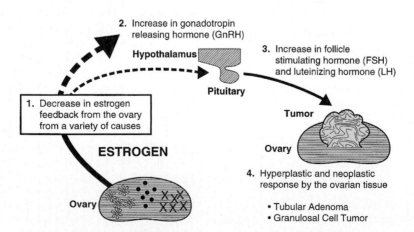

Figure 21-11. Decreased circulating estrogens release the hypothalamus–pituitary gland from negative feedback inhibition. The increased gonadotropin levels (LH and FSH) result in the mouse ovary being at greater risk of developing tubular adenomas in chronic studies.

BIBLIOGRAPHY

Coe FL, Favus MJ (eds): *Disorders of Bone and Mineral Metabolism.* New York: Raven Press, 1992.

Cook JC, Klinefelter GR, Hardisty JF, et al: Rodent Leydig cell tumorigenesis: A review of the physiology, pathology, mechanisms, and relevance to humans. *Crit Rev Toxicol* 29:169–261, 1999.

Harvey PW, Rush K, Cockburn A (eds): *Endocrine and Hormonal Toxicology.* Sussex, UK: Wiley, 1999.

Huff J, Boyd J, Barrett J (eds): *Cellular and Molecular Mechanisms of Hormonal Carcinogenesis: Environmental Influences,* New York. Wiley-Liss, 1996.

UNIT 5

TOXIC AGENTS

TOXIC EFFECTS OF PESTICIDES

Donald J. Ecobichon

KEY POINTS

- A pesticide can be defined as any substance or mixture of substances used to prevent, destroy, repel, or mitigate any pest.

- Pesticide exposures include (1) accidental and/or suicidal poisonings, (2) occupational (manufacturing, mixing/loading, application, harvesting, and handling of crops) exposure, (3) bystanders exposed to off-target drift from spraying operations, and (4) members of the general public who consume food items containing pesticide residues.

- Chemical insecticides in use today poison the nervous systems of the target organisms.

- A herbicide is any compound that is capable of killing or severely injuring plants.

- A fungicide is any chemical capable of preventing growth and reproduction of fungi.

INTRODUCTION

The U.S. Environmental Protection Agency (EPA) defines a pesticide as any substance or mixture of substances that is used to prevent, destroy, repel, or mitigate any pest. A pesticide also may be described as any physical, chemical, or biological agent that will kill an undesirable plant or animal pest. The term *pest* includes harmful, destructive, or troublesome animals, plants, or microorganisms. *Pesticide* is a generic name for agents that are classified more specifically on the basis of the pattern of use and the organism killed.

REGULATORY MANDATE

The Federal Insecticide, Fungicide, and Rodenticide Act (FIFRA) of 1947 grouped all pest control products under one law to be administered by the U.S. Department of Agriculture (USDA). In 1972, administrative authority was turned over to the EPA. The new law, along with subsequent amendments, defined the registration requirements and appropriate chemical, toxicologic, and environmental impact studies; label specifications; use restrictions; tolerances for pesticide residues on raw agricultural products; and responsibility for monitoring pesticide residue levels in foods. The U.S. Food and Drug Administration (FDA) is responsible for monitoring residue levels and for the seizure of foods that are not in compliance with the regulations, and the USDA monitors meat and poultry for pesticides as well as other chemicals. The Food Quality Protection Act (FQPA) of 1996 amended federal laws regarding pesticides to give special consideration to children. When data on pesticides are not adequate, pesticide tolerances for children must incorporate an additional 10-fold safety factor.

The typical spectrum of basic pesticide toxicity data required under FIFRA is summarized in Table 22-1. Extensive ancillary studies of environmental impacts on birds, mammals, aquatic organisms, plants, soils, environmental persistence, and bioaccumulation also are required. A schematic diagram showing the "information package" required to support a registration and the time span required to develop this database—from the point of patenting the newly synthesized chemical through to its marketing and user acceptability—is shown in Fig. 22-1.

Exposure

Populations of individuals may be identified as having exposure to a range of concentrations of a particular agent

Table 22-1
Basic Requirements Regarding Toxicity Data for New Pesticide Registrations

Acute
  Oral (rat)
  Dermal (rabbit)
  Inhalation (usually rat)
  Irritation studies
  Eye (rabbit)
  Skin (rabbit, guinea pig)
  Dermal sensitization (guinea pig)
  Delayed neurotoxicity (hen)
Subchronic
  90-day feeding study
  Rodent (rat, mouse)
  Nonrodent (dog)
  Dermal } Dependent on use pattern and
  Inhalation } potential for occupational exposure
  Neurotoxicity
Chronic
  One- or two-year oral study
  Rodent (usually rat)
  Nonrodent (dog)
  Oncogenicity study (rat or mouse)
Reproductive
  In vitro mutagenicity (microorganisms, etc.)
  Fertility/reproduction (rat, mouse, rabbit)
  Teratogenicity (rat, mouse, rabbit)

(Fig. 22-2): (1) accidental and/or suicidal poisonings that no amount of legislation or study can prevent, (2) occupational (manufacturing, mixing/loading, application, harvesting, and handling of crops) exposure, (3) exposure of bystanders to off-target drift from spraying operations, and (4) members of the general public who consume food items containing pesticide residues as a consequence of the illegal use or misuse of an agent, resulting in residue concentrations above established tolerance levels.

Minimal protection of certain parts of the body can reduce exposure to an agent markedly. Protection of the hands (5.6 percent of the body surface) by appropriate chemical-resistant gloves may reduce contamination by 33 percent (in forest spraying with a knapsack sprayer having a single-nozzle lance), 66 percent (in weed control using tractor-mounted booms equipped with hydraulic nozzles), or 86 percent (filling tanks on tractor-powered sprayers). Dermal absorption of pesticides varies, with the greatest uptake being in the scrotal region, followed

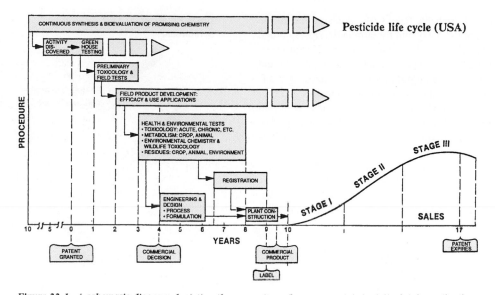

Figure 22-1. A schematic diagram depicting the generation of an appropriate toxicity database, the time frame for data acquisition, and the significant milestones in the life cycle of a pesticide in the United States. Stages I to III represent the sales of the pesticide once the commercial product enters the marketplace.

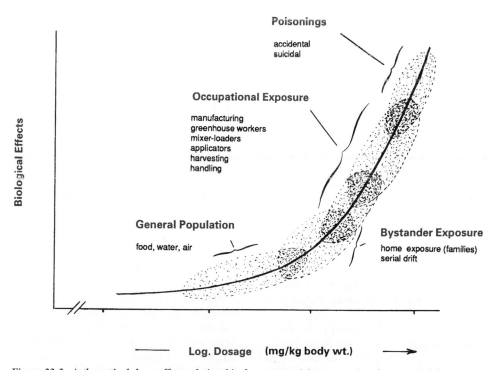

Figure 22-2. A theoretical dose–effect relationship for acute toxicity, comparing the potential for exposure in terms of occupation, level of exposure, and possible biological effects.

by the axilla, forehead, face, scalp, dorsal aspect of the hand, palm of the hand, and forearm in decreasing order.

The exposure of a bystander is more difficult to assess. Lower levels of exposure make residue analysis and the detection of meaningful biological changes more difficult. Greater variation in exposure estimates and biological effects can be anticipated. The adverse health effects may be subtle in appearance and nonspecific. The identification of pesticide-related adverse health effects in persons who inadvertently acquire low levels of pesticides daily from food and water is extremely difficult. Any biological effects resulting from such low-level exposure are unlikely to be distinctive. Any causal association with a chemical is tenuous and is confounded by lifestyle factors.

INSECTICIDES

All chemical insecticides in use today poison the nervous systems of the target organisms. The central nervous system (CNS) of insects is highly developed and is similar to that of mammals. The peripheral nervous system (PNS) of insects is not as complex as that of mammals. Insecticides are not selective and affect nontarget species as readily as target organisms. Potential sites of action of insecticides (Fig. 22-3) include interference with membrane transport of sodium, potassium, calcium, and chloride ions; inhibition of selective enzymatic activities; and contribution to the release and/or persistence of neurotransmitters at nerve endings.

Organochlorine Compounds

The organochlorine insecticides receive continued use in developing tropical countries because they are effective, inexpensive, and essential chemicals in agriculture, forestry, and public health. Low volatility, chemical stability, high lipid solubility, and slow rates of degradation contribute to their persistence in the environment, bioconcentration and biomagnification in food chains, and the acquisition of biologically active body burdens at higher trophic levels.

Signs and Symptoms of Poisoning The signs and symptoms of toxicity and the mechanisms of action of insecticides differ according to the chemical class (Table 22-2).

DDT poisoning affects CNS function in humans, but major pathologic changes are observed in the liver and reproductive organs. Hypertrophy of hepatocytes and subcellular organelles such as mitochondria, proliferation of smooth endoplasmic reticulum, centrolobular

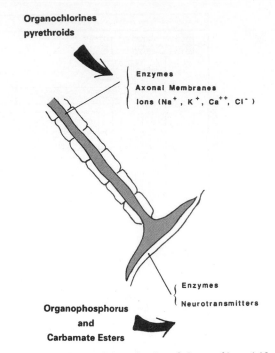

Figure 22-3. Potential sites of action of classes of insecticides on the axon and terminal portions of the nerve.

necrosis after exposure to high concentrations, and an increase in the incidence of hepatic tumors have been noted. In a study, DDT in male cockerels or rats reduced testicular size, and in female rats, the estrogenic effects on the oviduct and uterus contribute to problems in initiating and/or maintaining a pregnancy.

Site and Mechanism of Toxic Actions An insect or mammal poisoned with DDT-type agents displays periodic persistent tremoring and/or convulsive seizures that are suggestive of repetitive discharges in neurons. These repetitive tremors and seizures can be initiated by tactile and auditory stimuli.

At least four mechanisms, possibly all functioning simultaneously, could be involved in these effects of DDT (Fig. 22-4). DDT reduces potassium transport across the membrane. DDT alters the porous channels through which sodium ions pass. These channels activate (open) normally but are inactivated (closed) slowly, thus interfering with the active transport of sodium out of the nerve axon during repolarization. DDT inhibits neuronal adenosine triphosphatases (ATPase), particularly Na^+, K^+-ATPase and Ca^{2+}-ATPase, which play vital roles in neuronal repolarization. DDT also inhibits the

Table 22-2
Signs and Symptoms of Acute and Chronic Toxicity After Exposure to Organochlorine Insecticides

INSECTICIDE CLASS	ACUTE SIGNS	CHRONIC SIGNS
Dichlorodiphenylethanes		
DDT	Paresthesia (oral ingestion)	Loss of weight, anorexia
DDD (Rothane)	Ataxia, abnormal stepping	Mild anemia
DMC (Dimite)	Dizziness, confusion, headache	Tremors
Dicofol (Kelthane)	Nausea, vomiting	Muscular weakness
Methoxychlor	Fatigue, lethargy	EEG pattern changes
Methiochlor	Tremor (peripheral)	Hyperexcitability, anxiety
Chlorbenzylate		Nervous tension
Hexachlorocyclohexanes		
Lindane (γ-isomer)		
Benzene hexachloride		
(mixed isomers)		
Cyclodienes		
Endrin	Dizziness, headache	Headache, dizziness,
Telodrin	Nausea, vomiting	hyperexcitability
Isodrin	Motor hyperexcitability	Intermittent muscle twitching
Endosulfan	Hyperreflexia	and myoclonic jerking
Heptachlor	Myoclonic jerking	Psychological disorders,
Aldrin	General malaise	including insomnia,
Dieldrin	Convulsive seizures	anxiety, irritability
Chlordane	Generalized convulsions	EEG pattern changes
Toxaphene		Loss of consciousness
		Epileptiform convulsions
Chlordecone (Kepone)		Chest pains, arthralgia
Mirex		Skin rashes
		Ataxia, incoordination, slurred
		speech, opsoclonus
		Visual difficulty, inability to
		focus and fixate
		Nervousness, irritability, depression
		Loss of recent memory
		Muscle weakness, tremors of hands
		Severe impairment of spermatogenesis

ability of calmodulin, a calcium mediator in nerves, to transport calcium ions that are essential for the release of neurotransmitters. All these inhibited functions reduce the rate of depolarization and increase the sensitivity of neurons to small stimuli that would not elicit a response in a fully depolarized neuron.

The chlorinated cyclodiene-, benzene-, and cyclohexane-type insecticides differ from DDT (Table 22-2), although the overall appearance of an intoxicated individual is CNS stimulation. As is shown in Fig. 22-5, the cyclodiene compounds antagonize the action of the neu-rotransmitter gamma-aminobutyric acid (GABA) acting at the $GABA_A$ receptors, effectively blocking the GABA-induced uptake of chloride ions. The cyclodienes are also potent inhibitors of Na^+,K^+-ATPase and Ca^{2+},Mg^{2+}-ATPase, which are essential for the transport of calcium across membranes. Gamma-hexachlorocyclohexane (γ-HCH, lindane) neurotoxicity is related primarily to the blockade of chloride ion flux through the inotropic $GABA_A$ receptors. The inhibition of Ca^{2+},Mg^{2+}-ATPase in the synaptic membranes results in an accumulation of intracellular free calcium ions, which promotes the

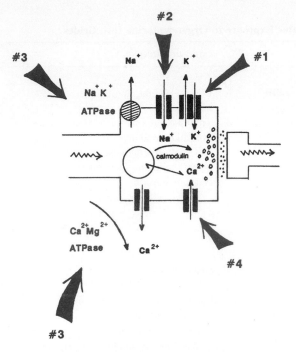

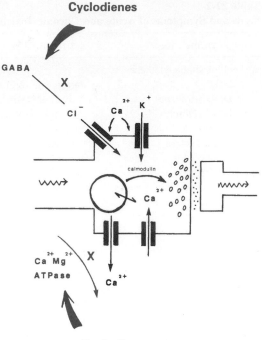

Cyclodienes

Cyclodienes

Figure 22-4. Proposed sites of action of DDT in (1) reducing potassium transport through pores, (2) inactivating sodium channel closure, (3) inhibiting sodium-potassium and calcium-magnesium ATPases, and (4) calmodulin-calcium binding with the release of neurotransmitter.

Figure 22-5. Proposed sites of action of cyclodiene-type organochlorine insecticides in chloride ion transport through inhibition of the GABA$_A$ receptor channel as well as inhibition of calcium-magnesium ATPase.

release of neurotransmitters from storage vesicles, the subsequent depolarization of adjacent neurons, and the propagation of stimuli throughout the CNS.

Biotransformation, Distribution, and Storage Biotransformation and degradation proceed exceptionally slowly. These highly lipophilic agents are sequestered in body tissue with a high lipid content. In the case of adipose tissue, the agents remain stored and undisturbed, as only small amounts equilibrate with blood and are degraded and/or excreted.

Anticholinesterase Agents

Today there are some 200 different organophosphorus ester insecticides and approximately 25 carbamic acid ester insecticides in the marketplace (Fig. 22-6), formulated into literally thousands of products. Although all the organophosphorus esters were derived from "nerve gases" (chemicals such as soman, sarin, and tabun), the insecticides used today are at least four generations of development away from those highly toxic chemicals.

Organophosphorus Esters

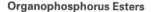

Carbamate Esters

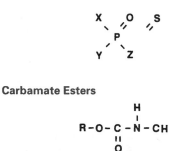

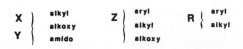

Figure 22-6. The basic backbone structures of the two types of anticholinesterase-class insecticides: the organophosphorus and carbamate esters.

Table 22-3
Signs and Symptoms of Anticholinesterase Insecticide Poisoning

NERVOUS TISSUE AND RECEPTORS AFFECTED	SITE AFFECTED	MANIFESTATIONS
Parasympathetic autonomic (muscarinic receptors) postganglionic nerve fibers	Exocrine glands	Increased salivation, lacrimation, perspiration
	Eyes	Miosis (pinpoint and nonreactive), ptosis, blurring of vision, conjunctival injection, "bloody tears"
	Gastrointestinal tract	Nausea, vomiting, abdominal tightness, swelling and cramps, diarrhea, tenesmus, fecal incontinence
	Respiratory tract	Excessive bronchial secretions, rhinorrhea, wheezing, edema, tightness in chest, bronchospasms, bronchoconstriction, cough, bradypnea, dyspnea
	Cardiovascular system	Bradycardia, decrease in blood pressure
	Bladder	Urinary frequency and incontinence
Parasympathetic and sympathetic autonomic fibers (nicotinic receptors)	Cardiovascular system	Tachycardia, pallor, increase in blood pressure
Somatic motor nerve fibers (nicotine receptors)	Skeletal muscles	Muscle fasciculations (eyelids, fine facial muscles), cramps, diminished tendon reflexes, generalized muscle weakness in peripheral and respiratory muscles, paralysis, flaccid or rigid tone
		Restlessness, generalized motor activity, reaction to acoustic stimuli, tremulousness, emotional lability, ataxia
Brain (acetylcholine receptors)	Central nervous system	Drowsiness, lethargy, fatigue, mental confusion, inability to concentrate, headache, pressure in head, generalized weakness
		Coma with absence of reflexes, tremors, Cheyne-Stokes respiration, dyspnea, convulsions, depression of respiratory centers, cyanosis

Signs and Symptoms of Poisoning Organophosphorus and carbamate ester insecticides elicit their toxicity through inhibition of acetylcholinesterase (AChE), the enzyme responsible for the destruction and termination of the biological activity of the neurotransmitter acetylcholine (ACh). With the accumulation of free, unbound ACh at the nerve endings of all cholinergic nerves, there is continual stimulation of electrical activity of the autonomic nervous system, the neuromusclar junction, and the CNS (Table 22-3).

There are additional and persistent signs of neurotoxicity. Frequently associated with exposure to high concentrations of insecticides, effects lasting for several months after exposure may involve neurobehavioral, cognitive, and neuromuscular functions such as persistently lowered vitality and ambition; defective autonomic regulation that leads to gastrointestinal and cardiovascular symptoms; premature decline in potency and libido; intolerance to alcohol, nicotine, and various medicines; and an impression of premature aging. These organoneurologic defects may develop and persist for some 5 to 10 years.

A second distinct manifestation of exposure to organophosphorus ester insecticides is a paralytic condition called the *intermediate syndrome*. Neurologic signs that appear 24 to 96 h after the acute cholinergic crisis include muscle weakness, primarily involving muscles innervated by the cranial nerves (neck flexors, muscles of respiration) as well as those of the limbs. Cranial nerve palsies are common. There is a distinct risk of death from the respiratory depression. The chemicals involved in the intermediate syndrome included fenthion, dimethoate, monocrotophos, and methamidophos.

A third syndrome, organophosphate-induced delayed neurotoxicity (OPIDN), is caused by tri-*o*-tolyl phosphate (TOTP, TOCP for tri-*o*-cresyl phosphate), mipafox, leptophos, omethoate, trichloronate, trichlorfon, parathion, methamidophos, fenthion, and chlorpyrifos. The initial flaccidity, which is characterized by muscle weakness in the arms and legs, giving rise to a clumsy shuffling gait, is replaced by spasticity, hypertonicity, hyperreflexia, clonus, and abnormal reflexes that are indicative of damage to the pyramidal tracts and a permanent upper motor neuron syndrome. A wallerian "dying-back" degeneration of large-diameter axons and their myelin sheaths occurs in distal parts of the peripheral nerves and long spinal cord tracts. The agents mentioned above inhibit a neuronal nonspecific carboxylesterase: neuropathic target esterase (NTE). If acute exposure to an appropriate organophosphorus ester results in >70 percent inhibition of NTE, the characteristic OPIDN usually follows 7 to 14 days after exposure and progresses from ataxia to moderate to severe muscular weakness and paralysis.

The signs and symptoms of acute intoxication by carbamate insecticides differ from those described for organophosphorus compounds in regard to the duration and intensity of the toxicity. Carbamate insecticides are reversible inhibitors of nervous tissue AChE and are biotransformed rapidly in vivo. There is little evidence of prolonged neurotoxicity, and carbamate ester insecticides do not inhibit NTE or elicit OPIDN-type neurotoxicity.

Site and Mechanism of Toxic Action   The reaction between an organophosphorus ester and the active site in the AChE protein (a serine hydroxyl group) results in the formation of a transient intermediate complex that partially hydrolyzes with the loss of the "Z" substituent group, leaving a stable, phosphorylated, and largely unreactive inhibited enzyme (Fig. 22-7). With many organophosphorus ester insecticides, an irreversibly inhibited enzyme is formed. Without intervention, the toxicity persists until sufficient quantities of "newly synthesized" AChE are available 20 to 30 days later to destroy excess acetylcholine.

In contrast, carbamic acid esters, which attach to the reactive site of AChE, undergo hydrolysis in two stages: The first stage is the removal of the "X" substituent (an aryl or alkyl group) with the formation of a carbamylated enzyme; the second stage is the decarbamylation of the inhibited enzyme with the generation of free, active enzyme (Fig. 22-7). The rate of dephosphorylation or de-

Organophosphorus Ester

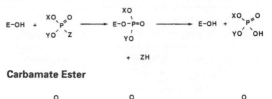

Carbamate Ester

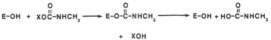

Figure 22-7. The interaction between an organophosphorus or carbamate ester with the serine hydroxyl groups in the active site of the enzyme acetylcholinesterase (E-OH). The intermediate, unstable complexes formed before the release of the "leaving" groups (ZH and XOH) are not shown. The dephosphorylation or decarbamoylation of the inhibited enzyme is the rate-limiting step to forming free enzymes.

carbamylation is exceedingly slow for organophosphorus esters and is very rapid for carbamate esters, which are considered reversible inhibitors. The organophosphates sarin, soman, tabun, DFP, mipafox, and leptophos bind tenaciously to the active site of AChE and NTE to produce an irreversibly inhibited enzyme through a mechanism known as *aging*. The aging process is caused by the dealkylation of the dialkylphosphorylated enzyme intermediates. The aging process is believed to fix an extra charge to the protein, causing some perturbation to the active site and thus preventing dephosphorylation.

Biotransformation, Distribution, and Storage   The organophosphorus and carbamate ester insecticides undergo extensive metabolism, which is highly species-specific and is dependent on the substituent chemical groups attached to the basic "backbone" structure of these esters. Both phase I (oxidative, reductive, hydrolytic) and phase II (transfer or conjugative reactions with glutathione, glucuronic acid, glycine) reactions are found in plant, invertebrate, and vertebrate species.

Pyrethroid Esters

Natural pyrethrum consists of a mixture of six esters, producing an effective contact and stomach poison mixture with both knockdown and lethality. Synthetic esters demonstrate selectivity toward certain insect species.

Signs and Symptoms of Poisoning   On the basis of the symptoms produced in animals that receive acute toxic

Table 22-4
Classification of Pyrethroid Ester Insecticides on the Basis of Chemical Structure and Observed Biological Activity

| | Signs and Symptoms | | |
SYNDROME	COCKROACH	RAT	CHEMICALS
Type I ("T" syndrome)	Restlessness Incoordination Prostration Paralysis	Hyperexcitation Sparring Aggressiveness Enhanced startle response Whole-body tremor Prostration	Allethrin Cismethrin Phenothrin Pyrethrin I Resmethrin Tetramethrin
Type II ("CS" syndrome)	Hyperactivity Incoordination Convulsions	Burrowing Dermal tingling Clonic seizures Writhing Profuse salivation	Acrinathrin Cycloprothrin Cyfluthrin Cyhalothrin Cyphenothrin Cypermethrin Deltamethrin Esfenvalerate Fenvalerate Flucynthrate Fluvalinate

doses, the pyrethroids fall into two distinct classes (Table 22-4). The type I poisoning syndrome, or *T syndrome,* is produced by esters that lack the α-cyano substituent and is characterized by restlessness, incoordination, prostration, and paralysis in the cockroach, in contrast to the rat, which exhibits sparring and aggressive behavior, an enhanced startle response, whole-body tremor, and prostration. The type II syndrome, or *CS* (choreoathetosis/salivation) *syndrome,* is produced by esters that contain the α-cyano substituent and elicits intense hyperactivity, incoordination, and convulsions in cockroaches, in contrast to rats, which display burrowing behavior, coarse tremors, clonic seizures, sinuous writhing (choreoathetosis), and profuse salivation without lacrimation. A few agents, such as fenpropanthrin, cause mixed type I and type II effects.

Although these insecticides are not highly toxic to mammals, pyrethrum can cause contact dermatitis, asthma-like attacks, anaphylactic reactions, and peripheral vascular collapse. Human toxicity associated with the natural pyrethrins stems from their allergenic properties. There has been little evidence of allergic-type reactions in humans exposed to synthetic pyrethroid esters.

Occupational exposure produces variable toxicity. Acute exposure to deltamethrin and fenvalerate can result in dizziness and a burning, itching, or tingling sensation of the exposed skin. The signs and symptoms disappear by 24 h after exposure. Spilling these agents on the head, face, and eyes can result in pain, lacrimation, photophobia, congestion, and edema of the conjunctiva and eyelids. Ingestion caused epigastric pain, nausea, vomiting, headache, dizziness, anorexia, fatigue, tightness in the chest, blurred vision, paresthesia, palpitations, coarse muscular fasciculations, and disturbances of consciousness. In severe poisonings, convulsive attacks with opisthotonos and loss of consciousness have occurred. No chronic toxicity has been reported.

Site and Mechanism of Toxicity Both type I and type II esters affect the activation (opening) and inactivation (closing) of the sodium channel, resulting in a hyperexcitable state. Type I esters hold sodium channels open for a relatively short period (milliseconds), whereas type II esters keep the channel open for a prolonged period (up to seconds). Pyrethroid esters also inhibit calcium channels and Ca^{2+},Mg^{2+}-ATPase.

Biotransformation, Distribution, and Storage There is little storage or accumulation of pyrethroid esters. Although pyrethroid esters are susceptible to hydrolysis by nonspecific carboxylesterases, the microsomal monooxygenase system found in the tissues of almost all species is involved extensively in the detoxification of pyrethroid esters in mammals and of some of these agents in insect and fish species. The importance of oxidative detoxification is demonstrated by the fact that the inclusion of piperonyl butoxide, a classic monooxygenase inhibitor, in preparations enhances the potency of pyrethroid esters 10- to 300-fold.

Avermectins

The avermectins were isolated from a culture of the actinomycete *Streptomyces avermitilis* and may be used for a wide range of ecto- and endoparasites of domestic and wild animals. The semisynthetic ivermectin, avermectins B1a and B1b, and emamectin (MK-244), a derivative of avermectin B1, are highly lipid-soluble, although dermal absorption accounts for less than 1.0 percent of the applied dose. Minimal oxidative biotransformation occurs. Ivermectin is the drug of choice in treating onchocerciasis (river blindness) in humans, because ivermectin treatment can limit the source of infection.

Avermectins have low water solubility and extensive nonspecific binding. These agents open GABA-insensitive chloride channels, reducing membrane resistance and increasing conductance inward.

Newer Chemical Insecticides

Three types of new agents are available in the marketplace: (1) the nitromethylene heterocycles, which were developed from the cyclodienes and cyclohexanes, (2) the nitroimino derivatives (chloronicotinyl and neonicotinoids), which are similar to nicotine, and (3) the phenylpyrazoles. These chemicals are highly specific for receptors in insect nervous systems, are effective at low application rates (8 to 10 g/ha), are not environmentally persistent, and show negligible toxicity for vertebrates. There have been no reports of toxicity in humans.

Nitromethylenes The nitromethylene heterocycle (NMH) insecticides are fast-acting neurotoxicants that are effective by both contact and oral ingestion. They are relatively safe to vertebrates and degrade rapidly in the environment. The NMHs act as neurotransmitter mimics, having both excitatory and depressant effects, eventually blocking postsynaptic nicotinic receptors.

Chloronicotinyl The nitroimino heterocycles, which are best known in the compound imidacloprid, have high potency in insects, with exceptionally low mammalian toxicity and a favorable persistence. Imidacloprid binds specifically to nicotinic ACh receptors in various insects' nervous systems and acts as a partial agonist.

Phenylpyrazoles The phenylpyrazole derivatives show extensive insecticidal, herbicidal, and miticidal properties. Fipronil blocks the passage of chloride ions through the GABA-regulated chloride channel, disrupting CNS activity. Fipronil is biotransformed to the corresponding sulfone, which is still a potent insecticide. This conversion can be blocked by piperonyl butoxide, a cytochrome P450 inhibitor.

BOTANICAL INSECTICIDES

Nicotine

Nicotine has been used as a contact insecticide, stomach poison, and fumigant. Extracted from the leaves of *Nicotiana tabacum* and *N. rustica,* nicotine is extremely toxic, is readily absorbed through the skin, and mimics or blocks, depending on the dose, the action of acetylcholine at all ganglionic synapses and at neuromuscular junctions. As an insecticide, nicotine blocks synapses associated with motor nerves.

Rotenoids

Rotenoid esters can be isolated from the plants *Derris eliptica, Lonchocarpus utilis,* and *L. urucu.* Rotenone, one of the alkaloids, can be used either as a contact poison or as a stomach poison. Since rotenone is unstable in light and heat, its toxicity can be lost after 2 to 3 days. Acute poisoning in animals is characterized by an initial respiratory stimulation followed by respiratory depression, ataxia, convulsions, and death from respiratory arrest. Rotenone blocks electron transport in mitochondria by inhibiting oxidation linked to $NADH_2$, resulting in nerve conduction blockade. Rotenone dust is highly irritating to the eyes (causing conjunctivitis), skin (causing contact dermatitis), upper respiratory tract (causing rhinitis), and throat (linked with pharyngitis).

HERBICIDES

A herbicide is any compound that is capable of killing or severely injuring plants. Herbicides may be classified by how and when the agents are applied. *Preplanting* her-

Table 22-5
Mechanisms of Action of Herbicides

MECHANISM(S)	CHEMICAL CLASSES
Inhibition of photosynthesis by disruption of light reactions and blockade of electron transport	Ureas, 1,3,5-triazines, 1,4-triazines, uracils, pyridazones, 4-hydroxybenzonitriles, N-arylcarbamates, acylanilides
Inhibition of respiration by blockade of electron transfer from NADH or blocking the coupling of electron transfer to ADP to form ATP	Dinitrophenols Halophenols
Growth stimulants, "auxins"	Aryloxyalkylcarboxylic acids, benzoic acids
Inhibitors of cell and nucleus division	Alkyl N-arylcarbamates
Inhibitors of protein synthesis	Dinitroanilines
Inhibition of carotenoid synthesis, protective pigments in chloroplasts that prevent chlorophyll from being destroyed by oxidative reactions	Chloracetamide, hydrazines, o-substituted diphenyl ethers
Inhibition of lipid synthesis	S-alkyl dialkylcarbamodithioates Aliphatic chlorocarboxylic acids
Inhibition of acetolase synthase	Sulfonylureas, imidazolines, triazolopyrimidines, sulfonamides
Inhibition of protoporphyrinogen oxidase	Diphenyl ethers, heterocyclic phenyl ethers (benzotriazoles, indolinones, benzisoxazoles, quinoxalindones, benzoxazines)
Inhibition of enolpyruvylshikimate-3-phosphate synthetase	Glyphosate
Inhibition of glutamine synthetase	Glufosinate
Unknown mechanisms, nonselective chemicals	Inorganic agents (copper sulfate, sulfuric acid, sodium chlorate, sodium borate) Organic agents (dichlobenil, benzoylpropethyl, chlorthiamid, bentazone)

bicides are applied to the soil before a crop is seeded. *Preemergent* herbicides are applied to the soil before the usual time of appearance of the unwanted vegetation. *Postemergent* herbicides are applied to the soil or foliage after the germination of the crop and/or weeds. Based on their mechanism of toxicity in plants, herbicides may be referred to as *selective* (toxic to some species), *contact* (act when impinging on the plant foliage), or *translocated* (absorbed via the soil or through the foliage).

Table 22-5 lists the mechanisms of herbicides representative of several chemical classifications and diverse structures. In general, these chemicals have relatively low acute toxicity, and subchronic and chronic studies have shown minimal significant biological effects. Low application rates minimize nontarget species toxicity and environmental contamination.

Most herbicides are dermal irritants, causing skin rashes and contact dermatitis. Subpopulations of individuals who are hypersensitive to dermal contact may present with moderate to severe urticaria that persists for 5 to 10 days after exposure. Individuals who are prone to allergic reactions may experience severe contact dermatitis, asthma-like attacks, and even anaphylactic reactions after dermal contact or inhalation. The herbicides discussed below can elicit a range of acute and chronic effects after exposure.

Chlorophenoxy Compounds

The chlorophenoxy compounds mimic the action of auxins, hormones that stimulate growth. Concerns over the formation of chlorinated dibenzofurans and dibenzodioxins, particularly 2,3,7,8-tetrachlorodibenzo-*p*-dioxin (TCDD), as a consequence of poorly monitored manufacturing practices or improper product storage have led to reduced use in some countries.

Accidental and/or occupational intoxications lead to acute skin, eye, and respiratory tract irritation; headache;

dizziness; nausea; acneiform eruptions; chloracne; severe muscle pain in the thorax, shoulders, and extremities; fatigue; nervousness; irritability; dyspnea; complaints of decreased libido; and intolerance to cold. Although chloracne is observed consistently in almost all incidents of chlorophenoxy herbicide exposure, this is not a specific effect because other halogenated aromatic compounds (polyhalogenated biphenyls, dibenzo-*p*-dioxins, dibenzofurans, and naphthalenes) can induce chloracne.

Bipyridyl Derivatives

Paraquat is still used in some 130 countries and is one of the most specific pulmonary toxicants known. A high mortality rate is encountered in poisonings. The signs and symptoms include lethargy, hypoxia, dyspnea, tachycardia, hyperpnea, adipsia, diarrhea, ataxia, hyperexcitability, and convulsions. Necropsy of exposed animals reveals hemorrhagic and edematous lungs, pulmonary fibrosis, centrilobular hepatic necrosis, and renal tubular necrosis. Lung weights increase significantly despite marked losses in body weight. The same histopathologic picture of pulmonary lesions is observed in mice, rats, dogs, and humans.

Paraquat has poor oral absorption and minimal metabolism by mammalian tissue and undergoes primarily renal excretion. Paraquat concentrates in lung owing to a unique diamine/polyamine transport system in the alveolar cells. Upon uptake, paraquat undergoes an NADPH-dependent one-electron reduction to a free radical, which can attack membrane lipids. Destruction of alveolar cells, invasion of the space by fibroblasts, loss of pulmonary elasticity, and inefficient gas (O_2, CO_2) exchange ensue.

The ingestion of commercial paraquat concentrates is invariably fatal and runs a time course of 3 to 4 weeks. The initial irritation and burning of the mouth and throat, severe gastroenteritis with esophageal and gastric lesions, abdominal and substernal chest pains, and bloody stools give way to dyspnea, anoxia, opacity in the lungs seen in chest x-rays, progressive fibrosis, coma, and death. Although pulmonary damage is extensive, paraquat also induces multiorgan toxicity with necrotic damage to the liver, kidneys, and myocardial muscle plus extensive hemorrhagic incidents throughout the body.

Diquat is a rapid-acting contact herbicide that is slightly less toxic than paraquat; it has poor absorption from the gastrointestinal tract. The major target organs are the gastrointestinal tract, liver, and kidneys, and in a study there was an increased incidence of cataracts. Diquat can form free radicals, and tissue necrosis is associated with superoxide-induced peroxidation as is ob-

served with paraquat. Diquat shows no special affinity for the lung.

Chloroacetanilides

Alachlor, acetochlor, amidochlor, butachlor, metalaxyl, metolachlor, and propachlor control annual grasses and broad-leaf weeds by interfering with protein synthesis and root elongation. All these agents show mutagenic activity mediated by metabolites. One example, acetochlor, is converted into a rat-specific metabolite that may be related to nasal tumors, thus posing no genetic or carcinogenic hazard to humans.

Phosphonomethyl Amino Acids

N-Phosphonomethyl glycine (glyphosate, Roundup, Vision) and *N*-phosphonomethyl homoalanine (glufosinate, Basta) have been used in attempted suicides in southeastern Asia. Both agents are broad-spectrum nonselective systemic herbicides for postemergent control of annual and perennial plants (grasses, sedges, broad-leaf weeds) and woody plants.

Glyphosate Glyphosate inhibits the enzyme 5-enolpyruvyl-shikimate-3-phosphate synthetase (EPSPS), an enzyme of the aromatic amino acid biosynthesis pathway that is essential for protein synthesis in plants. Although not a dermal irritant in animals, glyphosate is an ocular irritant in rabbits and humans. No carcinogenicity has been observed in mice, rats, or dogs.

Glyphosate is replacing paraquat as a suicidal agent in many countries. Mild intoxications are characterized by gastrointestinal symptoms (nausea, vomiting, diarrhea, abdominal pain) resulting from mucosal irritation and injury, with resolution within 24 h. In moderate intoxications, intestinal ulceration, esophagitis, and hemorrhage are seen, along with hypotension, some pulmonary dysfunction, acid-base disturbance, and evidence of hepatic and renal damage. Severe poisoning is characterized by pulmonary dysfunction, renal failure, cardiac arrest, repeated seizures, coma, and death.

Glufosinate Glufosinate irreversibly inhibits the plant enzyme glutamine synthetase, which decreases ammonia detoxification. Increased ammonia levels lead to impairment of photorespiration and photosynthesis.

Early clinical symptoms of glufosinate ammonium poisoning include nausea, vomiting, and diarrhea that is followed in 24 h by impaired respiration; seizures; muscle weakness (post–status epileptic myopathy); convulsions; and even death. For both glyphosate and gluphosphinate, concerns have been raised about whether polyoxyethyleneamine, the surfactant, may be responsible for death.

FUNGICIDES

Foliar fungicides are applied as liquids or powders to the aerial green parts of plants, producing a protective barrier on the cuticular surface and systemic toxicity in the developing fungus. *Soil fungicides* are applied as liquids, dry powders, or granules, acting through either the vapor phase or systemic properties. *Dressing fungicides* are applied to the postharvest crop (cereal grains, tubers, corms, etc.) as liquids or dry powders to prevent fungal infestation of the crop.

Fungicides may be described as protective, curative, or eradicative according to their mode of action. *Protective fungicides*, which are applied to the plant before the appearance of any phytopathic fungi, prevent infection either by sporicidal activity or by changing the physiologic environment on the leaf surface. *Curative fungicides* function by penetrating the plant cuticle and destroying the young fungal mycelium (the hyphae) growing in the epidermis of the plant. *Eradicative fungicides* control fungal development after the appearance of symptoms, usually after sporulation, by killing both the new spores and the mycelia.

An effective fungicide must have the following properties: (1) low toxicity to the plant but high toxicity to the particular fungus, (2) activity per se or the ability to convert itself (by plant or fungal enzymes) into a toxic intermediate, (3) ability to penetrate fungal spores or the developing mycelium to reach a site of action, and (4) formation of a protective, tenacious deposit on the plant surface that will be resistant to weathering by sunlight, rain, and wind. All commercially available compounds show some phytotoxicity and lack of persistence because of environmental degradation.

Most fungicides have low toxicity to mammals (Table 22-6). However, all fungicides are cytotoxic and most produce positive results in in vitro microbial mutagenicity test systems. Public concern has focused on the positive mutagenicity tests obtained with many fungicides and the fact that nearly 90 percent of all agricultural fungicides are carcinogenic in animal models.

Hexachlorobenzene

Hexachlorobenzene (HCB) causes a syndrome, called *black sore,* that is characterized by dermal blistering and epidermolysis, pigmentation and scarring, alopecia, photo-

sensitivity, hepatomegaly, porphyria, suppurative arthritis, osteomyelitis, and osteoporosis of the bones of the hands.

HCB has chemical stability, slow degradation and biotransformation, environmental persistence, bioaccumulation in adipose tissue, and the ability to induce cytochrome P450 and conjugative enzymes. Repeated exposure of animals results in hepatomegaly, porphyria, and focal alopecia with itching and eruptions, followed by pigmented scars, anorexia, irritability, ataxia, and tremors. In a study, hexachlorobenzene was particularly toxic to developing perinatal animals, causing hepatomegaly, hydronephrosis, and renomegaly.

Dithiocarbamates

The nomenclature of dimethyl- and ethylene-bisdithiocarbamate (EBDC) compounds arises from the metal cations with which they are associated; for instance, dimethyldithiocarbamic acid bound to iron or zinc is ferbam or ziram, respectively, whereas EBDC compounds associated with sodium, manganese, or zinc are nabam, maneb, or zineb, respectively. These chemicals have environmental stability, provide good foliar protection, and have low acute toxicity.

Although toxicity is negligible in animal feeding trials even at high doses, acceptance of these agents has been marred by reported adverse health effects. Maneb, nabam, and zineb have been reported to be teratogenic. Mancozeb has been associated with abnormally shaped sperm. Maneb has been associated with adverse reproductive outcomes in the pregnancy rate, the estrous cycle, and fetal development. These concerns, along with knowledge that the EBDC compounds degrade into ethylene thiourea (ETU), a known mutagen, teratogen, and carcinogen as well as an antithyroid compound, have raised suspicions about these agents and fostered requests for more in-depth studies.

FUMIGANTS

These agents are used to kill insects, nematodes, weed seeds, and fungi in soil as well as in silo-stored cereal grains, fruits and vegetables, clothes, and other consumables, with the treatment carried out in enclosed spaces because of the volatility of most of these products. Fumigants range from acrylonitrile and carbon disulfide to carbon tetrachloride, ethylene dibromide, chloropicrin, and ethylene oxide.

Phosphine

Used extensively as a grain fumigant, phosphine (PH_3) is released from aluminum phosphide (AlP) by the

Table 22-6
Acute Toxicity of Fungicides

COMMON NAME	CLASS	IRRITATION* (EYE/SKIN)	ORAL LD$_{50}$, RAT (mg/kg)
Anilazine	Triazine	I	2,710
Benomyl	Imidazole	I	>10,000
Captan	Phthalimide	I	8,400–15,000
Carboxin	Oxathiin	NI	3,820
Chinomethionate	Quinomethionate	NI	2,500–3,000
Chlorothalonil	Organochlorine	I	>10,000
Dichloropropene	Chlorinated alkene	I	130–713
Dinocap	Dinitrophenol	NI	980
Dodine	Aliphatic nitrogen	I	1,000
EPTC	Thiocarbamate	I	1,632
Etridiazole	Thiadiazole	NI	>1,000
Fenarimol	Pyrimidine	I	2,500
Hexachlorobenzene	Organochlorine	I	3,500
Imazalil	Imidazole	I	227–334
Iprodione	Dicarboximide	I	3,500
Maneb	Dithiocarbamate	I	5,000–8,000
Mancozeb	Dithiocarbamate	I	5,000–>11,200
Metalaxyl	Benzenoid	I	669
Metiram	Dithiocarbamate	I	6,180–>10,000
Nabam	Dithiocarbamate	I	395
Oxycarboxin	Oxathiin	NI	2,000
Pyrazophos	Phosphorothionate	NI	151–632
Quintozene	Organochlorine	I	1,710
Thiabendazole	Imidazole	NI	3,100–3,600
Thiophanate–Me	Dithiocarbamate	I	10,000
Thiram	Thiocarbamate	I	800–>1,900
Triallate	Thiocarbamate	I	800–2,165
Vinclozolin	Dicarboximide	I	>10,000
Zineb	Dithiocarbamate	I	7,600–8,900
Ziram	Dithiocarbamate	I	1,400

*KEY: I, irritant properties; NI, nonirritation.

natural moisture in the grain over a long period, giving continual protection during transhipment of the grain. Symptoms of PH$_3$ intoxication in adults include shortness of breath, cough and pulmonary irritation, nausea, headache, jaundice, and fatigue.

Ethylene Dibromide/ Dibromochloropropane

At relatively high (>200 ppm) concentrations, inhaled ethylene dibromide can cause pulmonary edema and inflammation in exposed animals. Repeated exposures to lower concentrations have produced centrolobular hepatic necrosis and proximal tubular damage in the kidneys. This chemical, along with 1,2-dibromo-3-chloropropane (DBCP), has had an adverse effect on testicular morphology and spermatogenesis in rats and humans.

RODENTICIDES

The black rat (*Rattus rattus*), the brown or Norway rat (*R. norvegicus*), and the house mouse (*Mus musculus*) pose particularly serious problems because they act as vectors for several human diseases.

To be effective yet safe, a rodenticide must (1) not be unpalatable to the target species and must be potent, (2) not induce bait shyness so that the animal will continue to eat it, (3) cause death in a manner that does not raise the suspicions of survivors, (4) make the intoxicated animal go out into the open to die (otherwise the rotting corpses create health hazards), and (5) be species-specific, with considerably lower toxicity to other animals that might inadvertently consume the bait or eat the poisoned rodent.

Accidental or intentional ingestion of most rodenticides poses a serious, acute toxicologic problem, and rodenticide poisoning is seen more frequently in children.

Zinc Phosphide

Widely used in developing nations because it is both cheap and effective, zinc phosphide hydrolyzes with water, producing PH_3 and causing widespread cellular toxicity with necrosis of the gut and injury to other organs, such as the liver and kidneys.

Signs of intoxication from accidental or suicidal poisonings include vomiting, diarrhea, cyanosis, tachycardia, rhales, restlessness, fever, and albuminuria several hours after exposure. Also, hypertension, pulmonary edema, dysrhythmias, and convulsions have been reported.

Fluoroacetic Acid and Derivatives

Sodium fluoroacetate and fluoroacetamide have extreme toxicity, which is facilitated by their ready absorption from the gastrointestinal tract. Fluoroacetate incorporates into fluoroacetyl–coenzyme A, which condenses with oxaloacetate to form fluorocitrate, which inhibits the enzyme aconitase and prevents the conversion of citrate to isocitrate in the tricarboxylic acid (Krebs) cycle. Inhibition of the Krebs cycle by fluorocitrate decreases glucose metabolism, cellular respiration, and tissue energy stores. These chemicals are uniquely effective in mice and rats because of the high metabolic rate in the tissues that are susceptible to inhibition.

In humans, gastrointestinal symptoms are seen initially some 30 to 100 min after ingestion. Initial nausea, vomiting, and abdominal pain are replaced by sinus tachycardia, ventricular tachycardia or fibrillation, hypotension, renal failure, muscle spasms, and CNS such symptoms as agitation, stupor, seizures, and coma. Histopathologic examination of postmortem samples has revealed cerebellar degeneration and atrophy. There are no known antidotes to fluoroacetate intoxication.

Anticoagulants

Coumadin (warfarin) antagonizes the actions of vitamin K in the synthesis of clotting factors II, VII, IX, and X. The onset of anticoagulation is delayed 8 to 12 h after the ingestion of warfarin owing to the half-lives of previously synthesized clotting factors. The safety of warfarin as a rodenticide rests with the fact that multiple doses are required before toxicity develops and the fact that single doses have little effect. The superwarfarins (brodifacoum, coumachlor, diphencoumarin) and the indanediones (diphacinone, chlorophacinone, pindone) differ from one another in terms of acute toxicity, rapidity of action, and acceptance by the rodent.

Human poisonings are rare. Nevertheless, after consumption over a period of days, bleeding of the gingiva and nose, bruising and hematomas developing at the knee and elbow joints and on the buttocks, gastrointestinal bleeding with dark tarry stools, hematuria accompanied by abdominal or low back pain, epistaxis, and cerebrovascular accidents occur. The signs and symptoms persist for many days after the cessation of exposure owing to the prolonged biological half-lives of the warfarins.

BIBLIOGRAPHY

Beadle JD (ed): *Progress in Neuropharmacology and Neurotoxicology of Pesticides and Drugs.* London: Royal Society of Chemistry, 1999.

Ecobichon DJ (ed): *Occupational Hazards of Pesticide Exposure. Sampling, Monitoring, Measuring.* Philadelphia, Taylor & Francis, 1998.

Krieger RI (ed): *Hayes' and Laws' Handbook of Pesticide Toxicology,* 3d ed. San Diego, CA: Academic Press, 2000.

Marrs TC, Balantyne B (eds): *Pesticide Toxicology.* New York: Wiley, 2002.

Whitford F: *The Complete Book of Pesticide Management: Science, Regulation, Stewardship, and Communication.* New York: Wiley, 2002.

C H A P T E R   2 3

TOXIC EFFECTS OF METALS

Robert A. Goyer and Thomas W. Clarkson

KEY POINTS

- Persons at either end of the life span—young children and elderly people—are more susceptible to toxicity from exposure to a particular level of metal than are most adults.
- Metals that provoke immune reactions include mercury, gold, platinum, beryllium, chromium, and nickel.
- *Complexation* is the formation of a metal ion complex in which the metal ion is associated with a charged or uncharged electron donor referred to as a *ligand.*
- *Chelation* occurs when bidentate ligands form ring structures that include the metal ion and the two ligand atoms attached to the metal.
- Metal-protein interactions include binding to numerous enzymes, the metallothioneins, proteins such as serum albumin and hemoglobin, and specific metal carrier proteins involved in the membrane transport of metals.

INTRODUCTION

The use of metals by humans influences environmental transport in air, water, soil, and food and alters the speciation or biochemical form of elements. Metals are redistributed naturally in the environment by both geologic and biological cycles (Fig. 23-1). Rainwater dissolves rocks and ores and physically transports material to streams and rivers, depositing and stripping materials from adjacent soil and eventually transporting those substances to the ocean to be precipitated as sediment or taken up in rainwater to be relocated elsewhere on earth. The biological cycles include bioconcentration by plants and animals and incorporation into food cycles. Human industrial activity may shorten the residence time of metals in ore greatly, form new compounds, and greatly enhance worldwide distribution by discharge to land, water, and the atmosphere.

DOSE–EFFECT RELATIONSHIPS

Relationships between sources of exposure, transport, and distribution to various organs and excretory pathways are shown in Fig. 23-2. The most precise definition of *dose* is the amount of metal within cells of organs that manifests a toxicologic effect. Results from single measurements may reflect recent exposure or longer-term or past exposure, depending on retention time in the particular tissue.

Blood, urine, and hair are the most accessible tissues in which to measure an exposure or dose. Blood and urine concentrations usually reflect recent exposure and correlate best with acute effects. An exception is urinary cadmium, which may reflect renal damage related to an accumulation of cadmium in the kidney. Speciation of toxic metals in urine also may provide diagnostic insights. For example, cadmium metallothionein in plasma or urine may be of greater toxicologic significance than is total cadmium. Finally, for most metals, hair is not a reliable tissue for measuring exposure because of metal deposits from external contamination that complicates analyses.

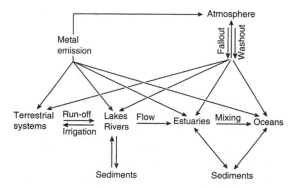

Figure 23-1. Routes for the transport of trace elements in the environment.

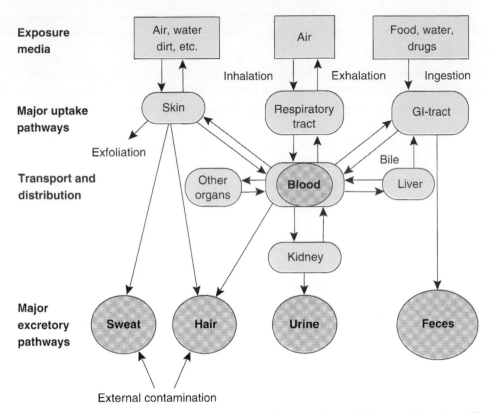

Figure 23-2. Metabolism after exposure to metals via skin absorption, inhalation, and ingestion. The arrows indicate how the metals are transported and distributed. Tissues that are particularly useful for biological monitoring are identified in shaded areas.

HOST FACTORS INFLUENCING THE TOXICITY OF METALS

A number of factors that influence the toxicity of metals are shown in Table 23-1. The interaction of toxic metals with essential metals occurs when the metabolism of a toxic metal is similar to that of the essential element. Ab-

Table 23-1
Factors Influencing the Toxicity of Metals

Interactions with essential metals
Formation of metal–protein complexes
Age and stage of development
Lifestyle factors
Chemical form or speciation
Immune status of host

sorption of toxic metals from the lung or gastrointestinal tract may be influenced by an essential metal, particularly if the toxic metal shares or influences a homeostatic mechanism, as occurs with lead and calcium and iron. Toxic metals may influence the role of essential metals as cofactors for enzymes or other metabolic processes (e.g., lead interferes with the calcium-dependent release of neurotransmitters).

Metalloprotein complexes that are involved in detoxification or protection from toxicity have been described for a few metals. Morphologically discernible cellular inclusion bodies are present with exposures to lead, bismuth, and a mercury-selenate mixture. Metallothioneins form complexes with cadmium, zinc, copper, and other metals, and ferritin and hemosiderin are intracellular iron-protein complexes. None of these proteins or metalprotein complexes have any known enzymatic activity.

Persons at either end of the life span—young children and elderly people—are more susceptible to toxicity from exposure to a particular level of metal than most adults are. The major pathway of exposure to many toxic metals in children is food, and children consume more calories per pound of body weight than adults do. Moreover, children have higher gastrointestinal absorption of metals, particularly lead. The rapid growth and rapid cell division that children's bodies experience provide opportunities for genotoxic effects.

Lifestyle factors such as smoking and alcohol ingestion may influence toxicity indirectly. Cigarette smoke contains some toxic metals, and cigarette smoking also may have pulmonary effects. Alcohol ingestion may affect toxicity indirectly by altering diet and reducing the intake of essential minerals.

For metals that produce hypersensitivity reactions, the immune status of an individual becomes an additional toxicologic variable. Metals that provoke immune reactions include mercury, gold, platinum, beryllium, chromium, and nickel. The clinical effects vary but usually involve any of four types of immune responses.

METAL-BINDING PROTEINS

Several kinds of metal-protein interactions may be considered. A protein may be the target of toxicity. Enzymes are the best-documented targets. A protein may play a protective role, reducing the toxicity of a metal. The metallothioneins are the best-known example. Nonspecific binding to proteins, such as serum albumin and hemoglobin, plays a role in metal transport in the bloodstream and in the distribution of metals between red blood cells and plasma. In addition, proteins with specific metal-binding properties are involved in the extracellular and intracellular transport of metals.

Specific Metal-Binding Proteins

The low-molecular-weight ($\sim$6000 Da) *metallothioneins* have high-affinity binding of several essential and nonessential metals, such as Cd, Cu, Hg, Ag, and Zn. The metallothioneins are highly inducible by a number of metals and other inducers.

Transferrin is a glycoprotein that binds most of the ferric iron in plasma. Transport of iron across cell membranes occurs by means of receptor-mediated endocytosis of ferric transferrin. This protein also transports Al and Mn.

Ferritin is primarily a storage protein for iron in the reticuloendothelial cells of the liver, spleen, and bone. Ferritin may serve as a general metal detoxicant, because it binds various toxic metals, including Cd, Zn, Be, and Al.

Ceruloplasmin is a copper-containing glycoprotein oxidase in plasma that converts ferrous iron to ferric iron, which then binds to transferrin. This protein also stimulates iron uptake by a transferrin-independent mechanism.

Membrane Carrier Proteins

A rapidly increasing number of carrier proteins are being discovered that transport metals across cell membranes and organelles inside cells. Although certain metals may be transported in free ionic forms, such as through calcium channels, many metals are transported as complexes with endogenous ligands on transport systems intended for the ligand itself.

Phosphate and sulfate transporters carry a number of metal oxyanions across the plasma membrane. Vanadate and arsenate are structurally similar to phosphate, whereas chromate, molybdate, and selenate are structurally similar to sulfate.

Amino acid and peptide transporters and organic solute carriers also accept metals as complexes with endogenous molecules such as amino acids, peptides, and bicarbonate. Cellular uptake of copper or zinc may occur in complexes with histidine; Methyl mercury is complexed with cysteine or glutathione. Zinc and lead may undergo uptake complexed.

Other examples of metal transporters include divalent cation transporters and ATP-activated membrane pumps. The human genome may contain as many as 9000 genes that code for transporter proteins, of which 2000 are involved with the transport of drugs and other xenobiotics. This rapidly expanding field is not sufficiently developed to identify polymorphisms of these protein carriers.

COMPLEXATION AND CHELATION THERAPY

Complexation is the formation of a metal ion complex in which the metal ion is associated with a charged or uncharged electron donor referred to as a *ligand*. The ligand may be monodentate, bidentate, or multidentate; that is, it may attach by using one, two, or more donor atoms. *Chelation* occurs when bidentate ligands form ring structures (*chelate* comes from the Greek word for "claw") that include the metal ion and the two ligand atoms attached to the metal. Metals may react with O-, S-, and N-containing ligands that are present in the form of OH, COOH, SH, NH_2, NH, and N.

Chelating drugs vary in their specificity for toxic metals. Ideal chelating agents should be water-soluble, resistant to biotransformation, able to reach sites of metal storage, capable of forming nontoxic complexes with toxic metals, and capable of being excreted from the body; they also should have a low affinity for essential metals, particularly calcium and zinc. Widely studied complexing agents include 2,3-dimercaptopropanol (BAL), 2,3-dimercaptosuccinic acid (succimer), calcium disodium ethylene diamine tetraacetic acid (EDTA), calcium disodium diethylene triamine pentaacetic acid, desferrioxamine, diethyldithiocarbamate (DTC), penicillamine, and *N*-acetylcysteine.

MAJOR TOXIC METALS WITH MULTIPLE EFFECTS

Arsenic (As)

The most common inorganic trivalent arsenic compounds are arsenic trioxide, sodium arsenite, and arsenic trichloride. Pentavalent inorganic compounds are arsenic pentoxide, arsenic acid, and arsenates, such as lead arsenate and calcium arsenate. Organic compounds also may be trivalent or pentavalent and even may occur in methylated forms as a consequence of biomethylation by organisms in soil, fresh water, and seawater. Inorganic arsenic is released into the environment from a number of anthropogenic sources, which include primary copper, zinc, and lead smelters; glass manufacturers that add arsenic to raw materials; and chemical manufacturers. Drinking water usually contains a few micrograms per liter or less. Seafoods contain several times the amount of arsenic found in other foods. Major sources of occupational exposure to arsenic in the United States include the manufacture of pesticides, herbicides, and other agricultural products. High exposure to arsenic fumes and dust may occur in the smelting industries.

Mechanisms of Toxicity Trivalent compounds of arsenic are the principal toxic forms, and pentavalent arsenic compounds have little effect on enzyme activity. Arsenic inhibits succinic dehydrogenase activity and uncouples oxidative phosphorylation; this process results in the stimulation of mitochondrial ATPase activity. Arsenic inhibits the energy-linked functions of mitochondria in two ways: competition with phosphate during oxidative phosphorylation and inhibition of energy-linked reduction of NAD. Inhibition of mitochondrial respiration results in decreased cellular production of ATP and increased production of hydrogen peroxide, which might cause oxidative stress through the production of reactive oxygen species.

Toxicology The ingestion of large doses (70 to 180 mg) of arsenic may be fatal. The symptoms of acute illness consist of fever, anorexia, hepatomegaly, melanosis, cardiac arrhythmia, and eventual cardiovascular failure. Other features include upper respiratory tract symptoms, peripheral neuropathy, and gastrointestinal, cardiovascular, and hematopoietic effects. Acute ingestion may be suspected from damage to mucous membranes, such as irritation, vesicle formation, and even sloughing. Sensory loss in the peripheral nervous system commonly appears 1 or 2 weeks after large exposures and consists of wallerian degeneration of axons. Anemia and leukopenia, particularly granulocytopenia, occur a few days after exposure and are reversible.

Chronic exposure to inorganic arsenic compounds may lead to neurotoxicity of both the peripheral and central nervous systems. Neurotoxicity usually begins with sensory changes, paresthesia, and muscle tenderness, followed by weakness, progressing from proximal to distal muscle groups. Peripheral neuropathy may be progressive, involving both sensory and motor neurons and leading to demyelination of long axon nerve fibers. Liver injury manifests initially as jaundice that may progress to cirrhosis and ascites.

Reproductive Effects and Teratogenicity High doses of inorganic arsenic compounds given to pregnant experimental animals produced various malformations in fetuses and offspring. However, those effects have not been noted in humans with excessive occupational exposures to arsenic compounds.

Carcinogenicity There is a causal association between inhalational exposure to arsenic and skin cancer and lung cancer. Additional studies indicate that arsenic causes cancer of internal organs from oral ingestion. In humans, chronic exposure to arsenic induces a series of characteristic changes in skin epithelium, proceeding from hyperpigmentation to hyperkeratosis. There actually may be two cell types of arsenic-induced skin cancer—basal cell carcinomas and squamous cell carcinomas—arising in keratotic areas.

Cadmium (Cd)

Cadmium is used in electroplating and galvanizing and as a cathode material for nickel-cadmium batteries. It also is used as a color pigment in paints and plastics. Cadmium is a by-product of zinc and lead mining and smelting.

Exposure For persons in the general population, the major source of cadmium is food. Plants readily take up cadmium from contaminated soil, water, and fertilizers. Mussels, scallops, and oysters may be a major source of dietary cadmium because shellfish accumulate cadmium from water in the form of cadmium-binding peptides. Meat, fish, fruit, and grains also contain significant levels of cadmium.

Workplace exposure to cadmium fumes and airborne cadmium is particularly hazardous. Occupations at risk include electrolytic refining of lead and zinc and occupations in other industries that employ thermal processes. Cigarettes are a major source of respirable cadmium.

Acute Toxicity Acute toxicity, in which nausea, vomiting, and abdominal pain occur, may result from the ingestion of relatively high concentrations of cadmium. Inhalation of cadmium fumes or other heated cadmium-containing materials may produce an acute chemical pneumonitis and pulmonary edema.

Chronic Toxicity The principal long-term effects of low-level exposure to cadmium are chronic obstructive pulmonary disease and emphysema and chronic renal tubular disease. There also may be effects on the cardiovascular and skeletal systems.

Chronic Pulmonary Disease Toxicity to the respiratory system is proportional to the time and level of exposure. Obstructive lung disease results from chronic bronchitis, progressive fibrosis of the lower airways, and accompanying alveolar damage that leads to emphysema. Dyspnea, reduced vital capacity, and increased residual volume are seen.

Nephrotoxicity Cadmium is toxic to renal tubular cells and glomeruli, impairing renal tubular and glomerular function and leading to proteinuria. The accumulation of cadmium in the kidneys to some extent without apparent toxic effect is possible because of the formation of cadmium-thionein. Cadmium bound to metallothionein in tissues is thought to be nontoxic. However, when the levels of cadmium exceed the critical concentration, it becomes toxic.

Other Toxicities Cadmium toxicity affects calcium metabolism, and associated skeletal changes probably related to calcium loss include bone pain, osteomalacia, and/or osteoporosis. Epidemiologic studies suggest that cadmium may be an etiologic agent for essential hypertension. Heart mitochondria may be the site of the cadmium-induced reduction in myocardial contractility. Epidemiologic studies in humans have suggested a relationship between abnormal behavior and/or decreased intelligence in children and adults exposed to cadmium.

Lead (Pb)

Lead is a ubiquitous toxic metal and is detectable in practically all phases of the inert environment and in all biological systems.

Exposure The principal route of exposure for the general population is food, and environmental sources include lead-based indoor paint in old dwellings, lead in contaminated drinking water, lead in air from the combustion of lead-containing industrial emissions, hand-to-mouth activities of young children living in polluted environments, lead-glazed pottery, and lead dust brought home by industrial workers on their shoes and clothes.

Toxicity The toxic effects of lead and the minimum blood lead level at which an effect is likely to be observed are shown in Table 23-2.

Table 23-2
Summary of Lowest Observed Effect Levels for Lead-Related Health Effects

EFFECT	Blood Lead Levels, $\mu g/dL$	
	ADULT	CHILDREN
Neurologic		
Encephalopathy (overt)	80–100	100–120
Hearing deficits	20	—
IQ deficits	10–15	—
In utero effects	10–15	—
Nerve conduction velocity ↓	40	40
Hematologic		
Anemia	80–100	80–100
U-ALA ↑	40	40
B-EP ↑	15	15
ALA-D inhibition	10	10
Renal		
Nephropathy	40	40–60
Vitamin D metabolism	<30?	—
Blood pressure		30?
Reproduction		
Males		40
Females		?

Neurologic, Neurobehavioral, and Developmental Effects in Children The symptoms of lead encephalopathy begin with lethargy, vomiting, irritability, loss of appetite, and dizziness, progressing to obvious ataxia and a reduced level of consciousness, which may progress to coma and death. Recovery often is accompanied by sequelae that include epilepsy, mental retardation, optic neuropathy, and blindness.

It has been difficult to discern whether specific neuropsychological deficits are associated with increased lead exposures. The most sensitive indicators of adverse neurologic outcomes are psychomotor tests and mental development indices, such as the Bayley Scales for infants, and broad measures of IQ. Children in the lower socioeconomic strata may begin to manifest language deficits by the second year of life. Increased blood lead levels in infancy and early childhood may be manifest in older children and adolescents as decreased attention span, reading disabilities, and failure to graduate from high school. An association between hearing thresholds and blood lead levels higher than 20 μg/dL has been found in teenagers.

Adults with occupational exposure may demonstrate abnormalities in measures of neurobehavior such as a slower response for pattern memory.

Mechanisms of Effects on the Developing Nervous System Possible mechanisms for lead effects on the nervous system are summarized in Table 23-3.

Lead impairs the timed programming of cell–cell connections during development, resulting in modification of neuronal circuitry. Lead induces precocious differentiation of the glia and causes alterations in the concentrations of the transmitters noradrenaline, dopamine, and possibly acetylcholine.

Lead impairs normal calcium homeostasis and uptake by calcium membrane channels and substitutes for calcium in calcium-sodium ATP pumps. Lead also blocks the entry of calcium into nerve terminals; it inhibits calcium uptake in brain mitochondria, with a decrease in energy production for the performance of brain functions. Also, lead interferes with calcium receptors that are coupled with second-messenger functions, affecting downstream effects.

Peripheral Neuropathy Peripheral neuropathy is a classic manifestation of chronic lead toxicity, particularly footdrop and wristdrop. Segmental demyelination and possibly axonal degeneration follow lead-induced Schwann cell degeneration.

Hematologic Effects Lead has multiple hematologic effects. In lead-induced anemia, the red blood cells are microcytic and hypochromic, and there are usually increased numbers of reticulocytes with basophilic stippling. The anemia results from two basic defects: shortened erythrocyte life span and impairment of heme synthesis.

A schematic presentation of the effects of lead on heme synthesis is shown in Fig. 23-3. There is inhibition of δ-aminolevulinic acid dehydratase (ALA-D), depression of coproporphyrinogen oxidase, and decreased ferrochelatase activity. This enzyme catalyzes the

Table 23-3
Mechanisms for Lead Effects on the Nervous System

Morphologic effects (neurodevelopmental)
   Impairment of timed programming of cell–cell connections
   Interference with neural cell adhesion molecules
   Altered migration of neurons during development
Pharmacologic effects (functional)
   Interferes with neurotransmitter function
Disrupts calcium metabolism
   Blocks voltage-dependent calcium membrane channels
   Substitutes for calcium in calcium–sodium ATP pump
   Competes for uptake by mitochondria
   Binds to second messenger calcium receptors (e.g., calmodulin, protein kinase C)

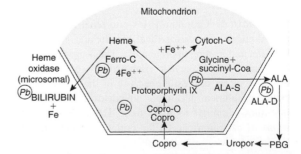

Figure 23-3. Scheme of heme synthesis showing sites where lead has an effect. CoA, coenzyme A; ALA-S, aminolevulinic acid synthetase; ALA, δ-aminolevulinic acid; ALA-D, aminolevulinic acid dehydratase; PBG, porphobilinogen; Uropor, uroporphyrinogen; Copro, coproporphyrinogen; Copro-O, coproporphyrinogen oxidase; Ferro-C, ferrochelatase; Cytoch-C, cytochrome-C; Pb, site for lead effect.

incorporation of the ferrous ion into the porphyrin ring structure. Failure to insert iron into protoporphyrin results in depressed heme formation. As a consequence, the increased production of δ-aminolevulinic acid (ALA) and decreased activity of ALA-D result in a marked increase in circulating blood levels and urinary excretion of ALA.

Renal Toxicity Acute lead nephrotoxicity is limited to functional and morphologic changes in proximal tubular cells. It is manifest clinically by decreases in energy-dependent transport functions, including aminoaciduria, glycosuria, and ion transport. The functional changes are thought to be related to an effect of lead on mitochondrial respiration and phosphorylation.

Other Toxic Effects Lead may affect blood pressure through changes in plasma renin and urinary kallikrein, alterations in calcium-activated functions of vascular smooth muscle cells, and changes in responsiveness to catecholamines. As an immunosuppressive agent, lead decreases immunoglobulins, peripheral B lymphocytes, and other components of the immunologic system. Retention and mobilization of lead in bone occur by the same mechanisms involved in regulating calcium influx and efflux. Lead also competes with calcium for gastrointestinal absorption. Lead toxicity has long been associated with sterility and neonatal deaths in humans. Lead, a 2B carcinogen, induces tumors of the respiratory and digestive systems. Epidemiologic studies suggest a relationship between occupational lead exposure and cancer of the lung, brain, and bladder among workers exposed to lead.

Mercury (Hg)

Mercury is the only metal that is in the liquid state at room temperature. *Mercury vapor* is much more hazardous than the liquid form. This element exists in three oxidation states: Hg^0, Hg^+, and Hg^{2+}. In addition, mercuric mercury can form a number of stable organic mercury compounds. Each oxidation state, as well as each organic species, has characteristic health effects.

Exposure The major sources of mercury (as mercury vapor) in the atmosphere are the natural degassing of the earth's crust and human activities. Mercury vapor resides in the atmosphere unchanged for months to a year and thus is distributed globally. Eventually, it is converted to a water-soluble form and returned to the earth's surface in rainwater.

At this stage, two important chemical changes may occur. The metal may be reduced back to mercury vapor and returned to the atmosphere, or it may be methylated by microorganisms present in sediments of bodies of fresh water and ocean water. The main product of this natural biomethylation is monomethyl mercury compounds, which usually are referred to generically as "methyl mercury." Methyl mercury enters an aquatic food chain involving plankton, herbivorous fish, and finally carnivorous fish. The consequence of biomethylation and bioconcentration can be human dietary exposure to methyl mercury.

Occupational exposures occur in the chlor-alkali industry, in the making of various scientific instruments and electrical control devices, in dentistry in the form of amalgam tooth filling, and in the extraction of gold.

Mercury levels in the general atmosphere and in drinking water are so low that they do not constitute an important source of exposure for the general population.

Metabolic Transformation Elemental or metallic mercury is oxidized to divalent mercury after absorption. Inhaled mercury vapor absorbed into red blood cells is transformed to divalent mercury, but a portion is transported as metallic mercury to more distal tissues, where biotransformation may occur.

Toxicology *Mercury Vapor* Inhalation of mercury vapor at extremely high concentrations may produce an acute, corrosive bronchitis and interstitial pneumonitis and, if not fatal, may be associated with central nervous system effects such as tremor and increased excitability. This condition has been termed the *asthenic-vegetative syndrome* or *micromercurialism*. Identification of the syndrome requires neurasthenic symptoms and three or more of the following clinical findings: tremor, enlargement of the thyroid, increased uptake of radioiodine in the thyroid, labile pulse, tachycardia, dermographism, gingivitis, hematologic changes, and increased excretion of mercury in urine. With increasing exposure, the symptoms become more characteristic, beginning with tremors of the fingers, eyelids, and lips, and may progress to generalized trembling of the entire body and violent chronic spasms of the extremities. This is accompanied by changes in personality and behavior, with loss of memory, increased excitability (erethism), severe depression, and even delirium and hallucination. Another characteristic feature of mercury toxicity is severe salivation and gingivitis.

There is growing concern that mercury vapor released from dental amalgams may cause various health effects.

An increase in urinary mercury and its accumulation in several organs, including the central nervous system and kidneys, have been related to the release of mercury from dental amalgams. However, this level of mercury exposure is believed to be below that which will produce any discernible health effect except in highly sensitive people.

Mercuric Salts Oral ingestion of bichloride of mercury causes severe abdominal cramps, bloody diarrhea, and suppression of urine. Corrosive ulceration, bleeding, and necrosis of the gastrointestinal tract usually are accompanied by shock and circulatory collapse. If a patient survives the gastrointestinal damage, renal failure occurs within 24 h owing to necrosis of the proximal tubular epithelium, followed by oliguria, anuria, and uremia. If the patient can be maintained by dialysis, regeneration of the tubular lining cells is possible.

Mercurous Mercury Mercurous compounds are less corrosive and less toxic than mercuric salts, presumably because they are less soluble.

Methyl Mercury Methyl mercury is the most important form of mercury in terms of toxicity. The major human health effects from exposure to methyl mercury are neurotoxic effects in adults and toxicity to the fetuses of mothers who are exposed to methyl mercury during pregnancy. The major source of exposure for the general population is the consumption of fish.

The clinical manifestations of neurotoxic effects are (1) paresthesia, a numbness and tingling sensation around the mouth, lips, and extremities, particularly the fingers and toes, (2) ataxia, a clumsy stumbling gait, and difficulty in swallowing and articulating words, (3) neurasthenia, a generalized sensation of weakness, fatigue, and inability to concentrate, (4) vision and hearing loss, (5) spasticity and tremor, and (6) coma and death.

Nickel (Ni)

Nickel is a respiratory tract carcinogen in workers in the nickel-refining industry. Allergic contact dermatitis is common among the general population.

Exposure Nickel is ubiquitous in nature, occurring mainly in the form of sulfide, oxide, and silicate minerals. Human exposure may occur through inhalation, ingestion, and dermal contact. The main route of occupational exposure to nickel is inhalation and to a lesser degree skin contact. For most of the general public,

exposure may result from food or from contact with everyday items such as nickel-containing jewelry, cooking utensils, and clothing fasteners.

Toxicity Nickel compounds are carcinogenic to humans. Risks were highest for lung and nasal cancers among workers heavily exposed to nickel sulfide, nickel oxide, and metallic nickel.

Dermatitis Nickel dermatitis accounts for 4 to 9 percent of cases of allergic dermatitis. Sensitization may occur from commonly used metal products such as coins and jewelry.

ESSENTIAL METALS WITH POTENTIAL FOR TOXICITY

This group includes eight metals generally accepted as essential: cobalt, copper, iron, magnesium, manganese, molybdenum, selenium, and zinc. All can produce some target organ toxicity (Table 23-4).

Copper (Cu)

For the general population, food and drinking water are potential sources of excess copper exposure. Copper exposures in industry are to particulates in miners and to metal fumes among workers in smelting operations, welding, and related activities.

Toxicity In humans, ingestion of drinking water with >3 mg Cu/L will produce gastrointestinal symptoms that include nausea, vomiting, and diarrhea. Ingestion of large amounts of copper salts, most frequently copper sulfate, may produce hepatic necrosis and death. Epidemiologic studies have not found any relationship between copper exposure and cancer. Individuals with glucose-6-phosphate deficiency may be at increased risk for the hematologic effects of copper.

Wilson's Disease Wilson's disease is characterized by the excessive accumulation of copper in the liver, brain, kidneys, and corneas. Serum ceruloplasmin is low, and serum copper that is not bound to ceruloplasmin is elevated. Urinary excretion of copper is high. Clinical abnormalities of the nervous system, liver, kidneys, and cornea are related to copper accumulation. The disorder sometimes is referred to as *hepatolenticular degeneration*. Patients with Wilson's disease have impaired biliary excretion of copper, which is believed to be the fundamental cause of copper overload. Reversal of abnormal

Table 23-4
Toxicity of Several Metals

METAL	CNS	GI TRACT	LUNG	KIDNEY	LIVER	HEART	BLOOD	SKIN
Aluminum	*		*					
Arsenic	*	*	*	*	*		*	
Beryllium			*					*
Bismuth				*	*			*
Cadmium	*	*	*	*	*	*		
Chromium	*		*	*	*			*
Cobalt	*	*	*			*		*
Copper		*					*	
Iron	*	*	*		*		*	
Lead	*	*		*			*	*
Manganese	*		*					
Mercury	*	*	*	*				
Nickel	*		*					*
Selenium		*		*				*
Zinc		*					*	

copper metabolism is achieved by liver transplantation, confirming that the basic defect is in the liver. Clinical improvement can be achieved with chelation therapy.

Iron (Fe)

Iron homeostasis is complex, mainly involving intake, stores, and loss. Generally, about 2 to 15 percent is absorbed from the gastrointestinal tract, whereas iron elimination accounts for only about 0.01 percent per day. During periods of increased iron need (childhood, pregnancy, and blood loss), absorption of iron is increased greatly. Absorbed iron is bound to the plasma protein transferrin for transfer to storage sites in hemoglobin, myoglobin and iron containing enzymes, and the iron storage proteins ferritin and hemosiderin. Normally, excess ingested iron is excreted, and some is contained within shed intestinal cells, in bile and urine, and even smaller amounts in sweat, nails, and hair.

Toxicity Acute iron poisoning from accidental or suicidal ingestion of iron-containing medicines is a common cause of acute iron toxicity. Severe toxicity occurs after the ingestion of more than 0.5 g of iron or 2.5 g of ferrous sulfate. The vomiting 1 to 6 h after ingestion is followed by signs of shock and metabolic acidosis, liver damage, and coagulation defects within the next couple of days. Late effects may include renal failure and hepatic cirrhosis. The mechanism of the toxicity is thought to begin with acute mucosal cell damage and absorption of ferrous ions directly into the circulation, which causes damage to capillary endothelial cells in the liver.

Chronic iron toxicity or iron overload in adults is a more common problem. The three basic ways in which excessive amounts of iron can accumulate in the body are (1) hereditary hemochromatosis resulting from abnormal absorption of iron from the intestinal tract, (2) excess dietary iron, and (3) regular blood transfusion in some refractory anemias (*transfusional siderosis*). The clinical effects of iron overload may include liver dysfunction, diabetes mellitus, endocrine disturbances, and cardiovascular effects. There is epidemiologic evidence for a relationship between iron levels and cardiovascular disease. Excess iron contributes to increased lipid peroxidation, with consequent membrane damage to mitochondria, microsomes, and other cellular organelles.

Zinc (Zn)

Zinc is a nutritionally essential metal. Excessive exposure to zinc is relatively uncommon. Zinc is present in most foodstuffs, water, and air. The zinc content of substances in contact with galvanized copper or plastic pipes may be increased. Seafoods, meats, whole grains, dairy products, nuts, and legumes are high in zinc. Even growing vegetables take up zinc from the soil.

Essentiality and Metabolism More than 200 metalloenzymes belonging to six major categories—including oxidoreductases, transferases, hydrolases, lyases, isomerases, and ligases—require zinc as a cofactor. Zinc induces the synthesis of metallothionein, which is a factor in regulating its absorption and storage. Zinc chelates with cysteine and/or histidine, forming "zinc fingers," which bind to specific DNA regions as well as various transcription factors, such as steroid hormone receptors and polymerase. Zinc stablizes membranes by binding ligands in membranes that maintain the normal structural geometry of the protein and lipid components. Zinc is essential for the development and normal function of the nervous system.

Toxicity Gastrointestinal distress and diarrhea have been reported after the ingestion of beverages standing in galvanized cans or from the use of galvanized utensils.

Metal fume fever resulting from the inhalation of freshly formed fumes of zinc presents 4 to 8 h after exposure. Chills and fever, profuse sweating, and weakness typically are seen. Attacks usually last 24 to 48 h and are most common on Mondays or after holidays. The pathogenesis is thought to result from endogenous pyrogen release caused by cell lysis.

Epidemiologic studies of workers in refining industries have not found any evidence of a relationship between zinc and cancer.

METALS RELATED TO MEDICAL THERAPY

Metals that are used to treat a number of human illnesses, including aluminum, bismuth, gold, lithium, and platinum, exert some toxicity (Table 23-4).

Aluminum (Al)

All aluminum compounds involve aluminum in the +3 valence state. This trivalent ion binds strongly to oxygen-donor ligands such as citrate and phosphate. Human exposure to aluminum comes from food and drinking water as well as from pharmaceuticals.

Toxicity In cases of human toxicity, the target organs are the lung, bone, and central nervous system. Aluminum also produces developmental effects in animals. In addition, aluminum from acid rain can kill fish by damaging their gills.

Lung and Bone Toxicity Occupational exposure to aluminum dusts can produce lung fibrosis in humans. Osteomalacia has been associated with excessive intake of aluminum-containing antacids in otherwise healthy individuals; this is assumed to be due to interference with intestinal phosphate absorption. Osteomalacia also can occur in uremic patients who are exposed to aluminum in the dialysis fluid. In these patients, osteomalacia may be a direct effect of aluminum on bone mineralization, as bone levels are high.

Neurotoxicity Aluminum has markedly different effects on animals at various times in the life span and in different species. In certain aluminum-sensitive species, such as cats and rabbits, increased aluminum induces subtle behavioral changes, including learning and memory deficits and poor motor function. These changes progress to tremor, incoordination, weakness, and ataxia. This is followed by focal seizures and death within 3 or 4 weeks of initial exposure.

Human Dementia Syndromes *Dialysis Dementia* A progressive, fatal neurologic syndrome has been reported in patients on long-term intermittent hemodialysis treatment for chronic renal failure. A speech disorder followed by dementia, convulsions, and myoclonus typically arises after 3 to 7 years of dialysis treatment and may be due to aluminum intoxication. The aluminum content of brain, muscle, and bone tissues increases in these patients. The syndrome may be prevented by avoiding the use of aluminum-containing oral phosphate binders and monitoring aluminum in the dialysate. Chelation therapy may slow or arrest the progression of the dementia.

Alzheimer's Disease A possible relationship between aluminum and Alzheimer's disease has been a matter of speculation for many decades. The elevated aluminum levels in Alzheimer brains may be a consequence and not a cause of the disease. The reduced blood-brain barrier in Alzheimer's patients might allow more aluminum into the brain. There are conflicting conclusions from epidemiologic studies examining the role of aluminum in Alzheimer's disease.

Lithium (Li)

Lithium (carbonate) is used in the treatment of depression. Lithium is present in many plant and animal tissues. It has some industrial uses in alloys, as a catalytic agent, and as a lubricant. Lithium hydride produces hydrogen on contact with water and is used in manufacturing electronic tubes, in ceramics, and in chemical synthesis.

Toxicokinetics Lithium compounds are absorbed readily from the gastrointestinal tract. Distribution is to total body water, with higher levels in kidney, thyroid, and bone compared with other tissues. Excretion is chiefly through the kidneys, with 80 percent of the filtered load reabsorbed. Lithium can substitute for sodium or potassium on several transport proteins.

Toxicity From the industrial point of view, except for lithium hydride, none of the other salts is hazardous, nor is the metal itself. Lithium hydride is intensely corrosive and may produce burns on the skin because of the formation of hydroxides.

The therapeutic use of lithium carbonate may produce unusual toxic responses. These responses include neuromuscular tremor and ataxia, blackout spells, seizures, slurred speech, coma, increased thirst, cardiac arrhythmia, hypertension, circulatory collapse, anorexia, nausea, vomiting, albuminuria, and glycosuria. Long-term sequelae from acute lithium poisoning include impaired memory, impaired attention and executive functions, and visuospatial deficits.

Chronic lithium nephrotoxicity and interstitial nephritis can occur with long-term exposure even when lithium levels remain within the therapeutic range.

Platinum (Pt)

Platinum is found in roadside dust in areas where traffic density is high because of its use in catalytic converters.

Allergenic Effects of Platinum Salts Platinum metal itself is generally harmless, but an allergic dermatitis can be produced in susceptible individuals. Skin changes are most common between the fingers and in the antecubital fossae. Symptoms of respiratory distress ranging from irritation to an asthmatic syndrome—with coughing, wheezing, and shortness of breath—have been reported after exposure to platinum dust. The skin and respiratory changes are termed *platinosis*. They are confined mainly to persons with a history of industrial exposure to soluble compounds such as sodium chloroplatinate. Platinum salt sensitization may persist for years after the cessation of exposure.

Antitumor Effects of Platinum Complexes *Cis*-dichlorodiammine platinum (II) (or cisplatin) and various analogs can inhibit cell division and have antibacterial properties as well. These compounds can react selectively with specific chemical sites in proteins and nucleic acids. They also exhibit neuromuscular toxicity and nephrotoxicity. Platinum complexes, particularly cisplatin, are effective antitumor agents and are used clinically for the treatment of cancers of the head and neck, certain lymphomas, and testicular and ovarian tumors. At therapeutically effective dosages, these complexes produce severe and persistent inhibition of DNA synthesis and little inhibition of RNA and protein synthesis. DNA polymerase activity and the transport of DNA precursors through plasma membranes are not inhibited.

Nephrotoxicity Cisplatin produces proximal and distal tubular cell injury, mainly in the corticomedullary region, where the concentration of platinum is highest. Tubular cell toxicity seems to be related directly to dose. Experimental studies suggest that the preadministration of bismuth subnitrate, a potent inducer of metallothionein in the kidney, reduces the nephrotoxicity of cisplatin without interfering with its anticancer effect.

BIBLIOGRAPHY

Goyer RA, Klaassen CD, Waalkes MP (eds): *Metal Toxicology.* San Diego, CA: Academic Press, 1995.

O'Dell BL, Sunde RA (eds): *Handbook of Nutritionally Essential Mineral Elements.* New York: Marcel Dekker, 1997.

Yasui M, Strong M, Ota K, Verity MA (eds): *Mineral and Metal Neurotoxicology.* Boca Raton, FL: CRC Press, 2000.

Zalups RK, Koropatnick J: *Molecular Biology and Toxicology of Metals.* New York: Taylor & Francis, 2000.

C H A P T E R 2 4

TOXIC EFFECTS OF SOLVENTS AND VAPORS

James V. Bruckner and D. Alan Warren

KEY POINTS

- The term *solvent* refers to a class of liquid organic chemicals with variable lipophilicity and volatility, small molecular size, and lack of charge.
- Absorption of inhaled volatile organic compounds occurs in the alveoli, with almost instantaneous equilibration with blood in the pulmonary capillaries.
- Solvents are absorbed readily from the gastrointestinal tract and across the skin.
- Most solvents produce some degree of central nervous system depression.

INTRODUCTION

Solvents are liquid organic chemicals with variable lipophilicity and volatility, small molecular size, and lack of charge. Solvents undergo ready absorption across the lung, skin, and gastrointestinal (GI) tract. In general, the lipophilicity of solvents increases with increasing molecular weight, whereas volatility decreases. Solvents frequently are used to dissolve, dilute, or disperse materials that are insoluble in water. Most solvents are refined from petroleum. Many, such as naphthas and gasoline, are complex mixtures that consist of hundreds of compounds.

Solvents are classified largely according to their molecular structure or functional group. Classes of solvents include aliphatic hydrocarbons, many of which are chlorinated (i.e., halocarbons); aromatic hydrocarbons; alcohols; ethers; esters/acetates; amides/amines; aldehydes; ketones; and complex mixtures that defy classification. Subtle differences in chemical structure can translate into dramatic differences in toxicity.

Nearly everyone is exposed to solvents during normal daily activities. Environmental exposures to solvents in air and groundwater have multiple exposure pathways (Fig. 24-1). Though it is not reflected in Fig. 24-1, household use of solvent-contaminated water may result in solvent intake from inhalation and dermal and oral absorption. In many cases, environmental risk assessment requires that risks be determined for physiologically diverse individuals who are exposed to several solvents by multiple exposure pathways.

The Occupational Safety and Health Administration (OSHA) has established legally enforceable Permissible

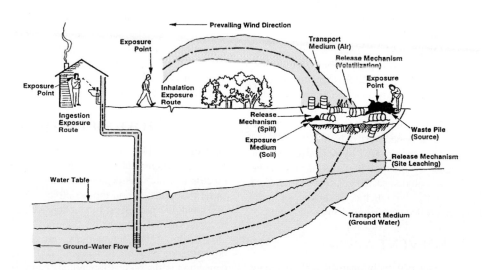

Figure 24-1. Solvent exposure pathways and media.

Exposure Limits (PELs) for over 100 solvents. The majority of existing PELs were adopted from the list of Threshold Limit Values (TLVs) published by the American Conference of Governmental Industrial Hygienists (ACGIH). Many current TLVs are more stringent than PELs but do not carry the weight of law. Whereas the ACGIH's TLVs for an 8-h work day and a 40-h work week are designed to be protective for a working lifetime, its Short-Term Exposure Limits (STELs) and ceiling values are designed to protect against the acute effects of high-level, short-term solvent exposures. If warranted, the ACGIH will assign a skin notation to a solvent, indicating that significant dermal exposure is possible.

Most solvent exposures involve a mixture of chemicals rather than a single compound. Our knowledge of the toxicity of solvent mixtures is rudimentary. Although the assumption that the toxic effects of multiple solvents are additive is made frequently, solvents also may interact synergistically or antagonistically.

Although some solvents are less hazardous than others, all solvents can have toxic effects. Most have the potential to induce narcosis and cause dermal and mucous membrane irritation. A number of solvents are animal carcinogens, but only a handful have been classified as known human carcinogens.

IS THERE A SOLVENT-INDUCED CHRONIC ENCEPHALOPATHY?

There has been considerable debate about whether chronic, low-level exposure to virtually any solvent or solvent mixture can produce a pattern of neurologic dysfunction referred to as *painter's syndrome, organic solvent syndrome, psychoorganic syndrome,* and *chronic solvent encephalopathy* (CSE). CSE is characterized by nonspecific symptoms (e.g., headache, fatigue, sleep disorders) with or without changes in neuropsychological function. A reversible form of CSE, the *neuroasthenic syndrome,* consists of symptoms only. The "mild" and "severe" forms are accompanied by objective signs of neuropsychological dysfunction that may or may not be fully reversible. Resolution of the controversial issue of CSE will come only through the conducting of well-designed and controlled clinical epidemiologic studies.

SOLVENT ABUSE

Many solvents are inhaled intentionally to achieve a state of intoxication with euphoria, delusions, and sedation as well as visual and auditory hallucinations. Solvent abuse is a unique exposure situation in that participants repeatedly subject themselves to vapor concentrations high enough to produce effects as extreme as unconsciousness. Solvents can be addicting and often are abused in combination with other drugs. Solvents are present in relatively inexpensive household and commercial products that are readily available to children and adolescents.

ENVIRONMENTAL CONTAMINATION

Most solvents enter the environment through evaporation (Fig. 24-1). The majority of the more volatile organic compounds (VOCs) volatilize when products containing them (e.g., aerosol propellants, paint thinners, cleaners, soil fumigants) are used as intended. Solvent loss into the atmosphere also occurs during production, processing, storage, and transport activities. Winds dilute and disperse solvent vapors across the world. Atmospheric concentrations of most VOCs are usually extremely low, though higher concentrations have been measured in urban areas, around petrochemical plants, and in the immediate vicinity of hazardous waste sites.

Solvent contamination of drinking water supplies is a major health concern. Although the majority of a solvent spilled onto the ground evaporates, some may permeate the soil and migrate until it reaches groundwater or impermeable material. All solvents are soluble in water to some extent. Concentrations diminish rapidly after VOCs enter bodies of water, primarily as a result of dilution and evaporation. VOCs in surface waters rise to the surface or sink to the bottom, according to their density. VOCs on the surface largely evaporate. VOCs on the bottom depend on solubilization in the water or on mixing by current or wave action to reach the surface. VOCs in groundwater tend to remain trapped until the water reaches the surface.

TOXICOKINETICS

Toxicokinetic (TK) studies delineate the uptake and disposition of chemicals in the body. Toxicity is a dynamic process in which the degree and duration of injury of a target tissue depend on the net effect of toxicodynamic (TD) and TK processes, interaction with cellular components, and tissue repair.

Volatility and lipophilicity are two important properties of solvents that govern their absorption and deposition in the body. Lipophilicity can vary from quite water-soluble (e.g., glycols and alcohols) to quite lipid-soluble (e.g., halocarbons and aromatic hydrocarbons). Many solvents have a relatively low molecular weight and are uncharged. Thus, they pass freely through membranes from areas of high concentration to low concentration by passive diffusion.

Absorption

Most systemic absorption of inhaled VOCs occurs in the alveoli, with some absorption occurring in the upper respiratory tract. Gases in the alveoli equilibrate almost instantaneously with blood in the pulmonary capillaries. The blood:air partition coefficient (PC) of a VOC may be defined as the ratio of concentration of a VOC achieved between two different media at equilibrium. More hydrophilic solvents have relatively high blood:air PCs, which favor extensive uptake. Since VOCs diffuse from areas of high concentration to low concentration, increases in respiration (to maintain a high alveolar concentration) and cardiac output/pulmonary blood flow (to maintain a large concentration gradient by removing capillary blood containing the VOC) enhance pulmonary absorption.

Solvents are well absorbed from the gastrointestinal (GI) tract. Peak blood levels are observed within minutes of dosing, although the presence of food in the GI tract can delay absorption. It usually is assumed that 100 percent of an oral dose of most solvents is absorbed systemically. The vehicle or diluent in which a solvent is ingested can affect the absorption and TK of the compound.

Absorption of solvents through the skin can result in both local and systemic effects. Solvents penetrate the stratum corneum by means of passive diffusion. Determinants of the rate of dermal absorption of solvents include the chemical concentration, surface area exposed, exposure duration, integrity and thickness of the stratum corneum, and lipophilicity and molecular weight of the solvent.

Transport and Distribution

Solvents absorbed into portal venous blood from the GI tract are subject to uptake/elimination by the liver and exhalation by the lungs during their first pass along this absorption pathway. Solvents that are well metabolized and quite volatile are eliminated most efficiently before they enter the arterial blood. Hepatic first-pass elimination depends on the chemical and the rate at which it arrives in the liver. Pulmonary first-pass elimination, in contrast, is believed to be a first-order process irrespective of the chemical concentration in the blood.

Solvents transported by the arterial blood are taken up according to the rate of tissue blood flow and the tissue:blood PC of the solvent. Relatively hydrophilic solvents solubilize to different extents in plasma. Lipophilic solvents do not bind to plasma proteins or hemoglobin but instead partition into hydrophobic sites in the molecules. Lipophilic solvents partition into phospholipids, lipoproteins, and cholesterol present in the blood.

Blood levels of solvents drop rapidly during the initial elimination phase. This redistribution phase is characterized by rapid diffusion of solvent from the blood into most tissues. Equilibration of adipose tissue is prolonged because of the small fraction of cardiac output (~3 percent) that supplies fat depots. Body fat increases the volume of distribution and total body burden of lipophilic solvents.

Metabolism

Biotransformation can modulate the toxicities of solvents. Many solvents are poorly soluble in water and must be converted to relatively water-soluble derivatives, which may be eliminated more readily in the largely aqueous urine and/or bile. Some solvents can undergo bioactivation to produce reactive metabolites that are cytotoxic and/or mutagenic.

Physiologic Modeling

Physiologically based toxicokinetic (PBTK) models are used to relate the administered dose to the tissue dose of the bioactive moiety or moieties. With knowledge of the physiology of the test animal and tissue, physiologically based toxicodynamic (PBTD) models can be developed. PBTK/PBTD models are well suited for species-to-species extrapolations, because human physiologic and metabolic parameter values can be entered and simulations of target tissue doses and effects in humans can be generated. Thus, solvent exposures necessary to produce the same target organ dose in humans as that found experimentally to cause unacceptable cancer or noncancer incidence in test animals can be determined with reasonable certainty in some cases.

POTENTIALLY SENSITIVE SUBPOPULATIONS

Endogenous Factors

Children Limited information is available on the toxic potential of solvents in children. Most age-dependent differences are less than an order of magnitude, usually varying no more than two- to threefold. The younger and more immature the subject, the more different its response from that of adults.

GI absorption of solvents varies little with age, because most solvents are absorbed by passive diffusion. Systemic absorption of inhaled VOCs may be greater in infants and children than it is in adults owing to the relatively high cardiac output and respiratory rates in children despite their lower alveolar surface area. Extracellular water expressed as a percentage of body weight is highest in newborns and gradually diminishes through childhood. Body fat content is high from ~1/2 year to 3 years of age and then steadily decreases until adolescence, when it increases again in females. Lipophilic solvents accumulate in adipose tissue, and so more body fat results in greater body burdens and slower clearance of chemicals.

Changes in xenobiotic metabolism during maturation may affect susceptibility to solvent toxicity. P450 isoforms develop asynchronously. Increased rates of metabolism, urinary excretion, and exhalation in children should hasten elimination and reduce body burdens of solvents. However, the net effect of immaturity on solvent disposition and toxicity is difficult to predict.

Elderly With aging, body fat usually increases substantially at the expense of lean mass and body water. Thus, relatively polar solvents tend to reach higher blood levels during exposures. Relatively lipid-soluble solvents accumulate in adipose tissue and are released slowly. Cardiac output and renal and hepatic blood flows are diminished in the elderly.

The elderly, like infants and children, may be more or less sensitive to the toxicity of solvents than young adults are. Greater organ system toxicity could be due to increased inflammatory damage or to age-related dysregulation of cytokines. Other major sources of variability and complexity in geriatric populations include inadequate nutrition, the prevalence of disease states, and the concurrent use of multiple medications.

Genetics Genetic polymorphisms for biotransformation occur at different frequencies in different ethnic groups. Polymorphisms for phase I and phase II xenobiotic metabolizing enzymes (specifically CYP2E1, 2D6, 1A1, and GSTM1) may affect the outcomes of solvent exposures in different racial groups. Disentangling the influences of genetic traits from those of socioeconomic status, lifestyles, and geographic setting is difficult.

Exogenous Factors

P450 Inducers and Inhibitors Preexposure to chemicals that induce or inhibit biotransformation enzymes can potentiate or reduce the toxicity of high doses of solvents that undergo metabolism. Inhibitors generally would be anticipated to enhance the toxicity of solvents that are metabolically inactivated and to provide protection against solvents that undergo metabolic activation.

Physical Activity Exercise increases alveolar ventilation and cardiac output/pulmonary blood flow. Polar solvents with relatively high blood:air PCs (e.g., acetone, ethanol, ethylene glycol) are absorbed very rapidly into the pulmonary circulation. Alveolar ventilation is rate-limiting for those chemicals. In contrast, pulmonary blood flow and metabolism are rate-limiting for the uptake of more lipophilic solvents. Heavy exercise can increase the pulmonary uptake of relatively polar solvents as much as fivefold in human subjects. Light exercise doubles the uptake of relatively lipid-soluble solvents, but no further increase occurs at higher workloads. Blood flow to the liver and kidneys diminishes with exercise, which may diminish the biotransformation of metabolized solvents and urinary elimination.

Diet The mere bulk of food in the stomach and intestines can inhibit systemic absorption of ingested chemicals. VOCs in the GI tract partition into dietary lipids, largely remaining there until the lipids are emulsified and digested. Food intake results in increased splanchnic blood flow, which favors GI absorption, hepatic blood flow, and biotransformation. Foods may contain certain natural constituents, pesticides, and other chemicals that may enhance or reduce solvent metabolism.

CHLORINATED HYDROCARBONS

Trichloroethylene

1,1,2-Trichloroethylene (TCE) is a widely used solvent for metal degreasing. Current data support weak associations between TCE exposure and multiple myeloma, Hodgkin's disease, and cancers of the prostate, skin, cervix, and kidney.

Metabolism Toxicities associated with TCE are mediated predominantly by metabolites rather than by the parent compound. Even the central nervous system

(CNS)-depressant effects of TCE are due in part to the sedative properties of the metabolite trichloroethanol (TCOH). After either oral or inhalational absorption, most of the TCE undergoes oxidation via cytochrome P450s, with a small proportion being conjugated with glutathione (GSH). Both metabolic pathways are implicated in the carcinogenicity of TCE: reactive metabolite(s) of the GSH pathway in kidney tumors in rats and oxidative metabolites in liver and lung tumors in mice.

Liver Cancer TCE induces liver cancer in B6C3F1 mice but not in rats. This differential susceptibility is due to the greater capacity of mice to metabolize TCE to an oxidative metabolite that stimulates peroxisome proliferation. Propagation results in an increased potential for oxidative DNA damage and decreased gap junctional intercellular communication, both of which have been implicated in neoplastic transformation.

Kidney Cancer TCE exposure by inhalation or the oral route results in kidney tumors in male but not female rats. The susceptibility of the male rat can be explained by its greater capacity for TCE metabolism through the GSH pathway. TCE-induced kidney tumors are believed to result from reactive metabolite(s) of this pathway that alkylates cellular nucleophiles, including DNA. The resulting DNA mutations lead to alterations in gene expression, which in turn lead to neoplastic transformation and tumorigenesis through a genotoxic pathway.

Alternatively, proximal tubular cell cytotoxicity and subsequent tumor formation through a nongenotoxic mode of action could be induced by reactive metabolites that cause oxidative stress, alkylation of cytosolic and mitochondrial proteins, marked ATP depletion, and perturbations in Ca^{2+} homeostasis. Tubular necrosis ensues, with subsequent reparative proliferation that can alter gene expression and in turn alter the regulation of cell growth and differentiation. In fact, somatic mutations in the von Hippel–Lindau (VHL) tumor suppressor gene may be a specific and susceptible target of TCE.

Chronic tubular damage may be a prerequisite to TCE-induced renal cell cancer. Reactive metabolite(s) of the GSH pathway may have a genotoxic effect on the proximal tubule of the human kidney, but the full development of a malignant tumor requires a promotional effect such as cell proliferation in response to tubular damage.

Lung Cancer Inhaled TCE is carcinogenic to the lung of the mouse but not to that of the rat. Oral TCE is not carcinogenic to the lung, probably because of hepatic metabolism that limits the amount of TCE reaching the organ. The primary target of TCE in the mouse lung is the nonciliated Clara cell. Toxicity to these cells is characterized by vacuolization and increases in cell replication in the bronchiolar epithelium. Clara cells of the mouse efficiently metabolize TCE to toxic metabolites. Clara cells in mouse lung are more numerous and have a much higher concentration of metabolizing enzymes than do those in the rat.

Tetrachloroethylene

Tetrachloroethylene (perchloroethylene, PERC) is used commonly as a dry cleaner, fabric finisher, degreaser, rug and upholstery cleaner, paint and stain remover, solvent, and chemical intermediate. The highest exposures usually occur in occupational settings through inhalation.

The systemic disposition and metabolism of PERC and TCE are quite similar. Both chemicals are well absorbed from the lungs and GI tract, distributed to tissues according to their lipid content, partially exhaled unchanged, and metabolized by P450s. PERC is oxidized by hepatic P450s to a much lesser degree than is TCE, though the two have a common major metabolite: trichloroacetic acid. GSH conjugation is a minor metabolic pathway quantitatively for TCE and PERC.

PERC's potential for causing cancer in humans is controversial. The many epidemiologic studies of cancer incidence and mortality in groups of persons who are occupationally exposed to PERC have been equivocal. Cigarette smoking and alcohol consumption are important confounders for esophageal cancer. Kidney cancer incidences did not appear to be elevated. Thus, the epidemiologic evidence gathered to date does not support a cause-and-effect relationship between either PERC or TCE and kidney cancer.

Methylene Chloride

Methylene chloride (dichloromethane, MC) has widespread use as a solvent in industrial processes, food preparation, degreasing agents, aerosol propellants, and agriculture. The primary route of exposure to this very volatile solvent is inhalation.

The TK of MC has been well characterized in humans and rodents. Inhaled MC reached near steady state in the blood of human subjects within 1 to 2 h of continuous exposure. MC was eliminated very rapidly from the body and did not accumulate over 5 days of exposure.

MC has limited systemic toxicity potential. High, repeated inhalation exposures produce slight, reversible changes in the livers of rodents. Persons subjected to high vapor levels manifest kidney injury occasionally. Carbon monoxide that is formed from MC binds to hemoglobin to produce dose-dependent increases in carboxyhemoglobin. Residual neurologic dysfunction in MC-exposed workers has been reported.

Occupational and environmental MC exposures are of concern primarily because of the carcinogenicity of MC in rodents and the potential of MC as a human carcinogen. Epidemiology studies of employees exposed to MC have revealed that cancer risks from occupational exposure to MC, if any, are quite small.

Carbon Tetrachloride

Carbon tetrachloride (CCl_4) is a classic hepatotoxin, but kidney injury is often more severe in humans. There does not appear to be a good animal model for kidney toxicity.

Early signs of hepatocellular injury in rats include dissociation of polysomes and ribosomes from rough endoplasmic reticulum, disarray of smooth endoplasmic reticulum, inhibition of protein synthesis, and triglyceride accumulation. CCl_4 undergoes metabolic activation, producing lipid peroxidation, covalent binding, and inhibition of microsomal ATPase activity. Single-cell necrosis, which is evident 5 to 6 h after dosing, progresses to maximal centrilobular necrosis within 24 to 48 h. Cellular regeneration is maximal 36 to 48 h after dosing. The rate and extent of tissue repair are important determinants of the ultimate outcome of liver injury.

Perturbation of intracellular calcium (Ca^{2+}) homeostasis appears to be part of CCl_4 cytotoxicity. Increased cytosolic Ca^{2+} levels may result from influx of extracellular Ca^{2+} caused by plasma membrane damage and from decreased intracellular Ca^{2+} sequestration. Elevation of intracellular Ca^{2+} in hepatocytes can activate phospholipase A_2 and exacerbate membrane damage. Elevated Ca^{2+} also may be involved in alterations in calmodulin and phosphorylase activity as well as changes in the activity of nuclear protein kinase C. Increased Ca^{2+} may stimulate the release of cytokines and eicosanoids from Kupffer cells, inducing neutrophil infiltration and hepatocellular injury. CCl_4 hepatotoxicity is obviously a complex, multifactorial process.

Chloroform

Chloroform ($CHCl_3$, trichloromethane) is used primarily in the production of the refrigerant chlorodifluo-

romethane. Measurable concentrations of $CHCl_3$ are found in municipal drinking water supplies. $CHCl_3$ is hepatotoxic and nephrotoxic. It can invoke CNS symptoms at subanesthetic concentrations similar to those of alcohol intoxication. Extremely high $CHCl_3$ exposures can sensitize the myocardium to catecholamines.

The metabolite phosgene covalently binds hepatic and renal proteins and lipids; this damages membranes and other intracellular structures, leading to necrosis and subsequent reparative cellular proliferation that promotes tumor formation in rodents by irreversibly "fixing" spontaneously altered DNA and clonally expanding initiated cells. The expression of certain genes, including *myc* and *fos,* is altered during regenerative cell proliferation in response to $CHCl_3$-induced cytotoxicity.

Although it is a rodent carcinogen, ingestion of $CHCl_3$ in small increments, similar to drinking water patterns in humans, fails to produce sufficient cytotoxic metabolite(s) per unit time to overwhelm detoxification mechanisms. Currently, $CHCl_3$ is classified as a probable human carcinogen (group B2).

AROMATIC HYDROCARBONS

Benzene

Benzene is derived primarily from petroleum and is used in the synthesis of other chemicals and as an important antiknock agent in unleaded gasoline. Inhalation is the primary route of exposure in industrial and everyday settings. Cigarette smoke is the major source of benzene in the home. Smokers have benzene body burdens that are 6 to 10 times higher than those of nonsmokers. Passive smoke can be a significant source of benzene exposure to nonsmokers. Gasoline vapor emissions and auto exhaust are the other key contributors to exposures in the general populace.

The hematopoietic toxicity of chronic exposure to benzene may manifest initially as anemia, leukopenia, thrombocytopenia, or a combination of these conditions. Bone marrow depression appears to be dose-dependent in both laboratory animals and humans. Continued exposure may result in marrow aplasia and pancytopenia, an often fatal outcome. Survivors of aplastic anemia frequently exhibit a preneoplastic state, termed *myelodysplasia,* that may progress to myelogenous leukemia.

There is strong evidence from epidemiologic studies that high-level benzene exposures result in an increased risk of acute myelogenous leukemia (AML) in humans. Evidence for increased risks of other cancers in such populations is less compelling.

Various potential mechanisms require the complementary actions of benzene and several of its metabolites for toxicity.

1. A number of benzene metabolites bind covalently to GSH, proteins, DNA, and RNA. This can result in disruption of the functional hematopoietic microenvironment through inhibition of enzymes, destruction of certain cell populations, and alteration of the growth of other cell types. Covalent binding of hydroquinones to spindle-fiber proteins inhibits cell replication.

2. Oxidative stress contributes to benzene toxicity. As the bone marrow is rich in peroxidase activity, phenolic metabolites of benzene can be activated there to reactive quinone derivatives. These active oxygen species can cause DNA damage, leading to cell mutation or apoptosis, respectively. Modulation of apoptosis may lead to aberrant hematopoiesis and neoplastic progression.

Toluene

Toluene is present in paints, lacquers, thinners, cleaning agents, glues, and many other products. Toluene also is used in the production of other chemicals. Gasoline, which contains 5 to 7 percent toluene by weight, is the largest source of atmospheric emissions and exposure of the general populace. Inhalation is the primary route of exposure, though skin contact occurs frequently. Toluene is a favorite of solvent abusers, who intentionally inhale high concentrations of this VOC.

Toluene is well absorbed from the lungs and GI tract. It accumulates rapidly in the brain and subsequently is deposited in other tissues according to their lipid content, with adipose tissue attaining the highest levels. Toluene is well metabolized, but a portion is exhaled unchanged.

The CNS is the primary target organ of toluene and other alkylbenzenes. Manifestations of exposure range from slight dizziness and headache to unconsciousness, respiratory depression, and death. Occupational inhalation exposure guidelines have been established to prevent significant decrements in psychomotor functions. Acute CNS effects are rapidly reversible upon the cessation of exposure. Subtle neurologic effects have been reported in some groups of occupationally exposed individuals. Severe neurotoxicity sometimes is diagnosed in persons who have abused toluene for a prolonged period. Clinical signs include abnormal electroencephalographic (EEG) activity, tremors, nystagmus, and cerebral atrophy as well as impaired hearing, vision, and speech. Magnetic resonance imaging has revealed permanent changes in brain structure that correspond to the degree of brain dysfunction.

Little is known about the mechanisms by which toluene and similar solvents produce acute or residual CNS effects.

Xylenes and Ethylbenzene

Large numbers of people are exposed to xylenes and ethylbenzene occupationally and environmentally. Xylenes and ethylbenzene, like benzene and toluene, are major components of gasoline and fuel oil. The primary uses of xylenes industrially are as solvents and synthetic intermediates. Most of the aromatics released into the environment evaporate into the atmosphere.

The TK and acute toxicity of toluene, xylenes, and other aromatic solvents are quite similar. Xylenes and the other aromatic solvents are well absorbed from the lungs and GI tract, distributed to tissues according to tissue blood flow and lipid content, exhaled to some extent, well metabolized by hepatic P450s, and largely excreted as urinary metabolites. Acute lethality of hydrocarbons (i.e., CNS depression) varies directly with lipophilicity. There is limited evidence that chronic occupational exposure to xylenes is associated with residual neurologic effects.

Xylenes and ethylbenzene have a limited capacity to affect organs other than the CNS adversely. Mild, transient liver and/or kidney toxicity have been reported occasionally in humans exposed to high vapor concentrations of xylenes. The majority of alkylbenzenes do not appear to be genotoxic or carcinogenic. Ethylbenzene and styrene are known animal carcinogens, but human data are limited.

ALCOHOLS

Ethanol

Many humans experience greater exposure to ethanol (ethyl alcohol, alcohol) than to any other solvent. Ethyl alcohol is used as a solvent in industry, in many household products and pharmaceuticals, and in intoxicating beverages. Frank toxic effects are less important occupationally than are injuries resulting from psychomotor impairment. Driving under the influence of alcohol is the major cause of fatal auto accidents. Blood alcohol level and the time necessary to achieve it are controlled largely by the rapidity and extent of ethanol consumption.

Ethanol is distributed in body water and to some degree in adipose tissue. The alcohol is eliminated by urinary excretion, exhalation, and metabolism. The blood level in an average adult decreases by ~15 to 20 mg/dL per hour. Thus, a person with a blood alcohol level of 120 mg/dL would require 6 to 8 h to reach negligible levels.

Ethanol is metabolized to acetaldehyde by three enzymes:

1. The major pathway involves alcohol dehydrogenase (ADH)-catalyzed oxidation to acetaldehyde. The acetaldehyde that is formed is oxidized rapidly by acetaldehyde dehydrogenase (ALDH) to acetate.
2. A second enzyme, catalase, utilizing H_2O_2 supplied by the actions of NADPH oxidase and xanthine oxidase, normally accounts for more than 10 percent of ethanol metabolism.
3. The third enzyme, CYP2E1, is the principal component of the hepatic microsomal ethanol oxidizing system (MEOS).

ALDH activity is usually sufficiently high to metabolize large amounts of acetaldehyde to acetate. Whites, blacks, and Asians have varying percentages of different ALDH isozymes, which affect the efficiency of acetaldehyde metabolism. Some 50 percent of Asians have inactive ALDH, and these persons may experience flushing, headache, nausea, vomiting, tachycardia, and hyperventilation upon the ingestion of ethanol.

Gender differences in responses to ethanol are well recognized. Females exhibit slightly higher blood ethanol levels than do men after the ingestion of equivalent doses. This phenomenon is due in part to more extensive ADH-catalyzed metabolism of ethanol by the gastric mucosa of males and to the smaller volume of distribution in women for relatively polar solvents such as alcohols. Also, women are more susceptible to alcohol-induced hepatotoxicity.

Fetal alcohol syndrome (FAS) is the most common preventable cause of mental retardation. The diagnostic criteria for FAS include (1) heavy maternal alcohol consumption during gestation, (2) pre- and postnatal growth retardation, (3) craniofacial malformations, including microcephaly, and (4) mental retardation. Less complete manifestations of gestational ethanol exposure are referred to as fetal alcohol effects or alcohol-related neurodevelopmental disorder. Overconsumption during all three trimesters of pregnancy can result in particular manifestations, depending on the period of gestation during which the insult occurs.

Human CYP2E1 is effective in the production of reactive oxygen intermediates from ethanol that cause lipid peroxidation. Also, ethanol induces the release of endotoxin from gram-negative bacteria in the gut. The endotoxin is taken up by Kupffer cells, causing the release of mediators that are cytotoxic to hepatocytes.

Alcohol-induced tissue damage results from both nutritional disturbances and direct toxic effects. Malabsorption of thiamine, diminished enterohepatic circulation of folate, degradation of pyridoxal phosphate, and disturbances in the metabolism of vitamins A and D can occur. Prostaglandins released from endotoxin-activated Kupffer cells may be responsible for a hypermetabolic state in the liver. With the increase in oxygen demand, the viability of centrilobular hepatocytes would be most compromised because of their relatively poor oxygen supply. Metabolism of ethanol via ADH and ALDH results in a shift in the redox state of the cell that can result in hyperlactic acidemia, hyperuricemia, and hyperglycemia.

Alcoholism can result in damage to extrahepatic tissues. Alcoholic cardiomyopathy is a complex process that may result from decreased synthesis of cardiac contractile proteins, attack of oxygen radicals, and antibody response to acetaldehyde-protein adducts. Heavy drinking appears to deplete antioxidants and increases the risk of both hemorrhagic and ischemic strokes. The brain and pancreas may be affected adversely in alcoholics.

The associations between alcohol and cancers came primarily from epidemiologic case-control and cohort studies. Ethanol and smoking act synergistically to cause oral, pharyngeal, and laryngeal cancers. It generally is believed that alcohol induces liver cancer by causing cirrhosis or other liver damage and/or by enhancing the bioactivation of carcinogens. Table 24-1 lists several mechanisms of ethanol-induced cancers.

Methanol

Methanol (methyl alcohol, wood alcohol) is found in a host of consumer products, including windshield washer fluid, and is used in the manufacture of formaldehyde and methyl *tert*-butyl ether (MTBE). Methanol can produce reversible sensory irritation and narcosis at airborne concentrations below those which produce organ system pathology. Serious methanol toxicity is associated most commonly with ingestion. Left untreated, acute methanol poisoning in humans is characterized by an asymptomatic period of 12 to 24 h followed by formic acidemia, ocular toxicity, coma, and in extreme cases death. Visual disturbances develop between 18 and 48 h after inges-

Table 24-1
Possible Mechanisms of Ethanol Carcinogenicity

Congeners, additives, and contaminants in alcoholic beverages influence carcinogenicity.

CYP2E1 induction by ethanol increases metabolic activation of procarcinogens.

Ethanol acts as a solvent for carcinogens, enhancing their absorption into tissues in the upper GI tract.

Ethanol affects the actions of certain hormones in hormone-sensitive tissues.

Immune function is suppressed by alcohol.

Absorption and bioavailability of nutrients are reduced by alcohol.

tion and range from mild photophobia and blurred vision to markedly reduced visual acuity and complete blindness.

The target of methanol in the eye is the retina, specifically the optic disk and optic nerve. Müller cells and rod and cone cells are altered functionally and structurally, because cytochrome oxidase activity in mitochondria is inhibited, resulting in a reduction in ATP.

Although methanol is metabolized in the liver, intraretinal conversion of methanol to formaldehyde and formate is critical. Metabolism of formate to CO_2 then occurs through a two-step tetrahydrofolate (THF)-dependent pathway. Susceptibility to methanol toxicity is dependent on the relative rate of formate clearance. A simplified scheme of methanol metabolism is presented in Fig. 24-2. In fact, formate acts as a direct ocular toxin,

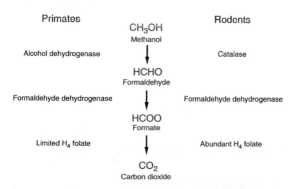

Figure 24-2. Scheme for the metabolism of methanol. Major enzymes are listed for primates (*left*) and rodents (*right*). Conversion of formate to CO_2 is rapid in rodents, but relatively slow in primates.

and the acidotic state potentiates formate toxicity because the inhibition of cytochrome oxidase increases as pH decreases.

GLYCOLS

Ethylene Glycol

Ethylene glycol (EG) is a major constituent of antifreeze, deicers, hydraulic fluids, drying agents, and inks and is used to make plastics and polyester fibers. The most important routes of exposure are dermal and accidental or intentional ingestion. EG is degraded rapidly in environmental media.

Acutely toxic to humans, EG is believed to cause over 100 deaths annually in the United States. Acute poisoning entails three clinical stages: (1) a period of inebriation, with the duration and degree depending on the dose, (2) the cardiopulmonary stage 12 to 24 h after exposure, characterized by tachycardia and tachypnea, which may progress to cardiac failure and pulmonary edema, and (3) the renal toxicity stage 24 to 72 h after exposure. Metabolic acidosis can become progressively more severe during stages 2 and 3.

Absorption from the GI tract of rodents is very rapid and virtually complete. Dermal absorption in humans appears to be less extensive. EG is distributed throughout the body extracellular fluid. As is shown in Fig. 24-3, EG is metabolized by NAD^+-dependent ADH to glycolaldehyde and then to glycolic acid. Glycolic acid is oxidized to glyoxylic acid by glycolic acid oxidase and lactic dehydrogenase. Glyoxylic acid may be converted to formate and CO_2 or oxidized by glyoxylic acid oxidase to oxalic acid. Metabolic acidosis in humans appears to be due largely to the accumulation of glycolic acid. Hypocalcemia can result from calcium chelation by oxalic acid to form calcium oxalate crystals. Deposition of these crystals in tubules of the kidney and small blood vessels in the brain is associated with damage of those organs. EG appears to have limited chronic toxicity potential.

Propylene Glycol

Propylene glycol (PG) is used extensively as a solvent, coolant, antifreeze, and component of hydraulic fluids. As PG is "generally recognized as safe" by the U.S. Food and Drug Administration (FDA), it is a constituent of many cosmetics and processed foods. Furthermore, it serves as a solvent/diluent for a substantial number of oral, dermal, and intravenous drug preparations.

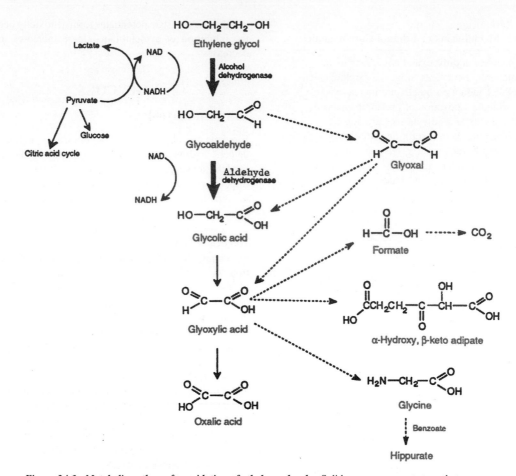

Figure 24-3. *Metabolic pathway for oxidation of ethylene glycol.* Solid arrows represent steps that are quantitatively the most important in humans. Broken arrows indicate minor conversions.

PG has a very low order of acute and chronic toxicity. Extremely high doses can cause CNS depression, metabolic acidosis, encephalopathy, and hemolysis in humans and rodents. PG is metabolized readily by alcohol dehydrogenase to lactaldehyde, which then is oxidized by aldehyde dehydrogenase to lactate. Excessive lactate is primarily responsible for the acidosis.

GLYCOL ETHERS

The glycol ethers include ethylene glycol monomethyl ether, also called 2-methoxyethanol (2-ME; CH_3—O—CH_2—CH_2—OH), ethylene glycol dimethyl ether (CH_3—O—CH_2—CH_2—O—CH_3), 2-butoxyethanol (2-BE; CH_3—CH_2—CH_2—CH_2—O—CH_2—CH_2—OH), and 2-ME acetate (CH_3—CO—O—CH_2—CH_2—O—CH_3). These solvents undergo rapid ester hydrolysis in vivo and exhibit the same toxicity profile as do unesterified glycols. The glycol ethers are metabolized to alkoxyacetic acids, which are regarded as the ultimate toxicants. Their acetaldehyde precursors also have been implicated.

Like glycol ether metabolism, glycol ether toxicity varies with chemical structure. With increasing alkyl chain length, reproductive and developmental toxicity decreases, whereas hematotoxicity increases.

Reproductive Toxicity

The reproductive toxicity of the glycol ethers is limited almost exclusively to reversible spermatotoxicity in males. Typical responses include testicular and seminiferous tubule atrophy, abnormal sperm head morphology, necrotic spermatocytes, decreased sperm motility and count, and infertility.

Developmental Toxicity

Developmental toxicity in rodents includes a variety of minor skeletal variations, hydrocephalus, exencephaly, cardiovascular malformations, dilatation of the renal pelvis, craniofacial malformations, and digit malformations. There are significant associations of glycol ether exposure with the induction of cleft lip and neural tube defects such as spina bifida.

Hematotoxicity

Some glycol ethers are hemolytic to red blood cells (RBCs). Typically, the osmotic balance of the cells is disrupted, they imbibe water and swell, their ATP concentration decreases, and hemolysis occurs. Humans are less susceptible than rodents are to glycol ether–induced RBC deformity and hemolysis.

FUELS AND FUEL ADDITIVES

Automotive Gasoline

Gasoline is a mixture of hundreds of hydrocarbons predominantly in the range of C_4 to C_{12}. Because its composition varies with the crude oil from which it is refined, the refining process, and the use of specific additives, generalizations about the toxicity of gasoline must be made carefully. Experiments conducted with fully vaporized gasoline may not be predictive of actual risk, since humans are exposed primarily to the more volatile components in the range of C_4 to C_5, which are generally less toxic than are higher-molecular-weight fractions. Gasoline additives have their own toxicities, and some are classified as known or probable human carcinogens (e.g., benzene and 1,3-butadiene). However, epidemiologic evidence associating gasoline exposure and cancer in humans is inconclusive.

The most extreme exposures are to those who sniff intentionally gasoline for its euphoric effects. This dangerous habit can cause acute and chronic encephalopathies that are expressed as both motor and cognitive impairment. Ingestion of gasoline during siphoning events typically is followed by a burning sensation in the mouth and pharynx as well as nausea, vomiting, and diarrhea resulting from GI irritation. Gasoline aspirated into the lungs may produce pulmonary epithelial damage, edema, and pneumonitis.

Methyl Tertiary-Butyl Ether

Methyl tertiary-butyl ether is used as an octane booster for gasoline. As a gasoline oxygenator, MTBE makes fuel combustion more complete, thus reducing pollutant emissions from automobile exhaust.

No significant epidemiologic association exists between MTBE exposure and the acute symptoms commonly attributed to MTBE. Those symptoms include headache; eye, nose, and throat irritation; cough; nausea; dizziness; and disorientation. Because three MTBE animal cancer bioassays indicate kidney and testicular tumors in male rats and liver adenomas, leukemia, and lymphoma in female rats, MTBE is classified as a possible human carcinogen (group C).

BIBLIOGRAPHY

Cameron RG, Feuer G, De la Iglesia FA (eds): *Drug Induced Hepatotoxicity.* Berlin: Springer-Verlag, 1996.
Karch SB: *Karch's Pathology of Drug Abuse.* Boca Raton, FL: CRC Press, 2002.

Patnaik P: *A Comprehensive Guide to the Hazardous Properties of Chemical Substances,* 2d ed. New York: Wiley, 1999.
Philip RB: *Ecosystems and Human Health: Toxicology and Environmental Hazards,* 2d ed. Boca Raton, FL: Lewis, 2001.

TOXIC EFFECTS OF RADIATION AND RADIOACTIVE MATERIALS

Naomi H. Harley

BASIC RADIATION CONCEPTS

    Alpha Particles

    Beta Particles, Positrons, and Electron
      Capture

    Gamma-Ray (Photon) Emission

**INTERACTION OF RADIATION WITH
MATTER**

    Alpha Particles

    Beta Particles

    Gamma Rays

      The Photoelectric Effect

      The Compton Effect

      Pair Production

**MECHANISMS OF DNA DAMAGE AND
MUTAGENESIS**

    Energy Deposition in the Cell Nucleus

    Direct and Indirect Ionization

    DNA Damage

**HUMAN STUDIES OF RADIATION
TOXICITY**

ENVIRONMENTAL EPIDEMIOLOGY

    The Environmental Studies

    Meta-Analysis of Environmental
      Epidemiology

    What Is Known about Radon Exposure
      in the Home

**NATURAL RADIOACTIVITY AND
RADIATION BACKGROUND**

    Local Environmental Releases

KEY POINTS

- The four main types of radiation are due to alpha particles, electrons (negatively charged beta particles or positively charged positrons), gamma rays, and x-rays.

- Alpha particles are helium nuclei (consisting of two protons and two neutrons) with a charge of +2 that are ejected from the nucleus of an atom.

- Beta particle decay occurs when a neutron in the nucleus of an element is effectively transformed into a proton and an electron, which is ejected.

- Gamma-ray emission occurs in combination with alpha, beta, or positron emission or electron capture. Whenever the ejected particle does not utilize all the available energy for decay, the excess energy is released by the nucleus as a photon or gamma-ray emission coincident with the ejection of the particle.

- Ionizing radiation loses energy when passing through matter by producing ion pairs (an electron and a positively charged atom residue).

- Radiation may deposit energy directly in DNA (direct effect) or may ionize other molecules closely associated with DNA—hydrogen or oxygen—to form free radicals that can damage DNA (indirect effect).

BASIC RADIATION CONCEPTS

Radiation may be due to loss of alpha particles, electrons (negatively charged beta particles or positively charged positrons), gamma rays, and x-rays. An atom can decay to a product element through the loss of a heavy (mass = 4) charged (+2) alpha particle (He^{2+}) that consists of two protons and two neutrons. An atom can decay through the loss of a negatively or positively charged electron (beta particle or positron). Gamma radiation results when the nucleus releases excess energy, usually after an alpha, beta, or positron transition. X-rays occur whenever an inner-shell orbital electron is removed and rearrangement of the atomic electrons results, with the release of the element's characteristic x-ray energy.

Alpha Particles

Alpha particles are helium nuclei (consisting of two protons and two neutrons) with a charge of +2 that are ejected from the nucleus of an atom. When an alpha particle loses energy, slows to the velocity of a gas atom, and acquires two electrons from the vast sea of free electrons present in most media, it becomes part of the normal background helium in the environment. The formula for alpha decay is

$$\underset{Z}{\overset{A}{X}} \rightarrow \underset{Z-2}{\overset{A-4}{Y}} + He^{2+} + gamma + Q_\alpha$$

Where Z = atomic number
        A = atomic weight

The energy available in this decay is Q_α and is equal to the mass difference of the parent and the two products. The energy is shared among the particles and the gamma ray if one is present.

An example of alpha decay is given by the natural radionuclide radium (^{226}Ra):

$$\underset{86}{\overset{226}{Ra}} \rightarrow \underset{84}{\overset{222}{Rn}} + alpha\ (5.2\ MeV)$$

The energy of alpha particles for most emitters is in the range of 4 to 8 MeV. More energetic alpha particles exist but are seen only in very short-lived emitters such as those formed by reactions occurring in particle accelerators.

Beta Particles, Positrons, and Electron Capture

Beta particle decay occurs when a neutron in the nucleus of an element is effectively transformed into a proton and an electron. Subsequent ejection of the electron occurs, and the maximum energy of the beta particle equals the mass difference between the parent and the product nuclei. A gamma ray also may be present to share the energy, Q_β:

$$\underset{Z}{\overset{A}{X}} \rightarrow \underset{Z+1}{\overset{A}{Y}} + beta + Q_\beta$$

An example of beta decay is given by the natural radionuclide lead (^{210}Pb):

$$\underset{82}{\overset{210}{Pb}} \rightarrow \underset{83}{\overset{210}{Bi}} + beta\ (0.015\ MeV) + gamma\ (0.046\ MeV)$$

Unlike monoenergetic alpha particles in alpha decay, beta particles are emitted with a continuous spectrum of energy from zero to the maximum energy available for the transition. The reason for this is that the total available energy is shared in each decay or transition by two particles: the beta particle and an antineutrino. The total energy released in each transition is constant, but the observed beta particles then appear as a spectrum. The residual energy is carried away by the antineutrino, which is a particle with essentially zero mass and charge that cannot be observed without extraordinarily complex instrumentation. The beta particle, by contrast, is observed readily with conventional nuclear counting equipment.

Positron emission is similar to beta particle emission but results from the effective nucleon transformation of a proton to a neutron and a positively charged electron. The atomic number decreases rather than increases, as it does in beta decay.

An example of positron decay is given by the natural radionuclide copper (^{64}Cu), which decays by beta emission 41 percent of the time, by positron emission 19 percent of the time, and by electron capture 40 percent of the time:

$$\underset{29}{\overset{64}{Cu}} \rightarrow \underset{28}{\overset{64}{Ni}} + positron\ (0.66\ MeV)$$

$$\begin{array}{ccc} 64 & & 64 \\ \text{Cu} & \rightarrow & \text{Zn} + \text{beta (0.57 MeV)} \\ 29 & & 30 \end{array}$$

$$\begin{array}{ccc} 64 & & 64 \\ \text{Cu} & \rightarrow & \text{Ni electron capture} \\ 29 & & 28 \end{array}$$

The energy of the positron appears as a continuous spectrum, similar to that in beta decay, in which the total energy available for decay is shared between the positron and a neutrino. In the case of positron emission, the maximum energy of the emitted particle is the mass difference of the parent and product nuclide minus the energy needed to create two electron masses (1.02 MeV), whereas the maximum energy of the beta particle is the mass difference itself. This is the case because in beta decay the increase in the number of orbital electrons resulting from the increase in atomic number of the product nucleus cancels the mass of the electron lost in emitting the beta particle. This does not happen in positron decay, and an orbital electron is lost as a result of the decrease in atomic number of the product and the loss of the electron mass in positron emission.

Electron capture competes with positron decay, and the resulting product nucleus is the same nuclide. In electron capture, an orbiting electron is acquired by the nucleus, and the transformation of a proton plus the electron to form a neutron takes place. In some cases, the energy available is released as a gamma-ray photon, but this is not necessary, and a monoenergetic neutrino may be emitted. If the 1.02 MeV required for positron decay is not available, positron decay is not kinetically possible and electron capture is the only mode observed.

Gamma-Ray (Photon) Emission

Gamma-ray emission is not a primary process except in rare instances, but it occurs in combination with alpha, beta, or positron emission or electron capture. Whenever the ejected particle does not utilize all the available energy for decay, the excess energy is released by the nucleus as photon or gamma-ray emission coincident with the ejection of the particle.

One of the rare instances of pure gamma-ray emission is technetium 99m (^{99m}Tc), which has a 6.0-h half-life and is used widely in diagnostic medicine for organ scans. Its decay product, ^{99}Tc, has a very long half-life (2.13×10^5 years), and as all ^{99}Tc ultimately is released to the environment, a background of this nuclide is emerging.

$$\begin{array}{ccc} 99m & & 99 \\ \text{Tc} & \rightarrow & \text{Tc} + \text{gamma (0.14 MeV)} \\ 43 & & 43 \end{array}$$

In many cases, the photon will not be emitted by the nucleus but the excess excitation energy will be transferred to an orbital electron. This electron then is ejected as a monoenergetic particle with energy equal to that of the photon minus the binding energy of the orbital electron. This process is known as internal conversion.

INTERACTION OF RADIATION WITH MATTER

Ionizing radiation, by definition, loses energy when passing through matter by producing ion pairs (an electron and a positively charged atom residue). A fraction of the energy loss raises atomic electrons to an excited state. The average energy needed to produce an ion pair, W, is numerically equal to 33.85 eV. This energy is roughly two times the ionization potential of most gases or other elements because it includes the energy lost in the excitation process. It is not clear what role the excitation plays, for example, in damage to targets in cellular DNA. Ionization, by contrast, can break bonds in DNA, causing strand breaks and easily understood damage.

All particles and rays interact through their charge or field with atomic or free electrons in the medium through which they are passing. There is no interaction with the atomic nucleus except at energies above about 8 MeV, which is required for interactions that break apart the nucleus (spallation). Very high energy cosmic-ray particles, for example, produce ^{3}H, ^{7}Be, ^{14}C, and ^{22}Na in the upper atmosphere through spallation of atmospheric oxygen and nitrogen.

Alpha Particles

The alpha particle is a heavy charged particle with a mass that is 7300 times that of the electrons with which it interacts. A massive particle interacting with a small particle has the interesting property that it can give a maximum velocity during energy transfer to the small particle of only two times the initial velocity of the heavy particle. The maximum energy that can be transferred per interaction is

$$E_{(\text{maximum electron})} = 4/7300 \, E_{(\text{alpha particle})} \qquad (1)$$

Although alpha particles can lose perhaps 10 to 20 percent of their energy in traveling 10 μm in tissue (1 cm in air), each interaction can impart only the small energy, given in the maximum, in Eq. (1). Thus, alpha particles are characterized by a high energy loss per unit path length and a high ionization density along the track length. This is called a *high linear-energy-transfer* (LET) or a *high-LET* particle.

The energy loss in matter, dE/dx or stopping power, for alpha energies between 0.2 and 10 MeV is given by

$$dE/dx = 3.8 \times 10^{-25} \, C \, NZ/E \, \ln\{548E/I\} \text{ MeV}/\mu\text{m}^{-1}$$
$$(2)$$

where N = number of atoms cm^{-3} in medium
Z = atomic number of medium
I = ionization potential of medium
E = energy of alpha particle
C = charge correction for alpha particles with energy below 1.6 MeV

A simple rule of thumb can be used to estimate the ionization potential of a compound or element:

$$I = 10(Z) \qquad (3)$$

When alpha particles are near the end of their range, the charge is not constant at +2 but can be +1 or even zero as the particle acquires or loses electrons. A correction factor, C, is needed for energies between 0.2 and 1.5 MeV to account for this effect. These factors vary from 0.24 at 0.2 MeV, 0.75 at 0.6 MeV, and 0.875 at 1.0 MeV, up to 1.0 at 1.6 MeV.

For the case of tissue, Eq. (2) reduces to

$$dE/dx_{\text{tissue}} = [0.126C/E] \ln\{7.99E\} \text{ MeV}/\mu\text{m}^{-1} \quad (4)$$

Example 1 Find the energy loss (stopping power) of a 0.6- and a 5-MeV alpha particle in tissue.

$$
\begin{aligned}
dE/dx &= 0.126(0.75)/0.6 \ln(7.99 \times 0.6) \\
&= 0.25 \text{ MeV}/\mu\text{m}^{-1} \\
&= 0.126(1.0)/5.0 \ln(7.99 \times 5.0) \\
&= 0.093 \text{ MeV}/\mu\text{m}^{-1}
\end{aligned}
$$

The significance of this energy loss is seen in the fact that it requires 33.85 eV to produce an ion pair; therefore, a 0.6-MeV alpha particle can produce $(0.25 \times 10^6$ eV/μm$^{-1})/(33.86$ eV/ion pair) = 7400 ion pairs in 1 μm, or enough damage to cause a double-strand break.

Beta Particles

The equations for beta particle energy loss in matter cannot be simplified, as in the case of alpha particles, because of three factors:

1. Even at low energies of a few tenths of an MeV, beta particles are traveling near the speed of light and relativistic effects (mass increase) must be considered.

2. Electrons are interacting with particles of the same mass in the medium (free or orbital electrons), and so large energy losses per collision are possible.

3. Radiative or bremsstrahlung energy loss occurs when electrons or positrons are slowing down in matter. Such a loss also occurs with alpha particles, but the magnitude of this energy loss is negligible.

Including the effects of these three factors, the energy loss for electrons and positrons has been well quantitated. Tabulations of energy loss in various media have been prepared with the ionization energy loss and the radiative loss detailed.

Gamma Rays

Photons do not have a mass or charge. The interaction between a photon and matter therefore is controlled by interaction of the electric and magnetic field of the photon with the electron in the medium. There are three modes of interaction with the medium.

The Photoelectric Effect The photon interaction with an orbital electron in the medium is complete, and the full energy of the photon is given to the electron.

The Compton Effect Part of the photon energy is transferred to an electron, and the photon scatters (usually at a small angle from its original path) with reduced energy. The governing expressions are

$$
\begin{aligned}
E' &= E \, 0.511/(1 + 1/a - \cos\theta) \qquad (5) \\
T &= Ea(1 - \cos\theta)/[1 + a(1 - \cos\theta)]
\end{aligned}
$$

where E, E' = initial and scattered photon energy in MeV
T = kinetic energy of electron in MeV
$a = E/0.511$
θ = angle of photon scatter from its original path

Pair Production Pair production occurs whenever the photon energy is greater than the rest mass of two electrons, $2(0.511 \text{ MeV}) = 1.02 \text{ MeV}$. The electromagnetic energy of the photon can be converted directly to an electron-positron pair, with excess energy above 1.02 MeV appearing as kinetic energy given to these particles.

The loss of photons and energy loss from a photon beam as it passes through matter are described by two coefficients. The attenuation coefficient determines the fractional loss of photons per unit distance (usually in normalized units of g/cm^2, which is the linear distance times the density of the medium). The mass energy absorption coefficient determines the fractional energy deposition per unit distance traveled. The loss of photons from the beam is given by

$$I/I_0 = \exp(-\mu/\rho d) \qquad (6)$$

where I = intensity of photon beam (numbers of photons)
     I_0 = beam intensity
     μ/ρ = attenuation coefficient in medium for energy considered (in m^2 kg^{-2})
     d = thickness of medium in superficial density units kg m^{-2} (thickness in meters times density in kg m^{-3})

Superficial density is convenient in that it normalizes energy absorption in different media. For example, air and tissue have approximately the same energy absorption per kg m^{-2}, whereas in the linear dimension, the energy absorption, say, per meter, is vastly different. The energy actually deposited in the medium per unit distance is calculated by using the mass energy absorption coefficient as opposed to the overall attenuation coefficient, and the energy loss is given by

$$\Delta E = (\mu_{\text{en}}/\rho)E_0 \qquad (7)$$

where ΔE = energy loss in medium per unit distance (in MeV m^2 kg^{-1})
     μ_{en}/ρ = mass energy absorption coefficient (m^2 kg^{-2})
     E_0 = initial photon energy

The values for μ_{en}/ρ as a function of gamma-ray energy are shown in Table 25-1 for air and muscle. Energy loss then can be expressed per unit linear distance by multiplying by the density of the medium (kg m^{-3}).

MECHANISMS OF DNA DAMAGE AND MUTAGENESIS

Energy Deposition in the Cell Nucleus

DNA is a double-helical macromolecule that consists of four repeating units: the purine bases adenine (A) and guanine (G) and the pyrimidine bases thymine (T) and cytosine (C). The bases are arranged in two linear arrays (or strands) held together by hydrogen bonds centrally and linked externally by covalent bonds to sugar-phosphate residues (the DNA "backbone"). Adenine base pairs naturally with thymine (A:T base pair) whereas guanine pairs with cytosine (G:C base pair), and so one DNA strand has the complementary sequence of the other. Damage to DNA may affect any one of its components, but it is the loss or alteration of base sequence that has genetic consequences.

Ionizing radiation loses energy and slows down by forming ion pairs (a positively charged atom and an electron). Different ionization densities result from gamma rays, beta particles, and alpha particles. Their track structure is broadly characterized as ranging from sparsely ionizing (or low-LET) to densely ionizing (high-LET) radiation. Each track of low-LET radiation, resulting from x-rays or gamma rays, consists of a few ionizations across an average-sized cell nucleus [e.g., an electron set in motion by a gamma ray crossing an 8-μm-diameter nucleus gives an average of about 70 ionizations, equivalent to about 5 mGy (500 mrad) absorbed dose]. Individual tracks vary widely around this value because of the stochastic nature of energy deposition, that is, variability of ion pairs per μm and path length through the nucleus. A high-LET alpha particle produces many thousands of ionizations and gives a relatively high dose to the cell. For example, a 4-MeV alpha-particle track yields on average about 30,000 ionizations (3 Gy, 300 rad) in an average-sized cell nucleus. However, within the nucleus, even low-LET gamma radiation will produce some microregions of relatively dense ionization over the dimensions of DNA structures because of the low-energy electrons set in motion.

Direct and Indirect Ionization

Radiation tracks may deposit energy directly in DNA (direct effect) or may ionize other molecules closely associated with DNA—hydrogen or oxygen—to form free radicals that can damage DNA (indirect effect). Within a cell, the indirect effect occurs over very short distances

Table 25-1
Mass Energy Absorption Coefficients for Air and Water

PHOTON ENERGY, MeV	AIR, $\mu_{en}/\rho(m^2\ kg^{-1})$	MUSCLE, STRIATE (ICRU), $\mu_{en}/\rho(m^2\ kg^{-1})$
0.01	0.46	0.49
0.015	0.13	0.14
0.02	0.052	0.055
0.03	0.015	0.016
0.04	0.0067	0.0070
0.05	0.0040	0.0043
0.06	0.0030	0.0032
0.08	0.0024	0.0026
0.10	0.0023	0.0025
0.15	0.0025	0.0027
0.20	0.0027	0.0029
0.30	0.0029	0.0032
0.40	0.0029	0.0032
0.50	0.0030	0.0033
0.60	0.0030	0.0033
0.80	0.0029	0.0032
1.00	0.0028	0.0031
1.50	0.0025	0.0028
2.00	0.0023	0.0026
3.00	0.0021	0.0023

on the order of a few nanometers. The diffusion distance of radicals is limited by their reactivity. Although it is difficult to measure accurately the different contributions made by the direct and indirect effects to DNA damage caused by low-LET radiation, evidence from radical scavengers introduced into cells suggests that about 35 percent is exclusively direct and 65 percent has an indirect (scavengeable) component.

Both direct and indirect effects cause similar early damage to DNA; this is the case because the ion radicals produced by direct ionization of DNA may react further to produce DNA radicals similar to those produced by water-radical attack on DNA.

DNA Damage

Ionization frequently disrupts chemical bonding in cellular molecules. If the majority of ionizations occur as single isolated events (low-LET radiation), the disrup-

tions are repaired readily by cellular enzymes. The average density of ionization by high-LET radiations is such that several ionizations may occur as the particle traverses a DNA double helix. Therefore, much of the damage from high-LET radiations, as well as a minority of the DNA damage from low-LET radiations, derives from localized clusters of ionizations that can disrupt the DNA structure severely. Although the extent of local clustering of ionizations in DNA from single tracks of low- and high-LET radiations will overlap, high-LET radiation tracks are more efficient at inducing larger clusters and thus more complex damage. Also, high-LET radiations induce some very large clusters of ionizations that do not occur with low-LET radiations; the resulting damage may be irreparable and also may have unique cellular consequences. When a cell is damaged by high-LET radiation, each track will produce large numbers of ionizations so that the cell will receive a relatively high dose, as was noted in the calculation above, and there

Table 25-2
Estimated Yields of DNA Damage in Mammalian Cells Caused by Low-LET Radiation Exposures

TYPE OF DAMAGE	YIELD (NUMBER OF DEFECTS PER CELL Gy^{-1})
Single-strand breaks	1000
Base damage*	500
Double-strand breaks	40
DNA protein cross-links	150

*Base excision enzyme-sensitive sites or antibody detection of thymine glycol.

will be a greater probability of correlated damage within a single DNA molecule. As a consequence, the irradiation of a population of cells or a tissue with a "low dose" of high-LET radiation results in a few cells being hit with a relatively high dose (one track) rather than in each cell receiving a small dose. In contrast, low-LET radiation is distributed more uniformly over the cell population. At doses of low-LET radiation in excess of about 1 mGy (for an average-size cell nucleus 8 μm in diameter), each cell nucleus is likely to be traversed by more than one sparsely ionizing track.

The interaction of ionizing radiation with DNA produces numerous types of damage. Table 25-2 lists some of the main damage products that can be measured after low-LET irradiation of DNA, with a rough estimate of their abundance. Attempts also have been made to predict the frequencies of different damage types from knowledge of radiation track structure, with certain assumptions about the minimum energy deposition (number of ionizations) required. Interactions can be classified according to the probability that they will cause a single-strand DNA alteration, a double-strand break, or more complex DNA damage (e.g., a double-strand break with adjacent damage). Good agreement has been obtained between these predictions and direct measurements of single-strand breaks. Although complex forms of damage are difficult to quantify with current experimental techniques, the use of enzymes that cut DNA at sites of base damage suggests that irradiation of DNA in solution produces complex damage sites that consist mainly of closely spaced base damage (measured as oxidized bases of abasic sites); double-strand breaks were associated with only 20 percent of the complex damage sites. It is expected that the occurrence of more complex types of damage will increase with increasing LET and that this category of damage will be less repairable than are the simpler forms of damage.

Some of the DNA damage caused by ionizing radiation is chemically similar to damage that occurs naturally in the cell. This "spontaneous" damage arises from the thermal instability of DNA as well as endogenous oxidative and enzymatic processes. Several metabolic pathways produce oxidative radicals within the cell, and these radicals can attack DNA to produce both DNA base damage and breakage, mostly as isolated events. The more complex types of damage caused by radiation may not occur spontaneously, because localized concentrations of endogenous radicals are less likely to be generated in the immediate vicinity of DNA.

HUMAN STUDIES OF RADIATION TOXICITY

There have been five major studies of the health detriment resulting from exposure of humans to ionizing radiation. Other studies of large worker populations exposed to very low levels of radiation and environmental populations exposed to radon are ongoing, but they are not expected to provide new data on risk estimates from ionizing radiation. These worker and environmental populations are studied to ensure that there is no inconsistency in the radiation risk data in extrapolating from the higher exposures. The basic studies on which the quantitative risk calculations are founded include radium exposures, A-bomb survivors, underground miners exposed to radon, patients irradiated with x-rays for ankylosing spondylitis, and children irradiated with x-rays for tinea capitis (ringworm).

The data from the five major studies are summarized in Table 25-3. This table shows the lifetime cancer risks that are significant, with the risks given in units of per gray (or per Sievert where appropriate for alpha emitters).

In the table, leukemia and cancers of the lung and female breast are the most critical. Osteogenic sarcoma is seen in the radium exposures. There is no clear linear dose response for ^{224,226}Ra. This has been attributed to the existence of an apparent threshold. The cancer risk to individual organs from different study groups is in general agreement regardless of radiation type or whole- or partial-body exposure.

ENVIRONMENTAL EPIDEMIOLOGY

The Environmental Studies

There are at least 24 published studies that attempt to define or detect the effect of radon exposure in the

Table 25-3
Lifetime Cancer Mortality per Gray from Five Major Epidemiologic Studies (in parentheses, risk per sievert for alpha emitters, $w_r = 20$)*

STUDY	ALL SITES	LEUKEMIA	LUNG	FEMALE BREAST	BONE	THYROID	SKIN
Atom bomb whole-body, gamma	0.05	0.005	0.0085	0.002	0.0005	0.0008	0.0002
Uranium miner bronchial epithelium, alpha			(0.04) 0.0020				
Ankylosing spondylitis, spinal x-ray		0.0011	0.0008 0.0028	0.0015			
Tinea capitis, head x-ray						0.0010§	0.0030‡
Radium ingestion, bone,* alpha (^{226}Ra)					0.004 (0.0002)		
Radium ingestion, bone,† alpha (^{224}Ra)					0.02 (0.0010)		

*The lifetime risk is calculated for an average skeletal dose of 10 Gy, assuming that the risk persists for 50 years. The risk is nonlinear and is about 0.01 Gy^{-1} at 100 Gy, for example.

†The lifetime risk is calculated for an average skeletal dose of 10 Gy. The risk is nonlinear and is about 0.01 Gy^{-1} for a skeletal dose of 1 Gy.

‡The mortality for skin cancer is estimated as 1 percent of the incidence; see text.

§Thyroid mortality for males and females. Estimated as 10 percent of incidence.

environment. The pattern emerging from the domestic studies indicates that the lung cancer risk from ^{222}Rn exposure is difficult to determine with accuracy or precision. This is due mostly to the high background lung cancer mortality caused by smoking.

Among the 24 published domestic studies, 13 are ecologic and 11 are case-control. Ecologic studies depend on relating the disease response of a population to some measure of a suspected causative agent. There usually are not enough data on all the variables involved in the disease to infer any reliable associations. Ecologic studies are the weakest type of epidemiologic exploration. Unless a biological marker for radon-induced lung cancer is found, it is unlikely that environmental epidemiology will be effective in assessing risk. The effects of radon in the environment are subtle compared with the overwhelming lung cancer mortality that results from smoking.

Meta-Analysis of Environmental Epidemiology

A meta-analysis combined the published information from the largest domestic studies into one study without actually having the raw data available. The results shown

in Fig. 25-1 reveal that essentially no study found statistically significant cancer deaths caused by radon, but the authors state that the combined trend in the relative risk with increasing exposure was statistically significant, with an estimated relative risk (RR) of 1.14 (95 percent CI = 1.0 to 1.3) at an exposure of 150 Bq m^{-3} (4 pCil^{-1}).

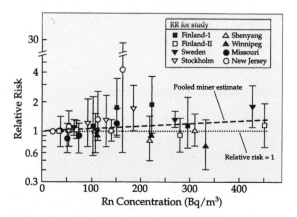

Figure 25-1. Meta-analysis of eight domestic radon case-control studies. $\sigma g = 2$ for size distributions.

What Is Known about Radon Exposure in the Home

Four concepts have emerged from current radon research:

1. Mining epidemiology indicates that short exposure to high levels of radon and daughters produces a clear excess of lung cancer.

2. Particle size can change the actual dose delivered by radon to bronchial tissue, with small particles giving a substantially higher dose per unit exposure. The use of open flames, electric motors, and the like, indoors produces a higher dose per unit exposure.

3. Smokers are at higher risk from radon per unit exposure than are nonsmokers.

4. Urban areas almost universally have low radon, and apartment dwellers removed from the ground source have particularly low radon exposure at home.

The miners' data show clearly that there is a risk of lung cancer from exposure to high concentrations of radon delivered over short periods. Comparable exposures delivered over a lifetime in the home have not produced statistically significant increases in lung cancer mortality except among smokers in one large study in Sweden. The risk can still exist, but the confounding effects of other carcinogens, such as smoking and urbanization, make it impossible to extract the more subtle impact of radon in existing studies.

NATURAL RADIOACTIVITY AND RADIATION BACKGROUND

Occupational, accidental, and wartime experiences have provided the bases for all the current radiation risk estimates. For many years, the radioisotopes deposited internally were compared with ^{226}Ra to evaluate the maximum permissible body burden for a particular emitter. The current limits for external and internal radiation are based on dose estimates that in turn can be related to cancer risks. One standard of comparison has always been exposure from the natural background.

A substantial dose is received annually from cosmic radiation and from external terrestrial radiation present from uranium, thorium, and potassium in the earth's crust. Internal emitters are present in the body as a consequence of dietary consumption and inhalation. For example, potassium is a necessary element in the body and is under homeostatic control. Radioactive ^{40}K constitutes a constant fraction of all natural potassium. Potassium delivers the largest internal dose from the diet of 0.15 mSv per year. However, the data are scanty on the

Table 25-4
Equivalent Dose Rates to Various Tissues from Natural Radionuclides Contained in the Body

RADIONUCLIDE	Equivalent Dose Rate, mSv yr^{-1} BRONCHIAL EPITHELIUM	SOFT TISSUE	BONE SURFACES	BONE MARROW
^{14}C	—	0.10	0.08	0.30
^{40}K	—	1.80	1.40	2.70
^{87}Rb	—	0.03	0.14	0.07
^{238}U-^{234}Th	—	0.046	0.03	0.004
^{230}Th	—	0.001	0.06	0.001
^{226}Ra	—	0.03	0.90	0.15
^{222}Rn	—	0.07	0.14	0.14
^{222}Rn daughters	24	—	—	—
^{210}Pb-^{210}Po	—	1.40	7.00	1.40
^{232}Th	—	0.001	0.02	0.004
^{228}Ra-^{224}Ra	—	0.0015	1.20	0.22
^{220}Rn	—	0.001	—	—
Total	24	3.50	11.00	5.00

Table 25-5

Estimated Total Effective Dose Rate for a Member of the Population in the United States and Canada from Various Sources of Background Radiation

SOURCE	LUNG	GONADS	BONE SURFACE	BONE MARROW	OTHER TISSUES	TOTAL
Total Effective Dose Rate, mSv yr^{-1}						
w_t*	0.12	0.25	0.03	0.12	0.48	1.0
Cosmic	0.03	0.07	0.008	0.03	0.13	0.27
Cosmogenic	0.001	0.002	—	0.004	0.003	0.01
Terrestrial	0.03	0.07	0.008	0.03	0.14	0.28
Inhaled	2.0	—	—	—	—	2.0
In body	0.04	0.09	0.03	0.06	0.17	0.40
Total	2.1	0.23	0.05	0.12	0.44	3.0

*Tissue weighting factor.

dietary intake of other radionuclides in the U.S. population. Given the usual distribution of intakes across a large population, it is probable that other emitters, notably ^{210}Pb, could deliver a significant dose to a fraction of the population.

The largest dose received by the population is from the inhaled short-lived daughters of radon. These daughters are present in all atmospheres because radon is released rather efficiently from the ^{226}Ra in rock and soil. The short-lived daughters, ^{218}Po, ^{214}Pb, and ^{214}Bi-^{214}Po, have an effective half-life of 30 min, but the 3.8-day parent radon supports their presence in the atmosphere.

Average outdoor concentrations in every state in the United States have been measured and summarized as 15 Bq m^{-3} and indoors as 40 Bq m^{-3}. A structure such as a house prevents the rapid upward distribution of radon into the atmosphere, and substantial levels can build up indoors. The source of radon is the ground; therefore, levels in living areas above the ground generally have one-third to one-fifth the concentrations measured in basements. An effective barrier across the soil-building interface also inhibits the entry of radon into buildings. Ventilation with outdoor air reduces indoor radon. For this reason, industrial buildings with more substantial foundations and higher ventilation rates tend to have lower radon concentrations than do single-family (or detached) houses. Apartments above ground level have radon concentrations about half the average of those in single-family dwellings.

It is of significance that an average radon concentration indoors of 40 Bq m^{-3} results in an equivalent dose to bronchial epithelium of 24 mSv/year or an effective

dose of 2 mSv per year. The equivalent doses for other major natural internal emitters are shown in Table 25-4.

It should be recognized that the actual dose accumulated by an individual depends on dietary habits, location (Denver, for example, at an altitude of 1.6 km, has double the average cosmic-ray exposure), and the dwelling. Table 25-5 provides estimated dose rates from various sources of background radiation. Figure 25-2 shows the average components of natural background in the United States.

Local Environmental Releases

Large- and small-scale accidents continue to release radioactivity into the environment. The accident at the

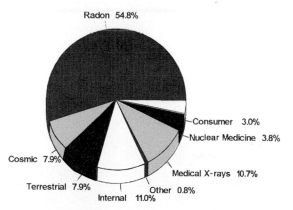

Figure 25-2. Contribution from natural background to effective dose of radiation in the U.S. population. Annual average effective dose, 3.6 mSv.

Table 25-6
Estimates of Radionuclide Released and Collective Effective Dose from Human-Made Environmental Sources of Radiation

SOURCE	^{3}H	^{14}C	NOBLE GASES	^{90}Sr	^{131}I	^{137}Cs	Collective Effective Dose* Person Sv — LOCAL AND REGIONAL	GLOBAL
Atmospheric nuclear testing	240,000	220		604	650,000	910		2,230,000
Local								
Semipalatinsk							4600	
Nevada							500†	
Australia							700	
Pacific test site							160†	
Underground nuclear testing			50		15		200	
Nuclear weapons fabrication								
Early practice							8000‡	
Hanford							15,000§	
Chelyabinsk							1000	10,000
Later practice							30,000¶	
Nuclear power production								
Milling and mining							2700	
Reactor operation	140	1.1	3,200		0.04		3700	
Fuel reprocessing	57	0.3	1,200	6.9	0.004	40	4600	
Fuel cycle							300,000¶	100,000
Radioisotope production and use	2.6	1.0	52		6.0		2000	80,000
Accidents								
Three Mile Island			370		0.0006		40	
Chernobyl					630	70		600,000
Kyshtym				5.4		0.04	2500	
Windscale		1.2			0.7	0.02	2000	
Palomares							3	
Thule							0	
SNAP 9A								2100
Cosmos 954				0.003	0.2	0.003		20
Ciudad Juarez							150	
Mohammedia							80	
Goiania						0.05	60	
Total							380,000	23,100,000
Total collective effective dose (Person Sv)								23,500,000

*Truncated at 10,000 years.
†External dose only.
‡From release of ^{131}I to the atmosphere.
§From releases of radionuclides into the Techa River.
¶Long-term collective dose from release of ^{222}Rn from tailings.

Windscale nuclear power reactor in 1957 was a local incident in Great Britain. The nearby population has been studied for over 30 years without the appearance of significant health effects. The nuclear power accident at Three Mile Island caused enormous financial damage, but the containment vessel was not breached and virtually no radioactivity escaped. In the accident at the Chernobyl nuclear power plant, containment failed and some radioactivity was spread widely over Europe. The United Nations Scientific Committee on the Effects of Atomic Radiation has summarized the committed dose from measurements made in the affected countries from various releases, and those findings are shown in Table 25-6.

Local exposures and doses from accidents can be anticipated to increase, as the use of radioactive materials industrially is widespread.

BIBLIOGRAPHY

Bushong SC: *Radiologic Science for Technologists: Physics, Biology, and Protection*, 7th ed. St. Louis: Mosby, 2001.

Forshier S: *Essentials of Radioation Biology and Protection.* Albany, NY: Delmar/Thomson, 2002.

UNSCEAR: *Sources and Effects of Ionizing Radiation.* Report of the United Nations Scientific Committee on the Effects of Atomic Radiation. New York: United Nations, 2000.

C H A P T E R   2 6

TOXIC EFFECTS OF TERRESTRIAL ANIMAL VENOMS AND POISONS

Findlay E. Russell

KEY POINTS

- Venomous animals produce poison in a highly developed secretory gland or group of cells and can deliver toxin during a biting or stinging act.

- Poisonous animals are those whose tissues, either in part or in their entirety, are toxic. Poisoning usually takes place through ingestion.

- The bioavailability of a venom is determined by its composition, molecular size, amount or concentration gradient, solubility, and degree of ionization and the rate of blood flow into that tissue as well as the properties of the engulfing surface itself.

- The distribution of most venom fractions is unequal, being affected by protein binding, variations in pH, and membrane permeability, among other factors.

- A venom may be metabolized in several or many different tissues.

- Because of their protein composition, many toxins produce an antibody response; this response is essential in producing antisera.

Venomous animals are capable of producing a poison in a highly developed secretory gland or group of cells and can deliver toxin during a biting or stinging act. Poisonous animals are those whose tissues, either in part or in their entirety, are toxic. These animals have no mechanism or structure for the delivery of their poisons, and poisoning usually takes place through ingestion.

PROPERTIES OF ANIMAL TOXINS

Venoms contain proteins, amines, lipids, steroids, glucosides, aminopolysaccharides, quinones, free amino acids, 5-hydroxytryptamine (5-HT), histamine, and other substances. Unfortunately, studying the chemistry, pharmacology, and toxicology of venoms requires taking the venoms apart. This has two shortcomings: First, a destructive process is used in attempting to understand what must have been a constructive one; second, the essential quality of the venom may be destroyed before suitable acquaintance with the full toxin has been achieved. Often the technology becomes so exacting that the end in regard to the venom's function is lost in our preoccupation with the means of the examination.

The bioavailability of a venom is determined by its composition, molecular size, amount or concentration gradient, solubility, and degree of ionization and the rate of blood flow into that tissue as well as the properties of the engulfing surface. The venom can be absorbed by active or passive transport, facilitated diffusion, or even pinocytosis. The venom then is transmitted into the vascular bed, sometimes directly and sometimes through lymphatic channels. The lymph circulation not only carries surplus interstitial fluid produced by the venom but also transports the larger molecular components and other particulates back to the bloodstream.

The receptor sites appear to have highly variable degrees of sensitivity. In the case of complex venom mixtures, there may be many receptor sites. There is also considerable variability in the sensitivity of those sites for different components in a venom.

The distribution of most venom fractions is unequal, being affected by protein binding, variations in pH, and membrane permeability, among other factors. Once a toxin reaches a particular site, its entry into that site is dependent on the rate of blood flow into that tissue, the mass of the structure, and the partition characteristics of the toxin between the blood and that particular tissue.

A venom also may be metabolized in several or many different tissues. Some venom components are metabolized in areas distant from the receptor site(s) and may never reach the primary receptor in a quantity sufficient to affect that site. The amount of toxin tissues can metabolize without endangering the organism also may vary.

Once a venom component is metabolized or in some way altered, the end substance is excreted, principally through the kidneys. The intestines play a minor role. Excretion may be complicated by the direct action of the venom on the kidneys.

ARTHROPODS

There are more than a million species of arthropods, which generally are divided into 25 orders. Medically, however, only about 10 orders are of significant venomous or poisonous importance. These orders include arachnids (scorpions, spiders, whipscorpions, solpugids, mites, and ticks), myriapods (centipedes and millipedes), insects (water bugs, assassin bugs, and wheel bugs), beetles (blister beetles), Lepidoptera (butterflies, moths, and caterpillars), and Hymenoptera (ants, bees, and wasps). Most arthropods do not have fangs or stings long or strong enough to penetrate human skin.

The number of deaths from arthropod stings and bites is not known. However, deaths from scorpion stings exceed several thousand a year, whereas spider bites probably do not account for more than 200 deaths a year worldwide. A common problem faced by physicians in dealing with suspected spider bites relates to the differential diagnosis. The arthropods most frequently involved in misdiagnoses were ticks (including their embedded mouth parts), mites, bedbugs, fleas (infected flea bites), Lepidoptera insects, flies, vesicating beetles, water bugs, and various stinging Hymenoptera. Among the disease states that were confused with spider or arthropod bites or stings were erythema chronicum migrans, erythema nodosum, periarteritis nodosum, pyoderma gangrenosum, kerion cell–mediated response to a fungus, Stevens-Johnson syndrome, toxic epidermal necrolysis, herpes simplex, and purpura fulminans.

As with the snake, a spider or any other arthropod may bite or sting and not eject venom. Finally, some arthropod venom poisonings give rise to the symptoms and signs of an existing undiagnosed subclinical disease. In some cases, stings or bites may induce stress reactions that bring the unrecognized disease to the surface.

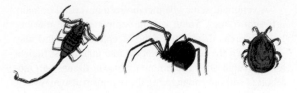

ARACHNIDA

Scorpions

Some of the more important scorpion species are noted in Table 26-1. The dangerous bark scorpion *Centruroides exilicauda,* so called because of its preference for hiding under the loose bark of trees or in dead trees or logs, often frequents human dwellings. Its general color is straw to yellowish-brown or reddish-brown, and it often is easily distinguishable from other scorpions in the same habitat by its long, thin telson, or tail, and thin pedipalps, or pincerlike claws.

Many scorpion venoms contain low-molecular-weight proteins, peptides, amino acids, nucleotides, and salts, among other components. The neurotoxic fractions generally are classified on the basis of their molecular size; the short-chain toxins composed of 30 to 40 amino acid residues with three or four disulfide bonds appear to affect potassium or chloride channels, whereas the long-chain toxins have 60 to 70 amino acids with four disulfide bonds and affect mainly sodium channels. The toxins can bind selectively to a specific channel of excitable cells, thus impairing the initial depolarization of the action potential in the nerve and muscle that results in their neurotoxicity.

Table 26-1
Medically Important Scorpions

GENUS	DISTRIBUTION
Androctonus species	North Africa, Middle East, Turkey
Buthus species	France and Spain to Middle East and north Africa, Mongolia, China
Buthotus species	Africa, Middle East, central Asia
Centruroides species	North, Central, South America
Heterometrus species	Central and southeast Asia
Leiurus species	North Africa, Middle East, Turkey
Mesobuthus species	Turkey, India
Parabuthus species	Southern Africa
Tityus species	Central and South America

The symptoms and signs of scorpion envenomation differ considerably, depending on the species. The sting of members of the family Vejovidae gives rise to localized pain, swelling, tenderness, and mild paresthesia. Systemic reactions are rare, although weakness, fever, and muscle fasciculations have been reported. Envenomations by some members of the genus *Centruroides* may or may not produce initial pain. However, the area becomes sensitive to touch, and merely pressing lightly over the injury elicits an immediate retraction. A poisoned child becomes tense and restless and shows abnormal and random head and neck movements. Often the child displays roving eye movements. Tachycardia is usually evident within 45 min, as well as some hypertension. Respiratory and heart rates are increased, and by 90 min the child may appear quite ill. Fasciculations may be seen over the face or large muscle masses, and the child may complain of generalized weakness and display some ataxia or motor weakness. Opisthotonos may occur. The respiratory distress may proceed to respiratory paralysis. Excessive salivation may further impair respiratory function. Slurring of speech may be present, and convulsions may occur. If death does not occur, the child usually becomes asymptomatic within 36 to 48 h.

In adults, the clinical picture is somewhat similar, but there are some differences. Almost all adults complain of immediate pain after the sting regardless of the *Centruroides* species involved. These adults are tense and anxious. They develop tachycardia and hypertension, and respirations are increased. They may complain of difficulties in focusing and swallowing, as may children. In some cases, there is some general weakness and pain on moving the injured extremity. Ataxia and muscle incoordination may occur. Most adults are asymptomatic within 12 h but may complain of generalized weakness for 24 h or more.

Spiders

Of the 30,000 or so species of spiders, at least 200 have been implicated in significant bites of humans. Some medically important spiders are listed in Table 26-2.

Spider venoms are very complex. From a neuroactive standpoint, the widow and grass spiders, with their neurotranmitter release and channel-affecting properties; the jumping spiders, with their Ca^{2+}–channel blocking activity; and the argiope and orb spinners, with their glutamate and Ca^{2+}–channel blocking activities appear to show much promise as tools in studying neurologic phenomena and perhaps for clinical use.

***Latrodectus* Species (Widow Spiders)** These spiders are commonly known as the black widow, brown widow, red-legged, hourglass, poison lady, deadly spider, red-

Table 26-2
Genera of Spiders for Which Significant Bites of Humans Are Known

GENUS	FAMILY	COMMON NAME	DISTRIBUTION
Aganippe species	Idiopidae	Trap-door spider	Australia
Agelenopsis	Agelenidae	Grass spider	North America
Aphonopelma species	Theraphosidiae	Tarantula	North America
Araneus species	Araneidae	Orbweaver	Worldwide
Arbanitis species	Idiopidae	Trap-door spider	Australia, East Indies
Argiope species	Araneidae	Argiope	Worldwide
Atrax species	Hexathelidae	Funnel-web spider	Australia
Bothriocyrtum species	Ctenizidae	Trap-door spider	California
Cheiracanthium species	Miturgidae	Running spider	Europe, north Africa, Orient, North America
Cupiennius species	Ctenidae	Banana spider	Central America
Drassodes species	Gnaphosidae	Running spider	Worldwide
Dyarcyops [=*Misgolas*]	Idiopidae	Trap-door spider	Australia
Dysdera	Dysderidae	Dysderid	Eastern hemisphere, Americas
Elassoctenus [=*Diallomus*]	Zordae	Ctenid	Australia
Filistata species	Filistatidae	Hackled-band spider	Temperate and tropical worldwide
Harpactirella species	Theraphosidae	Trap-door spider	South Africa
Heteropoda species	Sparassidae	Giant crab spider	East Indies, tropical Asia, south Florida
Isopoda species	Sparassidae	Giant crab spider	Australia, East Indies
Ixeuticus [=*Badumna*]	Desidae	Amaurobiid	New Zealand, southern California
Lampona species	Lamponidae	White-tailed spider	Australia, New Zealand
Latrodectus species	Theridiidae	Widow spider	Temperate and tropical regions worldwide
Liocranoides species	Tengellidae	Running spider	Appalachia
Loxosceles species	Loxoscelidae	Brown or violin spider	Americas, Africa, Europe, eastern Asia, Pacific Islands
Lycosa species	Lycosoidae	Wolf spider	Worldwide
Missulena species	Actinopodidae	Trap-door spider	Australia
Misumenoides species	Thomisidae	Crab spider	North and South America
Miturga species	Miturgidae	Running spider	Australia
Mopsus species	Salticidae	Jumping spider	Australia
Neoscona species	Araneidae	Orbweaver	Worldwide
Olios species	Sparassidae	Giant crab spider	North and South America
Pamphobeteus species	Theraphosidae	Tarantula	South America
Peucetia species	Oxyopidae	Green lynx spider	Worldwide
Phidippus species	Salticidae	Jumping spider	North and South America
Phoneutria species	Ctenidae	Hunting spider	Central and South America
Selenocosmia species	Theraphosidae	Tarantula	East Indies, India, Australia, tropical Africa
Steatoda species	Theridiidae	False black widow	Worldwide
Tegenaria	Agelenidae	Funnel-web spider	Worldwide
Ummidia	Ctenizidae	Trap-door spider	North and South America

bottom spider, T-spider, gray lady spider, and shoebutton spider. Widow spiders are found almost circumglobally in temperate and tropical climates. Although both male and female widow spiders are venomous, only the fe-

male has fangs large and strong enough to penetrate human skin. Their venom contains a family of proteins of about 1000 amino acid residues, latrotoxins. Alpha-latrotoxin is a presynaptic toxin that exerts its toxic effects on the vertebrate central nervous system in depolarizing neurons by increasing $[Ca^{2+}]_i$ and by stimulating exocytosis of neurotransmitters from nerve terminals.

Clinical Problem Bites by the black widow are described as sharp and pinprick-like, followed by a dull, occasionally numbing pain in the affected extremity and pain and cramps in one or several of the large muscle masses. Rarely is there any local skin reaction except during the first 60 min after the bite. Muscle fasciculations frequently can be seen within 30 min of the bite. Sweating is common, and the patient may complain of weakness and pain in the regional lymph nodes; lymphadenitis is observed frequently. Pain in the low back, thighs, or abdomen is a common complaint, and rigidity of the abdominal muscles is seen in most cases in which envenomation has been severe. Severe paroxysmal muscle cramps may occur, and arthralgia has been reported. Hypertension is common, particularly in the elderly, after moderate to severe envenomations.

Loxosceles **Species (Brown or Violin Spiders)** These spiders are variously known in North America as the fiddle-back spider or the brown recluse; the abdomen of these spiders varies in color from grayish through orange and reddish-brown to blackish and is distinct from the pale yellow to reddish-brown background of the cephalothorax. Both males and females are venomous.

Loxosceles venom may contain phospholipase, protease, esterase, collagenase, hyaluronidase, deoxyribonuclease, ribonuclease, dipeptides, dermonecrosis factor 33, dermonecrosis factor 37, and factors with sphingomyelinase D activity.

Clinical Problem The bite of this spider produces about the same degree of pain as does the sting of an ant. A local burning sensation may last for 30 to 60 min around the injury. Some bites produce no more than localized pain, slight redness, and minimal swelling. In more severe bites, pruritus over the area occurs, and the area becomes red, with a small blanched area surrounding the reddened bite site. Skin temperature usually is elevated over the lesion area. The reddened area enlarges and becomes purplish during the subsequent 1 to 8 h. Hemorrhages may develop throughout the area. A small bleb or vesicle forms at the bite site and increases in size. It subsequently ruptures, and a pustule forms. The red hemorrhagic area continues to enlarge, as does the pustule. The whole area may become swollen and painful, and lymphadenopathy is common.

In serious bites, systemic effects include fever, malaise, stomach cramps, nausea, vomiting, jaundice, spleen enlargement, hemolysis, hematuria, and thrombocytopenia. Fatal cases, while rare, usually are preceded by intravascular hemolysis, hemolytic anemia, thrombocytopenia, hemoglobinuria, and renal failure.

Steatoda **Species (Cobweb Spiders)** The cobweb spiders, *Steatoda* spp., are known variously as false black widow, combfooted, or cupboard spiders. Bites by *S. grossa* or *S. fulva* have been followed by local pain, often severe; induration; pruritus; and occasional breakdown of tissue at the bite site.

Cheiracanthium **Species (Running Spiders)** *Cheiracanthium punctorium, C. inclusum, C. mildei, C. diversum,* and *C. japonicum* are common biting spiders. The abdomen is convex and egg-shaped and varies in color from yellow, green, or greenish-white to reddish-brown. The chelicerae are strong, and the legs are long, hairy, and delicate. *Cheiracanthium* tends to be tenacious and sometimes must be removed from the bite area. The venom has a highly toxic 60-kDa protein and high concentrations of norepinephrine and serotonin.

The bite is sharp and painful, with the pain increasing during the first 30 to 45 h. A reddened wheal with a hyperemic border develops. Small petechiae may appear near the center of the wheal. Lymphadenitis and lymphadenopathy may develop. In Japan, *C. japonicum* produces more severe effects that include severe local pain, nausea, vomiting, severe pruritus, headache, chest discomfort, and shock.

Phidippus **Species (Jumping Spiders)** These spiders, variously known as crab spiders and eyebrow spiders, are usually less than 20 mm in length and have a somewhat rectangular cephalothorax that tends to blunt anteriorly. The abdomen is often oval or elongated. There is much variation in their coloring.

The bite of this spider produces a sharp pinprick of pain that usually lasts 5 to 10 min. An erythematous wheal 2 to 5 cm in diameter slowly develops. A dull, sometimes throbbing pain that rarely requires attention may develop over the injured part. A small vesicle may form at the bite site. Generally, swelling may be diffuse and often is accompanied by pruritus. The effects usually abate within 48 h.

Ticks

Tick paralysis is caused by the saliva of at least 60 species of ticks of the families Ixodidae and Argasidae and perhaps others. With respect to tick paralysis as opposed to tick toxicosis, one must consider the rickettsial, spirochetal, and microbacterial organisms transmitted by ticks (or mites) that cause neurologic disorders similar to those produced by the tick's saliva. Among the diseases caused by organisms transmitted by ticks are Lyme disease, Rocky Mountain spotted fever, babesiosis, leptospirosis, Q fever, ehrlichiosis, typhus, and tick-borne encephalitis, among others.

Tick bites often are not felt; the first evidence of envenomation may not appear until several days later, when small macules develop. The patient often complains of difficulty with gait, followed by paresis and eventually locomotor paresis and paralysis. Problems in speech and respiration may ensue and lead to respiratory paralysis if the tick is not removed. Since the tick is often in the hair, it may remain unseen, thus confusing the differential diagnosis. Removal of the tick usually results in a rapid and complete recovery, although regression of paralysis may resolve slowly.

The ticks that cause paralysis in humans and domestic animals may be the same, and it is the length of exposure to the feeding tick that determines the degree of poisoning. These comments are specific only for tick venom poisoning and not for allergic reactions, transmission of disease states, and other complications of tick bites.

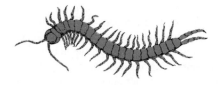

CHILOPODA (CENTIPEDES)

These elongated, many-segmented brownish-yellow arthropods are found worldwide. The first pair of legs behind the head are modified into poison jaws or maxillipeds. The venom is concentrated within the intracellular granules of the secretory cells and is moved by exocytosis into the lumen of the gland; from there, ducts carry the venom to the jaws.

The venoms of centipedes contain proteinases, esterases, 5-hydroxytryptamine, histamine, lipids, and polysaccharides. In humans, this venom produces immediate bleeding, redness, and swelling that often lasts for 24 h. Localized tissue changes and necrosis have been reported, and severe envenomations may cause nausea and vomiting, changes in heart rate, vertigo, and

headache. In the most severe cases, there can be mental disturbances.

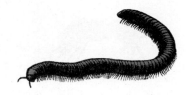

DIPLOPODA (MILLIPEDES)

These arthropods are cylindrical, wormlike creatures, mahogany to dark brown or black in color, bearing two pairs of jointed legs per segment and ranging in length from 20 to 300 mm.

The lesions produced by millipedes generally consist of a burning or prickling sensation and the development of a yellowish or brown-purple lesion; subsequently, a blister containing serosanguineous fluid forms, which may rupture. Eye contact can cause acute conjunctivitis, periorbital edema, keratosis, and much pain.

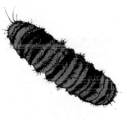

INSECTA

Lepidoptera (Caterpillars, Moths, and Butterflies)

The urticating hairs, or setae, of caterpillars are attached to unicellular poison glands at the base of each hair. The toxic material contains aristolochic acids, cardenolides, histamine, and a fibrinolytic protein. Coagulation defects such as prolonged prothrombin and partial thromboplastin times have been detected, and decreases in fibrinogen and plasminogen have been noted. The hemorrhagic syndrome cannot be classified as being either totally fibrinolytic or a syndrome such as disseminated intravascular coagulopathy.

Stings of *Megalopygidae, Dioptidae, Automeris,* and *Hermileucinae* species of Lepidoptera give rise to a bleeding diasthesis that often is severe and sometimes is fatal. In the more severe cases, there is localized pain as well as papules (sometimes hemorrhagic) and hematomas; on occasion, there also may be headache, nausea, vomiting, hematuria, lymphadenitis, and lymph-adenopathy.

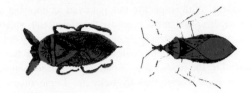

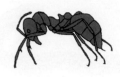

Formicidae (Ants)

The clinically important stinging ants are the harvester ants (*Pagonomyrmex*), fire ants (*Solenopsis*), and little fire ants (*Ochetomyrmex*). Harvester ants are large red, dark brown, or black, ranging in size from 6 to 10 mm and having fringes of long hairs on the posterior of the head. They are vicious stingers, and their venom is said to have strong cholinergic properties.

The venoms of ants vary considerably. The venoms of the Ponerinae, Pseudomyrmex, and Ecitoninae are proteinaceous in character. The Myrmecinae venoms are a mixture of amines, proteinaceous materials, histamine, hyaluronidase, and phospholipase A. Formicinae ant venom contains about 60% formic acid. Fire ants are unique in that although they are poor in polypeptides and proteins, they are rich in alkaloids that cause the formation of pruritic pustules and necrosis. The sting of the fire ant gives rise to a painful burning sensation, after which a wheal and localized erythema develop, leading in a few hours to a clear vesicle. Within 12 to 24 h, the fluid becomes purulent and the lesion turns into a pustule. It may break down or become a crust or a fibrotic nodule. In multiple stingings, there may be nausea, vomiting, vertigo, increased perspiration, respiratory difficulties, cyanosis, coma, and even death.

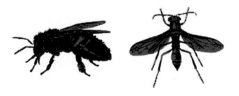

Apidae (Bees)

The most common stinging bees are *Apis mellifera mellifer* and the Africanized bee, *A. mellifer adansonii*. The venom contains apamine and melittin synergized by phospholipase A$_2$, hyaluronidase, histamine, dopamine, and a mast cell–degranulating peptide, among other components. It is said that 50 stings can lead to respiratory dysfunction, intravascular hemolysis, hypertension, myocardial damage, hepatic changes, shock, and renal failure. With 100 or more stings, death can occur.

Heteroptera (True Bugs)

The clinically most important of the true bugs are the Reduviidae (the reduviids): the kissing bug, assassin bug, wheel bug, or cone-nose bug. The most commonly involved species appear to be *Triatoma protracta, T. rubida, T. magista, Reduvius personatus,* and *Arilus cristatus*. The venom of these bugs has apyrase activity and is fairly rich in protease properties. It inhibits collagen-induced platelet aggregation.

The bites of *Triatoma* species are definitely painful and give rise to erythema, pruritus, increased temperature in the bitten part, localized swelling, and systemic reactions such as nausea and vomiting and angioedema. With some bites, the wound area sloughs, leaving a depression.

The water bugs are water-dwelling true bugs of which at least three families—Belostomatidae, Naucordiae, and Notonectidae—are capable of biting and envenomating humans. Water bug saliva contains digestive enzymes, neurotoxic components, and hemolytic fractions. Water bug bites give rise to immediate pain and some localized swelling.

There are some arthropods that are "poisonous" as opposed to "venomous"; that is, they have no mechanism for delivering their toxin, and the poison must come through their being crushed or eaten. These include, among others, the darkling beetles or stink bugs (*Eleodes*) and the blister beetles (*Epicauta*), for which cantharidin is known.

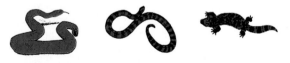

REPTILES

Lizards

The Gila monster (*Heloderma suspectum*) and the beaded lizard (*H. horridum*) are far less dangerous than generally is believed. Their venom is transferred from venom glands in the lower jaw through ducts that discharge their contents near the base of the larger teeth of the lower jaw. The venom then is drawn up along grooves in the teeth by capillary action. The venom has helothermine, serotonin, amine oxidase, phospholipase A, and proteolytic as well as hyaluronidase activities. Large doses of *Heloderma* venom produce a fall in systemic arterial pressure with a decrease in circulating blood volume, tachycardia, and respiratory distress; in lethal doses, there is a loss of ventricular contractility.

Snakes

Among the more than 3500 species of snakes, approximately 400 are sufficiently venomous to be dangerous to humans. Venomous species include the Elapidae, the Hydrophiodae, the Laticaudidae, the Viperidae, and certain Colubridae, of which the most clinically important are the boomslang and bird snake of Africa and the red-necked keelback of Asia. Some medically important venomous snakes and their general distribution are listed in Table 26-3.

Snake Venoms   The venoms of snakes are complex mixtures of proteins and peptides; inorganic cations such as

Table 26-3
Some Medically Important Snakes of the World

SCIENTIFIC AND COMMON NAMES	DISTRIBUTION
Crotalids	
Agkistrodon bilineatus—cantil	Mexico south to Guatemala and Nicaragua
Agkistrodon contortrix—copperhead	New York south to Florida and west to Nebraska and Texas
Agkistrodon halys—mamushi	Caspian Sea to Japan
Agkistrodon piscivorus—eastern cottonmouth	New York to Missouri
Calloselasma (Agkistrodon) rhodostoma—Malayan pit viper	Much of southeast Asia
Bothrops asper and/or *atrox*—fer-de-lance —barba amarillia —terciopelo	Southern Sonora to Peru and northern Brazil
Bothrops jararaca—jararaca	Brazil, Paraguay, and Argentina
Bothrops jararacussu—jararacussu	Brazil, Bolivia, Paraguay, and Argentina
Bothrops neuwiedi—jararaca pintada	Brazil, Bolivia, Paraguay, northern Argentina
Crotalus adamanteus—eastern diamondback rattlesnake	Southeastern United States
Crotalus atrox—western diamondback rattlesnake	Southwestern United States to central Mexico
Crotalus basiliscus—Mexican west-coast rattlesnake	Oaxaca and west coast of Mexico
Crotalus scutulatus—Mojave rattlesnake	Central California to New Mexico
Crotalus viridis helleri—southern Pacific rattlesnake	West Coast, southern California
Trimeresurus flavoviridis—habu	Amami and Okinawa islands
Trimeresurus mucrosquamatus—Chinese habu	Taiwan and southern China west through Vietnam and Laos to India
Viperids	
Bitis arietans—puff adder	Morocco and western Arabia through much of Africa
Bitis caudalis—horned adder	Angola south through Nambia into central and part of south Africa
Causus sp.—night adders	Most of Africa south of the Sahara
Cerastes cerastes—horned viper	Sahara, Arabian peninsula to Lebanon
Cerastes vipera—Sahara sand viper	Central Sahara to Lebanon
Daboi (Vipera) russelli—Russell's viper	Indian subcontinent, southeast China to Taiwan and parts of Indonesia

(continued)

Table 26-3
Some Medically Important Snakes of the World *(continued)*

SCIENTIFIC AND COMMON NAMES	DISTRIBUTION
Echis carinatus—saw-scaled viper	Southern India to northern and tropical Africa
Echis coloratus—saw-scaled viper	Eastern Egypt, western Arabian peninsula north to Israel
Vipera ammodytes—long-nosed viper	Italy through southeast Europe, Turkey, Jordan to northwest Iran
Vipera berus—European viper	British Isles through Europe to northern Asia
Vipera lebetina—Levantine viper	Cyprus through Middle East to Kashmir
Vipera xanthina—Near East viper	European Turkey and Asia Minor

Elapids
  Coral snakes (c.s.)

Calliophis species—Oriental c.s.	Southeast Asia, Orient
Micrurus alleni—Allen's c.s.	Atlantic Nicaragua to Panama
Micrurus corallinus—c.s.	Southern Brazil to Uruguay, northern Argentina
Micrurus frontalis—southern c.s.	Southwestern Brazil, northern Argentina, Uruguay, Paraguay, and Bolivia
Micrurus fulvius—eastern c.s.	Southeastern, southern United States and north central Mexico
Micrurus mipartitus—black-ringed c.s.	Venezuela and Peru to Nicaragua
Micrurus nigrocinctus—black-banded c.s.	Southern Mexico to northwest Colombia

  Cobras

Hemachatus haemachatus—Ringhals cobra	Southeastern and southern Africa
Naja atra—Chinese cobra	Thailand and South China to Taiwan
Naja haje—Egyptian or brown cobra	Africa and part of Arabian peninsula
Naja naja—Indian cobra	Most of Indian subcontinent
Naja nigricollis—spitting cobra	West Africa and southern Egypt to near the Cape
Naja nivea—Cape or yellow cobra	Nambia, Botswana south to the Cape
Naja oxiana—Central Asian cobra	Northern Pakistan to Iran, southern Russia
Naja philippinensis—Philippine cobra	Philippines
Naja sputatrix—Malayan cobra	Malayan peninsula and Indonesia
Ophiophagus hannah—king cobra	Indian subcontinent, China, and Philippines
Walterinnesia aegyptia—desert blacksnake or desert cobra	Egypt to Iran

Kraits and mambas

Bungarus caeruleus—Indian or blue krait	India, Pakistan, Sri Lanka, Bangladesh
Bungarus candidus—Malayan krait	Thailand, Malaysia, Indonesia
Bungarus multicinctus—many-banded krait	Southern China to Hainan, Taiwan
Dendroaspis polylepis—black mamba	Ethiopia and Somalia to Angola, Zambia, Nambia, southwest Africa

Australian elapids

Acanthophis antarcticus—common death adder	Most of Australia, Moluccas, New Guinea
Notechis scutatus—tiger snake	Southeastern Australia
Oxyuranus scutellatus—Taipan	Northern coastal Australia, parts of New Guinea
Pseudechis australis—mulga	Most of Australia except southeast and southern coast, New Guinea
Pseudonaja nuchalis—western brown snake	Most of Australia except east and southeast coast
Pseudonaja textilis—eastern brown snake	Eastern Australia

NOTE: The common names in this table are those generally employed as literature identifications for the snakes. However, these names may not be the ones used by people in the specific area where the snake abounds.

Table 26-4
Enzymes of Snake Venoms

Proteolytic enzymes	Phosphomonoesterase
Arginine ester hydrolase	Phosphodiesterase
Thrombin-like enzyme	Acetylcholinesterase
Collagenase	RNase
Hyaluronidase	DNase
Phospholipase A_2(A)	5′-Nucleotidase
Phospholipase B	NAD-nucleotidase
Phospholipase C	L-Amino acid oxidase
Lactate dehydrogenase	

sodium, calcium, potassium, and magnesium; and small amounts of metals: zinc, iron, cobalt, manganese, and nickel. Some snake venoms also contain carbohydrates (glycoproteins), lipids, and biogenic amines, whereas others contain free amino acids.

Enzymes The venoms of snakes contain at least 25 enzymes, although no single snake venom contains all of them (Table 26-4). Proteolytic enzymes catalyze the breakdown of tissue proteins and peptides. They also are known as peptide hydrolases, proteases, endopeptidases, peptidases, and proteinases. There may be several proteolytic enzymes in a single venom. Metals appear to be involved in the activity of certain venom proteases and phospholipases.

The crotalid venoms examined so far appear to be rich in proteolytic enzyme activity. Viperid venoms have lesser amounts, whereas elapid and sea snake venoms have little or no proteolytic activity. Venoms that are rich in proteinase activity are associated with marked tissue destruction.

Arginine ester hydrolase is found in many crotalid and viperid venoms and some sea snake venoms but is lacking in elapid venoms with the possible exception of *Ophiophagus hannah*. Some crotalid venoms contain at least three chromatographically separable arginine ester hydrolases. The bradykinin-releasing and possible bradykinin-clotting activities of some crotalid venoms may be related to esterase activity.

Thrombin-like enzymes are found in significant amounts in the venoms of the Crotalidae and Viperidae, whereas those of the Elapidae and Hydrophiodae contain little or no venom. The mechanism of fibrinogen clot formation by snake venom thrombin-like enzymes invokes the preferential release of fibrinopeptide A (or B); thrombin releases fibrinopeptides A and B. The proteolytic action of thrombin and thrombin-like snake venom

enzymes is shown in Table 26-5. This table also shows comparisons of ancrod (from *Calloselasma rhodostoma*), batroxobin (from *Bothrops moojeni*), crotalase (from *Crotalus adamanteus*), gabonase (from *Bitis gabonica*), and enzyme (from *Agkistrodon contortrix*).

Collagenase is a specific proteinase that digests collagen. This activity has been demonstrated in the venoms of a number of species of crotalids and viperids. The venom of *Crotalus atrox* digests mesenteric collagen fibers but not other protein.

Hyaluronidase catalyzes the cleavage of internal glycoside bonds in certain acid mucopolysaccharides, thus decreasing the viscosity of connective tissues and allowing other fractions of venom to penetrate the tissues.

Some venoms are rich sources of phospholipase A_2 (PLA_2), which catalyzes the Ca^{2+}-dependent hydrolysis of the 2-acyl ester bond, producing free fatty acids and lysophospholipid. PLA_2s are distributed widely in the venoms of elapids, vipers, crotalids, sea snakes, atractaspids, and several colubrids. Although the sequences of these enzymes are homologous and their enzymatic active sites are identical, they differ widely in their pharmacologic properties.

Phosphomonoesterase (phosphatase) is found in the venoms of all families of snakes except colubrids. It has the properties of an orthophosphoric monoester phosphohydrolase. There are two nonspecific phosphomonoesterases, and many venoms contain both acid and alkaline phosphatases, whereas other venoms contain one or the other.

Phosphodiesterase, which is found in the venoms of all families of poisonous snakes, is an orthophosphoric diester phosphohydrolase that attacks DNA, RNA, and derivatives of arabinose.

There are other enzymes for which the toxicologic contribution to snake venoms is not understood. These include acetylcholinesterase, RNase, DNase, 5′-nucleotidase, nicotinamide adenine dinucleotide (NAD) nucleotidase, L-amino acid, and lactate dehydrogenase.

Polypeptides Snake venom polypeptides are low-molecular-weight proteins that do not have enzymatic activity. Erabutoxin a, erabutoxin b, alpha-cobratoxin, crotactin, and crotamine are examples.

Toxicology In general, the venoms of rattlesnakes and other New World crotalids produce alterations in the resistances (and often the integrity) of blood vessels, changes in blood cells and blood coagulation mechanisms, direct or indirect changes in cardiac and pulmonary dynamics, and, with crotalids such as *C.*

Table 26-5
Proteolytic Action of Thrombin and Thrombin-Like Snake Venom Enzymes

ENZYME	Action on Human Fibrinogen		ACTIVATION OF FACTOR XIII	PROTHROMBIN FRAGMENT CLEAVAGE	PLATELET AGGGREGATION AND RELEASE	ACTIVATION OF FACTOR VIII	ACTIVATION OF FACTOR V
	FIBRINOPEPTIDES RELEASED	CHAIN DEGRADATION					
Thrombin	A − B	α(A)	Yes	Yes	Yes	Yes	Yes
Thrombin-like enzymes	A*	α(A)† or β(B)‡	No	Yes or no§	No	No	No
Agkistrodon c. contortrix venom	B	n.d.#	Incomplete	n.d.	No	n.d.	n.d.
Bitis gabonica venom	A + B	n.d.	Yes	n.d.	n.d.	n.d.	n.d.

*Includes ancrod, batroxobin, crotalase, and the enzyme from *T. okinavensis*.

†Ancrod [batroxobin degrades α(A) chain of bovine but not human fibrinogen].

‡Crotalase.

§Fragment I released by crotalase and *Agkistrodon contortrix* venom but not by ancrod or batroxobin.

#n.d. = not determined.

durrissus terrificus and *C. scutulatus,* serious alterations in the nervous system and changes in respiration. In humans, the course of the poisoning is determined by the kind and amount of venom injected; the site where it is deposited; the general health, size, and age of the patient; the type of treatment; and the pharmacodynamic principles noted earlier in this chapter. Clinical experience indicates that death in humans may occur in less than 1 h or after several days, with most deaths occurring between 18 and 32 h.

Hypotension or shock is the major therapeutic problem in North American crotalid bites. These effects appear to be caused by a decrease in circulating blood volume secondary to an increase in capillary permeability, which leads to the loss of fluid, protein, and to some extent erythrocytes. The severity of the hypotension is dose-related, and restoration of circulating fluid volume can be achieved with intravenous fluids.

Snakebite Treatment   The treatment of bites by venomous snakes is so highly specialized that almost every individual envenomation requires specific recommendations. However, three general principles for every bite should be kept in mind:

1. Snake venom poisoning is a medical emergency that requires immediate attention and the exercise of considerable judgment.
2. The venom is a complex mixture of substances, and the only adequate antidote is a specific or polyspecific antivenom.
3. Not every bite by a venomous snake ends in an envenomation. In almost 1000 cases of crotalid bites, 24 percent did not end in a poisoning. The incidence with the bites of cobras and perhaps other elapids is probably higher.

It would be difficult to detail specific treatments for the almost 400 snakes implicated in snake venom poisoning.

ANTIVENOM

Because of their protein composition, many toxins produce an antibody response; this response is essential in producing antisera. An antivenom consists of venom-specific antisera or antibodies concentrated from immune serum to the venom. Antisera contain neutralizing antibodies: one antigen (monospecific) or several antigens (polyspecific). Animals immunized with venom develop a variety of antibodies to the many antigens in the venom. The serum is harvested, partially or fully purified, and further processed before being administered to the patient. The antibodies bind to the venom molecules, rendering them ineffective. Antivenoms have been produced against most medically important snake, spider, scorpion, and marine toxins.

Antivenoms are available in several forms: intact IgG antibodies or fragments of IgG such as F(ab)$_2$ and Fab. The molecular weight of the intact IgG is about 150,000, whereas that of Fab is approximately 50,000. IgG has a volume of distribution much smaller than that of Fab and is too large for renal excretion. The elimination half-life of IgG is approximately 50 h. IgG probably is degraded by the reticuloendothelial system. Fab fragments have an elimination half-life of about 17 h and undergo renal excretion.

All antivenom products are produced through the immunization of animals, which increases the possiblity of hypersensitivity. The risks of anaphylaxis should always be considered when one is deciding whether to administer antivenom.

BIBLIOGRAPHY

Bon C, Goyffon M (eds): *Envenomings and Their Treatments.* Paris: Institut Pasteur, 1996.

Coombes JD (ed): *New Drugs from Natural Sources.* London: IBC Technical Services, 1997.

Meier J, White J: *Handbook of Clinical Toxicology of Animal Venoms and Poisons.* Boca Raton, FL: CRC Press, 1995.

Menez A (ed): *Perspectives in Molecular Toxinology.* New York: Wiley, 2002.

Russell FE, Nagabhushanam R: *The Venomous and Poisonous Marine Invertebrates of the Indian Ocean.* Enfield, NH: Science Publications, 1996.

CHAPTER 27

TOXIC EFFECTS OF PLANTS

Stata Norton

> **KEY POINTS**
> - Different portions of a plant (root, stem, leaves, seeds) often contain different concentrations of a chemical.
> - The age of a plant contributes to variability. Young plants may contain more or less of some constituents than do mature plants.
> - Climate and soil influence the synthesis of some chemicals.
> - Plants contain chemicals that may exert toxic effects on the skin, lung, cardiovascular system, liver, kidney, bladder, blood, central and peripheral nervous systems, bone, and reproductive system.
> - Contact dermatitis and photosensitivity are common skin reactions with many plants.
> - Gastrointestinal effects range from local irritation to emesis and/or diarrhea.
> - Cardiac glycosides in the leaves or seeds of many plants cause nausea, vomiting, and cardiac arrhythmias in animals and humans.

INTRODUCTION

Among the many species of plants that contain toxic chemicals, only a few are described here. Selection has been based on three considerations: frequency with which contact occurs, importance and seriousness of the toxic effect, and scientifically interesting nature of the action of the chemical.

The toxic effects of the same species of plant may vary with differences in the production of the toxic chemical by individual plants. The reasons for variability in the concentration of toxic chemicals are several:

1. Different portions of the plant (root, stem, leaves, seeds) often contain different concentrations of a chemical.
2. The age of a plant contributes to variability. Young plants may contain more or less of some constituents than mature plants do.
3. Climate and soil influence the synthesis of some chemicals.
4. Genetic differences within a species may alter the ability of individual plants to synthesize a chemical. Synthesis of related toxic chemicals often is found in taxonomically related species as a characteristic of a genus and sometimes as a familial characteristic.

TOXIC EFFECT BY ORGAN

Skin

Allergic Dermatitis Most people are familiar with dermatitis caused by some plants, such as poison ivy. Equally familiar is the allergenic response of many individuals in the form of "hay fever" or summer rhinitis.

Species of both *Philodendron* (family Araceae, arum family) and *Rhus* (Anacardiaceae, cashew family) cause allergic contact dermatitis. *Philodendron scandens* is a common houseplant, while *Rhus radicans* (poison ivy) is native to North America. In addition to poison ivy, the toxicodendron group of plants contains *R. diversiloba* (poison oak) and *R. vernix* (poison sumac). The active ingredients in *P. scandens* are resorcinols. In *R. radicans,* the allergenic component is a mixture of catechols called urushiol. Contact dermatitis also develops with repeated exposures to the sap of mango fruit, because the skin of the fruit contains oleoresins that cross-react with allergens of poison ivy.

Flower growers and other individuals who handle bulbs and cut flowers of daffodils, hyacinths, and tulips sometimes develop dermatitis from contact with the sap. The rashes are due to irritation from alkaloids (masonin, lycorin, and several related alkaloids) or to needle-like crystals of calcium oxalate in the bulbs. One alkaloid, tulipalin-A, which causes "tulip fingers," has allergenic properties.

The allergens of plants tend to be located in the outer cell layers of plant organs. In allergic contact dermatitis to chrysanthemums (*Dendranthema* species), the allergens are sesquiterpene lactones that are present in small hairs (trichomes) on the stems, on the undersides of leaves, and in flowering heads.

The major allergen in natural rubber latex from the rubber tree, *Hevea brasiliensis,* is prohevein, a chitin-binding polypeptide that is found in several plants. Individuals sensitive to latex rubber may be sensitized to several fruits containing a chitinase with a hevein-like domain, including banana, kiwi, tomato, and avocado.

Pollen from several genera in the family Asteraceae (for example, mugwort, *Artemisia vulgaris* in Europe, and ragweed, *Ambrosia artemisiifolia* in North America) contains allergens that cause summer rhinitis. Immunoglobulin antibodies produced by sensitized individuals cross-react with mugwort and ragweed pollen. The cross-reactive allergen has been identified as a highly conserved 14-kDa protein, profilin.

Contact Dermatitis Children may chew the leaves of the *Dieffenbachia* plant, and workers in greenhouses cut the plant in the course of their work. Contact of the eye or tongue with the juice results in pain and the rapid development of edema and inflammation, which may take days or weeks to subside. The toxicity is due to a combination of factors. The release of a histamine-like or serotonin-like chemical may be involved in the immediate pain. The needle-like crystals of irritating calcium oxalate crystals coated with a trypsin-like inflammatory protein, called raphides, are located in ampule-shaped ejector cells throughout the surface of the leaf. Slight pressure on these cells causes expulsion of the raphides.

Contact with the trichomes of species of *Urtica* (nettles) causes pain and erythema from penetration of the skin by the trichomes. In the stinging nettles, *Urtica urens* and *U. dioica* (family Urticaceae), the trichomes covering the leaves and stems consist of fine tubes with bulbs at the end that break off in the skin and release fluid containing histamine, acetylcholine, and serotonin, causing the acute response.

Several species of *Ranunculus* (buttercup) cause contact dermatitis. These plants contain ranunculin, which releases toxic protoanemonin, which also is present in *Anemone,* another genus of the buttercup family. Protoanemonin is converted readily to anemonin, which has marked irritant properties. Ingestion of plants containing protoanemonin may result in severe irritation of the gastrointestinal tract.

Photosensitivity Poisoning of livestock from *Hypericum perforatum* (St. John's wort) results in the development of edematous lesions of the skin, especially in areas not well covered with hair, including the ears, nose, and eyes. The toxic principle, hypericin, causes photosensitization, and lesions appear after exposure to sunlight. Photosensitivity is a rare event in humans who ingest St. John's wort.

Gastrointestinal System

Direct Irritant Effects The most common outcome of the ingestion of a toxic plant is gastrointestinal disturbance (nausea, vomiting, and diarrhea) from irritation of the mucous membranes. Many different kinds of chemicals are responsible for this. Some have found a place in medicine as mild purgatives, such as cascara sagrada ("sacred bark"). Cascara is obtained from the bark of *Rhamnus purshiana* (California buckthorn). The active ingredient is emodin.

Tung nut (*Aleurites fordii*) is grown widely around the world. The seeds, from which commercially useful oil is expressed, are the most toxic part. Ingestion of the ripe nuts causes abdominal pain, vomiting, and diarrhea. Outbreaks of poisoning are most common in children.

Buffalo bean or buffalo pea (*Thermopsis rhombifolia*) is a legume that grows wild in the western United States. Loss of life in livestock has been reported from consumption of the mature plant with seeds. Children develop nausea, vomiting, dizziness, and abdominal pain from eating the beans. The active toxic substances are quinolizidine alkaloids.

Aesculus hippocastanum (horse chestnut) and *A. glabra* (Ohio buckeye) are common trees with attractive panicles of flowers in the spring. The nuts from both trees contain a glucoside called esculin. When they are eaten by humans, the main effect is gastroenteritis. Esculin is absorbed poorly from the gastrointestinal tract of humans. In cattle, the glucoside may be hydrolyzed in the rumen, releasing the aglycone to cause systemic effects of a stiff-legged gait and, in severe poisoning, tonic seizures with opisthotonus.

Antimitotic Effects *Podophyllum peltatum* (May apple) contains the toxic purgative podophyllotoxin, especially in the foliage and roots. In low doses, mild purgation predominates. Overdose results in nausea and severe paroxysmal vomiting. Podophyllotoxin inhibits mitosis by binding to microtubules.

Colchicine is an antimitotic agent that blocks the formation of microtubules, causing subsequent failure of the mitotic spindle. Colchicine is the major alkaloid in the bulbs of *Colchicum autumnale* (autumn crocus, lily family). Severe gastroenteritis (nausea, vomiting, diarrhea, and dehydration) follows ingestion of the bulbs. Systemic effects may develop, including confusion, delirium, hematuria, neuropathy, bone marrow aplasia, and renal failure. Additional toxic effects may be due to lectins in the plant. These lectins are potent inducers of a gelatinase from mononuclear white blood cells. High circulating levels of gelatinase have been shown to be present in persons with circulatory shock.

Lectin Toxicity The seeds of *Wisteria floribunda* (family Leguminosae) contain a lectin with affinity for *N*-acetylglucosamine on mammalian neurons. Consumption of a few seeds can result in headache, nausea, and diarrhea within hours, followed by dizziness, confusion, and hematemesis.

Ricinus communis (castor bean) is a member of the family Euphorbiaceae. If the seeds are eaten, adults and children experience no marked symptoms of poisoning for several days. Loss of appetite, nausea, vomiting, and diarrhea develop gradually. Then gastroenteritis becomes severe, with persistent vomiting, bloody diarrhea, dehydration, and icterus in fatal cases. Death occurs in 6 to 8 days. The fatal dose for a child can be 5 to 6 seeds; it is about 20 seeds for an adult. Fatality is low in individuals who eat the seeds—less than 10 percent when a "fatal" dose is consumed—because the toxic protein is largely destroyed in the intestine. Death from castor beans is caused by two lectins, ricin I and ricin II, which inhibit protein synthesis. Similar toxic lectins are found in the seeds of *Abrus precatorius* (jequirity bean). Abrina, one of four isoabrins from the plant, has the highest inhibitory effect on protein synthesis.

Ricin-type lectins with both A and B chains are potentially deadly if they pass, even in small quantities, through the gastrointestinal tract. Plants that produce only A chains pose much less risk when ingested. Young shoots of pokeweed (*Phytolacca americana*) sometimes are used in the spring as a salad green. Mature leaves and berries may cause gastrointestinal irritation with nausea and diarrhea. The plant produces three isozymes of single-chain lectins (PAP, PAPII, and PAP-S) that can inhibit protein synthesis in cells by inactivating rRNA. Single-chain, ribosome-inhibiting proteins do not enter intact cells readily, but if the cell membrane has been breached by a virus, they may enter a cell. Lectins that bind strongly to the cells lining the small intestine and are endocytosed by them may be "nutritionally toxic" if they are consumed over a long period. Experimentally,

reduction in weight gain has been the major finding from the presence of high quantities of some lectins in the diet. A correlation between strength of binding to the brush border of the jejunum and effectiveness as an antinutrient has been reported.

Lung

In addition to the well-recognized involvement of the lung and airway tissues in allergic asthma in some individuals sensitized to plant allergens, the lung is affected directly by some plant chemicals.

Cough Reflex Workers who handle *Capsicum annum* (cayenne pepper) and *C. frutescens* (chili pepper) have an increased incidence of cough during the day. The major irritants in *Capsicum* are capsaicin and dihydrocapsaicin. Capsaicin-sensitive nerves in the airway are involved in the irritation and cough. The sensory endings of C fibers are part of the cough reflex, and the principal neurotransmitter for these fibers, the neuropeptide substance P, is depleted by capsaicin. Capsaicin activates a subtype of the vanilloid receptor found in the airway, spinal cord, dorsal root ganglion, bladder, urethra, and colon. Capsaicin can be irritating to the skin, and individuals who handle the peppers may experience irritation and vesication.

Cell Death In the laboratory, rats are highly susceptible to monocrotaline from seeds of *Crotalaria spectabilis* (showy rattlebox, legume family) and develop a condition resembling pulmonary hypertension. Monocrotaline is converted by rat liver into an active pyrrolic metabolite that is responsible for the cardiopulmonary lesions. Apoptosis of arterial endothelial cells may be involved early in the onset of pulmonary hypertension. In many other species, hepatitis is the primary toxicity.

Cardiovascular System

Cardioactive Glycosides Plants containing species with cardioactive glycosides include *Digitalis purpurea* (foxglove, Scrophulariaceae family), which contains digitalis; *Scilla maritima* (squill), which contains scillaren; *Convallaria majalis* (lily of the valley), which contains convallatoxin in the bulbs; *Asclepias* species (milkweeds), which contain 6′-O-(E-4-hydroxycinnamoyl) desglucouzarin; *Nereum oleander* (bay laurel), which contains oleandrin and nerium; and *Thevetia peruviana* (yellow oleander), which has thevetin A. Animals and humans who eat the leaves or seeds present with nausea, vomiting, and cardiac arrhythmias.

Action on Cardiac Nerves *Veratrum viride* (American hellebore, lily family), European hellebore (*Veratrum album*), and *V. californicum* have similar alkaloids, including protoveratrine, veratramine, and jervine. After ingestion, the alkaloids cause nausea, emesis, hypotension, bradycardia, and sometimes muscle spasm. The primary effect of the veratrum alkaloids on the heart is to cause a repetitive response to a single stimulus resulting from prolongation of the sodium current. Several species of *Zigadenus,* including *Z. nuttallii* (death camas), contain *Veratrum*-like alkaloids. The plants grow throughout North America, and the white bulbs may be mistaken for wild onions. All parts of the plant are toxic.

Aconitum species have been used in western and eastern medicine for centuries. The European plant *Aconitum napellus* (monkshood, Ranunculaceae family) is a perennial grown in gardens for its ornamental blue flowers. The roots of *A. kusnezoffii* (chuanwu) and *A. carmichaeli* (caowu) are in the Chinese materia medica. Poisoning may occur from intentional or accidental ingestion, and the concentration of the alkaloids— aconitine, mesaconitine, and hypoaconitine—varies, depending on species, place of origin, time of harvest, and processing procedure. The alkaloids cause a prolonged sodium current in cardiac muscle and nerve fibers with slowed repolarization. In addition to cardiac arrhythmias and hypotension, the alkaloids cause gastrointestinal upset, numbness of the mouth, and paresthesia in the extremities.

Grayanotoxins are produced exclusively by several genera of Ericaceae (heath family). They have been isolated from *Rhododendron ponticum* and *Kalmia angustifolia.* The grayanotoxins are present throughout the plants, including the leaves, flowers, pollen, and nectar. The toxin gets into honey from nectar collected by bees from the flowers. Poisoning from consumption of leaves or contaminated honey produces a syndrome consisting of marked bradycardia, hypotension, oral paresthesias, weakness, and gastrointestinal upset. In cases of severe poisoning, there is respiratory depression and loss of consciousness. Grayanotoxin I (acetylandromedol) slows both the opening and the closing of sodium channels in nerves.

Vasoactive Chemicals Mistletoe is a parasitic plant on trees that is poisonous. American mistletoe, *Phoradendron tomentosum,* is a member of the same family as European mistletoe (*Viscum album,* Loranthaceae family). Viscotoxins are basic polypeptides that produce hypotension, bradycardia, negative inotropic effects on heart muscle, and vasoconstriction of the vessels of skin and skeletal muscle. Serious poisoning from the plants is rare and includes gastrointestinal distress and hypotension.

Vasoconstriction is a primary toxic effect of *Claviceps purpurea* (ergot), a fungus that is parasitic on grains of rye. The main toxic effect of ergot alkaloids is vasoconstriction, primarily in the extremities, followed by gangrene. Abortion in pregnant women is also common after the ingestion of contaminated rye flour. The alkaloids, ergotamine and ergonovine, have been used in therapeutics.

The fungus *Acremonium coenophialum* grows symbiotically on the forage grass tall fescue (*Festuca arundinacea*) and produces some ergot alkaloids and other lysergic acid derivatives. The fungus causes "fescue toxicosis" in cattle that graze on infected plants. The condition in cattle includes decreased weight gain, decreased reproductive performance, and peripheral vasoconstriction. In the southwestern United States, *Stirpa robusta* (sleepy grass) also is infected with an *Acremonium* fungus. Horses that graze in areas where the infected perennial grass grows become somnolent, presumably as a result of ingesting lysergic acid amide, ergonovine, and related alkaloids produced by the fungus.

Liver

Hepatocyte Damage *Senecio* (ragwort or groundsel, aster family), *Crotalaria, Heliotropium,* and *Symphytum* have species containing the pyrrolizidine alkaloids responsible for hepatic venoocclusive disease. Animal species susceptible to pyrrolizidine alkaloids include rats, cattle, horses, and chickens, whereas guinea pigs, rabbits, gerbils, hamsters, sheep, and Japanese quail are resistant. Damage to hepatocytes may be due to the microsomal formation of pyrrole metabolites, with cross-linking of DNA strands by the metabolites. Resembling cirrhosis and some hepatic tumors, the clinical condition may be described as a Budd-Chiari syndrome, with portal hypertension and obliteration of small hepatic veins.

Inhibition of RNA Polymerase Many nonedible mushrooms may cause gastrointestinal distress, but most are not life-threatening. Most deaths from mushroom poisoning worldwide are due to liver damage after the consumption of *Amanita phalloides,* appropriately called "death cap." *A. ocreata* (death angel) is equally dangerous. *A. phalloides* contains two types of toxic chemicals: phalloidin and amatoxins. Phalloidin is a cyclic heptapeptide that combines with actin in muscle cells to interfere with muscle function; this contributes to some of the diarrhea that develops 10 to 12 h after ingestion. Readily absorbed amatoxins are bicyclic peptides, and the most toxic, alpha-amanitin, has a strong affinity for hepatocytes, where it binds to RNA polymerase II, thus inhibiting protein synthesis. Serious clinical signs begin about the third day after ingestion. Treatment in severe cases may require a liver transplant. Renal proximal tubular lesions are found in cases of severe amanita poisoning.

Block of Sphingolipid Biosynthesis Fumonisins are toxins produced by the fungus *Fusarium,* primarily *F. moniliforme* and *F. proliferatum* growing on corn. Ingestion by horses of corn contaminated with *Fusarium* mold causes "moldy corn poisoning," or equine leukoencephalomalacia. The signs in affected horses are lethargy, ataxia, convulsions, and death. Fumonisins are structurally similar to sphingosine, and their toxicity is related to their blockade of sphingolipid biosynthesis.

Lantadene Toxicity *Lantana camara* (Verbenaceae family) has been described as one of the 10 most noxious weeds in the world. Cattle, rabbits, and guinea pigs develop hyperbilirubinemia and cholestasis. One triterpenoid that induces hepatotoxicity is lantadene A.

Kidney and Bladder

Carcinogenic Chemicals Bracken fern (*Pteridium aquilinum*) grows worldwide and is the only higher plant known to cause epithelial and mesenchymal neoplasms of the bladder in animals under natural conditions of feeding. The carcinogen ptaquiloside alkylates adenines and guanines of DNA. Human consumption of bracken fern may lead to an increased incidence of esophageal and stomach cancers.

Kidney Tubular Degeneration Species of *Xanthium* (cocklebur, aster family) induce toxicosis in livestock (pigs, sheep, cattle, horses, and fowl) in pastures where two- and four-leaf seedlings are present. The clinical signs are depression and dyspnea. The pathologic findings include renal tubular necrosis and hepatic centrilobular necrosis.

Acute renal failure causes death in poisoning from *Cortinarius* species of woodland fungi, which are found especially in northern conifer forests. Species vary widely in habit and edibility. Renal biopsy in poisoned patients shows acute degenerative tubular lesions with inflammatory interstitial fibrosis.

Blood

Anticoagulants Fungal infections in sweet clover (*Melilotus alba*) silage and hay have caused serious toxicity and death in cattle. Deaths are from hemorrhages caused by dicumarol, a fungal metabolite. Dicumarol is an effective anticoagulant that causes prothrombin deficiency.

Cyanogenic Chemicals Cyanogens are constituents of several different kinds of plants. Amygdalin is present in the kernels of apples, cherries, peaches, and the bitter almond, *Prunus amygdalus,* var. *amara.* Amygdalin is not present in the seeds of the sweet almond, the nut used for food. In the stomach, amygdalin releases hydrocyanic acid, which combines with ferric ion in methemoglobin or cytochrome oxidase. The ingestion of several bitter almond seeds causes classic cyanide poisoning and asphyxiation.

Cassava is a staple food starch from *Manihot esculenta* (Euphorbiaceae family) that contains linamarin, a cyanogenic glucoside. During processing of the root for human consumption, the cyanogen is removed. However, if local processing is inadequate, chronic ingestion of linamarin in cassava may cause konzo, a form of tropical myelopathy with the sudden onset of spastic paralysis. Degeneration of the corticospinal motor pathway may be caused by the production of thiocyanate from linamarin and the stimulation of neuronal glutamate receptors by thiocyanate.

Central and Autonomic Nervous Systems

Excessive stimulation of neurons results in toxic signs that vary with the specific receptors involved. Permanent damage to the nervous system is a serious consequence of excessive neuronal stimulation.

Epileptiform Seizures The fleshy tubers of *Cicuta maculata* (water hemlock) may cause fatal poisoning, characterized by tonic-clonic convulsions. The toxic principle, cicutoxin, may be a potent blocker of potassium channels of neurons.

Several members of the mint family (Labiatae), such as pennyroyal (*Hedeoma*), sage (*Salvia*), and hyssop (*Hyssopus*), contain monoterpenes, which in high doses can cause tonic-clonic convulsions.

Excitatory Amino Acids Excitatory amino acids (EAAs) from plants may act on one or more glutamate receptor subtypes. The consequence of the ingestion of EAAs is excessive stimulation, which may result in the death of neurons. Kainic acid is present in the marine red alga *Digenia simplex.* Under some climatic conditions, the algae reproduce rapidly, causing a "red tide." Filter-feeding mussels eat the algae, and humans may be poisoned by eating those mussels. The green alga *Chondria aranta* produces domoic acid, a tricarboxylic amino acid, as does the marine diatom *Nitzschia pungens.* Consumption of domoic acid–containing mussles produces gastrointestinal distress, headache, hemiparesis, confusion, and seizures. Prolonged effects include severe memory deficits and sensorimotor neuronopathy.

The fungi *Amanita muscaria* (fly agaric) and *A. pantherina* (panther agaric) contain the EAA ibotenic acid and possibly its derivative muscimol. The effects are somewhat variable: central nervous system depression, ataxia, hysteria, and hallucinations. Myoclonic twitching and seizures sometimes develop.

EAAs also are found in flowering plants. The pea family (Leguminosae) contains several species that produce EAAs in the seeds. Willardiine, isolated from *Acacia willardiana, A. lemmoni, A. millefolia,* and *Mimosa asperata,* acts as an agonist on specific glutamate receptors. Other important EAAs are present in species of *Lathyrus.* The seeds of *Lathyrus sylvestris* (flat pea) contain 2,4-diaminobutyric acid and beta-*N*-oxalylamino-L-alanine, which induce an acute neurologic condition in sheep that begins with weakness and progresses to tremors and prostration and seizures. Chronic poisoning with seeds of *L. sativus* (chickling pea) induces lathyrism. Affected individuals have corticospinal motor neuron degeneration with severe spastic muscle weakness and atrophy but little sensory involvement.

Mannosidase Inhibitors Swainsonine, an indolizidine alkaloid found in *Swainsonia canescens, Astragalus lentiginosus* (spotted locoweed), and *Oxytropis sericea* (locoweed), causes aberrant behavior with hyperexcitability and locomotor difficulty. Swainsonine inhibits liver lysosomal and cytosomal alpha-mannosidase and Golgi mannosidase II, resulting in abnormal brain glycoproteins and the accumulation of mannose-rich oligosaccharides.

Motor Neuron Demyelination Anthracenones are found in the seeds of *Karwinskia humboldtiana,* family Rhamnaceae (buckthorn, coyotillo, and tullidora). In human and livestock poisonings, the clinical syndrome that develops after a latency period of several days is ascending flaccid paralysis, beginning with demyelination

of large motor neurons in the lower legs and leading to fatal bulbar paralysis.

Parasympathetic Stimulation Some mushrooms of the genera *Inocybe, Clitocybe,* and *Omphalatus* contain significant amounts of muscarine, and consumption of toxic species causes diarrhea, sweating, salivation, and lacrimation, all of which are referable to stimulation of parasympathetic receptors.

Parasympathetic Block The belladonna alkaloids (l-hyoscyamine, atropine, *d,l*-hyoscyamine, and scopolamine), which are present in several genera of plants of the family Solanaceae, are best known for their block of muscarinic receptors. Other plants containing anticholinergics include *Datura stramonium* (jimsonweed)—scopolamine; *Hyoscyamus niger* (henbane)—l-hyoscyamine; *Atropa belladonna* (deadly nightshade)—atropine; and *Duboisia myoporoides* (pituri)—l-hyoscyamine. Modest doses induce muscarinic block with tachycardia, dry mouth, dilated pupils, and decreased gastrointestinal motility. Large doses affect the central nervous system with confusion, bizarre behavior, hallucinations, and subsequent amnesia. Deaths are rare; recovery may take several days.

The brilliant orange-red seeds of *Solanum dulcamara* (woody nightshade, bittersweet) contain solanine, a glycoalkaloid that is responsible for the acute toxicity, including tachycardia, dilated pupils, and hot, dry skin, as in atropine poisoning.

Skeletal Muscle and Neuromuscular Junction

Neuromuscular Junction Block Block of the neuromuscular junction of skeletal muscle may result from either block of postsynaptic acetylcholine (nicotinic) receptors by an antagonist or from an agonist that causes excessive stimulation of the receptor followed by prolonged depolarization. Nicotine, for which the receptor is named, stimulates autonomic ganglia as well as the neuromuscular junction. An isomer of nicotine, anabasine ($C_{10}H_{14}N_2$), which is present in *Nicotiana glauca* (tree tobacco), produces prolonged depolarization of the junction. Consumption of the leaves of the plant has caused severe generalized muscle weakness and respiratory compromise after flexor muscle spasm and gastrointestinal irritation. Curare, the South American arrow poison, is a potent neuromuscular blocking agent for skeletal muscle and kills by stopping respiration. Paralysis is due to block of acetylcholine at the postsynaptic junction. Curare is obtained from tropical species of

Strychnos and *Chondrodendron*. In warm weather, blooms of the blue-green alga *Anabaena flosaquae* in pond water produce a neurotoxin, anatoxin A, that depolarizes and blocks both nicotinic and muscarinic receptors, causing death in animals that drink the pond water within minutes to hours from respiratory arrest.

Methyllycaconitine is a norditerpenoid that is present in *Delphinium barbeyi* (tall larkspur) and some related species. Poisoned cattle show muscle tremors, ataxia, and prostration and die from respiratory failure. The alkaloid has a high affinity for the acetylcholine receptor and causes death by blocking the action of acetylcholine at the neuromuscular junction.

Skeletal Muscle Damage Mature seeds of the poisonous species of *Thermopsis* (family Leguminosae) contain quinolizidine alkaloids, principally anagyrine and thermopsine. Young children who eat the seeds present with abdominal cramps, nausea, vomiting, and headache lasting up to 24 h.

Bone

Soft Tissue Calcification Consumption of *Solanum malacoxylon* (nightshade family, Solanaceae), which contains a water-soluble vitamin D–like substance, induces calcification of the entire vascular system, especially the heart and aorta. Joint cartilage, lungs, and kidneys also may be affected. Sheep and cows both are affected by ingestion of the plant. Consumption of *Cestrum diurnum* (day-blooming jasmine) and *C. laevigatum* also causes hypercalcemia and extensive soft tissue calcification in animals.

Reproductive System and Teratogenesis

Teratogens Birth defects that occur in cows and goats that graze on *Veratrum californicum* can be produced experimentally in chickens, rabbits, rats, mice, hamsters, and rainbow trout embryos. The alkaloids jervine, 11-deoxyjervine, and 3-*O*-glucosyl-11-deoxyjervine are responsible for the defects. The *Veratrum* alkaloids block cholesterol synthesis and thus the response of fetal target tissue to a gene locus [sonic hedgehog locus (Shh)], which plays a role in the developmental patterning of the head and brain. Blockade of cholesterol synthesis also results in the loss of midline facial structures. Malformations in the offspring involve cyclopia, exencephaly, and microphthalmia.

A cluster of fetal malformations characterized by deformation of the limbs and spinal cord is found in cattle grazing on *Lupinus caudatus* and *L. formosus* (lupines), *Nicotiana glauca* (tree tobacco), and *Conium maculatum* (poison hemlock) during sensitive gestational periods. The active alkaloids identified in these plants—anagyrine (*L. caudatus*), ammodendrine (*L. formosus*), anabasine (*N. glauca*), and coniine (*C. maculatum*)—may depress fetal movements during susceptible gestational periods and in this way cause malformations.

Abortifacients In addition to actions on the nervous system, swainsonine in the legumes *Astragalus* and *Oxytropus* frequently causes abortions when locoweeds are ingested by pregnant livestock. Two genera of tropical legumes, *Leucaena* and *Mimosa*, contain a toxic amino acid, mimosine. In large amounts in the foliage and seeds of *L. leucocephala*, *L. glauca*, and *M. pudica*, mimosine causes uncoordinated gait, goiter, and reproductive disturbances, including infertility and fetal death.

A lectin from bitter melon seeds (*Momordica charantia*, family Cucurbitaceae) has been shown to have antifertility, abortifacient, and embryotoxic actions. The lectins are alpha- and beta-momorcharins, single-chain glycoproteins that are known to induce midterm abortion in humans.

BIBLIOGRAPHY

Acamovic T, Stewart CS, Pennycott T: *Poisonous Plants and Related Toxins.* Wallingford, UK: CABI, 2003.

Garland T, Barr AC: *Toxic Plants and Other Natural Toxicants.* New York: CABI, 1998.

UNIT 6

ENVIRONMENTAL TOXICOLOGY

CHAPTER 28

AIR POLLUTION*

Daniel L. Costa

KEY POINTS

- Reducing-type air pollution, characterized by SO_2 and smoke, is capable of producing deleterious effects on human health.

- Photochemical air pollution arises from a series of complex reactions in the troposphere close to the earth's surface and includes a mixture of ozone, nitric oxides, aldehydes, peroxyacetyl nitrates, and a myriad of reactive hydrocarbon radicals.

- Indoor air can be even more complex than outdoor air, and outdoor air can permeate the indoor environment in spite of the reduced air exchange in buildings.

- Sick-building syndrome, including irritancy to the eyes, nose, and throat, occurs frequently but not always in new, poorly ventilated, or recently refurbished office buildings because of the outgassing of combustion products, volatile chemicals, biological materials and vapors, and emissions from furnishings.

AIR POLLUTION IN PERSPECTIVE

Air pollution is a reality of the twenty-first-century lifestyle, and unsatisfactory air quality plagues broad geographic areas. Most people in the western world face few episodes of extreme air pollution; instead, they experience prolonged periods of relatively low-level exposure to complex mixtures of photochemically transformed stationary and mobile emissions. We know most about the health effects of individual pollutants and use that knowledge to drive controls in situations where single pollutants dominate the situation. However, much less is understood about the realities of present-day patterns

*This article has been reviewed by the National Health and Environmental Effects Research Laboratory, U.S. Environmental Protection Agency, and approved for publication. Approval does not signify that the contents necessarily reflect the views and the policies of the Agency.

of diurnal and prolonged exposure and the ways in which mixtures of pollutants can affect human health.

Classically, air pollution has been distinguished on the basis of the chemical redox nature of its primary components. A reducing-type atmosphere has been associated with smelting and related combustion-based industries, in which SO_2 and smoke from incomplete combustion of coal accumulate as a chilled, acidic fog. This acidic mix reacts with surfaces, corroding metal and eroding masonry, as is characteristic of reductive chemistry. In contrast, photochemical air pollution with atmospheric reaction products of automobile exhaust consists of NO_x and many secondary photochemical oxidants, such as O_3, aldehydes, and electron-hungry hydrocarbon radicals. Today, most modern major metropolitan areas have atmospheres with both reducing and oxidant air pollutants.

People in most industrialized nations spend in excess of 80 percent of their time indoors at work, at school, and at home or traveling between those places in an automobile. Generally, the time spent indoors is disproportionately higher for adults, who have relatively less time to participate in outdoor activities, especially during the day, when outdoor pollutants are usually at the highest levels. Children and outdoor workers, by contrast, are much more likely to encounter outdoor air pollution at its worst; in fact, because of the relatively high activity levels of these subgroups compared with inactive office workers, their lungs may incur a considerably larger dose of any pollutant.

Indoor air can be even more complex than outdoor air. Outdoor air can permeate the indoor environment in spite of the reduced air exchange in buildings. Because the average insulated home has about one air change per hour, indoor concentrations of pollutants can range from 30 to 80 percent of those outdoors. When there are independent sources of contamination indoors, the ratio of an indoor pollutant to that outdoors can even exceed 1 (e.g., NO_2). The complexity of these multiple sources underscores the importance of appreciating the total exposure scenario in order to understand the nature of air pollution and its potential effects on humans (Fig. 28-1).

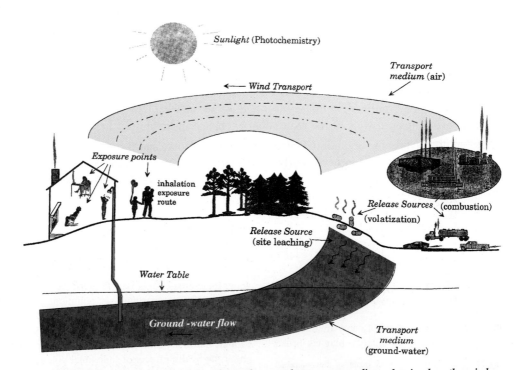

Figure 28-1. Illustration of contributors to the total personal exposure paradigm, showing how these indoor and outdoor factors interact.

EPIDEMIOLOGIC EVIDENCE OF HEALTH EFFECTS

Outdoor Air Pollution

The direction and design of population studies today, frequently referred to as panel or cohort studies, are largely person-based: Groups of people are studied (e.g., nursing home residents, schoolchildren) in their immediate environment, using noninvasive or minimally invasive clinical tools (pulmonary or cardiac function, symptoms, blood screenings, etc.) to correlate effects with ambient and/or personal environmental and air pollutant measures. These studies sacrifice the power of group numbers for more direct and individual data in an attempt to link biomarkers with exposure. These novel approaches are showing increasingly more subtle changes in cardiopulmonary function with exposure to very modest levels of air pollution.

Long-Term Exposures Epidemiologic studies of the chronic effects of air pollution are difficult to conduct because of the nature of the goal: outcomes associated with long-term exposures. The usual approach of retrospective, cross-sectional studies frequently is confounded

by unknown variables and inadequate historical exposure data. A good example of the problem of confounding is cigarette smoking. Without extensive control of both active and passive smoking, the ability to discern the impact of air pollution on a disease outcome such as chronic bronchitis and emphysema is impaired greatly because of the high background of disease attributable to smoking and the imprecision of most indexes of smoking exposure in this type of study. In contrast, prospective studies have the advantage of more precise control of confounding variables, such as the tracking of urinary cotinine as an index of tobacco smoke exposure, but they can be very expensive and require substantial time and dedication on the part of the investigators and the population under study. Depending on the study size and design, both exposure aspects and loss of subjects because of dropout are troublesome.

The role of air pollution in human lung cancer is also difficult to assess because the vast majority of respiratory cancers result from cigarette smoking. However, many compounds that occur as urban air pollutants have carcinogenic potency. Figure 28-2 gives estimates of the relative contributions of various chemicals to the lung cancer rate that is *not* associated with cigarette smoking, which,

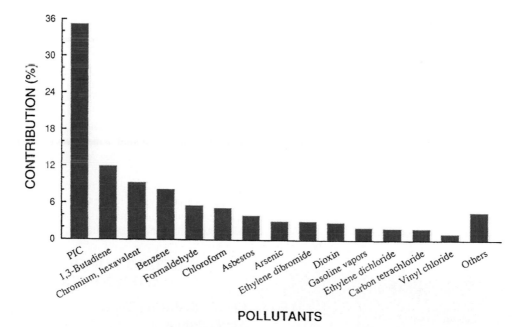

Figure 28-2. Relative contribution of individual airborne hazardous pollutants to lung cancer rates after removal of tobacco smoke cancer.   The total number of cancers from non-tobacco-smoke sources is estimated to be about 2000 per year.

for outdoor air, is estimated to be about 2000 cases per year. This compares with about 2000 cases per year for passive environmental tobacco smoke and about 100,000 cases per year for smokers. Volatile organic compounds (VOCs) and nitrogen-containing and halogenated organics account for most of the compounds that have been studied with animal and genetic bioassays. Most of these compounds are derived from combustion sources that range from tobacco to power plants to incinerators. Other potential carcinogens arise from mobile sources as products of incomplete combustion and their atmospheric transformation products as well as fugitive or accidental chemical releases. This contrasts with indoor air, where the sources are thought to derive largely from environmental tobacco smoke and radon, with some contribution from the off-gassed organics (e.g., adhesives, carpet polymers).

Indoor Air Pollution

There is growing awareness of the potential for indoor air pollution to elicit adverse health effects. Concern about indoor air remains controversial because many of the health problems associated with indoor air pollution generally involve nonspecific symptomatology and appear to involve a wide range of potential toxicants and sources. The responses to indoor air pollution also appear to be affected by ambient comfort factors such as temperature and humidity.

Sick-Building Syndromes This collection of ailments, defined by a set of persistent symptoms enduring at least 2 weeks (Table 28-1), occurs in at least 20 percent of those exposed and is typically of unknown specific etiology; however, it is relieved sometime after an affected individual leaves the offending building. Frequently but not always, this syndrome occurs in new, poorly ventilated,

Table 28-1
**Symptoms Commonly Associated with the
Sick-Building Syndromes**

Eye, nose, and throat irritation
Headaches
Fatigue
Reduced attention span
Irritability
Nasal congestion
Difficulty breathing
Nosebleeds
Dry skin
Nausea

or recently refurbished office buildings. The suspected causes include combustion products, household chemicals, biological materials and vapors, and emissions from furnishings. The perception of irritancy to the eyes, nose, and throat ranks among the predominant symptoms and can become intolerable with repeated exposures. The many factors that contribute to such responses are poorly understood but include host susceptibility factors such as personal stress and fatigue, diet and alcohol use, and other factors. Current biomarkers of response used in the laboratory include sensory irritancy to the eyes in volunteer test subjects and sometimes in animals as well.

Building-Related Illnesses This group of illnesses consists of well-documented conditions with defined diagnostic criteria and generally recognizable causes. These illnesses typically call for a conventional treatment regimen. Several of the biocontaminant-related illnesses (e.g., legionnaires' disease, hypersensitivity pneumonitis, humidifier fever) fall into this group, as do allergies to animal dander, dust mites, and cockroaches. Some toxic inhalants may be classified in this group, such as carbon monoxide. In many cases when the concentrations of CO, NO_2, and many VOCs result in less discernible or definable conditions, the responses may be mistaken for or considered to be sick-building syndromes, thus complicating the assessment of the situation. It should be noted that many inhalants, such as NO_2 and trichloroethylene (a VOC common to the indoor air arising from chlorinated water or dry-cleaned clothes), have been shown in animal toxicology studies to suppress immune defenses and allow opportunistic pathogens to proliferate in the lungs. The involvement of immunologic suppression is a particularly controversial yet important attribute of indoor pollution because of its insidious nature and its implications for all building-related illnesses. This is further complicated by the fact that complex indoor environments containing chemicals and biologicals also may lead to unexpected interactions that are virtually unstudied and thus are not appreciated in the assessment of indoor pollution.

POLLUTANTS OF OUTDOOR AMBIENT AIR

Classic Reducing-Type Air Pollution

Reducing-type air pollution, which is characterized by SO_2 and smoke, is capable of producing disastrous human health effects. Empiric studies in human subjects and animals have long stressed the irritancy of SO_2 and its role in these incidents, although the full potential for interactions among the copollutants in the smoky, sulfurous mix has not been replicated fully in the laboratory. Nevertheless, the irritancy of most S-oxidation products in the atmosphere is well documented, and there are both empiric and theoretical reasons to suspect that such products act to amplify the irritancy of fossil fuel emission atmospheres through chemical transformations and related interactions.

Sulfur Dioxide *General Toxicology* Sulfur dioxide is a water-soluble irritant gas that is absorbed predominantly in the upper airways and stimulates bronchoconstriction and mucus secretion in a number of species, including humans. The concentrations of SO_2 likely to be encountered in the United States are on average less than 0.1 ppm. Mandated use of cleaner (low-S) fossil fuels, emission control devices, and the use of tall emission stacks have been largely responsible for the reductions. However, occasional down-drafting of smokestack plumes or meteorological inversions near point sources result in low-ppm levels of SO_2 that may pose a hazard to some individuals. A 2-min exposure to 0.4 to 1.0 ppm can elicit bronchoconstriction in exercising asthmatic patients within 5 to 10 min. However, it is the low-level, long-term effects, which erode pulmonary defenses, that continue to worry some regulators. Studies have shown that SO_2 is itself capable of impairing macrophage-dependent bacterial killing in murine models. Exposed mice have a greater frequency and severity of infection, and this has been suggested to be linked to a diminished ability to generate endogenous oxidants for bacterial killing.

The penetration of SO_2 into the lungs is greater during mouth as opposed to nose breathing. An increase in the airflow rate further augments penetration of the gas into the deeper lung. As a result, persons who are exercising inhale more SO_2 and, as noted with asthmatics, are likely to experience greater irritation. Once deposited along the airway, SO_2 dissolves into surface-lining fluid as sulfite or bisulfite and is distributed readily throughout the body. It is thought that the sulfite interacts with sensory receptors in the airways to initiate local and centrally mediated bronchoconstriction.

Pulmonary Function Effects The basic pulmonary response to inhaled SO_2 is mild bronchoconstriction, which is reflected as a measurable increase in airflow resistance caused by narrowing of the airways. Concentration-related increases in resistance have been observed in guinea pigs, dogs, cats, and humans.

Sulfuric Acid and Related Sulfates

The conversion of SO_2 to sulfuric acid is favored in the environment. During oil combustion or the smelting of metal, sulfuric acid condenses downstream of the combustion processes with available metal ions and water vapor to form submicron sulfated fly ash. Photochemical environments in the lower troposphere also can promote acid sulfate formation through both metal-dependent and -independent mechanisms, but studies have shown that most of the oxidation of SO_2 occurs within diluted plumes drifting in the atmosphere. These sulfates may contribute to health hazards and acid rain (Fig. 28-3).

General Toxicology Sulfuric acid irritates respiratory tissues by virtue of its ability to protonate (H^+) receptor ligands and other biomolecules. This action can damage membranes directly or activate sensory reflexes that initiate inflammation.

Pulmonary Function Effects Sulfuric acid produces an increase in flow resistance in guinea pigs as a result of reflex airway narrowing, or bronchoconstriction, which impedes the flow of air into and out of the lungs. This process can be thought of as a defensive measure to limit the inhalation of air containing noxious gases. The magnitude of the response is related to both acid concentration and particle size. Small particles can penetrate deep into the lung, reaching receptors that stimulate bronchoconstriction and mucus secretion. The thicker mucus blanket of the nose may blunt (by dilution or neutralization by mucus buffers) much of the irritancy of the deposited acid, thus limiting its effects to mucous cell stimulation and a minor increase in nasal flow resistance. In contrast, the less shielded distal airway tissues, with their higher receptor density, can be expected to be more sensitive to the acid, as reflected by their responsiveness to the small particles reaching that area.

Asthmatic persons appear to be somewhat more sensitive to the bronchoconstrictive effects of sulfuric acid than are healthy individuals. Asthma generally is characterized by hyperresponsive airways, and so the tendency of those airways to constrict at low acid concentrations is expected, just as asthmatic airways are sensitive to nonspecific airway smooth muscle agonists (e.g., carbachol, histamine, exercise). The general correlation between airway responsiveness and inflammation that appears to be important in grading asthma severity and the risk of negative clinical outcomes also may be predictive of responses to environmental stimuli.

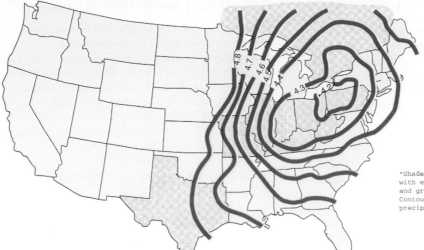

*Shaded areas indicate individual states
with emissions of 1,000 kilotonnes of SO$_2$
and greater.
Contours connect points of equal
precipitation pH.

Figure 28-3. Areas in 1988 where precipitation in the east fell below pH 5: acid rain.   The acidity of the air in the east is thought to result from air mass transport of fine sulfated particulate matter from the industrial centers of the midwest.

Effects on Mucociliary Clearance and Macrophage Function   Sulfuric acid alters the clearance of particles from the lung and thus can interfere with a major defense mechanism. The impact on mucus clearance appears to vary directly with the acidity ([H$^+$]) of the acid sulfate, with sulfuric acid having the greatest effect and ammonium sulfate having the smallest. Acidification of mucus is the primary metric to associate with population health effects affecting mucus rheology, viscosity, and secretion and ciliary function.

Chronic Effects   As might be expected, sulfuric acid induces effects along the airways that are quantitatively similar to those found with SO$_2$ at much higher concentrations. As a fine aerosol, sulfuric acid deposits deeper along the respiratory tract, and its high specific acidity imparts a greater injury effect on phagocytes and epithelial cells. Thus, a primary concern with regard to chronic inhalation of acidic aerosols is its potential to cause bronchitis, since this has been a problem in occupational settings in which employees are exposed to sulfuric acid mists (e.g., battery plants).

Sulfuric acid does not appear to stimulate a classic neutrophilic inflammation after exposure. Instead, disturbed eicosanoid homeostasis results in macrophage dysfunction and altered host defense. Therefore, it seems reasonable to postulate that chronic daily exposure of hu-mans to sulfuric acid at levels of about 100 $\mu g/m^3$ may lead to impaired clearance and mild chronic bronchitis. As this is less than an order of magnitude above haze levels of sulfuric acid, the possibility that chronic irritancy may elicit bronchitic-like disease in susceptible individuals appears to be reasonable.

Particulate Matter

Particulate matter (PM) in the atmosphere is a mélange of organic, inorganic, and biological materials whose compositional matrix can vary significantly, depending on local point sources. A large epidemiologic database contends that PM elicits both short- and long-term health effects at current ambient levels.

Metals   There have been many standard acute and subchronic rodent inhalation studies with specific metal compounds, often oxides or sulfates. Virtually any metal can be found at some concentration in ambient PM, and many of those metals have toxic or prooxidant potential. The most common are metals released during oil and coal combustion (e.g., transition and heavy metals), metals derived from the earth's crust as dust (e.g., iron, sodium, and magnesium), and metals released from engine wear. Metals derived from anthropogenic combustion sources tend to enrich the fine fraction (<2.5 μm) of PM, whereas coarse (2.5- to 10-μm) PM is made up of metal compounds of crustal origin (e.g., Fe_2O_3, SiO_2).

Solubility appears to play a role in the toxicity of many inhaled metals by enhancing metal bioavailability (e.g., nickel from nickel chloride versus nickel oxide), but insolubility also can be a critical factor in determining toxicity by increasing pulmonary residence time in the lung (e.g., insoluble cadmium oxide versus soluble cadmium chloride). Moreover, some metals, either in their soluble forms or when coordinated on the surface of silicate or bioorganic materials, can promote electron transfer to induce the formation of reactive oxidants. It is likely that these and other mechanisms are involved in the action of inhaled PM-associated metals.

Gas-Particle Interactions The coexistence of pollutant gases and particles in the atmosphere raises concern that these phases may interact chemically or physiologically to yield unpredictable outcomes. Many studies have shown that these generic interactions are feasible as mechanisms for altering the toxicity of either the particle or the gas.

Metal smelting and the combustion of coal can emit sulfuric acid that is associated physically with ultrafine metal oxide particles. These ultrafine particles are distributed widely and deeply in the lung and enhance the irritant potency beyond that predicted on the basis of the sulfuric acid concentration alone. Moreover, the combination of inert or chemically active particles with a toxic gas appears to be able to enhance the impact of the gas alone by altering dose distribution or through the formation of a more toxic product.

Another potential interaction may result from the ability of gaseous pollutants to influence the clearance of particles from the lung or alter the metabolism or cellular interactions with lung-deposited particles. Gaseous and particulate pollutants can interact through either chemical or physiologic mechanisms to enhance the immediate or associated long-term risks of complex polluted atmospheres.

Ultrafine Carbonaceous Matter Carbonaceous material often forms the core of fine PM. The organic materials, which can be of a semivolatile or nonvolatile nature, more often are dispersed within the structure of PM, forming layers or sheaths. Estimates of the carbonaceous content vary considerably but are considered nominally to be about 30 to 60 percent of the total mass of fine PM.

As an air pollutant, carbon in the ultrafine mode (<0.1 μm) has been suggested to be more toxic than the same substance in the larger range (2.5 μm). Diesel PM is made up of aggregated ultrafine carbon with small amounts of various combustion-derived complex polycyclic and nitroaromatic compounds and only a trace of metals. However, whole diesel exhaust also contains significant amounts of NO_x, CO, and SO_x as well as formaldehyde, acrolein, and other aldehyde compounds, which are known to be irritants. Diesel exhaust mix is inflammogenic and cytotoxic to airway cells.

Photochemical Air Pollution

Photochemical air pollution arises from a series of complex reactions in the troposphere close to the earth's surface and includes a mixture of ozone, nitric oxides, aldehydes, peroxyacetyl nitrates, and a myriad of reactive hydrocarbon radicals. If SO_2 is present, sulfuric acid PM also may be formed; likewise, the complex chemistry can generate organic PM, nitric acid vapor, and condensate. From the point of view of the toxicology of photochemical air pollutants, the gaseous hydrocarbon component is no longer listed collectively as a criteria pollutant, although individual compounds may fall into the category of hazardous air pollutants (most often associated with cancer). In general, the concentrations of the hydrocarbon precursors in ambient air generally do not reach levels high enough to produce acute toxicity. Their importance stems largely from their roles in the chain of photochemical reactions that leads to the formation of oxidant smog or haze.

The oxidant of the greatest toxicologic importance in the so-called photochemical soup is O_3. It is important to appreciate that atmospheric O_3 is not summarily undesirable. About 10 km above the earth's surface, there is sufficient short-wave ultraviolet (UV) light to directly split molecular O_2 to atomic $O^\bullet$, which then can recombine with O_2 to form O_3. This O_3 accumulates to several hundred ppm within a thin strip of the stratosphere and absorbs incoming short-wavelength UV radiation. The O_3 forms and decomposes and re-forms to establish a "permanent" barrier to UV radiation, which has become an issue of concern, as this barrier is threatened by various anthropogenic emissions (Cl_2 gas and certain fluorocarbons) that enhance O_3 degradation. The consequence is excess infiltration of UV light to the earth's surface and the potential for excess skin cancer risk and immune suppression.

The issue is different in the troposphere, where the accumulation of O_3 serves no known purpose and poses a threat to the respiratory tract. Near the earth's surface, NO_2 from combustion processes efficiently absorbs longer-wavelength UV light, from which a free O atom is cleaved, initiating the following simplified series of reactions:

$$NO_2 + h\nu(\text{UV light}) \rightarrow O^{\bullet} + NO^{\bullet} \qquad (1)$$
$$O^{\bullet} + O_2 \rightarrow O_3 \qquad (2)$$
$$O_3 + NO^{\bullet} \rightarrow NO_2 \qquad (3)$$

This process is inherently cyclic, with NO_2 regenerated by the reaction of the $NO^{\bullet}$ and O_3. In the absence of unsaturated hydrocarbons, this series of reactions will approach a steady state with no excess or buildup of O_3. The hydrocarbons, especially olefins and substituted aromatics, are attacked by the free atomic $O^{\bullet}$, resulting in oxidized compounds and free radicals that react with $NO^{\bullet}$ to produce more NO_2. Thus, the balance of the reactions shown in Eqs. (1) to (3) is upset, leading to buildup of O_3. This reaction is particularly favored when the sun's intensity is greatest at midday, utilizing the NO_2 provided by morning traffic. Aldehydes are major by-products of these reactions. Formaldehyde and acrolein account for about 50 percent and 5 percent, respectively, of the total aldehyde in urban atmospheres. Peroxyacetyl nitrate (CH_3COONO_2), often referred to as PAN, and its homologs also arise in urban air, most likely from the reaction of the peroxyacyl radicals with NO_2.

Chronic Exposures to Smog

Studies in animals and human populations have attempted to link degenerative lung disease with chronic exposure to photochemical air pollution. Cross-sectional and prospective field studies have suggested an accelerated loss of lung function in people living in areas of high pollution. However, as with many studies of this type, there are problems with confounding factors (meteorology, imprecise exposure assessment, and population variables). Recently, studies have been conducted in children living in Mexico City, which has oxidant and PM levels far in excess of those in any city in the United States. These studies have focused on the nasal epithelium as an exposure surrogate for pulmonary tissues, using biopsy and lavage methodologies to assess damage. Dramatic effects were found in exposed children, consisting of severe epithelial damage and metaplasia as well as permanent remodeling of the nasal epithelium. When children who migrated into Mexico City from cleaner, nonurban regions were evaluated, even more severe damage was observed, suggesting that the remodeling in the permanent residents imparted some degree of incomplete adaptation. Since the children were of middle-class ori-

gin, these observations probably were not confounded by poor diet. These dramatic nasal effects have raised concerns about the more fragile, deep lung tissues, where substantial deposition of oxidant air pollutants is thought to occur.

More recently, "sentinel" studies have been attempted in which animals live in the same highly polluted air to which people are exposed. The essential conclusion from most sentinel studies is that "pollution is unhealthy," since individual and mixed pollutant effects and interactions cannot be addressed easily.

Ozone *General Toxicology* Ozone is the primary oxidant of concern in photochemical smog because of its inherent bioreactivity and concentration. Current mitigation strategies for O_3 have been largely unsuccessful despite significant reductions in individual automobile emissions. These reductions have been offset by population growth, which brings with it additional vehicles. With the spread of suburbia and the downwind transport of air masses from populated areas to more rural environments, the geographic distribution of those exposed has spread, as has the temporal profile of potential exposure. In other words, O_3 exposures no longer are stereotyped as brief 1- to 2-h peaks. Instead, there are prolonged periods of exposure of 6 h or more at or near the National Ambient Air Quality Standards (NAAQS) level, and those exposures may occur either downtown or in the formerly cleaner suburban or rural areas downwind.

Ozone induces a variety of effects in humans and experimental animals at concentrations that occur in many urban areas. Those effects include morphologic, functional, immunologic, and biochemical alterations. Because of the low water solubility of ozone, a substantial portion of inhaled ozone penetrates deep into the lung, but its reactivity is such that about 17 percent and 40 percent are scrubbed by the nasopharynx of resting rats and humans, respectively. However, regardless of species, the region of the lung that is predicted to have the greatest O_3 deposition (dose per surface area) is the acinar region, from the terminal bronchioles to the alveolar ducts. Because O_3 penetration increases with increased tidal volume and flow rate, exercise increases the dose to the target area. Thus, it is important to consider the role of exercise in a study of O_3 or any inhalant before making cross-study comparisons, especially if that comparison is across species.

The acute morphologic response to O_3 involves epithelial cell injury along the entire respiratory tract, resulting in cell loss and replacement. Ciliated cells

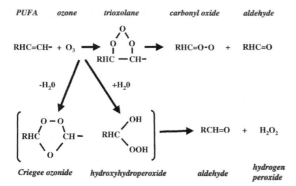

Figure 28-4. Major reactions pathways of O₃ with lipids in lung-lining fluid and cell membranes.

appear to be most sensitive to O₃, while Clara cells and mucus-secreting cells are the least sensitive.

As a powerful oxidant, O₃ attempts to extract electrons from other molecules. The surface fluid lining the respiratory tract and cell membranes that underlie the lining fluid contain a significant quantity of polyunsaturated fatty acids (PUFAs), either free or as part of the lipoprotein structures of the cell. The double bonds in these fatty acids have a labile, unpaired electron that is attacked easily by O₃ to form ozonides that ultimately recombine or decompose to lipohydroperoxides, aldehydes, and hydrogen peroxide. These pathways are thought to initiate the propagation of lipid radicals and autooxidation of cell membranes and macromolecules (Fig. 28-4).

Pulmonary Function Effects Exercising human subjects who are exposed to 0.12 to 0.4 ppm O₃ experience reversible concentration-related decrements in forced vital capacity (FVC) and forced expiratory volume in 1 second (FEV₁) after 2 to 3 h of exposure. Interestingly, the human lung dysfunction resulting from O₃ does not appear to be mediated vagally, but the response can be abrogated by analgesics such as ibuprofen and opiates, which function to reduce pain and inflammation. Thus, pain reflexes involving C-fiber networks are thought to be important in reductions in forced expiratory volumes. However, animal studies suggest that cardiac as well as lung function effects of O₃ have a significant parasympathetic component. It is widely thought that hyperreactive airways may predispose responses to other pollutants, such as sulfuric acid and aeroallergens, but such evidence is limited.

Ozone Interactions with Copollutants An approach simplifying the complexity of synthetic smog studies yet

addressing the issue of pollutant interactions involves the exposure of animals or humans to binary or tertiary mixtures of pollutants that are known to occur together in ambient air. These studies have had a number of permutations, but most have attempted to address the interactions of O₃ and nitrogen dioxide or O₃ and sulfuric acid. Depending on study design, there has been evidence supporting either augmentation or antagonism of lung function impairments, lung pathology, or other indexes of injury. This apparent conflict emphasizes the need to consider carefully the myriad of factors that may affect studies involving multiple determinants.

As the number of interacting variables increases, so does the difficulty of interpretation. Studies of complex atmospheres involving acid-coated carbon combined with O₃ at relevant levels show variable strength of evidence of interaction on lung function and macrophage receptor activities. The difficulty with any multicomponent study is the statistical separation of the interacting variables and responses from the individual or combined components. However, it is the complex mixture to which people are exposed that we wish to evaluate for its toxicologic potential. Creative approaches to understanding mixture responses will have to be addressed in the next decade.

Nitrogen Dioxide *General Toxicology* Nitrogen dioxide, like O₃, is a deep lung irritant that can produce pulmonary edema if it is inhaled at high concentrations. Potential life-threatening exposure is a real-world problem for farmers, as significant amounts of NO₂ can be liberated from silage. Typically, shortness of breath ensues rapidly with exposures nearing 75 to 100 ppm NO₂, with delayed edema and symptoms of pulmonary damage that are characterized collectively as silo-filler's disease. Nitrogen dioxide is also an important indoor pollutant, especially in homes with unventilated gas stoves or kerosene heaters. Under such circumstances, very young children and their mothers who spend considerable time indoors may be especially at risk. Sidestream tobacco smoke also can be a source of indoor NO₂.

Damage to the respiratory tract is most apparent in the terminal bronchioles. At high concentrations, the alveolar ducts and alveoli also are affected, with type I cells again showing their sensitivity to oxidant challenge. There is also damage to epithelial cells in the bronchioles, notably with loss of ciliated cells, as well as a loss of secretory granules in Clara cells. The pattern of injury of NO₂ is quite similar to that of O₃, but its potency is about an order of magnitude lower.

Inflammation of the Lung and Host Defense Unlike O_3, NO_2 does not induce significant neutrophilic inflammation in humans at exposure concentrations that approximate those in the ambient outdoor environment. There is some evidence for bronchial inflammation after 4 to 6 h at 2.0 ppm, which approximates the likely highest transient peak indoor levels of this oxidant. Exposures at 2.0 to 5.0 ppm have been shown to affect T lymphocytes, particularly $CD8^+$ cells and natural killer cells that function in host defenses against viruses. Although these concentrations may be high, epidemiologic studies variably show enhanced viral infection associated with NO_2 exposure, especially during seasonal use of unvented gas heating indoors. Susceptibility to infection appears to be governed more by the peak exposure concentration than by exposure duration. The effects are ascribed to suppression of macrophage function and clearance from the lung.

Other Oxidants Although a number of reactive oxidants have been identified in photochemical smog, most are short-lived because of their reaction with available VOCs, nitrogen oxides, and other reducing equivalents that have the effect of scrubbing them from the air before they can be breathed. One reactive, irritating constituent of the oxidant atmosphere is PAN, which is thought to be responsible for much of the eye-stinging activity of smog. More soluble and reactive than ozone, PAN decomposes rapidly in mucous membranes before it can get to tissues deep in the lungs. The cornea has many irritant receptors and responds readily, whereas the PAN absorbed into the thicker mucous fluids of the proximal nose and mouth presumably never reaches its target.

Aldehydes Various aldehydes in polluted air are formed as reaction products of the photooxidation of hydrocarbons. The two aldehydes of major interest are formaldehyde (HCHO) and acrolein ($H_2C{=}CHCHO$). These materials contribute to the odor as well as the eye and sensory irritations of photochemical smog. Formaldehyde accounts for about 50 percent of the estimated total aldehydes in polluted air, and acrolein, the more irritating of the two, may account for about 5 percent of the total. Acetaldehyde (CH_3CHO) and many other longer-chain aldehydes make up the remainder, but they are not as irritating because of their low concentration and lesser solubility in airway fluids. Formaldehyde and particularly acrolein are found in mainstream tobacco smoke (about 90 and 8 ppm, respectively, per drag) and are likely to be found in sidestream smoke as well. Formalde-

hyde is also an important indoor air pollutant and often can achieve higher concentrations indoors than outdoors if it is derived from outgassing by new upholstery or other furnishings.

Empiric studies have shown that formaldehyde and acrolein are competitive agonists for similar irritant receptors in the airways. Thus, irritation may be related not to "total aldehyde" concentration but to specific ratios of acrolein and formaldehyde. Their relative difference in solubility, with formaldehyde being somewhat more water-soluble and thus having more nasopharyngeal uptake, may distort this relationship under certain exposure conditions (e.g., exercise). However, acrolein is very reactive and may interact easily with many tissue macromolecules.

Formaldehyde Formaldehyde is a primary sensory irritant. Because it is very soluble in water, it is absorbed in mucous membranes in the nose, upper respiratory tract, and eyes. The dose–response curve for formaldehyde is steep: 0.5 to 1 ppm yields a detectable odor, 2 to 3 ppm produces mild irritation, and 4 to 5 ppm is intolerable to most people. Formaldehyde is thought to act through sensory nerve fibers that signal through the trigeminal nerve to reflexively induce bronchconstriction through the vagus nerve. The general pattern of the irritant response and its rapid recovery is similar to that produced by higher concentrations of SO_2. Also like SO_2, the introduction of formaldehyde through a tracheal cannula to bypass nasal scrubbing greatly augments the irritant response, indicating that deep lung irritant receptors also can be activated by this vapor.

Formaldehyde, like SO_2, can interact with water-soluble salts such as submicron sodium chloride and with carbon-based particles during inhalation and produce irritancy beyond that expected for the gas alone.

Two aspects of formaldehyde toxicology have brought it from relative obscurity to the forefront of attention in recent years. One is its presence in indoor atmospheres as an offgassed product of construction materials such as plywood and improperly installed urea-formaldehyde foam insulation. This irritant vapor has the potential to cause respiratory effects at commonly experienced exposure levels. Formaldehyde is also a weak allergen. The second finding is the nasal cancer that has been induced with formaldehyde vapor in rodents. Recent epidemiology studies have not found an increased incidence of nasal cancer in exposed workers.

Acrolein Acrolein is an unsaturated aldehyde that is more irritating than formaldehyde. Concentrations below

1 ppm cause irritation of the eyes and the mucous membranes of the respiratory tract. The mechanism of increased pulmonary flow resistance after acrolein appears to be mediated through a cholinergic reflex. Atropine (a muscarinic blocker) and aminophylline, isoproterenol, and epinephrine (sympathetic agonists) partially or completely reversed the changes, whereas the antihistamines pyrilamine and tripelennamine had no effect.

Carbon Monoxide Carbon monoxide is classed toxicologically as a chemical asphyxiant because its toxic action stems from its formation of carboxyhemoglobin, preventing oxygenation of the blood for systemic transport (see Chap. 11).

Analysis of data from air-monitoring programs in California indicates that 8-h average values can range from 10 to 40 ppm of CO. Depending on the location in a community, CO concentrations can vary widely. Concentrations predicted inside the passenger compartments of motor vehicles in downtown traffic were almost three times those for central urban areas and five times those expected in residential areas. Occupants of vehicles traveling on expressways had CO exposures somewhere between those in central urban areas and those in downtown traffic. Concentrations above 87 ppm have been measured in underground garages, tunnels, and buildings over highways.

No overt human health effects have been demonstrated for COHb levels below 2 percent, but levels above 40 percent can be fatal as a result of asphyxia. At COHb levels of 2.5 percent resulting from about 90-min exposure to about 50 ppm CO, there is an impairment of time-interval discrimination; at approximately 5 percent COHb, there is an impairment of other psychomotor faculties. Cardiovascular changes also may be produced by exposures sufficient to yield COHb in excess of 5 percent.

WHAT IS AN ADVERSE HEALTH EFFECT?

The goal of air-quality management is clearly to avoid or, at worst, limit negative impacts of air pollution on public health. However, one must appreciate the distinction between risk to an individual and risk to a population. Clearly, risk to an individual can be beyond an acceptable limit and can put that person's health in jeopardy, but this response may be lost in a population index. In contrast, risk to a population is the summation of individual risks such that there is a shift in the normal distribution, putting unspecified individuals at risk. These two forms of risk are clearly related, but most often, the

population risk is considered most appropriate and most reasonably quantifiable.

The American Thoracic Society issued a position paper that attempted to define an adverse effect related to air pollution. This statement considers seven broad areas: biomarkers, quality of life, physiologic impacts, symptoms, clinical outcomes, mortality, and population health versus individual risk. The summary conclusion states that caution should be exercised in evaluating the many new biomarkers of effect (especially cell and molecular markers), as there is a need for validation that *small* changes in these markers represent a progression along a course to disease or permanent impairment. Admittedly, in the clinical environment, many of these markers may appear as salient features of a disease or injury, but the health implications of minor changes in these biomarkers remains uncertain. A common thread through all these subject areas is the influential role of susceptibility, which can take the form of hyperresponsiveness or loss of reserve. What was a minor reversible effect may now be a dysfunction that cannot be reversed or compensated (Fig. 28-5). An obvious example would be cardiopulmonary-compromised individuals who function with little or no reserve.

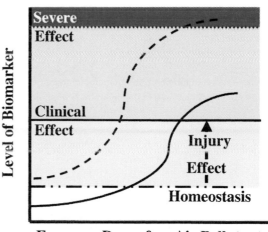

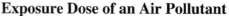

Exposure Dose of an Air Pollutant

Figure 28-5. Schematic illustration of the elements of a dose response to an air pollutant(s) by a susceptible versus a healthy individual. The hypothetical susceptible individual has both a *loss of reserve* and an *inability to maintain homeostasis*. The *leftward shift in the slope* of the dose–response curve also suggests an increase in responsiveness. These response elements of the susceptible individual may contribute to apparent sensitivity to challenge and the likelihood of progressing from subtle to severe effects.

CONCLUSIONS

This chapter relates the breadth and complexity of the problem of air pollution, from the development of credible databases to supporting regulatory action and decision making. The classic and still most important air pollutants provide a foundation for understanding and appreciating the nuances of the issues and strategies for air pollution control and protection of public health.

BIBLIOGRAPHY

American Thoracic Society: What constitutes an adverse health effect of air pollution? *Am J Respir Crit Care Med* 161:665–673, 2000.

Hayes SM, Gobbell RV, Ganick NR (eds): *Indoor Air Quality: Solutions and Strategies.* New York: McGraw-Hill, 1995.

Holgate ST, Samet JM, Koren H, Maynard RL (eds): *Air Pollution and Health.* London: Academic Press, 1999.

Swift DL, Foster WM (eds): *Air Pollutants and the Respiratory Tract.* New York: Marcel Dekker, 1998.

CHAPTER 29

ECOTOXICOLOGY

Ronald J. Kendall, Todd A. Anderson, Robert J. Baker,
Catherine M. Bens, James A. Carr, Louis A. Chiodo,
George P. Cobb III, Richard L. Dickerson, Kenneth R. Dixon,
Lynn T. Frame, Michael J. Hooper, Clyde F. Martin,
Scott T. McMurry, Reynaldo Patino, Ernest E. Smith, and
Christopher W. Theodorakis

KEY POINTS

- Ecotoxicology is the study of the fate of toxic substances and their effects on an ecosystem.
- Chemodynamics is in essence the study of the release, distribution, degradation, and fate of chemicals in the environment.
- A chemical can enter any of four matrices: the atmosphere by evaporation, the lithosphere by adsorption, the hydrosphere by dissolution, or the biosphere by absorption, inhalation, or ingestion (depending on the species). Once in a matrix, a toxicant can enter another matrix by these methods.
- The *biological availability* (bioavailability) of a chemical is the portion of the total quantity of the chemical present that is potentially available for uptake by organisms.
- Pollution may result in a cascade of events, beginning with effects on homeostasis in individuals and extending through populations, communities, ecosystems, and landscapes.
- Terrestrial toxicology is the science of exposure to and effects of toxic compounds in terrestrial ecosystems.
- Aquatic toxicology is the study of the effects of anthropogenic chemicals on organisms in the aquatic environment.

INTRODUCTION TO ECOTOXICOLOGY

Ecotoxicology is the study of the fate of toxic substances and their effects on an ecosystem and is based on scientific research that employs both field and laboratory methods. Environmental toxicology as it relates to ecotoxicology requires an understanding of how chemicals can affect individuals, populations, communities, and ecosystems. Ecotoxicology builds on the science of toxicology and the principles of toxicologic testing, although its emphasis is more on the population, community, and ecosystem levels. Unlike standard toxicologic tests, which attempt to define the cause-and-effect relationship with certain concentrations of toxicant exposure at a sensitive receptor site, ecotoxicologic testing attempts to evaluate cause-and-effect relationships at higher levels of organization, particularly on populations.

A critical component in ecotoxicologic testing is the integration of laboratory and field research. Knowledge acquired in the laboratory is integrated with what occurs under field conditions and is critical to understanding the complex set of parameters with which an organism must deal in order to reproduce or survive after toxicant exposure. Laboratory testing often limits the complexity of stress parameters. It therefore is difficult to interpret potential ecotoxicologic effects resulting from laboratory studies without data from pertinent field investigations. For these reasons, integrating laboratory and field research ensures that ecotoxicologic testing methods produce relevant data. Moreover, society's interest in the relationship of the environment and potential environmental toxicant stressors in human health implications is increasing.

CHEMICAL MOVEMENT, FATE, AND EXPOSURE

To characterize chemical behavior, it is necessary to measure a chemical in different environmental compartments (e.g., air, soil, water, and biological systems), understand the movement and transport of the chemical within and among those compartments, and follow the chemical as it is metabolized, degraded, stored, or concentrated in each compartment, even if it is in very low concentrations.

Chemodynamics

Chemical transport occurs both within environmental compartments (intraphase) and between them (interphase), and comprehension of chemodynamics is critical to understanding and interpreting environmental toxicology data. Often a chemical is released into one environmental compartment and then partitioned among environmental compartments and involved in movement and reactions within each compartment. Then it is partitioned between each compartment and the biota that reside in that compartment, and finally it reaches an active site in an organism at a high enough concentration and for a long enough period to induce an effect. Chemodynamics is in essence the study of chemical release, distribution, degradation, and fate in the environment.

Chemodynamics also can describe the movement of a chemical or its absorption into organisms. Detoxification mechanisms such as partitioning into adipose tissue, metabolism, and accelerated excretion can reduce significantly, eliminate, or in some cases increase the toxic action of a chemical. Thus, an appreciation of chemodynamics aids in the prediction of chemical concentrations in compartments.

Single-Phase Chemical Behavior

Once a synthetic chemical enters the environment, it is acted on primarily by natural forces such as temperature, wind and water-flow directions and velocities, incident solar radiation, atmospheric pressure and humidity, and the concentration of the chemical in one of four matrices: atmosphere (air), hydrosphere (water), lithosphere (soil), and biosphere (living organisms). Intraphase movement consists of mass transfer, diffusion, or dispersion within a single phase. Contaminant persistence is a function of the stability of a chemical in a phase and its transport within that phase. Stability is a function of the physicochemical properties of a particular chemical and the kinetics of its degradation in the phase.

Air The primary routes for a contaminant's entry into the atmosphere are evaporation, stack emissions, and other matrices. Wind currents transport airborne contaminants much more rapidly than does diffusion. Atmospheric stability affects the amount of turbulence and thus the degree of vertical mixing in the atmosphere. The stability of the atmosphere is considered neutral when the convective forces—heat transfer from warm ground surfaces and radiative cooling from the top of the cloud layer—are equal.

Water Contaminants enter the hydrosphere through direct application, spills, wet and dry deposition, and interphase movement. In addition, chemicals enter the hydrosphere through direct dissolution of lighter-than-water spills in the form of slicks or from pools on the bottoms of channels, rivers, or other waterways. Chemical movement in the hydrosphere occurs through diffusion, dispersion, and bulk flow of the water.

In areas away from the boundaries of other media (i.e., air and soil), transport in water is dominated by turbulence. Even in seemingly still water, water is moving constantly in vertical and horizontal eddies. This mode of transport is defined as *eddy diffusion*. In addition, a contaminant can be transported rapidly by bulk flow (also referred to as *advection*) in streams and rivers.

Soil Chemicals enter the lithosphere by processes similar to those for the hydrosphere. Soils have varying porosities because of their differing composition, but the pores invariably are filled with either gas or fluids. Chemical movement in the soil occurs by means of diffusion in these fluids or the movement of water through the voids between soil particles. The direction of diffusion is from areas of high concentration to areas of low concentration. Contaminants leave the soil by interphase transport or decomposition. Transformation of contaminants (such as through microbial degradation) can be significant in soil because of the density and diversity of microorganisms in this compartment.

Chemical Transport between Phases

Once it is released, a chemical can enter any of the four matrices: the atmosphere by evaporation, the lithosphere by adsorption, the hydrosphere by dissolution, or the biosphere by absorption, inhalation, or ingestion (depending on the species). Once it is in a matrix, a contaminant can enter another matrix by these methods.

Chemical Behavior and Bioavailability

In the environment, only a portion of the total quantity of a chemical present is potentially available for uptake by organisms. This concept is referred to as the *biological availability* (bioavailability) of a chemical. Chemical bioavailability in various environmental compartments ultimately dictates toxicity.

The behavior and bioavailability of contaminants in the water column have been shown to be related directly to their water solubility. However, the presence of certain constituents in water may affect the apparent water solubility of toxicants. Dissolved organic carbon may increase the transport and mobility of organic contaminants in the water column but also may reduce their bioavailability.

The awareness that many aquatic contaminants settle into sediments has prompted studies of metals and organics to characterize their fate and disposition within those sediments. Deposition is a combination of physical, chemical, and biological processes that ultimately may change the form of a xenobiotic. Many metals are reduced abiotically or biotically as they are incorporated into sediments, changing their bioavailability. Organic chemicals residing in the sediment matrix also undergo a variety of abiotic and biotic transformations.

In soils, sorption also controls the bioavailability of contaminants. Tight sorption or sequestration of contaminants with increasing residence time in soil, often referred to as "aging," also has been documented. Although the amount of a contaminant in soil remains fairly constant, the fraction of the contaminant available to soil organisms decreases significantly with time.

BIOMARKERS

A fundamental challenge in environmental toxicology is relating the presence of a chemical in the environment to a valid prediction of the ensuing hazard to potential biological receptors. Adverse health effects in biological receptors begin with exposure to a contaminant and can progress to damage or alteration in the function of an organelle, cell, or tissue. Exposure of wildlife by contact with contaminated environmental media is defined as an *external dose,* whereas internalization of the contaminated media through inhalation, ingestion, or dermal absorption results in an *internal dose.* The amount of an internal dose necessary to elicit a response or health effect is referred to as the *biologically effective dose.*

Traditionally, environmental risk was assessed by the determination of chemical residue in samples of environmental media, combined with comparison to the toxicity observed in species in contact with the media. A biomarker-based approach provides a direct measure of toxicant effects in the affected species. Biomarkers can be broadly categorized as markers of exposure, effects, or susceptibility. Growing awareness of the possibility of using wildlife as sentinels for human environmental disease has created a demand for biomarkers that are nonlethal and correlate with adverse effects in humans.

Dosing with an adequate concentration of a toxicant produces a continuum of responses that begins with exposure and may result in the development of a disease. These events begin with external exposure, followed by the establishment of an internal dose and leading to the delivery of a contaminant to a critical site. This is followed by reversible or irreversible adverse alterations to the critical site, resulting in the development of recognizable disease states. A clearer understanding of a chemically induced disease state in a species leads to an increase in the number of specific and useful biomarkers that may be extrapolated to other species. However, in many cases, the exact mechanism by which a toxicant induces injury is not well understood, and nonspecific indicators of disease must be used.

Biomarkers of Exposure

The presence of a xenobiotic or its metabolite(s) or the product of an interaction between a xenobiotic agent and a target molecule or cell that is measured within a compartment of an organism can be classified as a biomarker of exposure. In general, biomarkers of exposure are used to predict the dose received by an individual, which then can be related to changes that result in a disease state.

Biomarkers of Effect

Biomarkers of effect are defined as measurable biochemical, physiologic, behavioral, or other alterations in an organism that, depending on their magnitude, can be recognized as an established or potential health impairment or disease.

Less specific biomarkers also are well validated, but they have wider applications and tend to respond to broader classes of chemicals. These assays require either additional biomarker studies or chemical residue analysis to link the causative agent to the adverse effect. For example, the induction of cytochrome P450 1Al enzymes in fish liver generally is recognized as a useful biomarker of the exposure of fish to anthropogenic contaminants, but these results are not compound-specific, as they may be induced by various polynuclear and halogenated aromatic hydrocarbons as well as by hypoxia.

Biomarkers of Susceptibility

Biomarkers of susceptibility are endpoints that are indicative of an altered physiologic or biochemical state that may predispose an individual to the impacts of chemical, physical, and infectious agents. These biomarkers can be useful in extrapolating human disease states from wildlife sentinels.

Biomarker Interpretation

Caution must be used in interpreting biomarker results and extrapolating from one species to another. The same chemical may induce different proteins in one species compared with another, and the same enzyme may have different substrate specificities in different species. Extrapolation of results requires a thorough knowledge of comparative physiology and biochemistry.

ENDOCRINE AND DEVELOPMENTAL DISRUPTORS

A number of compounds, both natural and anthropogenic, cause alterations in the endocrine system. Profound endocrine effects both in individuals and at the population level have been documented after exposure to high levels of certain compounds. Endocrine-disrupting compounds (EDCs) may have significant effects on pregnancy, sexual differentiation and development, and male–female behavioral patterns.

Endocrine disruption initially was observed in wildlife species and has received much attention in both the lay and the scientific press. Studies of EDCs in wildlife are an important tool in determining the risk posed by the environment. Table 29-1 lists a number of studies in various species, the causative agents (if known), and the effects observed.

Mechanisms of Endocrine Toxicity and Sensitive Life Stages

It is evident that EDCs may interact with multiple targets. There is evidence for EDCs acting at every level of hormone synthesis, secretion, transport, site of action, and metabolism. Some examples of known mechanisms for EDCs include the following.

Receptor-Mediated Effects of EDCs A xenobiotic compound may exert effects at the receptor level through multiple mechanisms beyond the classic ligand-receptor interaction. Xenobiotics may act on the endocrine system by affecting transcription and signal transduction and can act through receptor-mediated or non-receptor-mediated mechanisms.

Effects of EDCs on Hormone Synthesis and Metabolism A compound may alter levels of critical endogenous hormones adversely by inducing or inhibiting biosynthetic or metabolic enzyme activities. Some phy-

toestrogens can interact with the 17β-dehydrogenase that regulates estradiol and estrone levels, suggesting that they can modulate overall estrogen levels in addition to acting as a ligand for the estrogen receptor.

Effects on Hormone Secretion and Transport It has been known for many years that Cd^{2+} is a nonselective Ca^{2+} blocker that can disrupt Ca^{2+}-dependent exocytosis in hypothalamic neurosecretory neurons and pituitary endocrine cells.

TERRESTRIAL AND AQUATIC ECOTOXICOLOGY

Ecosystems are composed of groups of all types of organisms that function together as well as interact with the physical environment. In turn, ecosystems collectively constitute landscapes. Cycling and flow of materials maintain varying levels of connectivity within ecologic systems such that disturbances to one component may be realized at another seemingly distinct component. In general, ecologic systems are in a constant state of communication, and this can facilitate the large-scale effects of pollution.

Ecotoxicology includes all aspects of aquatic and terrestrial systems in an attempt to elucidate the effects on biota after contaminant exposure. Studies in aquatic and terrestrial toxicology rely heavily on interdisciplinary scientific exploration. Pollution may result in a cascade of events, beginning with effects on homeostasis in individuals and extending through populations, communities, ecosystems, and landscapes. This complexity and the potential for large-scale effects extending through ecosystems result in a challenging research environment for environmental toxicologists.

Toxicity Tests

Acute and chronic toxicity tests are designed to determine the short- and long-term effects of chemical exposure on a variety of endpoints, including survival, reproduction, and physiologic and biochemical responses. Because of the complex possibilities in typical field conditions, acute and chronic toxicity testing provides a critical foundation for evaluating the exposures and effects encountered in the field and for linking cause and effect in the case of specific chemicals. Results derived from acute and chronic tests can be used to determine the pathologic effects of contaminants, provide the data necessary to analyze the effects discovered in field tests, identify the potential effects to be aware of

Table 29-1
Studies of Endocrine Disruption in Representative Wildlife Species

SPECIES	COMPOUND	EFFECTS
Invertebrates		
Molluscs	Tributyltin	Imposex
Insects	DDE	Metabolic masculinization
Fish		
White sucker (*Catostomus commersoni*)	Kraft mill effluent	Delayed maturation, induction of vitellogenin in male fish, reduced gonad size and development, altered sex steroid concentrations
Trout (*Salmo gairderi*)	Municipal sewer effluent (containing alkylphenols and conjugated estrogens)	Feminization of male fish, including induction of plasma vitellogenin
Amphibians		
African clawed frog (*Xenopus laevis*)	Estrogens	Sexual imprinting (100% females)
Reptiles		
Red-eared slider (*Trachemys scripta*)	Estrogens, pesticides	Sex reversal, gonadal aberrations, altered sex steroid concentrations
American alligator (*Alligator mississippiensis*)	Estrogens, pesticides	Sex reversal, gonadal and phallus malformations, altered sex steroid concentrations
Birds		
Herring gulls (*Larus argentatus*)	PCBs, pesticides	Masculinization, altered gonadal structure
American bald eagle (*Haliaeetus leucocephalus*)	PCBs, dioxins, pesticides	Eggshell thinning, brain asymmetry
Mammals		
Beluga whale (*Delphinptenus leucas*)	Organochlorines, metals	Tumors, immune suppression, impaired reproduction
Mink (*Mustela vision*)	PCBs, dioxins	Impaired reproduction, fetal mortality

KEY: DDE, 1,1-dichloro-2,2-bis(*p*-chlorophenyl) ethylene; PCBs, polychlorinated biphenyls.

in field conditions, and provide dose–response data for comparison to exposure levels in the field.

Sublethal Effects

Mortality represents a nonreversible endpoint of interest in ecotoxicology. However, documenting die-offs can be challenging, as success is affected by search efficiency and rapid disappearance of carcasses. Also, many contaminants exist in smaller, nonlethal amounts or in relatively unavailable forms so that acute mortality is unlikely. Thus, understanding and monitoring the sublethal effects of contaminant exposure in aquatic and terrestrial

systems are of great interest. Biochemical and physiologic measurement endpoints have been developed or adapted from other sources and used with various plant and animal sentinels to assess exposure and effect in many different species. Strategies for monitoring sublethal effects include monitoring immune function, certain biomarkers, genotoxicity, and reproductive endpoints. Even though these effects may not result in immediate mortality, they can affect fecundity and behavioral traits such as predator avoidance capability, parenting ability, and foraging behavior, all of which ultimately may have effects on population structure and function. These changes may occur at earlier times or at lower doses than does overt mortality, providing an early-warning indicator of toxic effects.

Population and Community Effects

One of the major objectives of ecotoxicology is the detection and prevention of pollutant effects on population structure and function. These effects may be determined by the collection of empiric data or simulated with the use of population models. With empiric data collection, natural populations are sampled to determine the effects of environmental contamination on the density, abundance, or biomass of indigenous organisms. The pattern of population response to pollution may provide information about the mechanism of population effect, such as changes in adult mortality, juvenile recruitment, food availability, and so on.

Alternatively, the effects of pollutants on populations can be predicted or simulated by using mathematical models. These models use empiric data such as abundance, age distribution, and age-specific mortality and fecundity to predict the effects of pollutant exposure on the abundance of individuals and the rate of population change.

Any effects on populations ultimately may be manifest as effects on communities, which are collections of interacting populations. Environmental contaminants can affect the structure of communities as well as the interactions of species within them. The trophic structure of communities is related to the relative abundance of species that feed on various food items or have various foraging methods. Changes in species/trophic composition may come about by direct or indirect mechanisms. The direct effects involve the loss of some species as a result of an increase in pollution-induced mortality or reduced reproductive output. Alternatively, community structure may change through indirect mechanisms. For example, a species may be absent from a community because the organisms on which it feeds have been exterminated by pollutant exposure. Indirect effects also may be affected by changes in dynamic interactions between species, for example, predator-prey interactions and competition for food. These types of perturbations in community structure and dynamics ultimately may compromise the stability, sustainability, and productivity of affected ecosystems.

Chemical Interactions and Natural Stressors

There is increasing interest in understanding the interactive effects of exposure to multiple contaminants as well as the interactions between contaminants and inherent stressors (e.g., nutritional stress, disease, predation, climate, water quality). The effects of some chemicals are antagonized or exacerbated by interaction with other pollutants in the environment. Effects also have been found for the interaction between temperature and chemical exposure. Cold stress has been shown to augment the effects of exposure to pesticides. Toxicity, accumulation, and metabolism of aquatic contaminants may be influenced by water temperature because the metabolism of fish is dependent on ambient temperature. Other environmental variables, such as salinity and pH, also may affect the uptake and toxicity of aqueous chemicals. Conversely, exposure to pollutants may affect an organism's ability to tolerate natural environmental variables.

Trophic-Level Transfer of Contaminants

Although contaminant exposure may occur through inhalation, dermal contact, or ingestion from preening or grooming behavior, significant exposure also occurs through food-chain transport. Species that normally are not in direct contact with contaminated media may become exposed through the ingestion of contaminated prey, promoting accumulation or magnification of contaminants into higher trophic levels.

Genotoxicity

Ecogenotoxicology studies the effects of pollutants or chemicals on the genetic material of organisms. Although it is possible to damage the genetic material of an organism without any subsequent effect on that individual, it is also possible that mutations in the DNA will result in somatic effects such as cancers. If these effects occur in germinal tissues, this also can result in heritable effects.

The field of evolutionary toxicology deals with other types of multigenerational effects that may not occur through direct interaction of contaminants with the DNA molecule. Selection for pollutant-resistant genotypes as well as reductions in population size or recruitment may reduce genetic variability in affected populations. An elevated mutation rate also may alter a population's genetic structure.

Terrestrial Ecotoxicology

Terrestrial toxicology is the science of the exposure to and effects of toxic compounds in terrestrial ecosystems.

Acute and Chronic Toxicity Testing Terrestrial organisms typically are exposed to contaminants through the ingestion of contaminated media, although inhalation and dermal absorption of contaminants do occur. Thus, toxicity tests for terrestrial species usually are designed to test the effects of a chemical dose that is administered orally. Methods for measuring endpoints in toxicity tests include LD_{50} and LC_{50}, ED_{50} and EC_{50}, and reproductive tests (fertility, egg hatchability, neonate survival).

Field Testing Field studies address exposure to contaminants and the resulting effects on organisms outside the highly controlled environment of the laboratory. Field studies may be designed specifically to address questions suggested by laboratory studies or to test modeled or predicted exposure and effects based on site contaminant levels.

Field studies are conducted in complex ecologic systems where plants and animals are affected by numerous natural stressors (e.g., nutrient restriction, disease, predation) that might confound the measurement of contaminant exposure and effects. Issues of habitat use, home range size, foraging characteristics, and other factors must be considered in designing a field study. Field studies have provided information on the impacts of contaminants on wildlife abundance and survival, acute mortality, food-chain relationships, reproduction, and behavior.

Field studies often are designed to examine populations of organisms living on contaminated sites, which then are compared with other populations living on noncontaminated reference sites. Although some control is available over other factors, such as the test species and habitat type, study design is still subject to the local conditions dictated by the contaminated site.

The use of enclosures has greatly enhanced control over many of the environmental factors that can complicate field studies. Enclosure studies incorporate a variety of outdoor, open-air facilities to enclose test organisms during toxicologic testing. The purpose of using enclosures is to simulate natural field conditions while maintaining a level of control over experimental conditions. In essence, enclosure-based experiments can be used to bridge the gap between laboratory and field investigations.

Aquatic Ecotoxicology

Aquatic toxicology is the study of the effects of anthropogenic chemicals on organisms in the aquatic environment. Certain chemicals are not volatile in air but are soluble in water (e.g., metals), and so aquatic organisms may be exposed to chemicals through routes that are not present in their terrestrial counterparts. Also, many contaminants are degraded readily in an aerobic environment; the aquatic environment frequently contains little or no oxygen, and so some contaminants can persist in aquatic ecosystems for a long time.

Acute and Chronic Toxicity Testing In aquatic toxicity tests, fish, invertebrates, or algae are exposed to aqueous chemicals in the laboratory by being immersed in a solution of a contaminant. The endpoints of aquatic toxicity tests are recorded as LC_{50} and EC_{50} (lethal and effective concentrations).

Toxicity tests have been used to measure the toxic effects of individual chemicals or contaminated water collected from the field. Single-chemical tests typically are used for the purposes of chemical registry, whereas testing of contaminated water is used commonly for environmental monitoring purposes and to verify compliance with permitting requirements. In these tests, the water to be tested is collected on site and test organisms are exposed to various concentrations diluted with clean water.

Sublethal Effects In the aquatic environment, concentrations of contaminants in the water or sediment may not be high enough to elicit mortality but still may induce sublethal effects on the health of aquatic organisms. This type of damage can lead to tumors or infections and parasitic infestations. Unlike cancers, infectious and parasitic diseases are not induced directly by contaminant exposure, but such exposure may increase the occurrence and severity of these infections. If significant numbers of individuals are affected, this ultimately could have effects at the population level.

Field Studies Aquatic field studies can be classified as either manipulative or observational. In manipulative studies, previously unexposed organisms are used and the experimenter determines the level of contamination to which they are exposed. In contrast, in observational studies, the level of contamination to which the organisms are exposed is not under the control of the experimenter.

Biomonitoring involves sampling aquatic organisms in the natural environment as an indication of the impact of anthropogenic contamination. Endpoints are assessed by exposing caged organisms to contaminated water, sediment, or both and noting mortality and reproductive impairments. These types of tests are termed *ambient toxicity tests.*

Evidence of overt toxicity is more difficult to determine in indigenous populations except during fish kills and other episodes of massive mortality. Consequently, endpoints other than mortality are documented more commonly in biomonitoring studies such as studies of tissue concentrations of the contaminants of concern. These data are useful in determining whether chemicals present in the water or sediment are in a form that is bioavailable to aquatic organisms, determining possible health risks to humans who might consume those organisms, or modeling accumulation and effects in organisms at higher trophic levels.

The most efficacious methods of biomonitoring integrate multiple endpoints at various levels of biological organization. For example, the *sediment quality triad* approach incorporates analysis of sediment chemical concentrations, acute toxicity, and invertebrate community structure to assess the level of sediment contamination. Concordance between all three endpoints is taken as strong evidence that there are contaminants present in the sediment that could have detrimental effects on the aquatic ecosystem. Integrated approaches such as these are necessary to evaluate environmental contamination in natural settings accurately, because the aquatic environment is too complex to be assessed accurately through the use of one endpoint alone.

ECOTOXICOLOGIC MODELING

Modeling in ecotoxicology allows prediction of the effects of toxic compounds on the environment, which can be characterized by various ecosystems (forests, grasslands, lakes, wetlands, etc.). Because the dynamics of real systems are quite complex, an understanding of the impacts of toxicants on a system can be enhanced by modeling that system.

Once the system has been defined, it is possible to identify stimuli or disturbances from exogenous toxic substances, called *inputs,* from outside the system. These inputs operate on the system to produce a response called the *output*. The modeling process involves three steps: (1) identification of system components and boundaries, (2) identification of component interactions, and (3) characterization of those interactions by using quantitative abstractions of mechanistic processes. Models can be used to obtain qualitative or quantitative information about the interactions between variables of interest in a complex system.

ECOLOGIC RISK ASSESSMENT

With the growth of environmental toxicology has come the need to assess and quantify the impact of toxic chemicals on organisms, their populations, and communities in ecosystems. The U.S. Environmental Protection Agency issued a framework for conducting ecologic risk assessment that allows for the assessment of the impact of toxic chemicals as well as other stressors on ecologic systems. In the problem-formulation phase, the potential pathways and species that may be affected by the toxic substance are considered and a conceptual model is developed that describes routes of exposure, biota of concern, and anticipated effect endpoints. The actual risk of chemicals to wildlife or other biota then is determined by using exposure data and toxic effects of the chemicals of interest. In the risk-characterization phase, exposure and effect data accumulated in the analysis phase are combined and the risk potential is characterized. On the basis of the resulting risk, risk management steps can be taken.

The key to understanding ecologic risk assessment in ecotoxicology is to consider more than just chemical toxicity. It is necessary to consider ecologic risk assessment in the context of exposure and other issues, such as sublethal effects and ecosystem impacts.

ENVIRONMENTAL TOXICOLOGY AND HUMAN HEALTH

Links between wildlife and human health serve as a premise for extrapolation in risk assessment. Humans share many cellular and subcellular mechanisms with wildlife species. Humans and wildlife also overlap in their physical environment and therefore are exposed to many of the same contaminants.

There are obvious challenges and concerns in the extrapolation of wildlife data to humans. When there are contaminant-specific alterations in wildlife health, concerns about coordinate adverse effects in humans tend to focus on susceptible developmental periods, including the in utero, neonatal, pubertal, lactational, and menopausal stages. There is also a real concern about an increased risk of various cancers caused by environmental contaminants. Unfortunately, linking known contaminant exposures to an affected human population is difficult, particularly when effects are not identified for many years. By the time human effects are identified, the causative agent may not be present or detectable.

As with wildlife, some human health effects may be reversible whereas others may involve irreversible changes. Particularly because of the longevity of humans, chronic low-dose exposures may result in a health risk, predisposing elderly individuals to chronic disease processes. Wildlife may not be affected in the same ways because of the generally shorter life span of animals.

Regardless of species, the process of risk assessment requires four steps: hazard identification, dose–response assessment, exposure assessment, and risk characterization. Often these processes are difficult in human populations, and extrapolations are required, including qualitative interspecies extrapolation from test animal to human and quantitative extrapolation from high dose to low dose. When human data are of low quality or are not available, wildlife sentinels can serve a useful role in assessing human risk.

The interconnections between ecologic health and human health should not be overlooked. The indirect effects of environmental pollution may in the end be more important than the direct effects for human health. The environment is thought to act as a buffer for both toxicants and disease. However, even a buffer has its limits. In the future, it is important that researchers focus on closing the artificial gap that views "environmental" and "human" health issues separately.

BIBLIOGRAPHY

Crane M: *Predictive Ecotoxicology.* New York: Wiley, 2002.

Dell'Omo G: *Behavioral Ecotoxicology.* New York: Wiley, 2002.

Hoffman DJ: *Handbook of Ecotoxicology,* 2d ed. Boca Raton, FL: CRC Press, 2002.

Kendall RJ, Dickerson RL, Giesy JP, Suk WA (eds): *Principles and Processes for Evaluating Endocrine Disruption in Wildlife.* Pensacola, FL: SETAC Press, 1998.

UNIT 7

APPLICATIONS OF TOXICOLOGY

CHAPTER 30

FOOD TOXICOLOGY

Frank N. Kotsonis, George A. Burdock, and W. Gary Flamm

KEY POINTS

- Food is an exceedingly complex mixture of nutrient and nonnutrient substances.
- A substance listed as generally recognized as safe achieves that determination on the basis of safety, as shown through scientific procedures or through experience based on common use.
- An estimated daily intake is based on two factors: the daily intake of the food in which a substance will be used and the concentration of that substance in that food.
- Food hypersensitivity (allergy) refers to a reaction involving an immune-mediated response, including cutaneous reactions, systemic effects, and even anaphylaxis.
- The vast majority of food-borne illnesses in developed countries are attributable to microbiological contamination of food.

UNIQUENESS OF FOOD TOXICOLOGY

The nature of food is responsible for the uniqueness of food toxicology. Because most food cannot be produced commercially in a definable environment under strict quality controls, food generally cannot meet the rigorous standards of chemical identity, purity, and good manufacturing practice that are met by most consumer products. The fact that food is harvested from the soil, the sea, or inland waters or is derived from land animals, which are subject to the unpredictable forces of nature, makes the constancy of raw food unreliable. Food in general is more complex and variable in composition than are all the other substances to which humans are exposed, and humans are exposed more to food than to any other chemicals.

Nature and Complexity of Food

Food is an exceedingly complex mixture of nutrient and nonnutrient substances whether it is consumed in the "natural" (unprocessed) form or as a highly processed ready-to-eat microwaveable meal. Nonnutrient substances (substances other than carbohydrates, proteins, fats, and vitamins/minerals) often are characterized in the popular literature as being contributed by food processing, but nature provides the vast majority of nonnutrient constituents. For instance, in Table 30-1, one can see that even among "natural" (or minimally processed) foods, there are far more nonnutrient than nutrient constituents. Many of these nonnutrient substances are vital for the growth and survival of a plant, including hormones and naturally occurring pesticides. Nonnutrient substances also are added during processing; many are flavor additives.

Table 30-1
Nonnutrient Substances in Food

FOOD	NUMBER OF IDENTIFIED NONNUTRIENT CHEMICALS
Cheddar cheese	160
Orange juice	250
Banana	325
Tomato	350
Wine	475
Coffee	625
Beef (cooked)	625

SAFETY STANDARDS FOR FOODS, FOOD INGREDIENTS, AND CONTAMINANTS

The Food, Drug and Cosmetics Act

The FD&C Act presumes that traditionally consumed foods are safe if they are free of contaminants. For the U.S. Food and Drug Administration (FDA) to ban foods, it must have clear evidence that death or illness can be traced to the consumption of a particular food. The FD&C Act permits the addition of a substance to food to accomplish a specific technical effect if that substance is determined to be generally recognized as safe (GRAS). The act requires that scientific experts base a GRAS determination on the adequacy of safety, as shown through scientific procedures or through experience based on common use. If a food contains an unavoidable contaminant even with the use of current good manufacturing practices, it may be declared unfit as food if the contaminant may render it injurious to health. Foods containing *unavoidable* contaminants are not banned automatically, but the FDA has set some informal limits (called action levels) on the tolerable quantity of unavoidable contaminants.

In addition to allowing GRAS substances to be added to food, the act provides for a class of substances that are regulated food additives, which must be approved and regulated for their intended conditions of use by the FDA. Two distinct types of color additives have been approved for food use: those requiring certification by FDA chemists and those exempt from certification. Most certified colors approved for food use bear the prefix FD&C (such as FD&C Blue No. 1). Such color additives consist of structures that cannot be synthesized without a variety of impurities and therefore must be monitored carefully and certified as safe before they are used in food products. Food colors that are exempt from certification are derived primarily from natural sources.

Methods Used to Evaluate the Safety of Foods, Ingredients, and Contaminants

Safety Evaluation of Direct Food and Color Additives The safety of any substance added to food must be established on the basis of specific intended conditions of use or uses in food.

Exposure: The Estimated Daily Intake Exposure most often is referred to as an estimated daily intake (EDI)

Table 30-2
Assignment of Concern Level

STRUCTURE CATEGORY A	STRUCTURE CATEGORY B	STRUCTURE CATEGORY C	CONCERN LEVEL
<0.05 ppm in the total diet (<0.0012 mg/kg/day) or	<0.025 ppm in the total diet (<0.00063 mg/kg/day) or	<0.0125 ppm in the total diet (<0.00031 mg/kg/day) or	I
≥0.05 ppm in the total diet (≥0.0012 mg/kg/day) or	≥0.025 ppm in the total diet (≥0.00063 mg/kg/day) or	≥0.0125 ppm in the total diet (≥0.00031 mg/kg/day) or	II
≥1 ppm in the total diet (≥0.025 mg/kg/day)	≥0.5 ppm in the total diet (≥0.0125 mg/kg/day)	≥0.25 ppm in the total diet (≥0.0063 mg/kg/day)	III

and is based on two factors: the daily intake (I) of the food in which the substance will be used and the concentration (C) of the substance in that food. In estimates of consumption and/or exposure, one also must consider other sources of consumption for the proposed intended use of the additive if it already is used in food for another purpose, occurs naturally in foods, or is used in nonfood sources (e.g., drugs, toothpaste, lipstick).

Before a food additive is approved, regulatory agencies require evidence that it is safe for its intended use(s) and that its EDI is less than its acceptable daily intake (ADI), which generally is based on the results from animal toxicology studies.

Assignment of Concern Level (CL) and Required Testing

Structures of functional groups in food additives are assigned to categories (A, B, and C) on the basis of their relative harmful nature (category A is least harmful; category C is most harmful). Based on structure assignment and calculated exposure, a concern level (CL) for a certain additive can be assigned (Table 30-2). An additive with a higher concern level (CLIII) is more likely to be dangerous than one with a lower concern level (CLI). Once the CL is established, a specific test battery is prescribed, as shown in Table 30-3.

Safety Determination of Indirect Food Additives

Indirect food additives are substances that are not added directly to food but enter food by migrating from surfaces that contact food. These surfaces may be packaging materials (cans, paper, plastic) or surfaces used in processing, holding, or transporting food. The level of overall consumption of these materials determines the testing required by the FDA to allow certain foods to be packaged in certain ways.

Safety Requirements for GRAS Substances

The FD&C act regards foods as GRAS when they are added to other food, for example, green beans in vegetable soup. It also regards a number of food ingredients as GRAS. A list of examples of substances regarded as GRAS is given in Table 30-4. It is important to reemphasize that GRAS substances, though *used* like food additives, are *not* food additives; this allows GRAS substances to be exempt from the premarket clearance restrictions applied to food additives.

Transgenic Plant (and New Plant Varieties) Policy

The FDA requires tests to be done on new plant varieties to make sure that any new proteins produced in a plant by genetic engineering are nontoxic and nonallergenic.

Dietary Supplements

Dietary supplements have a special status within the law and the regulations; supplements are regarded as foods or food-type substances but not as food additives and not as drugs. Whereas a food ingredient must have *demonstrated safety,* a supplement ingredient must have *no history of unsafe use,* a much easier standard to meet. An unapproved health claim cannot be made for a dietary supplement, as it then would be regarded as a "drug" and would be subject to the rigorous drug application process with demonstrations of safety and effectiveness.

Carcinogenicity as a Special Problem

The Delaney clause of the FD&C Act prohibits the approval of regulated food additives "found to induce cancer when ingested by man or animals." It must be

Table 30-3
Tests for Each Concern Level

CONCERN LEVEL	TESTS REQUIRED
I	Short-term feeding study (at least 28 days in duration) Short-term tests for carcinogenic potential that can be used to determine priority for conduction of lifetime carcinogenicity bioassays and may assist in the evaluation of results from such bioassays, if conducted
II	Subchronic feeding study (at least 90 days in duration) in a rodent species Subchronic feeding study (at least 90 days in duration) in a nonrodent species Multigeneration reproduction study (minimum of two generations with a teratology phase) in a rodent species Short-term tests for carcinogenic potential
III	Carcinogenicity studies in two rodent species A chronic feeding study at least 1 year in duration in a rodent species (may be combined with a carcinogenicity study) Long-term (at least 1 year in duration) feeding study in a nonrodent species Multigenerational reproduction study (minimum of two generations) with a teratology phase in a rodent species Short-term tests for carcinogenic potential

emphasized that the Delaney prohibition applies only to the approval of food additives, color additives, and animal drugs; it does not apply to unavoidable contaminants or GRAS substances. To be a carcinogen under the Delaney clause, a food or color additive must be demonstrated to induce cancer directly when ingested by humans or animals.

SAFETY OF FOOD

Adverse Reactions to Food or Food Ingredients

Food hypersensitivity (allergy) refers to a reaction involving an immune-mediated response. An allergic re-

Table 30-4
Examples of GRAS Substances and Their Functionality

CFR NUMBER	SUBSTANCE	FUNCTIONALITY
	Substances Generally Recognized as Safe 21 CFR 182	
182.2122	Aluminum calcium silicate	Anticaking agent
182.5065	Linoleic acid	Dietary supplement
	Direct Food Substances Affirmed as Generally Recognized as Safe 21 CFR 184	
184.1005	Acetic acid	Several
184.1355	Helium	Processing aid
	Indirect Food Substances Affirmed as Generally Recognized as Safe 21 CFR 186	
186.1025	Caprylic acid	Antimicrobial
186.1374	Iron oxides	Ingredient of paper and paperboard

Table 30-5
Symptoms of IgE-Mediated Food Allergies

Cutaneous	Urticaria (hives), eczema, dermatitis, pruritus, rash
Gastrointestinal	Nausea, vomiting, diarrhea, abdominal cramps
Respiratory	Asthma, wheezing, rhinitis, bronchospasm
Other	Anaphylactic shock, hypotension, palatal itching, swelling including tongue and larynx, methemoglobinemia*

*An unusual manifestation of allergy reported to occur in response to
  soy or cow milk protein intolerance in infants.

action may be manifest by one or more of the symptoms listed in Table 30-5. Cutaneous reactions and anaphylaxis are the most common symptoms associated with food allergy. Any protein in food may act as an allergen; some of the allergenic components of common food allergens are listed in Table 30-6. Food idiosyncrasies may resemble hypersensitivity but do not involve immune mechanisms. Examples of such reactions and the foods that probably are responsible for them are given in Table 30-7.

Anaphylactoid reactions historically are thought of as reactions mimicking anaphylaxis (and other "allergic-type" responses) through the direct application of histamine. Ingestion of some types of fish that have been acted on by certain microorganisms to produce histamine may result in an anaphylactoid reaction. Sulfite-induced bronchospasm (sometimes leading to asthma) first was noticed as an acute sensitivity to metabisulfites sprayed on restaurant salads and used in wine.

Also referred to as "false food allergies," pharmacologic food reactions are characterized by exaggerated responses to pharmacologic agents in food (Table 30-8).

Metabolic food reactions are distinct from other categories of adverse reactions in that the foods are more or less commonly eaten and demonstrate toxic effects only when eaten to excess or when improperly processed (Table 30-9).

TOLERANCE SETTING FOR SUBSTANCES IN FOODS

Pesticide Residues

Pesticides intended for use on food crops must be approved under the FD&C Act. An additional 10-fold safety

Table 30-6
Known Allergenic Food Proteins

FOOD	ALLERGIC PROTEINS
Cow's milk	Casein
	β-Lactoglobulin
	a-Lactalbumin
Egg whites	Ovomucoid
	Ovalbumin
Egg yolks	Livetin
Peanuts	Ara h II
	Peanut I
Soybeans	β-Conglycinin (7S fraction)
	Glycinin (11S fraction)
	Gly mIA
	Gly mIB
	Kunitz trypsin inhibitor
Codfish	Gad cl
Shrimp	Antigen II
Green peas	Albumin fraction
Rice	Glutelin fraction
	Globulin fraction
Cottonseed	Glycoprotein fraction
Peach, guava, banana, mandarin, strawberry	30-kDa protein
Tomato	Several glycoproteins
Wheat	Gluten
	Gliadin
	Globulin
	Albumin
Okra	Fraction I

factor must be applied for infants and children to take into account potential pre- and postnatal toxicity.

Drugs Used in Food-Producing Animals

The pharmacokinetic and biotransformation characteristics of both the animal and the human must be considered in an assessment of the potential human health hazard of an animal drug. Safety assessment is concerned primarily with residues that occur in animal food products (milk, cheese, etc.) and edible tissues (muscle, liver, etc.).

Unavoidable Contaminants

Certain substances are unavoidable in food because their widespread industrial applications or their presence

Table 30-7
Idiosyncratic Reactions to Foods

FOOD	REACTION	MECHANISM
Fava beans	Hemolysis, sometimes accompanied by jaundice and hemoglobinuria; also, pallor, fatigue, nausea, dyspnea, fever and chills, abdominal and dorsal pain	Pyramidene aglycones in fava bean cause irreversible oxidation of GSH in G-6-PD-deficient erythrocytes by blocking NADPH supply, resulting in oxidative stress of the erythrocyte and eventual hemolysis
Chocolate	Migraine headache	Phenylethylamine-related (?)
Beets	Beetanuria: passage of red urine (often mistaken for hematuria)	Excretion of beetanin in urine after consumption of beets
Asparagus	Odorous, sulfurous-smelling urine	Autosomal dominant inability to metabolize methanthiol of asparagus and consequent passage of methanthiol in urine
Red wine	Sneezing, flush, headache, diarrhea, skin itch, shortness of breath	Diminished histamine degradation: deficiency of diamine oxidase (?) Histamines present in wine
Choline- and carnitine-containing foods	Fish odor syndrome: foul odor of body secretions	Choline and carnitine metabolized to trimethylamine in gut by bacteria, followed by absorption but inability to metabolize to odorless trimethylamine N-oxide
Lactose intolerance	Abdominal pain, bloating, diarrhea	Lactase deficiency
Fructose-containing foods	Abdominal pain, vomiting, diarrhea, hypoglycemia	Reduced activity of hepatic aldolase B toward fructose-1-phosphate

in the earth's crust have resulted in their becoming a persistent and ubiquitous contaminant in the environment. Examples are heavy metals, which cause varied symptoms ranging from neurologic effects to cancer; the N-nitroso substances found in nitrate-cured meats and some beverages, which cause cancer; and food-borne mycotoxins (toxins elaborated by fungi), such as the carcinogenic and hepatotoxic aflatoxins and the hyperestrogenic mycotoxin zearalenone (Table 30-10).

Table 30-8
Pharmacologic Reactions to Food

FOOD	REACTION	MECHANISM
Cheese, red wine	Severe headache, hypertension	Tyramine from endogenous or ingested tyrosine
Nutmeg	Hallucinations	Myristicin
Coffee, tea	Headache, hypertension	Methylxanthine (caffeine) acting as a noradrenergic stimulant
Chocolate	Headache, hypertension	Methylxanthine (theophylline) acting as a noradrenergic stimulant

Table 30-9
Metabolic Food Reactions

FOOD	REACTION	MECHANISM
Lima beans, cassava roots, millet (sorghum) sprouts, bitter almonds, apricot and peach pits	Cyanosis	Cyanogenic glycosides releasing hydrogen cyanide on contact with stomach acid
Cabbage family, turnips, soybeans, radishes, rapeseed, and mustard	Goiter (enlarged thyroid)	Isothiocyanates, goitrin, or S-5-vinyl-thiooxazolidone interferes with utilization of iodine
Unripe fruit of the tropical tree *Blighia sapida*, common in Caribbean and Nigeria	Severe vomiting, coma, and acute hypoglycemia sometimes resulting in death, especially among the malnourished	Hypoglycin A, isolated from the fruit, may interfere with oxidation of fatty acids so that glycogen stores have to be metabolized for energy, with depletion of carbohydrates, resulting in hypoglycemia
Leguminosae, Cruciferae	Lathyritic symptoms: neurologic symptoms of weakness, leg paralysis, and sometimes death	L-2-4-Diaminobutyric acid inhibition of ornithine transcarbamylase of the urea cycle, inducing ammonia toxicity
Licorice (glycyrrhizic acid)	Hypertension, cardiac enlargement, sodium retention	Glycyrrhizic acid mimicking mineralocorticoids
Polar bear and chicken liver	Irritability, vomiting, increased intracranial pressure, death	Vitamin A toxicity
Cycads (cycad flour)	Amyotrophic lateral sclerosis (humans), hepatocarcinogenicity (rats and nonhuman primates)	Cycasin (methylazoxymethanol); primary action is methylation, resulting in a broad range of effects from membrane destruction to inactivation of enzyme systems

SUBSTANCES FOR WHICH TOLERANCES MAY NOT BE SET

The substances in this section are regarded as (1) *avoidable* or of such a level of hazard that a safe level cannot be set; therefore, the FDA has determined that food containing such substances is banned, or (2) beyond the control of the FDA and therefore not subject to regulation (for example, substances produced in the home).

Toxins in Fish, Shellfish, and Turtles

In general, seafood toxins under FDA policy have a zero tolerance, with any detectable level considered cause for regulatory action. Saxitoxin is found in shellfish; it blocks neural transmission at neuromuscular junctions by interfering with ion channels, leading to paresthesia and muscular weakness without hypotension. Domoic acid also is found in shellfish; it is an analog of glutamine, a neurotransmitter, and leads to damage to the hippocampus and other brain areas, causing various neurologic symptoms. Ciguatera originally is made by dinoflagellates, is passed down the food chain, and is biotransformed into the active form by fish; it then is consumed by humans and causes gastrointestinal disorders, neurologic symptoms, or death. Tetrodotoxin, another potent neurotoxin, is consumed by humans who eat improperly prepared pufferfish. It causes paralysis of the central nervous system and peripheral nerves by blocking the movement of all monovalent cations, leading to muscular

Table 30-10
Selected Mycotoxins Produced by Various Molds

MYCOTOXIN	SOURCE	EFFECT	COMMODITIES CONTAMINATED
Aflatoxins B$_1$, B$_2$, G$_1$, G$_2$	*Aspergillus flavus, parasiticus*	Acute aflatoxicosis, carcinogenesis	Corn, peanuts, and others
Aflatoxin M$_1$	Metabolite of AFB$_1$	Hepatotoxicity	Milk
Fumonisins B$_1$, B$_2$, B$_3$, B$_4$, A$_1$, A$_2$	*Fusarium moniliforme*	Carcinogenesis	Corn
Trichothecenes	*Fusarium, Myrothecium*	Hematopoietic toxicity, meningeal hemorrhage of brain, "nervous" disorder, necrosis of skin, hemorrhage in mucosal epithelia of stomach and intestine	Cereal grains, corn
T-2 toxin	*Trichoderma*		Corn, barley, sorghum
Trichodermin	*Cephalosporium*		
Zearalenones	*Fusarium*	Estrogenic effect	Corn, grain
Cyclopiazonic acid	*Aspergillus, Penicillium*	Muscle, liver, and splenic toxicity	Cheese, grains, peanuts
Kojic acid	*Aspergillus*	Hepatotoxic?	Grain, animal feed
3-Nitropropionic acid	*Arthrinium sacchari, saccharicola, phaeospermum*	Central nervous system impairment	Sugarcane
Citreoviridin	*Penicillium citreoviride, toxicarium*	Cardiac beriberi	Rice
Cytochalasins E, B, F, H	*Aspergillus and Penicillium*	Cytotoxicity	Corn, cereal grain
Sterigmatocystin	*Aspergillus versiolar*	Carcinogenesis	Corn
Penicillinic acid	*Penicillium cyclopium*	Nephrotoxicity, abortifacient	Corn, dried beans, grains
Rubratoxins A, B	*Penicillium rubrum*	Hepatotoxicity, teratogenic	Corn
Patulin	*Penicillium patulatum*	Carcinogenesis, liver damage	Apple and apple products
Ochratoxin	*A. ochraceus, P. viridicatum*	Balkan nephropathy, carcinogenesis	Grains, peanuts, green coffee
Ergot alkaloids	*Cladosporium purpurea*	Ergotism	Grains

paralysis, respiratory distress, and sometimes death. Chelonitoxin is found in sea turtles and causes necrosis of the myocardium and pulmonary edema.

Microbiological Agents

Although the United States probably has the safest and cleanest food supply in the world, most U.S. food-related illness results from microbial contamination.

Botulism is due to botulism toxin produced by *Clostridium botulinum* and *C. butyricum* in improperly canned foods. The toxin interferes with acetylcholine at peripheral nerve endings, leading to respiratory distress and respiratory paralysis. *C. perfringens* food poisoning occurs when meat has been contaminated with intestinal contents at slaughter and then roasted and stored inadequately, allowing *C. perfringens* to grow and elaborate its toxin. The toxin causes death of enterocytes and severe fluid loss from diarrhea. *Bacillus cereus* makes two toxins; one causes vomiting and is elaborated in improperly prepared rice, and the other causes vomiting and can be present in various foods. *Staphylococcus aureus* produces a wide variety of toxins and is part of the normal flora of human skin. Foods usually are contaminated after cooking by persons handling them and then keeping the foods at room temperature for several hours. Cattle are natural resevoirs of *Escherichia coli;* outbreaks of *E. coli* are associated with improperly prepared beef as well as unpasteurized juices and raw vegetables fertilized with manure. Bovine spongiform encephalopathy (BSE, or mad cow disease) is transmitted by an infectious protein called a prion; it is present in diseased cows and is transmitted to humans in meat that is handled improperly. BSE manifests clinically as neurologic deterioration that leads to death.

CONCLUSIONS

Food consists of hundreds of thousands of chemical substances in addition to the macro- and micronutrients that are essential to life. The federal law defining food safety in the United States, the FD&C Act, provides a workable scheme for establishing the safety of foods, food ingredients, and contaminants. It is important to emphasize that the vast majority of food-borne illnesses in developed countries are attributable to microbiological contamination of food. Thus, the overwhelming concern for food safety in the United States remains directed toward preserving the microbiological integrity of food.

BIBLIOGRAPHY

Belitz HD, Grosch W: *Food Chemistry.* Berlin: Springer-Verlag, 1999.

Eisenbrand G (ed): *Food Allergies and Intolerances.* New York: VCH Publishers, 1996.

Kotsonis F, Mackey M (eds): *Nutritional Toxicology.* New York: Taylor & Francis, 2001.

Lund BM, Baird-Parker TC, Gould GW (eds): *The Microbiological Safety and Quality of Food.* Gaithersburg, MD: Aspen Publishers, 2000.

Metcalf DD, Sampson HA, Simon RA: *Food Allergy: Adverse Reactions to Food and Food Additives.* Oxford: Blackwell Science, 2002.

Omaye ST: *Food and Nutritional Toxicology.* Boca Raton, FL: CRC Press, 2002.

Shils ME (ed): *Modern Nutrition in Health and Disease.* Baltimore: Williams & Wilkins, 1999.

ANALYTIC/FORENSIC TOXICOLOGY

Alphonse Poklis

KEY POINTS

- Analytic toxicology involves the application of the tools of analytic chemistry to the qualitative and/or quantitative estimation of chemicals that may exert adverse effects on living organisms.

- Forensic toxicology involves the use of toxicology for the purposes of the law; by far the most common application is to identify any chemical that may serve as a causative agent in inflicting death or injury on humans or in causing damage to property.

- A toxicologic investigation of a poison death involves (1) obtaining the case history in as much detail as possible and gathering suitable specimens, (2) conducting suitable toxicologic analyses that are based on the available specimens, and (3) interpreting the analytic findings.

- A toxicologist as an expert witness may provide objective testimony and opinion. Objective testimony usually involves a description of analytic methods and findings. When a toxicologist testifies about the interpretation of analytic results, that toxicologist is offering an "opinion."

ANALYTIC TOXICOLOGY

Analytic toxicology applies the tools of analytic chemistry to the qualitative and/or quantitative estimation of chemicals in living organisms. Forensic toxicology uses toxicology for the purposes of the law; the most common application is to identify any chemical that may serve as a causative agent in inflicting death or injury on humans or in causing damage to property.

A systematic approach and reliance on the practical experience of generations of forensic toxicologists can be used in conjunction with the sophisticated tools of analytic chemistry to provide the data needed to understand the hazards of toxic substances more completely.

In 1873, in his *Elements de Toxicologie,* Chapuis described a system for classifying toxic agents into several categories: gases, volatile substances, corrosive agents, metals, anions and nonmetals, nonvolatile organic substances, and miscellaneous. Closely related to that descriptive classification is the method for separating a toxic agent from the matrix in which it is embedded. The agent of interest may exist in the matrix in a simple solution or may be bound to protein and other cellular constituents; before analysis can be done, the agent must be isolated. Each type of material has a different analytic method by which it can be isolated.

ANALYTIC ROLE IN FORENSIC TOXICOLOGY

The duties of a forensic toxicologist in postmortem investigations include the qualitative and quantitative analysis of drugs or poisons in biological specimens collected at autopsy and the interpretation of the analytic findings in regard to the physiologic and behavioral effects of the detected chemicals on the deceased at the time of death.

Establishing the cause of death rests with the medical examiner, coroner, or pathologist, but success in arriving at the correct conclusion often depends on the combined efforts of the pathologist and the toxicologist. The cause of death in cases of poisoning cannot be proved beyond contention without a toxicologic analysis that establishes the presence of the toxicant in the tissues and body fluids of the deceased person. Additionally, a toxicologist can furnish valuable evidence about the circumstances surrounding a death. Such cases commonly involve demonstrating the presence of intoxicating concentrations of ethanol in victims of automotive or industrial accidents or intoxicating concentrations of carbon monoxide in fire victims to determine whether the deceased person died as a result of a fire or was dead before the fire started.

TOXICOLOGIC INVESTIGATION OF A POISON DEATH

The toxicologic investigation of a poison death can be divided into three steps: (1) obtaining the case history in as much detail as possible and gathering suitable specimens, (2) conducting suitable toxicologic analyses on the basis of the available specimens, and (3) interpreting the analytic findings. Specific questions may be answered, such as the route of administration, the dose administered, and whether the concentration of the toxicant present was sufficient to cause death or alter the decedent's actions enough to cause his or her death.

CRIMINAL POISONING OF THE LIVING

Over the last few decades, forensic toxicologists have become more involved in the analysis of specimens obtained from living victims of criminal poisonings. Generally, this increase in testing has resulted from two types of cases: (1) administration of drugs to incapacitate victims of kidnapping, robbery, or sexual assault and (2) poisoning as a form of child abuse.

Although alcohol often is still a primary factor in cases of alleged sexual assault, common drugs of abuse and other psychoactive drugs often are involved (Table 31-1). Of particular concern are the many potent inductive agents that are administered medically before general anesthesia. Many of these drugs, such as benzodiazepines and phenothiazines, are available through illicit sources or can be purchased legally in foreign countries. When administered surreptitiously, they cause sedation and incapacitate the victim while also producing amnesia about the events that occurred while the victim was drugged without causing severe central nervous system depression. These cases often present a difficult analytic challenge to toxicologists because the drug usually has been eliminated from the body by the time the victim can bring forth an allegation.

Poisoning as a form of child abuse involves the deliberate administration of toxic or injurious substances to a child. Common agents used to poison children intentionally have included syrup of ipecac, table salt, laxatives, diuretics, antidepressants, sedative-hypnotics, and narcotics. The poison may be given to an infant to stop its crying or may be force-fed to older children as a form of punishment. Sophisticated gas chromatography/mass spectroscopy testing methods may be required to detect these agents.

FORENSIC URINE DRUG TESTING

Concern about the potentially adverse consequences of substance abuse both for the individual and for society has led to the widespread use of urine analysis for the

Table 31-1
Distribution of Drugs of Abuse Encountered in Urine Specimens in 578 Cases of Alleged Sexual Assault

RANK	DRUG/DRUG GROUP	INCIDENCE	PERCENT OF CASES*
1.	No drugs found	167	29
2.	Ethanol	148	26
3.	Benzodiazepines	70	12
4.	Marijuana	67	12
5.	Amphetamines	41	7
6.	Gamma-hydroxybutyrate	24	4
7.	Opiate (morphine/codeine)	20	4
8.	Other drugs	13	3

*Percentages do not add to 100 percent because of rounding.
SOURCE: Data from ElSohly MA et al: Analysis of flunitrazepam metabolites and other substances in alleged cases of sexual assault. Presentation at the 50th Anniversary Meeting of the American Academy of Forensic Sciences; San Francisco, CA, February 13, 1997.

detection of controlled or illicit drugs. Forensic urine drug testing (FUDT) differs from other areas of forensic toxicology in that urine is the only specimen analyzed and testing is performed for a limited number of drugs. Initial testing is performed with immunoassays on high-speed, large-throughput analyzers. A confirmation analysis in FUDT-certified laboratories then is performed.

Many individuals who are subject to regulated urine testing have devised techniques to mask their drug use either by physiologic means such as the ingestion of diuretics or by attempting to adulterate a specimen directly with bleach, vinegar, or other products that interfere with the initial immunoassay tests. Thus, specimens are tested routinely for adulteration by checking urinary pH, creatinine, and specific gravity and noting any unusual color or smell. Recently, a mini-industry has developed to sell various products that are alleged to "fool drug testers" by interfering with the initial or confirmatory drug test. Thus, FUDT laboratories now routinely test not only for drugs of abuse but also for a wide variety of chemical adulterants. In most instances, a positive test result for adulteration has as serious a consequence as does a positive drug test.

HUMAN PERFORMANCE TESTING

Forensic toxicology activities also include the determination of the presence of ethanol and other drugs and chemicals in blood, breath, or other specimens and the evaluation of their role in modifying human performance and behavior. The most common application of human performance testing is to determine driving under the influence of ethanol (DUI) or drugs (DUID). The threshold blood alcohol concentration (BAC) for diminished driving performance in many individuals is as low as 0.04 g/dL, the equivalent of the ingestion of two beers within an hour's time. The statutory definition of DUI in the United States is a BAC of either 0.08 or 0.10 g/dL, depending on the particular state law. These concentrations are consistent with diminished performance of complex driving skills in the vast majority of individuals.

During the last decade, there has been growing concern about the deleterious effects of drugs other than ethanol on driving performance. The highest drug-use accident rates are associated with the use of illicit or controlled drugs such as cocaine, benzodiazepines, marijuana, and phencyclidine. Proving that drug use was important in a driving accident is difficult, and both legal and scientific problems concerning drug concentrations and driving impairment have to be resolved. No protocols for determining DUID have been generally defined in legal terms.

COURTROOM TESTIMONY

A forensic toxicologist often is called on to testify in legal proceedings. The toxicologist is referred to as an "expert witness." An expert witness may provide two types of testimony: objective testimony and "opinion." Objec-

Table 31-2

Most Commonly Encountered Drugs and Methods for Analysis in Emergency Toxicology

RANK	DRUG/DRUG GROUP	SPECIMEN	ANALYTIC METHOD
1.	Drugs of abuse (amphetamines, cocaine, opiates, phencyclidine)	Urine	Immunoassays
2.	Ethanol	Serum	GC
3.	Benzodiazepines	Urine/serum	Immunoassay/GC/MS
4.	Acetaminophen, salicylates	Serum	Immunoassay or HPLC
5.	Tricyclic antidepressants	Serum	Immunoassay or HPLC
6.	Ibuprofen	Urine/serum	TLC/HPLC
7.	Dextropropoxyphene	Urine	Immunoassay
8.	Fluoxetine	Urine/serum	TLC/HPLC
9.	Barbiturates (50% phenobarbital)	Urine/serum	Immunoassay/GC
10.	Diphenhydramine	Urine	TLC

KEY: GC, gas chromatography; GC/MS, gas chromatography/mass spectrometry; HPLC, high-pressure liquid chromatography; TLC, thin-layer chromatography.

tive testimony by a toxicologist usually involves a description of his or her analytic methods and findings. When a toxicologist testifies about the interpretation of his or her analytic results or those of others, that toxicologist is offering an opinion. An expert witness is called to provide informed assistance to the jury. The jury, not the expert witness, determines the guilt or innocence of the defendant.

ANALYTIC ROLE IN CLINICAL TOXICOLOGY

Analytic toxicology in a clinical setting plays a role very similar to its role in forensic toxicology. As an aid in the diagnosis and treatment of toxic incidents as well as in monitoring the effectiveness of treatment regimens, it is useful to identify the nature of the toxic exposure clearly and measure the amount of the toxic substance that has been absorbed. Frequently, this information, together with the clinical state of the patient, permits a clinician to relate the signs and symptoms observed to the anticipated effects of the toxic agent. A cardinal rule in the treatment of poisoning cases is to remove any unabsorbed material, limit the absorption of additional poison, and hasten the elimination of the poison. The clinical toxicology laboratory serves an additional purpose in this phase of the treatment by monitoring the amount of the toxic agent remaining in circulation or measuring what is excreted. The most commonly encountered intoxicants in emer-

gency toxicology testing and the rapid methodologies to detect their presence in serum and/or urine specimens are described in Table 31-2.

Primary examples of the usefulness of emergency toxicology testing are the rapid quantitative determination of acetaminophen, salicylate, alcohols, and glycol serum concentrations in instances of suspected overdose. Ethanol is the agent most commonly encountered in emergency toxicology. Although few fatal intoxications occur with ethanol, serum values are important in the assessment of behavioral and neurologic function. Intoxications from accidental or deliberate ingestion of other alcohols or glycols—such as methanol from windshield deicer or paint thinner, isopropanol from rubbing alcohol, and ethylene glycol from antifreeze—often are encountered in emergency departments.

The utilization of the analytic capabilities of a clinical toxicology laboratory has increased enormously in recent years. Typically, the laboratory performs testing not only for the emergency department but also for a wide variety of other medical departments, as drugs and toxic agents may be a consideration in diagnosis.

ANALYTIC ROLE IN THERAPEUTIC MONITORING

Historically, the administration of drugs for long-term therapy was based largely on experience. If a drug seemed ineffective, the dose was increased; if toxicity developed, the dose was decreased or the frequency of dosing was altered. The factors responsible for individual variability in responses to drug therapy include the rate and extent of drug absorption, distribution and binding in body tissues and fluids, the rate of metabolism and excretion, pathologic conditions, and interaction with other drugs. Monitoring of the plasma or serum concentration at regular intervals will detect deviations from the average serum concentration, which in turn may suggest that one or more of these variables have to be identified and corrected.

In a given patient, when the various factors are assumed to be constant, the administration of the same dose of a drug at regular intervals eventually produces a steady-state condition (Fig. 31-1). Monitoring of steady-state drug concentrations assures that an effective concentration is present. Appropriate situations for therapeutic drug monitoring are listed in Table 31-3.

Because the nature of drugs is varied, many different analytic techniques may be applied. Virtually all the tools of the analyst may be used for specific applications of analytic toxicology. Drugs that are monitored commonly during therapy, their usual effective therapeutic serum concentrations, "panic values" (serum concentrations associated with potentially serious toxicity), and typical analytic methodologies applied to serum measurements are described in Table 31-4.

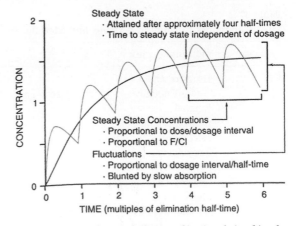

Figure 31-1. Fundamental pharmacokinetic relationships for the repeated administration of drugs. The blue line is the pattern of drug accumulation during the repeated administration of a drug at intervals equal to its elimination half-time, when drug absorption is 10 times as rapid as elimination. As the relative rate of absorption increases, the concentration maxima approach 2 and the minima approach 1 during steady state. The black line depicts the pattern during the administration of an equivalent dosage by continuous intravenous infusion. Curves are based on the one-compartment model. Average concentration (Css) when steady state is attained during intermittent drug administration is $Css = F \times dose/Cl \times T$, where F = fractional bioavailability of the dose and T = dosage interval (time). By substitution of the infusion rate for $F \times dose/T$, the formula provides the concentration maintained at steady state during continuous intravenous infusion.

Table 31-3
Appropriate Use of Therapeutic Drug Monitoring

USE	EXAMPLES
Optimize efficacy while minimizing toxicity	
Optimal SDC* for clinical effect	
Routine, prophylactic peak serum	Aminoglycosides
Poor patient response	Antiarrhythmics, antidepressants
Suspected toxicity	
Resolve complicating factors	
Patient characteristics	Age, smoking, noncompliance
Disease	Renal failure, hepatic disorders
Drug interactions	Induction or inhibition of drug metabolism
Sudden change in physiologic state	Improved cardiac function on lidocaine therapy increases clearance
Dosage regimen design	
Individualize future dosing (single SDC)	
Pharmacokinetic profiling (multiple SDC)	Ideal dosage for aminoglycosides
Follow-up SDC	Single steady-state lidocaine
Verify therapy	Medicolegal lithium

*SDC, serum drug concentration.

Table 31-4
Drugs Commonly Indicated for Therapeutic Monitoring

THERAPEUTIC USE DRUG	EFFECTIVE SERUM RANGE mg/L	PANIC VALUE = OR > mg/L	ANALYTIC METHODOLOGY
Antiarrhythmic			
Digoxin	0.0005–0.002	0.0024	Immunoassay
Procainamide	4–10	12	Immunoassay
NAPA	5–30	40	Immunoassay
Anticonvulsant			
Carbamazepine	4–12	15	Immunoassay
Gabapentin	2–15	20	GC
Lamotrigine	0.5–8	10	HPLC
Phenobarbital	15–30	50	Immunoassay
Phenytoin	10–20	40	Immunoassay
Tropiramate	2–10	Undetermined	GC
Valproic acid	50–100	200	GC
Antidepressants			
Amitriptyline	0.08–0.250	0.5	HPLC
Desipramine	0.125–0.30	0.4	HPLC
Nortriptyline	0.08–0.250	0.5	HPLC
Antimicrobials			
Tobramycin	0.5–1.5 (trough)	2	Immunoassay
	5–10 (peak)	12	
Vancomycin	5–10 (trough)		Immunoassay
	30–40 (peak)	90	
Immunosuppressant			
Cyclosporine	0.1 (trough, whole blood)		HPLC
Neonatal apnea			
Caffeine	8–20	50	HPLC

KEY: GC, gas chromatography; HPLC, high-pressure liquid chromatography.

ANALYTIC ROLE IN BIOLOGICAL MONITORING

It has become apparent that monitoring a worker directly can be a better indicator of exposure than is simply monitoring the environment, because it can show what actually has been absorbed. This is biological monitoring. Often environmental exposures are to a mixture of compounds and/or to compounds that are converted into physiologically important metabolites. Thus, analytic methods must be capable of separating a family of chemical agents and their major metabolites (Fig. 31-2). Additionally, methods must be sufficiently specific and

sensitive to measure minute concentrations of the compounds in complex biological matrices.

In addition to the measurement of the chemical or its metabolites in the body fluids, hair, or breath of a worker, other, more indirect methods may be employed. Substances that interact with macromolecules may form adducts that persist for long periods. Those adducts can be sampled periodically and potentially can serve as a means of integrating exposure to certain substances over long periods. For example, adducts of ethylene oxide with DNA or hemoglobin have been studied in workers. Another approach that is useful in biological monitoring is to measure changes in normal metabolites that are

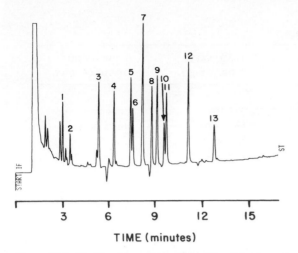

Figure 31-2. Capillary gas chromatographic separation of chlorinated hydrocarbon pesticides added to human serum at concentrations ranging from 1 to 4 ng/mL. Peak number 1, a-lindane; 2, c-lindane; 3, heptachlor; 4, internal standard; 5, heptachlor epoxide; 6, oxychlordane; 7, c-chlordane; 8, a-chlordane; 9, *trans*-nonachlor; 10, dieldrin; 11, *p,p*9-DDE; 12, *p,p*-DDD; 13, *p,p*9-DDT. (Separation based on the method of Saady JJ, Poklis A: Determination of chlorinated hydrocarbon pesticides by solid phase extraction and capillary GC with electron capture detection. *J Anal Toxicol* 14:301–304, 1990.)

induced by xenobiotics. Although monitoring the alteration of the urinary excretion of these metabolites may not indicate exposure to specific substances, this technique can be used in a generic fashion to flag a potentially harmful exposure. The early recognition of a toxicologic problem may permit the protection of a worker before irreversible effects occur.

SUMMARY

The analytic techniques initiated by forensic toxicologists have continued to expand in complexity and improve in reliability. Forensic toxicologists continue to be concerned about conducting unequivocal identification of toxic substances in a manner that allows the results to withstand a legal challenge. The problems of substance abuse, designer drugs, the increased potency of therapeutic agents, and widespread concern about pollution and the safety and health of workers present challenges to analysts' skills. As these challenges are met, analytic toxicologists continue to play a significant role in the expansion of the discipline of toxicology.

BIBLIOGRAPHY

Brandenberger H, Maes RAA: *Analytical Toxicology for Clinical, Forensic, and Pharmaceutical Chemists.* New York: De Gruyter, 1997.

Flanagan RJ: *Basic Analytical Toxicology.* Geneva: World Health Organization, 1995.

LeBeau M, Andollo W, Hearn WL, et al: Recommendations for toxicological investigation of drug-facilitated sexual assaults. *J Forensic Sci* 44:227–230, 1999.

Shaw LM: *The Clinical Toxicology Laboratory: Contemporary Practice of Poisoning Evaluation.* Washington, DC: AACC Press, 2001.

CLINICAL TOXICOLOGY

Louis R. Cantilena, Jr.

CLINICAL STRATEGY FOR TREATMENT OF THE POISONED PATIENT
   Clinical Stabilization
   Clinical History in the Poisoned Patient
      Physical Examination
      Laboratory Evaluation

Radiographic Examination
Prevention of Further Poison Absorption
Enhancement of Poison Elimination

SUMMARY

KEY POINTS

- Clinical toxicology encompasses expertise in the specialties of medical toxicology, applied toxicology, and clinical poison information.
- Important components of the initial clinical encounter with a poisoned patient include stabilization of the patient, clinical evaluation (history, physical, laboratory, radiology), prevention of further toxin absorption, enhancement of toxin elimination, administration of an antidote, and supportive care with clinical follow-up.

CLINICAL STRATEGY FOR TREATMENT OF THE POISONED PATIENT

The following general steps are important components of the initial clinical encounter with a poisoned patient:

1. Stabilization of the patient
2. Clinical evaluation (history, physical, laboratory, radiology)
3. Prevention of further toxin absorption
4. Enhancement of toxin elimination
5. Administration of an antidote
6. Supportive care and clinical follow-up

Clinical Stabilization

The first priority in the treatment of a poisoned patient is stabilization. Assessment of the vital signs and the effectiveness of respiration and circulation are the initial concerns. Some toxins and drugs can cause seizures early in the course of presentation. The steps and clinical procedures incorporated in the stabilization of a critically ill poisoned patient are numerous and include assessment and, if appropriate, support of ventilation, circulation, and oxygenation.

Clinical History in the Poisoned Patient

The primary goal of taking a medical history in poisoned patients is to determine, if possible, the substance ingested or the substance to which the patient has been exposed as well as the extent and time of exposure. In the case of intentional self-poisoning, patients may not provide any history or may give incorrect information to increase the chance that they will bring harm to themselves. Information sources commonly employed in this setting include family members, emergency medical technicians who were at the scene, a pharmacist who sometimes can provide a list of prescriptions recently filled, and an employer who can disclose what chemicals are available in the work environment.

Table 32-1
Clinical Features of Toxic Syndromes

	BLOOD PRESSURE	PULSE	TEMPERATURE	PUPILS	LUNGS	ABDOMEN	NEUROLOGIC
Sympatho-mimetic	Increased	Increased	Slightly increased	Mydriasis	NC	NC	Hyperalert, increased reflexes
Anticho-linergic	Slightly increased or NC	Increased	Increased	Mydriasis	NC	Decreased bowel sounds	Altered mental status
Cholinergic	Slightly decreased or NC	Decreased	NC	Miosis	Increased bronchial sounds	Increased bowel sounds	Altered mental status
Opioid	Decreased	Decreased	Decreased	Miosis	NC or rales (late)	Decreased bowel sounds	Decreased level of consciousness

NC, no change.

In estimating the level of exposure to a poison, one generally should maximize one's estimate of the possible dose received. That is, one should assume that the entire contents of the prescription bottle were ingested, that the entire bottle of liquid was consumed, or that the highest possible concentration of an airborne contaminant was present in the case of a patient poisoned by inhalation.

With an estimate of dose, a toxicologist can refer to various information sources to determine what the range of expected clinical effects from the exposure may be. The estimation of expected toxicity greatly assists in the triage of poisoned patients. Estimating the timing of the exposure to the poison is frequently the most difficult aspect of the clinical history in the setting of the treatment of a poisoned patient.

Taking an accurate history in a poisoned patient can be very difficult. Despite diligent efforts, using both direct and external sources for the medical history information, a clinical toxicologist sometimes is left without a clear indication of the exposure history. In this setting, the treatment proceeds empirically for an "unknown ingestion" poisoning. This type of treatment is discussed later in this chapter.

Physical Examination A thorough physical examination is required to assess the patient's condition and to categorize the patient's mental status and, if it is altered, determine possible additional causes, such as trauma and central nervous system infection. Whenever possible, a clinical toxicologist categorizes the patient's physical examination parameters into broad classes referred to as *toxic syndromes*: collections of clinical signs that, taken together, probably are associated with exposure to certain classes of toxicologic agents. Categorization of the patient's presentation into toxic syndromes allows the initiation of rational treatment based on the most likely category of toxin responsible even if the exact nature of the toxin is unknown. Table 32-1 lists the clinical features of the major toxic syndromes.

Laboratory Evaluation Table 32-2 lists drugs, special laboratory tests, and other chemical substances that typ-

Table 32-2
Toxins and Special Laboratory Tests Commonly Measured in a Hospital Setting on a Stat Basis

Acetaminophen	Methemoglobin
Acetone	Osmolality
Carbamazepine	Phenobarbital
Carboxyhemoglobin	Phenytoin
Digoxin	Procainamide
Ethanol	Quinidine
Ethyl alcohol	Salicylates
Gentamicin	Theophylline
Iron	Tobramycin
Lithium	Valproic acid

ically are available for immediate measurement in a hospital facility. As one can see, the number of agents for which detection is possible in the rapid-turnaround clinical setting is extremely limited compared with the number of agents that can poison patients. This emphasizes the importance of recognizing clinical syndromes for poisoning and of the clinical toxicologist being able to initiate general treatment and supportive care for a patient with poisoning from an unknown substance.

For substances that can be measured on a rapid-turnaround basis in an emergency department setting, the quantitative measurement often can provide both prognostic and therapeutic guidance.

Predictive relationships of drug plasma concentration and clinical outcome and/or suggested concentrations that require therapeutic interventions are available for several agents, including salicylates, acetaminophen, lithium, digoxin, iron, phenobarbital, and theophylline. Some authors have identified "action levels," or toxic threshold values, for the measured plasma concentrations of various drugs or chemicals. Generally, these values represent mean concentrations of the respective substances that have been shown retrospectively to produce a significant harmful effect.

Because of the limited clinical availability of "diagnostic" laboratory tests for poisons, toxicologists utilize specific, routinely obtained clinical laboratory data, especially the anion gap and the osmol gap, to determine which poisons may have been ingested. An abnormal anion or osmol gap suggests a differential diagnosis for significant exposure. Both calculations are used as diagnostic tools when the clinical history suggests poisoning and the patient's condition is consistent with exposure to agents known to cause elevations of these parameters (metabolic acidosis, altered mental status, etc.).

The anion gap is calculated as the difference between the serum Na ion concentration and the sum of the serum Cl and HCO_3 ion concentrations. A normal anion gap is <12. When there is laboratory evidence of metabolic acidosis, the finding of an elevated anion gap suggests systemic toxicity from a relatively limited number of agents, which are listed in Table 32-3.

The second calculated parameter from clinical chemistry values is the osmol gap. The osmol gap is calculated as the numeric difference between the measured serum osmolarity and the serum osmolarity calculated from the clinical chemistry measurements of the serum sodium ion, glucose, and blood urea nitrogen (BUN) concentrations. The normal osmol gap is <10 mOsm. An elevated osmol gap in the setting of a poisoned patient suggests the presence of an osmotically active substance in

Table 32-3
Differential Diagnosis of Metabolic Acidosis with Elevated Anion Gap: "AT MUD PILES"

A	Alcohol (ethanol ketoacidosis)
T	Toluene
M	Methanol
U	Uremia
D	Diabetic ketoacidosis
P	Paraldehyde
I	Iron, isoniazid
L	Lactic acid
E	Ethylene glycol
S	Salicylate

the plasma that is not accounted for by the Na, glucose, or BUN concentration. Table 32-4 lists several substances that, when ingested, can be associated with an elevated osmol gap in humans.

Radiographic Examination The use of clinical radiographs to visualize drug overdose or poison ingestions is relatively limited. Generally, plain radiographs can detect a significant amount of ingested oral medication that contains ferrous or potassium salts. In addition, certain formulations that have an enteric coating and certain types of sustained-release products are radiopaque as well.

The most useful radiographs ordered in a case of overdose or poisoning include the chest and abdominal radiographs and the computed tomography (CT) study of the head. The abdominal radiograph has been used to detect recent lead paint ingestion in children and ingestion of halogenated hydrocarbons, such as carbon tetrachloride or chloroform, that may be visualized as a radiopaque liquid in the gut lumen. Finally, abdominal plain radiographs have been helpful in settings where foreign bodies are detected in the gastrointestinal tract, such as would be seen in a "body packer," or one who smuggles illegal substances by swallowing latex or plastic storage vesicles filled with cocaine or another substance. Occasionally,

Table 32-4
Differential Diagnosis of Elevated Osmol Gap

Ethanol
Ethylene glycol
Isopropanol
Methanol

these storage devices rupture and the drug is released into the gastrointestinal tract, with serious and sometimes fatal results.

Plain radiography and other types of diagnostic imaging in clinical toxicology also can be extremely valuable in the diagnosis of toxin-induced pathology. An example is the detection of the drug-induced noncardiac pulmonary edema associated with serious intoxication with salicylates and opioid agonists. Another example of the use of radiologic imaging in clinical toxicology is CT of the brain. Significant exposure to carbon monoxide (CO) has been associated with CT lesions of the brain consisting of low-density areas in the cerebral white matter and the basal ganglia.

Prevention of Further Poison Absorption   During the early phases of poison treatment or intervention for a toxic exposure by the oral or the topical route, a significant opportunity exists to prevent further absorption of the poison by minimizing the total amount that reaches the systemic circulation. For toxins presented by the inhalation route, the main intervention to prevent further absorption consists of removing the patient from the environment where the toxin is found and providing adequate ventilation and oxygenation for the patient. For topical exposures, clothing containing the toxin must be removed and the skin must be washed with water and mild soap. The three primary methods for preventing continued absorption of an oral poison are induction of emesis with syrup of ipecac, gastric lavage, and oral administration of activated charcoal.

Currently, syrup of ipecac is the only agent used for the induction of emesis in the treatment of a potentially toxic ingestion. Home use of syrup of ipecac upon the advice of a poison information center remains the most widely used poison treatment intervention. A shorter time interval between ingestion and the administration of syrup of ipecac is more efficacious for gastric emptying.

Gastric lavage involves placing an orogastric tube into the stomach and aspirating fluid and then cyclically instilling fluid and aspirating until the effluent is clear. Unfortunately, gastric lavage is limited by the risk of aspiration during the lavage procedure and growing evidence that its effectiveness may be more limited than originally was thought.

For many years, orally administered activated charcoal has been incorporated routinely into the initial treatment of a patient poisoned by the oral route. The term *activated* means that the charcoal has been specially processed to be more efficient at adsorbing toxins.

Enhancement of Poison Elimination   Several methods are available to enhance the elimination of specific poisons or drugs once they have been absorbed into the systemic circulation. The primary methods employed today include alkalinization of the urine, hemodialysis, hemoperfusion, hemofiltration, plasma exchange or exchange transfusion, and serial oral activated charcoal.

The use of urinary alkalinization results in enhancement of the renal clearance of weak acids. The basic principle is to increase the pH of urinary filtrate to a level sufficient to ionize the weak acid and prevent reabsorption of the molecule by the renal tubules by infusing a basic solution into the blood. Although potentially there are similar advantages to be gained from acidification of the urine to enhance the clearance of weak bases, this method is not used because acute renal failure and acid-base and electrolyte disturbances are associated with acidification.

The dialysis technique, either peritoneal dialysis or hemodialysis, relies on passage of the toxic agent through a semipermeable dialysis membrane so that it can be removed subsequently. Hemodialysis incorporates a blood pump to pass blood next to a dialysis membrane; this allows agents that are permeable to the membrane to pass through and reach equilibrium. Some drugs are bound to plasma proteins and therefore cannot pass through the dialysis membrane; others are distributed mainly to the tissues and therefore are not concentrated in the blood, making dialysis impractical. Drugs and toxins for which hemodialysis has been shown to be clinically effective in the treatment of poisoning by these agents is shown in Table 32-5.

The technique of hemoperfusion is similar to hemodialysis except that no dialysis membrane or dialysate is involved in the procedure. The patient's blood is pumped through a perfusion cartridge, where it is in direct contact with adsorptive material (usually activated

Table 32-5
Agents for Which Hemodialysis Has Been Shown to Be Effective as a Treatment Modality for Poisoning

Amphetamines	Isoniazid
Antibiotics	Meprobamate
Boric acid	Paraldehyde
Bromide	Phenobarbital
Calcium	Potassium
Chloral hydrate	Salicylates
Fluorides	Strychnine
Iodides	Thiocyanates

charcoal or Amberlite resin). Protein binding does not interfere significantly with removal by hemoperfusion.

The technique of hemofiltration is relatively new in clinical toxicology applications. As in the case of hemodialysis, the patient's blood is delivered through hollow fiber tubes and an ultrafiltrate of plasma is removed by hydrostatic pressure from the blood side of the membrane. The perfusion pressure for the technique is generated either by the patient's blood pressure (for arteriovenous hemofiltration) or by a blood pump (for venovenous hemofiltration). Needed fluid and electrolytes removed in the ultrafiltrate are replaced intravenously with sterile solutions.

The use of either plasma exchange or exchange transfusions has been relatively limited in the field of clinical toxicology. Although these techniques afford the potential advantage of the ability to remove high-molecular-weight and/or plasma protein–bound toxins, their clinical utility in poison treatment has been limited. Plasma exchange, or pheresis, involves removal of plasma and replacement with frozen donor plasma, albumin, or both with intravenous fluid. Exchange transfusion involves replacement of a patient's blood volume with donor blood. The use of this technique in poison treatment is relatively uncommon and is confined mostly to an inadvertent drug overdose in a neonate or premature infant.

Serial oral administration of activated charcoal, also referred to as multiple-dose activated charcoal (MDAC), has been shown to increase the systemic clearance of various drug substances. The mechanism for the observed augmentation of nonrenal clearance caused by repeated doses of oral charcoal is thought to be transluminal efflux of drug from blood to the charcoal passing through the gastrointestinal tract. The activated charcoal in the gut lumen serves as a "sink" for toxin. A concentration gradient is maintained, and the toxin passes continuously into the gut lumen, where it is adsorbed to charcoal. In addition, MDAC is thought to produce its beneficial effect by interrupting the enteroenteric-enterohepatic circulation of drugs. The technique involves continuing oral administration of activated charcoal beyond the initial dosage every 2 to 4 h. An alternative technique is to give a loading dose of activated charcoal through an orogastric tube or nasogastric tube, followed by a continuous infusion intragastrically. A list of agents for which MDAC has been shown to be an effective means of enhanced body clearance is given in Table 32-6.

Use of Antidotes in Poisoning   A relatively small number of specific antidotes are available for clinical use in

Table 32-6

Agents for Which Multiple-Dose Activated Charcoal Has Been Shown to Be Effective as a Treatment Modality for Poisoning

Carbamazepine
Dapsone
Phenobarbital
Quinine
Theophylline

the treatment of poisoning. The U.S. Food and Drug Administration (FDA) has created incentives for sponsors to develop drugs for rare diseases or conditions through the Orphan Drug Act.

The mechanism of action of various antidotes is quite different. For example, a chelating agent or Fab fragments specific to digoxin work by physically binding the toxin, preventing the toxin from exerting a deleterious effect in vivo, and, in some cases, facilitating body clearance of the toxin. Other antidotes pharmacologically antagonize the effects of the toxin. Atropine, an antimuscarinic, anticholinergic agent, is used to pharmacologically antagonize at the receptor level the effects of organophosphate insecticides that produce lethal cholinergic, muscarinic effects. Certain agents exert their antidote effects by reacting chemically with biological systems to increase a patient's detoxifying capacity for the toxin. For example, sodium nitrite is given to patients poisoned with cyanide to cause the formation of methemoglobin, which serves as an alternative binding site for the cyanide ion, thus making it less toxic to the body.

Supportive Care of a Poisoned Patient   The supportive care phase of poison treatment is very important. Not only are there certain poisonings that have delayed toxicity, there also are toxins that exhibit multiple phases of toxicity. Close clinical monitoring can detect these later-phase poisoning complications and allow prompt medical intervention.

Another important component of this phase of poison treatment is the psychiatric assessment. For intentional self-poisonings, a formal psychiatric evaluation of the patient should be performed before discharge. In many cases, it is not possible to perform a psychiatric interview during the early phases of treatment and evaluation. Once the patient has been stabilized and is able to communicate, a psychiatric evaluation should be obtained.

SUMMARY

Clinical toxicology encompasses expertise in the specialties of medical toxicology, applied toxicology, and clinical poison information. The clinical science has evolved significantly to the present state of the discipline over the last 50 years or more. The incorporation of evidence-based, outcome-driven practice recommendations has improved the critical evaluation of treatment modalities and methods for poison treatment significantly. A careful diagnostic approach to a poisoned patient is essential, as the important medical history often is absent or unreliable. Skillful use of antidotes is an important component of the practice of medical toxicology. Continued research will increase the repertoire of effective treatments for poisoning and ultimately improve clinical practice.

BIBLIOGRAPHY

Ellenhorn MJ (ed): *Ellenhorn's Medical Toxicology, Diagnosis and Treatment of Poisoning,* 2d ed. Philadelphia: Williams & Wilkins, 1997.

Goldfrank NR, Flomenbaum NE, Lewin NA, et al (eds): *Goldfrank's Toxicologic Emergencies,* 6th ed. Stamford, CT: Appleton & Lange, 1998.

Tintinalli JE, Kelen GD, Stapczynski JS (eds): *Emergency Medicine: A Comprehensive Study Guide,* 5th ed. New York: McGraw-Hill, 2000.

OCCUPATIONAL TOXICOLOGY

Peter S. Thorne

KEY POINTS

- Occupational toxicology is the application of the principles and methodology of toxicology to chemical and biological hazards encountered at work.
- In occupational environments, exposure often is used as a surrogate for dose.
- Occupational exposure limits correspond to the levels of exposure below which the probability of impairing the health of exposed workers is acceptable.
- Diseases that arise in occupational environments involve exposure primarily through inhalation, ingestion, or dermal absorption.

INTRODUCTION

Occupational toxicology applies the principles and methodology of toxicology to chemical and biological hazards encountered at work. The objective of an occupational toxicologist is to prevent adverse health effects in workers that arise from the work environment. Because that environment often presents exposures to complex mixtures, an occupational toxicologist also must recognize exposure combinations that are particularly hazardous.

It often is difficult to establish a causal link between a worker's illness and that worker's job. First, the clinical expressions of occupationally induced diseases often are indistinguishable from those arising from nonoccupational causes. Second, there may be a long interval between exposure and the expression of disease. Third, diseases of occupational origin may be multifactorial, with personal or other environmental factors contributing to the disease process.

WORKPLACES, EXPOSURES, AND STANDARDS

Determinants of Dose

Dose is defined as the amount of a toxicant that reaches the target tissue over a defined time span. In occupational environments, exposure often is used as a surrogate for dose. The response to a toxic agent is dependent on both host factors and dose. Figure 33-1 illustrates the pathway from exposure to subclinical disease or to an adverse health effect and suggests that there are important modifying factors: contemporaneous exposures, genetic susceptibility, age, gender, nutritional status, and behavioral factors. These modifying factors can influence whether a worker remains healthy, develops subclinical disease that is repaired, or progresses to illness. As is illustrated in Fig. 33-1, the dose is a function of exposure concentration, duration, and frequency. Individual and environmental characteristics also can affect dose. Table

33-1 indicates determinants of dose for exposure through the inhalation and dermal routes.

Occupational Exposure Limits

Workplace exposure limits exist for chemical, biological, and physical agents to promote worker health and safety. For chemical and biological agents, exposure limits are expressed as acceptable ambient concentration levels (occupational exposure limits) or concentrations of a toxicant, its metabolites, or a specific marker of its effects (biological exposure indexes).

Occupational exposure limits are established as standards by regulatory agencies or as guidelines by research groups and trade organizations. In the United States, the Occupational Safety and Health Administration under the Department of Labor promulgates legally enforceable standards known as permissible exposure limits. The National Institute for Occupational Safety and Health, under the Centers for Disease Control and Prevention, publishes recommended exposure limits that frequently are updated and generally are more stringent than permissible exposure limits.

The American Conference of Governmental Industrial Hygienists is a trade organization that annually pub-

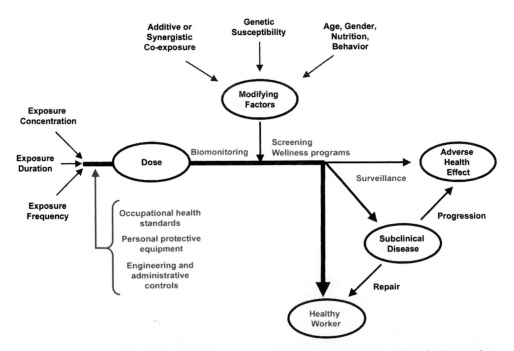

Figure 33-1. Pathway from exposure to disease, showing modifying factors and opportunities for intervention.

Table 33-1
Determinants of Toxicant Dose

Inhalation exposure
　Airborne concentration
　Particle size distribution
　Respiratory rate
　Tidal volume
　Other host factors
　Duration of exposure
　Chemical, physical, and biological properties of
　　the hazardous agent
　Effectiveness of personal protective devices

Dermal exposure
　Concentration in air, droplets, or solutions
　Degree and duration of wetness
　Integrity of skin
　Percutaneous absorption rate
　Region of skin exposed
　Surface area exposed
　Preexisting skin disease
　Temperature in the workplace
　Vehicle for the toxicant
　Presence of other chemicals on skin

lishes occupational exposure limits for chemicals and physical agents. These limits take the form of threshold limit values (TLVs) and biological exposure indexes (BEIs). They are developed as guidelines and are not enforceable standards.

Occupational exposure limits correspond not to exposure conditions devoid of health risk but to the level of exposure below which the probability of impairing the health of exposed workers is acceptable. To determine that the risks from an occupational hazard are acceptable, it is necessary to characterize the hazard, identify the potential diseases or adverse outcomes, and establish the relationship between exposure intensity or dose and the adverse health effects.

OCCUPATIONAL DISEASES

Routes of Exposure

Diseases arising in occupational environments involve exposure primarily through inhalation, ingestion, or dermal absorption. Exposures leading to occupational infections may arise through inhalation or ingestion of microorganisms or from needlesticks in health care workers

and insect bites among those who work outdoors. Additionally, poisonings from toxic plants or venomous animals can occur through skin inoculation (e.g., zookeepers, horticulturists, and commercial skin divers). Table 33-2 presents a list of the major occupational diseases and examples of the agents that cause them.

Occupational Respiratory Diseases

Occupational lung diseases (e.g., coal workers' pneumoconiosis, asbestosis, and occupational asthma) are largely responsible for the creation of the occupational regulatory framework. Table 33-3 lists the crude U.S. death rate and annual deaths and illustrates that although the death rates are fairly low, about 3600 deaths per year are attributable to asbestos, silica, coal dust, and other pneumoconiotic dusts and 343 result from hypersensitivity pneumonitis. However, fatalities are just the tip of the iceberg. Hypersensitivity pneumonitis rarely is fatal but often is debilitating. Moreover, there are 11,000 yearly hospital discharges related to cases of asbestosis and 13,500 resulting from coal workers' pneumoconiosis.

Toxic gas injuries often are characterized by leakage of both fluid and osmotically active proteins from the vascular tissue into the interstitium and airways. The vapors of anhydrous ammonia combine with water in the tissues of the eyes, sinuses, and upper airways and form ammonium hydroxide, quickly producing liquefaction necrosis. Chemicals with lower solubility, such as nitrogen dioxide, act more on the distal airways and alveoli and take longer to induce tissue damage.

Occupational asthma occurs when airways constrict in response to a stimulus present in the workplace. Stimuli include plastic and rubber polymers, reactive dyes, acid anhydrides, biocides and fungicides, metals, latex, and some enzymes. Exposure to plants, animals, and fungi also may induce asthma.

Other Occupational Diseases

Occupational toxicants may induce diseases in a variety of sites distant from the lung or skin. These diseases include tumors attributable to a variety of chemical classes. Nervous system damage can be central, peripheral, or both. It may be acute, as with some organophosphate exposures, or chronic, as with organomercury poisoning and acrylamide-induced neuropathy. Injury affecting the immune system may arise from the immunosuppressive effects of chemicals or from hypersensitivity leading to respiratory or dermal allergy or systemic hypersensitivity reactions. Autoimmune syndromes have been

Table 33-2
Examples of Occupational Diseases and the Toxicants That Cause Them

ORGAN SYSTEM OR DISEASE GROUP	DISEASE	CAUSATIVE AGENT
Lung and airways	Acute pulmonary edema, bronchiolitis obliterans	Nitrogen oxides, phosgene
	Allergic rhinitis	Pollens, fungal spores
	Asphyxiation	Carbon monoxide, hydrogen cyanide, inert gas dilution
	Asthma	Toluene diisocyanate, α-amylase, animal urine proteins
	Asthma-like syndrome	Swine barn environments, cotton dust, bioaerosols
	Bronchitis, pneumonitis	Arsenic, chlorine
	Chronic bronchitis	Cotton dust, grain dust, welding fumes
	Emphysema	Coal dust, cigarette smoke
	Fibrotic lung disease	Silica, asbestos
	Hypersensitivity pneumonitis	Thermophilic bacteria, avian proteins, pyrethrum, *Penicillium, Aspergillus*
	Metal fume fever	Zinc, copper, magnesium
	Mucous membrane irritation	Hydrogen chloride, swine barn environments
	Organic dust toxic syndrome	"Moldy" silage, endotoxin
	Upper respiratory tract inflammation	Endotoxin, peptidoglycan, glucans, viruses
Cancer	Acute myelogenous leukemia	Benzene, ethylene oxide
	Bladder cancer	Benzidine, 2-naphthylamine, 4-biphenylamine
	Gastrointestinal cancers	Asbestos
	Hepatic hemangiosarcoma	Vinyl chloride
	Hepatocellular carcinoma	Aflatoxin, hepatitis B virus
	Mesothelioma, lung carcinoma	Asbestos, arsenic, radon, bis-chloromethyl ether
	Skin cancer	Polycyclic aromatic hydrocarbons, ultraviolet irradiation
Skin	Allergic contact dermatitis	Natural rubber latex, isothiazolins, poison ivy, nickel
	Chemical burns	Sodium hydroxide, hydrogen fluoride
	Chloracne	TCDD,* polychlorinated biphenyls
	Irritant dermatitis	Sodium dodecyl sulfate
Nervous system	Cholinesterase inhibition	Organophosphate insecticides
	Neuronopathy	Methyl mercury
	Parkinsonism	Carbon monoxide, carbon disulfide
	Peripheral neuropathy	N-Hexane, trichloroethylene, acrylamide
Immune system	Autoimmune disease	Vinyl chloride, silica
	Hypersensitivity	See entries for allergic rhinitis, asthma, hypersensitivity pneumonitis, allergic contact dermatitis
	Immunosuppression	TCDD,* lead, mercury, pesticides

(continued)

Table 33-2

Examples of Occupational Diseases and the Toxicants That Cause Them (*continued*)

ORGAN SYSTEM OR DISEASE GROUP	DISEASE	CAUSATIVE AGENT
Renal disease	Indirect renal failure	Arsine, phosphine, trinitrophenol
	Nephropathy	Paraquat, 1,4-dichlorobenzene, mercuric chloride
Cardiovascular disease	Arrhythmias	Acetone, toluene, methylene chloride, trichloroethylene
	Atherosclerosis	Dinitrotoluene, carbon monoxide
	Coronary artery disease	Carbon disulfide
	Cor pulmonale	Beryllium
	Systemic hypotension	Nitroglycerine, ethylene glycol dinitrate
Liver disease	Fatty liver (steatosis)	Carbon tetrachloride, toluene
	Cirrhosis	Arsenic, trichloroethylene
	Hepatocellular death	Dimethylformamide, TCDD*
Reproductive system	Male	Chlordecone (Kepone), dibromochloropropane, hexane
	Female	Aniline, styrene
	Both sexes	Carbon disulfide, lead, vinyl chloride
Infectious diseases	Arboviral encephalidites	Alphavirus, Bunyavirus, Flavivirus
	Aspergillosis	*Aspergillus niger, A. fumigatus, A. flavus*
	Cryptosporidiosis	*Cryptosporidium parvum*
	Hepatitis B	Hepatitis B virus
	Histoplasmosis	*Histoplasma capsulatum*
	Legionellosis	*Legionella pneumophila*
	Lyme disease	*Borrelia burgdorferi*
	Psittacosis	*Chlamydia psittaci*
	Tuberculosis	*Mycobacterium tuberculosis hominis*

*TCDD, 2,3,7,8-tetrachlorodibenzo-*p*-dioxin.

Table 33-3

Crude U.S. Death Rates (1987–1996) and Deaths in 1996 Attributed to Selected Occupational Lung Diseases

DISEASE	DEATH RATE PER MILLION	DEATHS (1996)	INSPECTOR SAMPLES EXCEEDING PEL
Asbestosis	4.83	1176	3.9%
Coal workers' pneumoconiosis	9.16	1417	7.4%
Silicosis	1.40	212	13.6%
Byssinosis	0.07	9	24.9%
Other pneumoconioses*	1.60	316	
Neoplasms of the pleura	2.62	510	
Hypersensitivity pneumonitis	0.17	343	

*This includes aluminosis, berylliosis, stannosis, siderosis, and fibrosis from bauxite, graphite fibers, wollastonite, cadmium, portland cement, emery, kaolin, antimony, and mica.

PEL, permissible exposure limit.

SOURCE: U.S. Bureau of Labor Statistics.

associated with occupational exposures to crystalline silica and vinyl chloride.

Occupational diseases of the cardiovascular system include atherosclerosis, a variety of arrhythmias, problems with coronary blood supply, systemic hypotension, and right ventricular hypertrophy usually caused by pulmonary hypertension. Liver diseases include carbon tetrachloride–induced fatty liver. Occupational diseases of the reproductive system can be gender- and organ-specific or affect both sexes. Exposures to infectious agents are aspects of a variety of occupations (veterinarians, health care workers, biomedical researchers, and farmers).

Both industrial and nonindustrial indoor environments may pose occupational hazards as a result of the presence of chemical or biological agents. Problems with ventilation and the use of synthetic building materials has led to problems associated with occupancy in buildings. Volatile and semivolatile chemicals are released from manufacturing process materials, building materials, floor coverings, furniture, cleaning products, biocides, and microorganisms. In some cases, the occupied space of a building may be clean and dry but local amplification sites for molds, such as damp closets and subfloors, may develop. Airborne viruses, bacteria, and fungi are responsible for a variety of building-related illnesses.

TOXICOLOGIC EVALUATION OF OCCUPATIONAL AGENTS

Evaluation of Occupational Risks

To recommend an acceptable exposure level to an industrial chemical, one must attempt to define the risk associated with adverse effects in the most sensitive populations exposed. One then must decide what proportion of exposed subjects may develop an adverse effect at the proposed acceptable exposure level.

Establishing Causality In complex occupational environments, it may be difficult to establish a causal relationship between a toxic substance and a disease. A matrix was developed to evaluate the weight of evidence for a causal association between a toxicant and an occupational disease (Fig. 33-2). Evidence from well-conducted in vitro studies, animal studies, human challenge studies (intentional clinical exposure to humans), case reports, and epidemiologic investigations is evaluated. This evaluation is guided by seven criteria (shown in blue). If a chemical was studied thoroughly in animals, humans, and in vitro studies and produced clear and convincing evidence of an exposure–response

	Assessment of Exposure to Specific Agents	Consideration or Control of Confounders	Evidence of a Dose–Response Relationship	Consistent Results From Different Studies	Objective Clinical Data	Endpoints Related to Human Pathology	Appropriate Subjects or Models
In Vitro Studies							
Animal Studies							
Human Challenge Studies							
Case Studies							
Epidemiology Studies							

For each type of study listed in the first column weight the quality of data from existing studies based on the criteria listed in the column headings as follows:

0 No evidence or condition is not met
1 Equivocal evidence or condition is partially met
2 Some evidence or condition is mostly met
3 Clear evidence or condition is convincingly met

Figure 33-2. Matrix for assessing the strength of an association between a toxicant and an occupational disease.

relationship in controlled studies that used appropriate models and relevant endpoints, that would constitute compelling evidence of a causal relationship between that chemical and that disease.

Animal Toxicology Testing for Establishing Acceptable Levels of Exposure

Animal studies provide valuable data from which to estimate the level of exposure at which the risk of health impairment is acceptable. The duration of tests necessary to establish an acceptable level for occupational exposure is primarily a function of the type of toxic action suspected. It generally is recognized that for systemically acting chemicals, subacute and short-term toxicity studies usually are insufficient for proposing occupational exposure limits. Subacute and short-term toxicity tests usually are performed to find out whether a compound exhibits immunotoxic properties and cumulative characteristics and to aid in the selection of the doses for long-term exposures. Studies designed to evaluate reproductive effects and teratogenicity also should be considered.

Information derived from exposure routes similar to those sustained by workers is clearly the most relevant. The choice of what studies to perform using which routes of administration must be evaluated scientifically for each toxicant. Important considerations include its target sites and mechanism of action, its metabolism, the nature of its adverse effects, and how workers are exposed to the toxicant.

Worker Health Surveillance

The primary objective of occupational toxicology is to prevent the development of occupational diseases. The monitoring of exposures to toxicants in the workplace may play an important role in detecting excessive exposures before the occurrence of significant biological disturbances and health impairment. When a new chemical is being used on a large scale, the careful clinical surveillance of workers and monitoring of workplaces should be instituted. Evaluation of the validity of the proposed occupational exposure limit derived from animal experiments through workplace surveillance is the major aim.

Epidemiologic studies designed to assess exposure–response relationships can be carried out by using a variety of variables for assessing the exposure and health changes. It is evident that the assessment of the health risk resulting from exposure will have more validity if it results from exposure–response studies in which both the target dose and the critical biological changes are monitored. Of course, the use of such parameters requires knowledge of the fate of the chemical in the organism and its mechanism of action.

Because early biomarkers of effect are subtle and individual variations exist in the response to a chemical insult, the results generally require a statistical comparison between a group of exposed workers and a similar group of workers who have not received the exposure of interest. If exposures are high enough to induce an adverse effect, it is expected that these studies may permit the establishment of the relationship between integrated exposure (intensity $\times$ time) and frequency of abnormal results and, consequently, a redefinition of the occupational exposure limit.

In cases in which a surveillance program was not instituted before the introduction of a new chemical, it is more difficult to establish the efficacy of the exposure limit. In this situation, evaluation depends on retrospective cohort studies or case-control studies or on cross-sectional studies of workers who already have sustained exposure.

Case reports of isolated overexposures resulting from specific incidents such as containment breaches, chemical spills, and vessel or pipe ruptures can provide useful information. Such observations may indicate whether human symptomatology is similar to that found in animals and may suggest functional or biological tests that may prove useful for routine monitoring of exposed workers.

Linkage of Animal Studies and Epidemiologic Studies

In the field of occupational toxicology, perhaps more than in other areas of toxicology, close cooperation between those conducting animal studies and those conducting studies of workers is essential for examining the risks associated with overexposure to chemicals and other toxicants.

Several occupational carcinogens have been identified clearly through combined epidemiologic and experimental approaches. For example, the carcinogenicity of vinyl chloride first was demonstrated in rats, and a few years later, epidemiologic studies confirmed the same carcinogenic risk for humans. This observation stimulated several investigations of the metabolism of vinyl chloride in animals and its mutagenic activity in in vitro systems, leading to a better understanding of its mechanism of carcinogenicity.

Studies of the metabolic handling of occupational toxicants in animals are instrumental in the characterization of reactive intermediates and may suggest unsuspected risks or indicate new methods of biological monitoring. Conversely, clinical observations of workers may stimulate studies of the metabolism or the mechanism of toxicity of a toxicant in animals, revealing the health significance of a biological disturbance.

Arsenic is one of the very few compounds for which there are limited data of predictive value from animal studies that can be applied to human health effects. Inorganic arsenic has been shown conclusively to cause human cancers of many organs but not to cause cancer in animals. This demonstrates that an occupational toxicologist cannot rely solely on animal or epidemiologic studies. A combined approach is necessary to identify, elucidate, and prioritize risks and to develop interventions and techniques for worker health surveillance.

EXPOSURE MONITORING

Two important applications of occupational toxicologic investigations are compared below: environmental monitoring and biological monitoring.

Environmental Monitoring for Exposure Assessment

A critical element in establishing occupational exposure limits is the accurate and uniform assessment of exposure. The methodology for exposure assessment must be tailored specifically to the agent under study and the environment in which it appears. To assess airborne exposures, personal samples taken in the breathing zone generally are used. Repeated random sampling is usually the best approach to developing unbiased measures of exposure.

Although one cannot assess dose directly through exposure monitoring, that type of monitoring has distinct advantages over biological monitoring, which cannot provide route-specific exposure data. Environmental monitoring techniques are generally less expensive and less invasive than are techniques involving the collection and analysis of biological samples such as blood and urine. Spatial, temporal, and work practice associations can be established by means of air monitoring and can suggest better interventions and engineering controls.

Biological Monitoring for Exposure Assessment

Biological monitoring of exposure assesses health risk through the evaluation of the internal dose, or the amount of chemical stored in one or several body compartments or in the whole body. The greatest advantage of using biological measurements is that the biological parameter of exposure is related more directly to the adverse health effects than is the case with environmental measurements. Therefore, biological monitoring may offer a better estimate of the risk than can be determined from ambient monitoring. Biological monitoring accounts for uptake by all exposure routes.

Several factors can influence uptake. Personal hygiene habits vary from one person to another, and there is some degree of individual variation in the absorption rate of a chemical through the lungs, skin, or gastrointestinal tract. Because of its ability to encompass and evaluate the overall exposure (regardless of the route of entry), biological monitoring also can be used to test the overall efficacy of personal protective equipment such as respirators, gloves, and barrier creams. Another consideration with biological monitoring is the fact that nonoccupational exposures (hobbies, residential exposures, dietary habits, smoking, second jobs) also may be expressed in the biological level.

Relationships between air monitoring and biological monitoring may be modified by factors that influence the fate of an occupational toxicant in vivo. Metabolic interactions can occur when workers are exposed simultaneously to chemicals that are biotransformed through identical pathways or modify the activity of the biotransformation enzymes. Furthermore, metabolic interferences may occur between occupational toxicants and alcohol, tobacco, food additives, prescription drugs, natural product remedies, or recreational drugs.

In summary, environmental monitoring and biological monitoring should not be regarded as opposites but as complementary elements in an occupational health and safety program.

CONCLUSION

The working environment will always present the risk of overexposure of workers to various toxicants. Recognition of these risks should not be delayed until epidemiologic studies have defined hazardous levels. A combined experimental, clinical, and epidemiologic approach is the most effective for evaluating the potential risks. One then can promulgate scientifically based occupational health standards, apply effective workplace controls to ensure adherence to those standards, and institute worker health surveillance programs to identify unexpected effects in susceptible individuals.

BIBLIOGRAPHY

ACGIH: *2000 TLVs and BEIs: Threshold Limit Values for Chemical Substances and Physical Agents and Biological Exposure Indices.* Cincinnati, OH: American Conference of Governmental Industrial Hygienists, 2000.

DiNardi SR (ed): *The Occupational Environment—Its Evaluation and Control.* Fairfax, VA: American Industrial Hygiene Association, 1997.

Greenberg MI, Hamilton RJ (eds): *Occupational, Industrial and Environmental Toxicology.* St. Louis: Mosby, 1997.

Salthammer T (ed): *Organic Indoor Air Pollutants—Occurrence, Measurement, Evaluation.* Weinheim, Germany: Wiley/VCH, 1999.

Stacey NH: *Occupational Toxicology.* London: Taylor & Francis, 2002.

C H A P T E R   3 4

REGULATORY TOXICOLOGY

Richard A. Merrill

KEY POINTS

- To justify government regulation of human exposure to a substance, it must be determined that that substance is capable of harming persons who may be exposed to it and that humans are likely to be exposed to it in ways that could be harmful.

- Regulations ensure consistency and are more easily enforced than guidelines, but they are more rigid because they restrict the agency, and the procedures for their adoption are cumbersome.

THE RELATIONSHIP BETWEEN THE DISCIPLINE OF TOXICOLOGY AND REGULATORY INSTITUTIONS

The most obvious connection between regulation and toxicology is that regulators whose job is to protect health rely heavily on toxicologic principles and experimental data for evaluations of problems that present the need for a decision. Whether the decision is to assign priorities among a group of compounds or to approve a new substance or restrict the use of an old one, the findings of toxicologic investigations are likely to be influential and often decisive.

Regulators are not merely consumers of experimental results but also shape toxicologic science in ways that may be unexpected. Regulatory demands have provided a major impetus for improvements in toxicologic methods and have stimulated a demand for major toxicologic studies. Such studies constitute a major part of the discipline's research agenda. Thus, communication between government officials and laboratory scientists flows in both directions. Government testing standards are influenced strongly by the prevailing consensus among toxicologists, many of whom work in regulatory agencies.

REGULATORY PROGRAMS THAT RELY ON TOXICOLOGY

An Overview of Approaches to Toxic Chemical Regulation

Current federal programs for controlling human exposure to toxic chemicals are concerned with the "burden of proof," which is the responsibility for demonstrating whether a substance is safe or hazardous. The range of possible approaches can be observed by comparing laws such as the Food Additives Amendment, which requires users of new substances to prove *lack of* hazard *before* humans can be exposed, with laws such as the Occupational Safety and Health Act (1970), which requires regulators to show that a substance *is* hazardous *before* exposures can be restricted. The approach chosen by Congress powerfully influences an agency's ability to require comprehensive toxicologic investigation of compounds and thus affects the quality of data on which decisions ultimately are based.

Typology of Regulatory Approaches

At least two issues must be resolved to justify government action to regulate human exposure to a substance. First, it must be determined that the substance is capable of harming persons who may be exposed. Second, it must be determined that humans are likely to be exposed to the substance in ways that could be harmful. Most laws under which chemicals are regulated mandate or permit consideration of other criteria as well, such as the *magnitude* of the risk posed by a substance and the *consequences and costs* of regulating it.

Agencies Involved

At the federal level, four agencies are chiefly responsible for regulating human exposure to chemicals: the U.S. Food and Drug Administration (FDA), the U.S. Environmental Protection Agency (EPA), the Occupational Safety and Health Administration (OSHA), and the Consumer Product Safety Commission (CPSC).

Summary of Current Approaches

For noncarcinogenic chemicals, regulators generally have embraced a standard safety assessment formula built around the concept of the *acceptable daily intake* (ADI). The ADI for a chemical is derived by applying a safety factor—usually 100—to the human equivalent of the lowest "no observed effect level" (NOEL) revealed in animal experiments. When estimated human exposure to a chemical falls below the ADI, it—or the quantity of it that results in that exposure—is adjudged "safe."

However, this traditional approach to conventional toxicants has not been considered appropriate for carcinogens. Regulators in many countries have operated on the premise that carcinogens as a class cannot be assumed to have "safe" or threshold doses and that any chemical shown convincingly in animal studies to cause cancer should be considered a potential human carcinogen. As research has begun to illuminate the different mechanisms by which chemicals may cause cancer, however, regulatory agencies cautiously have accepted the possibility that "safe" thresholds may be established for particular carcinogens.

No Risk   The traditional approach is epitomized by the Delaney clause, which is part of the Food Additives Amendment. The amendment requires that any food additive be found "safe" before the FDA may approve its use. The Delaney clause stipulates that a food additive may not be considered "safe" if it has been shown to induce cancer in humans or experimental animals.

Negligible Risk   Because the risk posed even by a carcinogenic substance depends on the dose as well as the potency, it may be possible to reduce human exposure to such low levels that any associated risk is small enough to ignore. In 1996, Congress amended the provisions of the Food, Drug and Cosmetics (FD&C) Act applicable to pesticide residues on food, adopting a standard that is understood to permit a tolerance for a carcinogenic pesticide if the estimated cancer risk is extremely small, on the order of 1 in 1 million.

PROGRAMS FOR REGULATING CHEMICAL HAZARDS

Food and Drug Administration

The oldest of the major health regulation laws, the FD&C Act, was enacted in 1938 and covers food for humans and animals, human and veterinary drugs, medical devices, and cosmetics.

Food The Food and Drug Act forbids the marketing of any food containing "any *added* poisonous or deleterious *substance which may render it injurious* to health," and the marketing of foods containing *nonadded* toxicants that make them *"ordinarily injurious* to health." Environmental contaminants are also of concern to regulators. The FDA authorizes the establishment of tolerances for "added poisonous or deleterious substances" that cannot be avoided through good manufacturing practice. In setting such tolerances, the FDA weighs three factors: (1) the health effects of the contaminant, which usually are estimated on the basis of animal data, (2) the ability to measure the contaminant, and (3) the effects of various tolerance levels on the price and availability of the food.

Human Drugs Preclinical studies in animals play an important role in the FDA's evaluation of human drugs. The current law requires premarket approval, for both safety and efficacy, of all new drugs. Investigation of therapeutic agents in humans has long been accepted, and the primary evidence of safety (as well as effectiveness) accordingly comes from clinical studies, not laboratory studies. However, animal studies are the sole source of information about a substance's biological effects before human trials are begun, and their results influence not only the decision whether to expose human subjects but also the design of clinical protocols.

Medical Devices The regulatory scheme for medical devices involves three tiers of control, the most restrictive of which is premarket approval similar to that required for new drugs. To obtain FDA approval of a so-called class III device, the sponsor must demonstrate safety and efficacy. The bulk of the data supporting such applications is derived from clinical studies but also includes toxicologic studies of any constituents likely to be absorbed by the patient.

Cosmetics The basic safety standard for cosmetics is similar to that for food ingredients: No product may be marketed if it contains "a poisonous or deleterious substance which may render it injurious to health." The case law establishes that this language also bars the distribution of a product that poses any significant risk of more than transitory harm when used as intended, but it places on the FDA the burden of proving a violation.

Environmental Protection Agency

Toxicologic evidence plays a central role in the EPA activities of regulation of pesticides, industrial chemicals, and drinking water supplies; hazardous waste control; and regulation of toxic pollutants of water and of air.

Pesticides No pesticide may be marketed unless it has been registered by the EPA. The Federal Insecticide, Fungicide, and Rodenticide Act (FIFRA) specifies that a pesticide shall be registered if it is effective, bears proper labeling, and "when properly used. . . . will not generally cause unreasonable adverse effects on the environment." A pesticide is scrutinized closely if the EPA concludes that it induces cancer in experimental mammalian species or humans. Even if a pesticide is shown convincingly to be a carcinogen, however, the law allows it to be registered if the EPA concludes that its economic benefits outweigh the risk.

Industrial Chemicals The Toxic Substances Control Act (TSCA) covers all chemical substances manufactured or processed in or imported into the United States except for substances already regulated under other laws. The TSCA empowers the EPA to restrict or even ban the manufacture, processing, distribution, use, or disposal of a chemical substance when there is a reasonable basis to conclude that any such activity poses an "unreasonable risk of injury to health or environment." If the EPA suspects that a chemical *may* pose an unreasonable risk but lacks sufficient data to take action, the TSCA empowers it to require testing to develop the necessary data. Finally, the TSCA requires the manufacturer of a new chemical substance to notify the agency 90 days before production or distribution. This notice must include any known health effects data. However, the EPA is not empowered to require that manufacturers routinely conduct testing of all new chemicals to permit an evaluation of their risks.

Hazardous Wastes Several statutes administered by the EPA regulate land disposal of hazardous materials (those which are ignitable, corrosive, reactive, or toxic). In 1976, the Resource Conservation and Recovery Act (RCRA) established a comprehensive federal scheme for regulating hazardous waste. RCRA directs the EPA to regulate the activities of generators, transporters, and those who treat, store, or dispose of hazardous wastes to "protect human health and the environment."

Toxic Water Pollutants   In 1972, the Federal Water Pollution Control Act required the EPA to publish a list of toxic pollutants for which effluent standards (discharge limits) would be established. In establishing standards for any listed pollutant, the EPA was to provide an *"ample margin of safety,"* a difficult criterion to meet for most toxic pollutants. Modifications of this act have allowed the EPA to take into account economic cost and technologic feasibility in setting limits.

Drinking Water   The 1974 Safe Drinking Water Act (SDWA) was enacted to ensure that public water supply systems "meet minimum national standards for the protection of public health." The EPA is required to regulate any contaminants "which may have an adverse effect on human health." For each contaminant of concern, the agency must prescribe a maximum contaminant level or a treatment technique for its control.

Toxic Air Pollutants   Section 112 of the Clean Air Act (CAA) provides a list of 189 hazardous air pollutants that the EPA may modify by adding or deleting items. The EPA must establish national emissions standards for sources that emit any listed pollutant. The EPA requires an "ample margin of safety," taking into account achievable goals, for carcinogens.

Occupational Safety and Health Administration

The 1970 Occupational Safety and Health Act requires employers to provide employees with safe working conditions and empowers OSHA to prescribe mandatory occupational safety and health standards. Manufacturers of food additives, drugs, and pesticides must demonstrate the safety of their products before marketing, but no employer need obtain advance approval of processes or materials or conduct tests to ensure that its operations will not jeopardize workers' health. OSHA first must discover that a material already in use threatens workers' health before it may attempt to control exposure. Standards for toxic chemicals typically set maximum limits on employee exposure and prescribe changes in employer procedures or equipment to achieve that level.

Consumer Product Safety Commission

The Consumer Product Safety Commission was created in 1972 by the Consumer Product Safety Act, with authority to regulate or ban products that pose an unreasonable risk of injury or illness to consumers. The CPSC also administers the Federal Hazardous Substances Act (FHSA), which authorizes the CPSC to regulate, primarily through prescribed label warnings, products that are toxic, corrosive, combustible, or radioactive or that generate pressure.

REGULATORY CONTROLS OVER TOXICOLOGY

Modern toxicology has developed in substantial part in response to the information needs of contemporary regulation. Regulatory agencies often prescribe the specific objectives and design of studies that are conducted to satisfy regulatory requirements. The pressure to protect animals used in research has produced additional laws and regulations. An agency such as the FDA or the EPA, which must confirm the safety of new substances before marketing, can dictate the kinds of tests that manufacturers must conduct to gain approval. By contrast, an agency that has no premarket approval function has less leverage. The agency's power to withhold approval when it has doubts about a product's safety gives it the practical leverage necessary to demand whatever tests its scientific reviewers believe are necessary.

Any time a regulatory agency wants to provide guidance for private behavior, it confronts a choice between establishing standards that have the force of law and merely conveying its current best judgment of what conduct will satisfy the law. Regulations ensure consistency and are more easily enforced than guidelines, but they are more rigid because they restrict the agency, and the procedures for their adoption are cumbersome.

FDA and EPA Testing Standards

This section is intended to acquaint the reader with the principal federal programs that specify standards for toxicity testing, focusing on the FDA and the EPA.

Food and Drug Administration The FDA exercises premarketing approval authority over several classes of compounds, of which the most important, for current purposes, are new human drugs and direct additives to food.

Toxicologic Testing Requirements for Human Drugs In 1962, Congress expressly authorized the FDA to exempt investigational drugs from the premarket approval requirement so that they could be shipped for use in clinical testing, subject to conditions the agency believed were appropriate to protect human subjects. One condition that the FDA established was that an investigational drug first must have been evaluated in preclinical studies. Almost invariably, a drug's sponsor will consult agency personnel to get a precise understanding of what sorts of toxicologic studies are expected.

Testing Requirements for Food Additives The Food Additives Amendment and the Color Additive Amendments require premarket approval of new additives to human foods. Both laws assume that laboratory studies in animals will provide the principal data for assessing safety. In 1982, the FDA first codified the tests necessary for various food additives in *Toxicological Principles for the Safety Assessment of Direct Food Additives and Color Additives Used in Food,* known thereafter as the "Red Book." The Red Book describes the types of tests the FDA believes are necessary to evaluate an additive's safety. The agency's requirements, which are in the form of guidelines rather than regulations, are calibrated to the purposes for which an additive will be used, estimated levels of human exposure, and the results of sequential studies.

Environmental Protection Agency The EPA's premarket approval authority over pesticides places it, like the FDA, in a position where it can dictate the design and conduct of studies of such compounds.

Toxicology Requirements for Pesticides FIFRA clearly contemplates the submission of toxicologic studies, as well as other types of investigations, to support the EPA's evaluation of a pesticide. The statute also requires the EPA to "publish guidelines specifying the kinds of information which will be required to support the registration of a pesticide."

Testing of Industrial Chemicals The primary means by which the EPA may mandate health effects testing of new or existing industrial chemicals is a provision in TSCA that states that the administrator "shall by rule require that testing be conducted to develop data with respect to the health and environmental effects for which there is an insufficiency of data and experience" to permit the assessment of whether a substance presents an unreasonable risk. The statute creates an Interagency Testing Committee (ITC) with members from EPA, OSHA, Council for Environmental Quality, National Institute for Occupational Safety and Health, National Institute for Environmental Health Sciences, National Cancer Institute, National Science Foundation, and the Department of Commerce to recommend a list of chemicals that should be tested, and then the EPA must either initiate testing or publish its reasons for not doing so.

Interagency Testing Criteria and Programs

Both the FDA and the EPA, along with the White House Office of Science and Technology Policy, continue to work to achieve internal consistency in testing standards. The National Toxicology Program (NTP) was established in 1978 as an administrative umbrella for coordinating federal efforts to improve test methods and coordinate toxicologic studies then under way. An NTP committee that includes representatives of all four regulatory agencies is responsible for selecting chemicals to be tested at public expense. Attention continues to be focused on improving health risk assessment research techniques.

Animal Welfare Requirements

Researchers who conduct studies funded by federal agencies must comply with the Animal Welfare Act (AWA), and some also may be subject to restrictions imposed by the Public Health Service (PHS). The AWA is administered by the Animal and Plant Health Inspection Service (APHIS), which is part of the U.S. Department of Agriculture. The AWA requires all covered research facilities to register with APHIS and agree to comply with applicable AWA standards. Each facility must file an annual report that includes the following:

1. Assurances that alternatives to painful procedures were considered in the design of the studies conducted there
2. A summary and brief explanation of all exceptions to the standards and regulations that were approved by the Institutional Animal Care and Use Committee
3. The common names and the numbers of animals used in three research categories: (a) research involving no pain, distress, or use of pain-relieving

drugs, (b) research involving pain and distress and in which pain-relieving drugs were used, and (c) research involving pain or distress in which no pain-relieving drugs were used because of adverse effects on the procedures, results, or interpretation

4. The common names and the numbers of animals bred, conditioned, or held for research purposes but not yet used

Pursuant to the AWA, APHIS has established specific requirements for the humane handling, care, and transportation of dogs and cats, guinea pigs and hamsters, rabbits, nonhuman primates, marine mammals, and other warm-blooded animals.

The AWA requires each research facility to establish an Institutional Animal Care and Use Committee (IACUC) composed of three or more members, one of whom must be a veterinarian and one of whom must represent community interests and may not be affiliated with the institution. At least one member of the IACUC must review and approve the animal care and use components of all proposed research activities. Prerequisites to approval include the avoidance or minimization of discomfort, distress, and pain; the use of pain-relieving drugs where appropriate; the consideration of pain-free alternatives; and euthanization when an animal otherwise would experience severe or chronic pain or distress that cannot be relieved. The IACUC also is responsible for conducting semiannual inspections of the facility itself and of the program for the humane care and use of animals.

The PHS Policy on Humane Care and Use of Laboratory Animals by Awardee Institutions applies to research using all vertebrates and requires each facility to submit an annual report, called an "Assurance," that is evaluated by the National Institutes of Health (NIH) Office for Protection from Research Risks (OPRR) to determine the sufficiency of animal care. The PHS policy imposes two primary obligations on researchers: Each institution must adopt a Program for Animal Care and Use and must establish an IACUC. The IACUC must be made up of at least five members, including a veterinarian, an animal research scientist, a nonscientist, and a person who is not affiliated with the facility in any other capacity. The IACUC must review all applications for research funding and review the institution's programs to ensure compliance with NIH standards.

Scientists working with no federal funding who expect their research to be submitted to the FDA or the EPA are not subject to the AWA and PHS policies but must comply with the animal protection provisions of those agencies' regulations.

BIBLIOGRAPHY

Gad SC (ed): *Regulatory Toxicology.* London: Taylor & Francis, 2001.

Holcomb ML (ed): *International Toxicology: Worldwide Regulatory Toxicology Support.* Eugene, OR: International Toxicology, 1995.

Self-Assessment Questions and Answers

Each question below contains four suggested answers. Choose the ONE BEST response to each question.

1. Absorption across the skin:
   a. occurs equally well across the skin from all parts of the body.
   b. occurs predominantly by active transport across the stratum corneum.
   c. involves passive diffusion across the dried, keratin-filled cells of the stratum corneum.
   d. occurs predominantly via passive diffusion across the hair follicles, sweat ducts, and sebaceous glands.

2. Xenobiotics elicit toxicity generally by all the following mechanisms EXCEPT:
   a. interference with cellular energy metabolism.
   b. interference with intracellular calcium concentration homeostasis.
   c. interference with normal receptor-toxicant interactions.
   d. interference with renal excretion.

3. Mechanisms that contribute to transmembrane movement of toxicants include all the following EXCEPT:
   a. the process of passive diffusion.
   b. the process of active transport.
   c. the process of biotransformation.
   d. the process of filtration.

4. A properly executed assessment of risk considers all the following EXCEPT:
   a. evaluation of data from human exposures.
   b. evaluation of data from laboratory animal studies.
   c. evaluation of public perception of risks versus benefits.
   d. evaluation of data regarding chemical production.

5. Which of the following statements BEST characterizes synergism?
   a. Synergism occurs if two chemicals with a similar action, when given together, produce an effect that is greater in magnitude than the sum of the effects when the chemicals are given individually.
   b. Synergism occurs if a xenobiotic that lacks an effect of its own increases the effect of a second, active xenobiotic.
   c. Synergism occurs if two chemicals with the same effect, when given together, produce an effect that is equal in magnitude to the sum of the effects when the chemicals are given individually.
   d. Synergism occurs if two drugs with the same effect, when given together, produce an effect that is equal in magnitude to the effect of only one of the drugs given individually.

6. Absorption of an inhaled gas is usually:
   a. not dependent on dissolution of toxicant in the blood.
   b. dependent on degree of ionization.
   c. not dependent on blood flow.
   d. dependent on the blood-gas partition ratio.

7. Toxicants may move across biological membranes by all the following mechanisms EXCEPT:
   a. aqueous diffusion.
   b. aqueous hydrolysis.
   c. lipid diffusion.
   d. special carrier transport.

8. Toxicology may be defined as the study of:
   a. the degradation of biological warfare agents.

b. the cost of toxicity testing.

c. the adverse effects of chemicals on living systems.

d. the regulation of chemicals in the home.

9. Which of the following reactions is NOT considered a phase II biotransformation?

a. glucuronidation.

b. acetylation.

c. sulfation.

d. epoxide hydration.

10. The therapeutic index (TI) may be defined by all the following statements EXCEPT:

a. The TI is a less useful expression than is the margin of safety.

b. A high TI means that the chemical is generally safe to use.

c. A low TI means the chemical is probably dangerous to use.

d. A high TI means the ED_{50} far exceeds the LD_{50}.

11. Which of the following statements describes the process of active transport?

a. The chemical moves from an area of high concentration to an area of low concentration.

b. The chemical moves with an electrochemical gradient through a carrier-mediated process.

c. The chemical moves across the membrane through an energy-consuming process.

d. Administration of metabolic inhibitors that block energy production stimulates transport.

12. In comparing an idiosyncratic reaction and an allergic reaction, it is important to remember that allergic reactions induced upon exposure to a toxicant:

a. will consist of immunologically mediated effects that follow a previous exposure to the toxicant.

b. will occur frequently in the general population.

c. will seldom present any threat to mortality.

d. will clearly demonstrate a dose–response relationship.

13. In considering dose–response data, efficacy typically is considered a measure of:

a. the concentration of chemical needed to produce a maximal response.

b. the all-or-nothing response to a chemical.

c. the maximal effect produced by a chemical.

d. the slope of the dose–response curve.

14. Biotransformation reactions generally produce a product that is:

a. more likely to distribute intracellularly.

b. more likely to produce unwanted effects.

c. less lipid-soluble than the original chemical.

d. more lipid-soluble than the original chemical.

15. Particles approximately 1 μm in diameter typically deposit in the:

a. alveolus.

b. bronchus.

c. trachea.

d. nasopharyngeal region.

16. Which of the following statements regarding the justification of animal toxicity testing is false?

a. A lack of toxicity in the rat or mouse means a chemical is safe for other species, including humans.

b. Exposure to a high dose of the chemical is a necessary and valid method of discovering possible hazards in humans.

c. Description of the toxic effects a chemical can produce is invaluable in ascertaining risk to humans.

d. Effects produced by the chemical in laboratory animals, when properly qualified, are applicable to humans.

17. Induction of xenobiotic biotransformation by exposure to a toxicant will:

a. result in irreversible changes in enzyme activity.

b. result in increased amounts of enzymes in the endoplasmic reticulum.

c. result in decreased amounts of enzymes in the nucleus.

d. require 3 to 4 months to reach completion.

18. Toxicity testing of a potential new insulation agent will:

a. unequivocally predict chemically induced allergic-type reactions.

b. require the use of at least two primate species.

c. not add much cost to the development of the product.

d. extend over different time periods, depending on the projected human use.

19. Cytochrome P450 monooxygenases catalyze all the following reactions EXCEPT:

a. sulfation.

b. hydroxylation.

c. O-dealkylation.

d. epoxidation.

20. Xenobiotics that undergo enterohepatic circulation are subject to:

a. uptake into adipose tissue, uptake into hepatic tissue, and biliary excretion.

b. uptake into intestinal cells, intestinal excretion, and fecal elimination.

c. uptake into enterocytes, secretion into blood, uptake into hepatocytes, and biliary excretion.

d. uptake into enterocytes, uptake into hepatocytes, secretion into blood, and biliary excretion.

21. Which of the following statements is false?

a. Glucuronide conjugates are excreted readily by the kidneys.

b. A lipid-soluble xenobiotic metabolite will sequester in fatty tissue.

c. Acidification of the urine may help trap acidic drugs in urine.

d. For a weakly acidic drug ($pK_a = 3$) at equilibrium, the ratio of nonionized to ionized drug (HA/A^-) equals 1 when the pH of the medium is 3.

22. Which of the following definitions is NOT correct?

a. Teratogenesis studies chemical-induced derangement of cell growth and cell reproduction.

b. Physiologically based toxicokinetic modeling utilizes mass-balance equations to estimate all tissue effects and is generally a fairly accurate predictor of xenobiotic distribution.

c. Mutagenesis studies chemical-induced formation of damaged genetic material.

d. Reproductive toxicity is concerned with the effects of toxicants on fertility, rate of conception, and embryonic or fetal toxicity.

23. Which of the following statements about the hepatic microsomal cytochrome P450 monooxygenase system is false?

a. The cytochrome P450 monooxygenase system requires NADPH and molecular oxygen.

b. The cytochrome P450 monooxygenase system is involved with exogenous chemicals only.

c. The cytochrome P450 monooxygenase system includes N- and O-dealkylations.

d. The cytochrome P450 monooxygenase system catalyzes aliphatic and aromatic hydroxylations.

24. Which of the following definitions is NOT correct?

a. Volume of distribution is a proportionality constant that relates plasma concentration to the total amount of a chemical in the body.

b. Clearance is the volume of a particular fluid from which a chemical has been removed.

c. The time required for the concentration to decrease by 50 percent is the elimination half-life.

d. Glucuronidation involves the conjugation of a chemical with glutathione.

25. **A toxicant's distribution to a specific tissue does NOT:**

a. depend on blood flow and the size of the organ.

b. depend on the solubility of the chemical in that tissue.

c. depend on the concentration gradient between blood and tissue.

d. increase for xenobiotics that are bound to plasma proteins.

26. **Which of the following is a CORRECT statement about the membrane transport of a xenobiotic?**

a. Generally, only small amounts of an ionized chemical passively diffuse into cells.

b. Phagocytosis refers to the expulsion of a solid chemical into the cell.

c. The size of the absorbing surface area influences simple diffusion.

d. Active, energy-requiring, carrier-mediated transport is saturable.

27. **Biotransformation of xenobiotics is an important defense mechanism for living systems because it:**

a. always increases the aqueous solubility of the parent xenobiotic.

b. always abolishes a toxicant's activity.

c. always occurs in order for all toxicants to undergo elimination.

d. is performed by enzymes that are found in most body tissues.

28. **Conjugation reactions:**

a. always yield an inactive metabolite.

b. tend to decrease the molecular weight of many toxicants.

c. tend to yield more water-soluble products.

d. include hydroxylation and glucuronidation.

29. **Which one of the following definitions is NOT correct?**

a. The therapeutic index is equal to LD_{50} or TD_{50} divided by ED_{50}.

b. The efficacy of a drug is similar to the potency of that drug.

c. An agonist is a chemical that binds to a receptor and elicits a response.

d. An antagonist is a chemical that binds to a receptor and does not elicit a response.

30. **Which of the following statements regarding biotransformation reactions is CORRECT?**

a. Esterases add water to the parent chemical, forming an acid and an alcohol.

b. Epoxide hydrolase removes water from chemicals containing an epoxide.

c. Glucuronidation involves conjugation with glucuronic acid.

d. Ethanol generally is oxidized to acetaldehyde by alcohol dehydrogenase.

31. **High-energy cofactors that are NOT involved in phase II reactions include:**

a. UDP-glucuronic acid.

b. S-adenosylmethionine.

c. phosphoadenosine phosphosulfate.

d. amino acids such as taurine and glycine.

32. **Which of the following assumptions is NOT generally acceptable for toxicity testing?**

a. The effects produced by a chemical in laboratory animals, when properly qualified, are applicable to humans.

b. A lack of toxicity in the rat or mouse means a chemical is safe for other species, including humans.

c. Exposure to a high dose of a chemical is a necessary and valid method of discovering possible hazards in humans.

d. The description of the toxic effects a chemical can produce is invaluable in ascertaining risk to humans.

33. Oogenesis includes:

a. conversion of spermatogonia into spermatids.

b. conversion of an oogonium into four ova.

c. conversion of spermatids into spermatozoa.

d. conversion of an oogonium into one ovum and three polar bodies.

34. Which of the following definitions is correct?

a. Mitosis requires nondisjunction for proper cell division.

b. Translation requires conversion of RNA codons into amino acids during protein synthesis.

c. Transcription requires separation of RNA strands with subsequent synthesis of new DNA.

d. Replication requires separation of DNA strands with subsequent synthesis of new RNA.

35. The process of teratogenesis:

a. is induced by all chemicals that have been tested so far.

b. is induced during the embryonic period only.

c. is involved in the induction of malformed organisms.

d. is involved in the induction of neoplasms in the developed organism.

36. The correct sequential chronological steps in carcinogenesis are:

a. bioactivation, progression, promotion, initiation.

b. initiation, bioactivation, progression, promotion.

c. initiation, promotion, progression, bioactivation.

d. bioactivation, initiation, promotion, progression.

37. Which of the following terms does NOT describe a mutagenic effect?

a. chromatid deletion.

b. mitosis.

c. polyploid.

d. nondisjunction.

38. Chemicals may accentuate the carcinogenic process by all the following mechanisms EXCEPT:

a. inhibiting covalent binding with macromolecules.

b. inhibiting DNA repair processes.

c. stimulating the proliferation of cells with DNA damage.

d. stimulating the uptake of the carcinogen.

39. The process of decision point carcinogen testing:

a. is limited to the evaluation of promoters of carcinogenicity.

b. evaluates only in vitro tests for carcinogenicity.

c. requires evaluation of all possible tests for carcinogenesis.

d. evaluates a number of systematic, sequential tests for carcinogenicity.

40. During mutagenesis, a +2 frameshift mutation:

a. involves the deletion of two base pairs from DNA.

b. involves the deletion of two ribose units from DNA.

c. involves the insertion of two ribose units into DNA.

d. involves the insertion of two base pairs into DNA.

41. **Histogenesis:**
    a. involves the formation of tissues from undifferentiated cells.
    b. involves the segregation of cells, cell groups, and tissues into organs.
    c. occurs at the same time for all tissues in the organism.
    d. is seldom sensitive to the action of carcinogens.

42. **Which one of the following definitions is NOT correct?**
    a. Procarcinogens require metabolic activation before becoming genotoxic.
    b. Promoters generally exert no direct genotoxic action.
    c. Cocarcinogens are fully active genotoxic agents.
    d. Direct-acting genotoxic chemicals tend to be electrophilic organic compounds that interact with DNA.

43. **Teratogenesis may be caused by all the following mechanisms EXCEPT:**
    a. alterations in DNA caused by ionizing radiation.
    b. chromosomal abnormalities caused by advancing maternal age.
    c. alterations in RNA caused by ionizing radiation.
    d. nutritional deficiencies.

44. **Methylation of bases on DNA may:**
    a. lead to base recognition errors that lead to point mutations.
    b. cause DNA polymerase to act more quickly.
    c. induce DNA ligase.
    d. lead to cross-linking of mRNA.

45. **All the following statements are correct EXCEPT:**
    a. Exposure to teratogens during the period from fertilization to implantation generally results in prenatal death.
    b. Exposure to teratogens during the period of organogenesis typically results in major morphologic abnormalities.
    c. Exposure to teratogens during the fetal period typically results in life-threatening morphologic abnormalities.
    d. Exposure to teratogens during the fetal period typically results in physiologic defects.

46. **In males, the blood-testes barrier:**
    a. is a poor anatomic barrier to toxic chemicals in adults.
    b. is more effective than the blood-brain barrier in all species.
    c. is found only in laboratory rodents.
    d. is poorly differentiated in utero and at birth.

47. **In the process of carcinogenesis, initiation is the:**
    a. formation of new proteins.
    b. presence of clearly evident neoplasms in rodents.
    c. process by which a normal cell is converted to a neoplastic cell.
    d. reaction catalyzed by DNA polymerase.

48. **Explanations for the difficulty of assessing the reproductive hazards of chemicals include all the following statements EXCEPT:**
    a. In vitro tests are excellent predictors of human toxicity.
    b. The quality of human data may be poor.
    c. Complications may result from toxic effects on the endocrine system.
    d. The reproductive system is complex.

49. **Aerosols include all the following EXCEPT:**
    a. mists.
    b. smoke.
    c. dusts.
    d. vapor.

50. In inhalation toxicology, forced expiratory volume may be defined as:

  a. maximal inspiration and exhalation.

  b. volume of air exhaled per unit time.

  c. volume of air that is exchanged during restful breathing.

  d. residual volume plus vital capacity.

51. Toxicants can cause all the following adverse effects EXCEPT:

  a. an increase in forced expiratory volume.

  b. bronchoconstriction leading to dyspnea and asthma.

  c. an increase in bronchial and tracheal secretions.

  d. emphysema.

52. Which of the following statements regarding testing of potential mutagens is false?

  a. Positive controls are always included.

  b. Most tests evaluate phenotypic changes and attempt to draw conclusions regarding the actual gene damage.

  c. Evaluation for aneuploidy involves determination of the gain or loss of complete sets of chromosomes.

  d. Evaluation of chromosomal damage involves looking for evidence of alteration in chromosomal structure and number.

53. Excision repair mechanisms that are involved in DNA repair:

  a. are saturable and error-free.

  b. are nonsaturable and error-free.

  c. are saturable and error-prone.

  d. are nonsaturable and error-prone.

54. Which of the following definitions is incorrect?

  a. Chronic bronchitis involves excessive mucus production and a recurrent cough.

  b. Asthma is characterized by open airways and easy gas exchange.

  c. Fibrosis involves alveolar macrophages, fibroblast proliferation, and excess collagen synthesis.

  d. Emphysema is characterized by enlarged airspaces resulting from destruction of alveolar walls.

55. Glaucoma generally is defined as:

  a. decreased intraocular pressure.

  b. increased intraocular pressure.

  c. decreased vitreous humor production.

  d. increased vitreous humor production.

56. Tests of neurotoxicant-induced actions include all the following EXCEPT:

  a. muscle function.

  b. reflexes.

  c. behavior.

  d. electrodermatogram.

57. Which of the following tests is NOT used to measure toxicity in the eye?

  a. Draize test.

  b. cultures of corneal cells.

  c. cultures of proximal tubular cells.

  d. intraocular pressure.

58. Photoallergy testing:

  a. requires initial treatment with the test chemical and exposure to UV light followed by a challenge dose of chemical and UV light.

  b. requires initial treatment with the test chemical and exposure to UV light that is not followed by a challenge dose of chemical.

  c. generally uses the white rabbit.

  d. generally uses the hairless mouse.

59. Chemically induced hepatotoxicity may result from:

  a. stimulation of biliary excretion.

  b. stimulation of biotransformation.

c. stimulation of bile production.

d. stimulation of hepatic blood flow.

60. Chemicals can cause cardiac toxicity by all the following mechanisms EXCEPT:

a. impairment of normal ion movement into and out of heart cells.

b. derangement of normal electrical signaling.

c. stimulation of sinusoidal membrane function.

d. impairment of energy production.

61. Which of the following effects does NOT apply to damage to the heart?

a. positive inotropic response.

b. arrhythmias.

c. myocardial depression.

d. vasoconstriction.

62. Cataractogenesis results from:

a. deposition of chemicals in the retina.

b. deposition of chemicals in the iris.

c. deposition of chemicals in the lens.

d. deposition of chemicals in the aqueous humor.

63. Renal clearance may be defined as the:

a. volume of plasma completely cleared of the chemical in its passage through the liver.

b. volume of plasma completely cleared of the chemical in its passage through the kidney.

c. volume of plasma completely cleared of the chemical during its passage through the lungs.

d. concentration of the chemical that is cleared completely during the filtration of plasma on its passage through the kidney.

64. In primary irritation testing:

a. the test animal is always given an analgesic.

b. the test chemical is placed on normal and abraded skin under a patch for 24 h.

c. the test animal is usually the rat.

d. the skin is evaluated only once.

65. Acid rain:

a. can stimulate lacrimation by irritating sensory nerve endings.

b. can stimulate urination by irritating sensory nerve endings.

c. can induce myelinopathy by irritating sensory nerve endings.

d. can induce glaucoma by irritating sensory nerve endings.

66. The skin:

a. is a fairly permeable barrier to environmental toxicants.

b. is not responsive to UV light.

c. is in a constant state of change as stratum corneum cells typically are replaced monthly.

d. is fairly static as stratum corneum cells typically are not replaced with any regularity.

67. Electroencephalograms:

a. indicate the chemical to which an animal or human has been exposed.

b. are always useful in predicting the site of brain damage.

c. record the electrical activity of the brain.

d. record the movement of the eye after stimulation with light.

68. In the eye:

a. the retina is the layer that brings blood to the rod and cone cells.

b. the lens is the layer that controls pupil diameter.

c. the iris is the white layer that surrounds the eye.

d. the ciliary body is involved in aqueous humor production.

69. Acute dermal irritation may be defined as:

a. wheal and flair reactions induced very shortly after cutaneous exposure to chemicals.

b. reversible chemical-induced changes in sebaceous gland secretions.

c. a local reversible inflammation of normal living skin that occurs shortly after a single exposure of the skin to a toxicant.

d. a toxic effect resulting from DNA damage.

70. The blood-brain barrier:

a. is a semipermeable barrier that excludes molecules greater than 40 kD.

b. is found around all parts of the brain and spinal cord.

c. is formed by having keratinocytes surround the neurons.

d. is not an effective barrier.

71. Axons:

a. are involved in receiving messages from other nerve cells.

b. are short extensions of the cell body of the neuron.

c. are fairly tolerant of the toxic effects of chemicals.

d. are involved in the synthesis and release of neurotransmitters.

72. The autonomic nervous system normally does NOT function to:

a. control heart rate.

b. stimulate breathing.

c. stimulate skeletal muscle contractions.

d. control pupil diameter.

73. Testing of the potential of chemicals to induce eye irritation:

a. is needed to ensure the safety of all cosmetic products.

b. requires the Draize test as the usual testing protocol.

c. requires simultaneous testing of two species and three dose levels for the chemical.

d. is quite humane for laboratory animals.

74. Which of the following morphologic descriptions of nerve damage is accurate?

a. Loss of the white layer around myelinated neurons indicates a myelinopathy.

b. Nissl substance is increased markedly in neuronopathy.

c. Damage to the cell body is called axonopathy.

d. Loss of white layer around myelinated neurons indicates a transmission defect.

75. Toxicants may damage the central nervous system by all the following mechanisms EXCEPT:

a. alteration of neurotransmitter function.

b. injury to myelin-producing cells.

c. stimulation of neuron regeneration.

d. promotion of axonal damage.

76. The primary response in humoral immunity is:

a. An antigen binds to T cells to induce antibody formation.

b. An antigen binds to B cells to induce antibody formation.

c. Interleukins bind to the antigen and stimulate macrophages.

d. Macrophages are stimulated by antigens to induce antibody formation.

77. Which of the following is NOT a common environmental pollutant?

a. metals.

b. pesticides.

c. solvents.

d. water.

78. Which one of the following statements is correct?

a. Food additives are substances that normally are consumed as food.

b. Dermal exposures often result from solvents because of their ubiquitous use by humans.

c. Herbicides are used widely to control insect populations in agriculture.

d. The testis is the male reproductive organ that is the major site of toxicity for mercury-containing compounds.

79. The immune system is composed of all the following EXCEPT:

a. serum albumin.

b. interleukins.

c. T lymphocytes.

d. B lymphocytes.

80. Allergy may be defined as

a. a decreased responsive state resulting from a second exposure to a toxicant.

b. a decreased responsive state acquired through a previous exposure to a toxicant.

c. an increased responsive state acquired through a previous exposure to a toxicant.

d. an increased responsive state resulting from a second exposure to a toxicant.

81. Which one of the following statements is NOT correct?

a. Metals generally exert toxicity during the period of fetal development in utero called gestation.

b. Most solvents are highly toxic to the immune system.

c. Nutritional food additives include vitamins, minerals, and amino acids.

d. Fungicides are substances that can prevent and destroy fungal growth.

82. Which of the following definitions of pesticides is NOT correct?

a. Insecticides are chemicals that kill insects.

b. Fumigants are chemicals that kill fungi.

c. Herbicides are chemicals that kill plants.

d. Fertilizers are chemicals that kill plants.

83. Which of the following metals is correctly paired with the target enzyme system?

a. iron—renal reabsorption carriers.

b. arsenic—enzymes of phase II biotransformation.

c. lead—enzymes of hemoglobin synthesis.

d. mercury—maturation of oogonia.

84. Which of the following chemicals is NOT a pesticide?

a. ethylene glycol.

b. dithiocarbamates.

c. ethylene dibromide.

d. diazinon.

85. Which of the following agents induces nephrotoxicity?

a. parathion.

b. n-hexane.

c. arsenic trioxide.

d. mercuric chloride.

86. Maintenance of an adequate food supply absolutely requires the use of food additives, including all the following EXCEPT:

a. growth-promoting hormones.

b. appearance-enhancing agents.

c. preservatives.

d. processing aids.

87. Pesticide uses include all the following EXCEPT:

a. the killing of rodents.

b. the prevention of weed growth in a field.

c. the retardation of fungal growth on picked fruits and vegetables.

d. the removal of toxicity tests from required testing.

88. Which of the following statements about organochlorine insecticides is NOT correct?

a. Organochlorine insecticides are highly persistent in the environment.

b. Organochlorine insecticides are not bioaccumulated readily in the food chain.

c. Organochlorine insecticides are suspected human carcinogens.

d. Organochlorine insecticides include DDT, lindane, and kepone.

89. **Which of the following statements about pesticides is true?**

a. Pesticide use is a relatively modern phenomenon.

b. Pesticide use has brought only good things to humans.

c. Pesticide cost is clearly less than the benefits for all humans.

d. Pesticides possess an inherent degree of toxicity to some living organisms.

90. **Toxic effects of metals include all the following EXCEPT:**

a. carcinogenicity.

b. neurotoxicity.

c. damage to the gastrointestinal tract.

d. diabetes.

91. **Iron:**

a. inhibits the synthesis of hemoglobin.

b. causes nephrosis on acute exposure.

c. accumulates in the mitochondria and leads to cell necrosis.

d. does not affect the gastrointestinal tract.

92. **The American Conference of Government Industrial Hygienists (ACGIH):**

a. established the TLV.

b. established the ADI.

c. established the RDA.

d. established the GRAS list.

93. **Organophosphates are:**

a. herbicides.

b. solvents.

c. insecticides.

d. fumigants.

94. **Inhalational toxicity of solvents:**

a. depends on vapor pressure.

b. depends on concentration in the lungs.

c. depends on their aqueous solubility.

d. depends on the volume of the liquid that has been spilled.

95. **Among over 2800 approved food additives:**

a. most are used in such small quantities that they are not mentioned on the label.

b. sugar and salt are seldom used.

c. coloring agents are the most commonly used agents.

d. all are not generally recognized as safe.

96. **Which of the following statements regarding the testing of mutagens is NOT correct?**

a. Evaluation of chromosomal damage involves looking for evidence of alteration in chromosomal structure and number.

b. Most tests evaluate phenotypic changes and attempt to draw conclusions about the actual gene damage.

c. Positive controls always are included.

d. Evaluation for aneuploidy involves determination of the gain or loss of complete sets of chromosomes.

97. **Which of the following properties of chemicals does NOT influence transport across the blood-testes barrier?**

a. blood-gas partition coefficient.

b. molecular weight.

c. water/lipid partition coefficient.

d. degree of ionization.

98. **Which of the following statements regarding toxicity from solvents is false?**

a. Billions of pounds are used annually as solubilizers, dispersants, or diluents.

b. Occupational and home/recreational exposures occur frequently.

c. Users often fail to take adequate precautions.

d. These chemicals are always extremely toxic.

99. Which of the following solvents is correctly paired with a specific toxicity?

   a. hexane—neurotoxicity.

   b. methanol—nephrotoxicity.

   c. benzene—blood dyscrasias.

   d. ethylene glycol—reproductive toxicity.

100. Toxicants that affect the lung include:

   a. mercury.

   b. ethacrynic acid.

   c. paraquat.

   d. cadmium.

101. Which of the following problems is NOT considered a typical result from long-term chronic exposure to pulmonary toxicants?

   a. carcinoma.

   b. fibrosis.

   c. emphysema.

   d. bronchoconstriction.

102. A virtually safe dose may be defined as:

   a. the dose that has an associated risk of carcinogenicity of 1 in 100,000.

   b. the dose to which an individual may be exposed daily with statistical assurance that cancer will not develop.

   c. an extrapolation from all available data that provides a level of exposure that will not induce harm in workers.

   d. the dose at which an effect was not observed.

103. Which of the following statements regarding pesticides is false?

   a. Pesticides may be used during preplanting, growth, harvesting, handling, and storage of food crops.

   b. Pesticides may not be present in foods at levels that exceed the maximum residue limit tolerance.

   c. Pesticides are found in foods at levels that are considerably below their ADIs, according to a recent survey by the FDA.

   d. Pesticides can never be used safely under normal use conditions.

104. Autoimmunity may be defined as:

   a. an increased responsive state acquired through previous exposure to an antigen.

   b. a specific acquired immunity in which T lymphocytes are involved.

   c. a specific humoral or cell-mediated immune response against the constituents of one's own body.

   d. a specific acquired immunity in which interleukins control the process of foreign body destruction.

105. Which of the following definitions is NOT correct?

   a. Toxicology is the study of the adverse effects of chemicals on living systems.

   b. Environmental toxicology evaluates the movement of toxicants through the biophase, as well as toxicant effects on living systems.

   c. Teratogenesis is the process of malformations and birth defects that may be induced by toxicants.

   d. Mutagenesis is the process of aberrant cell growth and division.

106. Which one of the following functions is NOT performed by the kidney?

   a. excretion of wastes via the bile.

   b. maintenance of acid-base balance.

   c. maintenance of electrolyte balance.

   d. production of certain endocrine hormones.

107. Which of the following is NOT a toxic effect on blood vessels?

   a. increased capillary permeability after lead or mercury.

   b. vasoconstriction.

   c. arrhythmias.

   d. degenerative changes such as atherosclerosis.

108. Myocardial depression may be defined as:

   a. a toxicant-induced reduction in the heart's ability to contract and pump blood throughout the body.

   b. toxicant-induced damage to blood vessels.

   c. toxicant-induced CNS stimulation followed by depression.

   d. a toxicant-induced increase in blood pressure.

109. Excision repair mechanisms:

   a. are saturable and error-prone.

   b. are nonsaturable and error-prone.

   c. are saturable and error-free.

   d. are nonsaturable and error-free.

110. The therapeutic index:

   a. describes the potency of a chemical in producing a specified response.

   b. describes the ability of a chemical to block a specified response to another chemical.

   c. describes the ratio of the therapeutic effect with a toxic response to the same chemical.

   d. describes the change in response to a chemical as the dose is increased.

111. Which of the following is NOT a mechanism for teratogenesis?

   a. alterations in RNA caused by ionizing radiation.

   b. chromosomal abnormalities caused by advancing maternal age.

   c. interference in RNA function by antibiotic agents.

   d. nutritional deficiencies.

112. Physiologically based toxicokinetic modeling:

   a. effectively ignores some tissues of the body.

   b. is a mathematical description of the distribution of a toxicant in either the whole organism or a specific part.

   c. accurately predicts the influence of disease states and species variation.

   d. does not require knowledge of whether a toxicant's distribution into a tissue is perfusion-limited.

113. Bioactivation may be defined as:

   a. the process of producing a chemical that is more readily excreted from the body.

   b. the process of producing a more toxic chemical by allowing it to interact with DNA.

   c. the process by which biotransformation enzymes produce a more reactive chemical.

   d. the process by which a chemical stimulates the synthesis of new proteins.

114. If a cell replicates while DNA damage is present, permanent alterations can occur by:

   a. transitions of pyrimidines to purines, resulting in genetic rearrangements.

   b. mispairing of deoxyribose groups, leading to point mutations.

   c. Errors in replication, leading to positive frameshift mutations.

   d. Errors in translation, leading to negative frameshift mutations.

115. Which of the following structures of the kidney is least affected by toxicants?

   a. glomerulus.

   b. convoluted tubules.

   c. loop of Henle.

   d. ureter.

116. Which of the following statements BEST characterizes potentiation?

   a. Potentiation occurs if a xenobiotic that lacks an effect of its own increases the effect of a second, active xenobiotic.

   b. Potentiation occurs if two chemicals with the same effect, when given together, produce an effect that is equal in magnitude to the sum of the effects when the chemicals are given individually.

c. Potentiation occurs if two chemicals with the same effect, when given together, produce an effect that is greater in magnitude than the sum of the effects when the chemicals are given individually.

d. Potentiation occurs if two drugs with the same effect, when given together, produce an effect that is equal in magnitude to the effect of only one of the drugs given individually.

117. **Which of the following physicochemical properties of a toxicant is very important to its passive diffusion across membranes?**

a. molecular weight.

b. water solubility.

c. physical state (i.e., solid, liquid, gas).

d. cost.

118. **Which of the following biotransformation reactions is incorrectly paired with the enzyme that normally catalyzes that reaction?**

a. glucuronidation—UDP-glucuronosyltransferase.

b. sulfoxidation—cytochrome P450 monooxygenase.

c. deamination—epoxide hydrolase.

d. hydroxylation—cytochrome P450–dependent hydroxylase.

119. **Which of the following mechanisms is NOT involved in liver injury?**

a. lipid peroxidation.

b. hepatitis.

c. renal excretion.

d. bioactivation.

120. **Which of the following statements is NOT true?**

a. The cornea is the transparent covering of the eye.

b. The lens is responsible for controlling the diameter of the pupil in response to light.

c. Cataractogenesis is the formation of lenticular opacities.

d. Glaucoma refers to increased intraocular pressure.

121. **Which of the following terms may NOT be used to describe particulates in air?**

a. sedimentation.

b. homogeneous.

c. heterogeneous.

d. monodispersed.

122. **Which of the following is NOT a component of the immune system?**

a. interleukins.

b. lymphocytes.

c. macrophages.

d. enterocytes.

123. **Which of the following is NOT a criterion for a chemical to be called a neurotransmitter?**

a. The chemical must cause the same response as stimulation of the nerve.

b. Synthesis of the chemical must be able to occur in the nerve.

c. The chemical must be present in all nerves.

d. The nerve must possess the ability to terminate the action of the chemical.

124. **Which of the following is NOT a mechanism of teratogenesis?**

a. interference with mitosis.

b. interference with the functions of RNA.

c. interference with the functions of DNA.

d. interference with reproductive behavior.

125. **Which of the following factors has little influence on biotransformation reactions?**

a. exposure to other chemicals that might induce or inhibit biotransformation enzyme function.

b. the differences in expression of enzymes that may be found in various species and strains of animals.

c. the sex and age of the experimental animals.

d. the processes of hepatic blood flow and hepatic uptake.

126. Epigenetic carcinogens:

a. are often chemicals that do not react directly with DNA to produce a response.

b. require bioactivation to the ultimate carcinogen.

c. act directly with DNA to induce neoplasia.

d. include genotoxic carcinogens and promotors.

127. Which of the following is NOT a cause of human developmental defects?

a. environmental chemicals such as anticoagulants and organic mercury.

b. radiation such as that which comes from white light in classrooms.

c. viral infections, such as those from syphilis and rubella viruses.

d. chromosomal aberrations from unknown causes.

128. Assessment of exposure to toxicants includes:

a. ignoring the dose–response relationship.

b. characterization of the risk of an adverse effect.

c. development of management options.

d. determination of the exposure level and the population at risk.

129. Which one of the following is an oxidant-type air-polluting chemical?

a. ozone.

b. heavy metals.

c. sulfur oxides.

d. hexanes.

130. Inorganic mercury after acute exposure causes:

a. inhibition of hemoglobin synthesis.

b. garlic odor, dermatitis, and dementia.

c. gastrointestinal irritation and loss of renal function.

d. corrosive destruction of the stomach and hepatic necrosis.

131. Which of the following pesticides is NOT correctly paired with its primary use?

a. organophosphates—herbicides.

b. organochlorines—insecticides.

c. warfarin—rodenticide.

d. dithiocarbamates—herbicides.

132. Which of the following food additives represents 93 percent of total food additive use?

a. butylated hydroxytoluene (BHT) and butylated hydroxyanisole (BHA).

b. vitamins.

c. yeast and leavening agents.

d. salt, sucrose, dextrose, and corn syrup.

133. During the normal process of reproduction, oogenesis:

a. begins at puberty and continues throughout adult life.

b. is the period of time during which a mother nurses her young.

c. is a complex process involving the production of a fertilizable ovum.

d. occurs daily throughout reproductive life.

134. Which of the following is a toxic effect on the nervous system?

a. nephropathy.

b. cardiomyopathy.

c. retinopathy.

d. axonopathy.

135. The Draize test for ocular toxicity determines:

a. corneal opacity, lens opacity, and retinal opacity.

b. corneal opacity, redness of conjunctivae, and chemosis.

c. pupillary reflex, corneal thickness, and fluorescein staining.

d. pupillary reflex, pigmentation, and the presence of cells in the aqueous humor.

136. Which of the following enzymes does NOT catalyze a phase II biotransformation reaction?
a. epoxide hydrolase.
b. glucuronosyltransferase.
c. sulfotransferase.
d. N-acetyltransferase.

137. Absorption of a chemical from the gastrointestinal tract is NOT influenced by:
a. an individual's dietary patterns.
b. the plasma half-life of the drug.
c. the pH of the stomach.
d. stress.

138. Which of the following is the quantitatively least important route of toxicant excretion from the body?
a. bile.
b. tears.
c. intestine.
d. exhalation.

139. Which of the following mechanisms is NOT involved in the genesis of liver injury?
a. bioactivation of the chemical to a highly reactive intermediate.
b. derangements in hepatic blood flow.
c. potentiation of a chemical's action by the presence of a second chemical.
d. cirrhosis.

140. Which of the following is NOT a major route for toxicant absorption into the blood?
a. dermal.
b. oral.
c. renal.
d. ocular.

141. Which of the following abbreviations is correctly defined?
a. GRAS: generally reacts as acid in solution.
b. NOEL: National Oil and Energy League.
c. TSCA: Toxic Substances Control Act.
d. FDCA: Federal Drug and Cosmetic Act.

142. The blood-testes barrier:
a. is very effective in a newborn animal.
b. is a poor anatomic barrier to chemicals in adult animals.
c. is more effective than the blood-brain barrier.
d. protects Sertoli, Leydig, and seminiferous tubular cells.

143. Quantitative risk assessment:
a. is always influenced by political and financial concerns.
b. ascertains the quality of the available experimental data.
c. readily places little importance on animal data when scanty human data are available.
d. readily ignores all data that may contain flaws from their collection.

144. Translation involves:
a. conversion of DNA into RNA.
b. conversion of RNA into protein.
c. conversion of protein into RNA.
d. conversion of DNA into new DNA.

145. Polyploidy occurs when a cell contains:
a. multiple copies of specific RNA.
b. multiple copies of specific DNA.
c. multiple copies of the nucleus of the cell.
d. multiple copies of all chromosomes.

146. Which of the following tests is NOT used to determine potential carcinogenicity?
a. limited bioassays.
b. chronic bioassays.

c. short-term in vitro tests.

d. In vitro and in vivo tests for reporters.

147. **Which of the following is NOT a critical period in embryogenesis?**

a. proliferation.

b. differentiation.

c. organogenesis.

d. teratogenesis.

148. **Primary irritation testing:**

a. determines the effect of a toxicant on renal function.

b. determines the effect of a toxicant on pulmonary function.

c. determines the effect of a toxicant on normal and abraded skin.

d. determines the effect of a toxicant on cardiac function.

149. **Which of the following is NOT a general mechanism by which a chemical can induce toxicity?**

a. interference with cellular energy production.

b. interference with distribution throughout the body.

c. interference with membrane functions.

d. interference with normal receptor-ligand interactions.

150. **Agonists are chemicals that:**

a. bind to a membrane receptor and prevent a response.

b. bind to a membrane receptor and initiate a response.

c. are always poorly bound to a receptor.

d. exert a response in all tissues in the body.

151. **Which of the following mechanisms does NOT apply to percutaneous toxicity?**

a. biliary excretion of the toxicant.

b. integrity of the skin to the toxicant.

c. physicochemical properties of the toxicant.

d. vehicle used to dissolve the toxicant.

152. **Toxicant effects on the nervous system do NOT include:**

a. alteration in neurotransmission.

b. nephropathy.

c. axonopathy.

d. demyelination.

153. **Now that you know that all chemicals are toxic, which of the following corollary statements is FALSE?**

a. It is the dose that determines a remedy from a poison.

b. Exposure limits may be set for all chemicals that will instill confidence that we are safe from chemicals.

c. We cannot maintain our standard of living without exposure to chemicals.

d. Life begins with perfect chemistry.

154. **Which of the following statements regarding the distribution of xenobiotics to tissues is FALSE?**

a. Distribution depends on blood flow and the size of the organ.

b. Distribution depends on the solubility of the chemical in that tissue.

c. Distribution depends on the concentration gradient between blood and tissue.

d. Distribution is increased for xenobiotics that are bound to plasma proteins.

155. **Which of the following statements is NOT correct?**

a. Food additives normally are not considered foods themselves.

b. Dermal exposures result from solvents because of their ubiquitous use by humans.

c. Metals have luster, conduct heat and electricity, and ionize positively in solution.

d. Rodenticides are used widely to control insect populations in agriculture.

ANSWERS

1. c.	**40.** d.	**79.** a.	**118.** c.
2. d.	**41.** a.	**80.** c.	**119.** c.
3. c.	**42.** c.	**81.** b.	**120.** b.
4. d.	**43.** c.	**82.** d.	**121.** a.
5. a.	**44.** a.	**83.** c.	**122.** d.
6. d.	**45.** c.	**84.** a.	**123.** c.
7. b.	**46.** d.	**85.** d.	**124.** d.
8. c.	**47.** c.	**86.** b.	**125.** d.
9. d.	**48.** a.	**87.** d.	**126.** a.
10. d.	**49.** d.	**88.** b.	**127.** b.
11. c.	**50.** b.	**89.** d.	**128.** d.
12. a.	**51.** a.	**90.** d.	**129.** a.
13. c.	**52.** c.	**91.** c.	**130.** c.
14. c.	**53.** c.	**92.** a.	**131.** a.
15. a.	**54.** b.	**93.** c.	**132.** d.
16. a.	**55.** b.	**94.** b.	**133.** c.
17. b.	**56.** d.	**95.** a.	**134.** d.
18. d.	**57.** c.	**96.** d.	**135.** b.
19. a.	**58.** a.	**97.** a.	**136.** a.
20. c.	**59.** b.	**98.** d.	**137.** b.
21. c.	**60.** c.	**99.** a.	**138.** b.
22. a.	**61.** d.	**100.** c.	**139.** d.
23. b.	**62.** c.	**101.** d.	**140.** c.
24. d.	**63.** b.	**102.** a.	**141.** c.
25. d.	**64.** b.	**103.** d.	**142.** d.
26. b.	**65.** a.	**104.** c.	**143.** b.
27. d.	**66.** c.	**105.** d.	**144.** b.
28. c.	**67.** c.	**106.** a.	**145.** d.
29. b.	**68.** d.	**107.** c.	**146.** d.
30. a.	**69.** c.	**108.** a.	**147.** d.
31. d.	**70.** a.	**109.** a.	**148.** c.
32. b.	**71.** d.	**110.** c.	**149.** b.
33. d.	**72.** c.	**111.** a.	**150.** b.
34. b.	**73.** b.	**112.** b.	**151.** a.
35. c.	**74.** a.	**113.** c.	**152.** b.
36. d.	**75.** c.	**114.** c.	**153.** b.
37. b.	**76.** b.	**115.** d.	**154.** d.
38. a.	**77.** d.	**116.** a.	**155.** d.
39. d.	**78.** b.	**117.** a.	

INDEX

NOTE: Pages in **boldface** refer to major discussions; page numbers followed by *f* indicate figures; those followed by *t* indicate tables.

Polychlorodibenzofurans (PCDFs), chloracne and, 298*t*

Polychloronaphthalenes (PCNs), chloracne and, 298*t*

Polyethylene glycols, biotransformation, 91*t*

Polyhalogenated biphenyls, thyroid toxicity of, 322

Polyhalogenated dibenzofurans, chloracne and, 298*t*

Polymorphonuclear neutrophils (PMNs), 178, 178*f*

Polymyxin, as contact allergen, 294*t*

Polypeptides, in snake venom, 393

Poly(ADP-ribose)polymerase (PARP), in excision repair, 40

Poor metabolizers, 72

Population effects, in terrestrial and aquatic ecotoxicology, 425

Porphyrin derivatives, phototoxicity of, 297*t*

Postemergent herbicides, 343

Postreplication repair, 40

Potash, caustic, ocular toxicity of, 260

Potassium channel blockade, cardiotoxicity and, 270

Potassium dichromate, as contact allergen, 294*t*

Potassium hydroxide, ocular toxicity of, 260

Potassium perchlorate, aplastic anemia and, 167*t*

Potency, efficacy versus, 17, 17*f*

Potentiation, 11

Pott, Percival, 4

Practolol, hematotoxicity of, 173*t*

Prazosin, cellular dysregulation and, 33*t*

Prednisolone, cardiotoxicity of, 278*t*

Prednisone
  cardiotoxicity of, 278*t*
  reproductive toxicity of, 309*t*

Preemergent herbicides, 343

Pregnancy. *See also* Developmental toxicology
  ethanol during, 239, 368
  pharmacokinetics and metabolism in, 151–152

Preimplantation period, 149

Prenatal exposure. *See* Developmental toxicology; Pregnancy

Preplanting herbicides, 342–343

Presystemic elimination, 23, 63

Probit units, 13

Procainamide
  autoimmunity and, 191*t*
  cardiotoxicity of, 273*t*, 276*t*
  hematotoxicity of, 173*t*
  neutropenia and, 170*t*
  therapeutic monitoring of, 445*t*

Procarbazine, reproductive toxicity of, 310*t*

Procaterol, cardiotoxicity of, 274*t*

Progesterone
  biotransformation, 90*f*
  cardiotoxicity of, 277*t*
  vascular toxicity of, 282*t*

Progestins, cardiotoxicity of, 277*t*, 278

Programmed cell death. *See* Apoptosis

Progression stage of cancer, 116, 117*t*
  bases for, 119–120, 120*f*, 121*t*
  cell and molecular mechanisms of, 118*t*
  reversibility of, molecular basis of, 119

Proguanil, biotransformation, 85*t*

Prokaryotes, gene mutations in, assays for, 139

Proliferation, tissue repair and, 41

Promethazine, as photoallergen, 298*t*

Promotion stage of cancer, 116, 117*t*
  bases for, 119–120, 120*f*, 121*t*
  cell and molecular mechanisms of, 117, 118*t*
  reversibility of, molecular basis of, 118–119

Propafenone
  biotransformation, 86*t*
  cardiotoxicity of, 273*t*

Propidine, biotransformation, 86*t*

β-Propiolactone, biotransformation, 95*f*

Propofol
  biotransformation, 90*f*
  cardiotoxicity of, 275*t*

Propranolol
  biotransformation, 85*t*, 86*t*, 90*f*
  cardiotoxicity of, 273*t*

N-Propylajmaline, biotransformation, 86*t*

Propyl chloride, cardiotoxicity of, 280*t*

Propylene glycol, as contact allergen, 294*t*

Propylene glycol (PG), 369–370

Propyl hydroxybenzoate, cross-reactivity of, 295*t*

Propylthiouracil
  aplastic anemia and, 167*t*
  autoimmunity and, 191*t*
  neutropenia and, 170*t*

Prostaglandin H synthetase (PHS), 76–77, 77*f*

Protease inhibitors, nephrotoxicity of, 211*t*

Protective fungicides, 345

Protein(s)
  food, allergenic, 435, 435*t*
  molecular repair of, 39
  plasma
    as storage depot, 66, 66*f*
    toxicant binding to, 24
  recombinant DNA-derived, immunosuppression by, 187
  synthesis of, tissue repair and, 42

Proteinases, nephrotoxicity and, 216

Protein toxins, detoxication of, 25

Proteolytic enzymes, of snake venoms, 390, 393, 393*t*, 394*t*

Proteomics, in immunotoxicology, 192

clearance and, 101
elimination and, 100–101
half-life and, 101–102
one-compartment, 99, 100*f*
saturation toxicokinetics and, 102
two-compartment, 99–100
definition of, 98
physiologic, 102–107
basic model structure for, 103
compartments and, 103, 103*f*, 104–107,
105*f*, 106*f*
parameters for, 103–104
Toxicologists, 7
Toxicology
areas of, 7–8
definition of, 7
Toxicology and Applied Pharmacology, 5
Toxicology Data Network (TOXNET), 54
Toxicology testing. *See also* Bioassays
for terrestrial and aquatic ecotoxicology, 423–424
Toxic responses, **17–18**
individual differences in, 18
selective toxicity and, 17
species differences in, 17–18
Toxic Substances Control Act (TSCA), 464
Toxic syndromes, 448, 448*t*
Toxins, definition of, 8*t*
TOXNET (Toxicology Data Network), 54
Transcription, dysregulation of, 29
Transdermal drug delivery, 291
Transferrin, 351
Transforming growth factor-*β* (TGF-*β*)
fibrogenesis and, 43
in immune regulation, 183*t*
Transfusional siderosis, 357
Transgenic animals
as carcinogenesis models, 127*t*, 127–128
gene mutation assays using, 125–126, 140
in immunotoxicology, 192
Transgenic plant policy, 433
Transport, of solvents, 363
Transport parameters, in physiologic toxicokinetic
model, 104
Tranylcypromine, biotransformation, 85*t*
Trees, contact urticaria and, 299*t*
Tree tobacco toxicity, 403
Triallate, 346*t*
Triamterene, nephrotoxicity of, 211*t*
Triatoma envenomations, 390
Triazolam, biotransformation, 86*t*
Tribromosalicylanilide, as photoallergen, 298*t*

Tributyltin, 424*t*
Trichlorethylene, ocular toxicity of, 263
Trichlorfon, 340
Trichlorocarbanilide, as photoallergen, 298*t*
Trichloroethane, cardiotoxicity of, 280*t*
1,1,1-Trichloroethane, cardiotoxicity of, 280*t*
Trichloroethanol, biotransformation, 90*f*
Trichloroethylene (TCE), 364–365
autoimmunity and, 191*t*
biotransformation, 87*t*
cardiotoxicity of, 280*t*
neurotoxicity of, 244*t*
Trichlorofluoroethane, cardiotoxicity of, 280*t*
Trichlorofluoromethane, cardiotoxicity of, 280*t*
Trichloromethane (chloroform), 366
biotransformation, 87*t*
cardiotoxicity of, 280*t*
cytosolic calcium elevation and, 36*t*
nephrotoxicity of, 217
Trichloromonofluoromethane, cardiotoxicity of, 280*t*
Trichloronate, 340
Trichodermin, 438*t*
Trichothecenes, 438*t*
immunosuppression by, 188*t*
Triclosan, as photoallergen, 298*t*
Tricyclic antidepressants (TCADs)
cardiotoxicity of, 272
cellular dysregulation and, 32*t*, 33*t*
reproductive toxicity of, 306*t*
Triethyltin, neurotoxicity of, 247*t*
Trifluoperazine, aplastic anemia and, 167*t*
Trifluorobromomethane, cardiotoxicity of, 280*t*
Trifluoroiodomethane, cardiotoxicity of, 280*t*
Trifluperidol, biotransformation, 86*t*
Trihexachlorodibenzofuran (TCDF), chloracne and, 298*t*
Triiodothyronine, cardiotoxicity of, 278*t*, 279
Trimethadione
aplastic anemia and, 167*t*
biotransformation, 86*t*
Trimethoxypsoralen, phototoxicity of, 297*t*
Trimethyltin, neurotoxicity of, 241*t*
Trimetrexate, biotransformation, 91*t*
Trinitroglycerin, biotransformation, 96*f*
Tri-*o*-cresyl phosphate (TOCP), 340
neurotoxicity of, 245
Tri-*o*-tolyl phosphate (TOTP), 340
Triparanol, adrenocortical toxicity of, 319, 320
Tripelennamine
aplastic anemia and, 167*t*
biotransformation, 90*f*
Triphenylmethane dyes, as contact allergen, 294*t*